Pediatric Rheumatology Comes of Age: Part II

Editors

YUKIKO KIMURA
LAURA E. SCHANBERG

RHEUMATIC DISEASE CLINICS OF NORTH AMERICA

www.rheumatic.theclinics.com

Consulting Editor

MICHAEL H. WEISMAN

February 2022 • Volume 48 • Number 1

ELSEVIER

1600 John F. Kennedy Boulevard • Suite 1800 • Philadelphia, Pennsylvania, 19103-2899
http://www.theclinics.com

RHEUMATIC DISEASE CLINICS OF NORTH AMERICA Volume 48, Number 1
February 2022 ISSN 0889-857X, ISBN 13: 978-0-323-84880-0

Editor: Lauren Boyle
Developmental Editor: Karen Solomon

Rheumatic Disease Clinics of North America (ISSN 0889-857X) is published quarterly by Elsevier Inc., 360 Park Avenue South, New York, NY 10010-1710. Months of issue are February, May, August, and November. Business and editorial offices: 1600 John F. Kennedy Boulevard, Suite 1800, Philadelphia, PA 19103-2899. Periodicals postage paid at New York, NY and additional mailing offices. Subscription prices are USD 366.00 per year for US individuals, USD 1020.00 per year for US institutions, USD 100.00 per year for US students and residents, USD 431.00 per year for Canadian individuals, USD 1040.00 per year for Canadian institutions, USD 100.00 per year for Canadian students/residents, USD 470.00 per year for international individuals, USD 1040.00 per year for international institutions, and USD 230.00 per year for foreign students/residents. To receive student/ resident rate, orders must be accompanied by name of affiliated institution, date of term, and the *signature* of program/residency coordinator on institution letterhead. Orders will be billed at individual rate until proof of status received. Foreign air speed delivery is included in all *Clinics* subscription prices. All prices are subject to change without notice. **POSTMASTER:** Send address changes to *Rheumatic Disease Clinics of North America,* Elsevier Health Sciences Division, Subscription Customer Service, 3251 Riverport Lane, Maryland Heights, MO 63043. **Customer Service: 1-800-654-2452 (US and Canada). From outside of the US and Canada: 314-447-8871. Fax: 314-447-8029. For print support, e-mail: JournalsCustomerService-usa@elsevier.com. For online support, e-mail: JournalsOnlineSupport-usa@elsevier.com.**

Reprints. For copies of 100 or more of articles in this publication, please contact the Commercial Reprints Department, Elsevier Inc., 360 Park Avenue South, New York, New York, 10010-1710; Tel.: +1-212-633-3874, Fax: +1-212-633-3820, and E-mail: reprints@elsevier.com.

Rheumatic Disease Clinics of North America is covered in *MEDLINE/PubMed (Index Medicus), Current Contents/Clinical Medicine, Science Citation Index, ISI/BIOMED,* and *EMBASE/Excerpta Medica.*

Contributors

CONSULTING EDITOR

MICHAEL H. WEISMAN, MD
Adjunct Professor of Medicine, Stanford University, Distinguished Professor of Medicine, Emeritus, David Geffen School of Medicine at UCLA, Professor of Medicine Emeritus, Cedars-Sinai Medical Center, Los Angeles, California, USA

EDITORS

YUKIKO KIMURA, MD
Professor of Pediatrics, Hackensack Meridian School of Medicine, Pediatric Rheumatology Division Chief, Joseph M. Sanzari Children's Hospital, Hackensack University Medical Center, Co-Chair, CARRA Registry and Research Oversight Committee, Co-PI, CARRA Registry, Hackensack, New Jersey, USA

LAURA E. SCHANBERG, MD
Professor of Pediatrics, Division of Pediatric Rheumatology, Duke University School of Medicine, Duke Clinical Research Institute, Co-Chair, CARRA Registry and Research Oversight Committee, Co-PI, CARRA Registry, Durham, North Carolina, USA

AUTHORS

ALISHA M. AKINSETE, MD
Fellow, Division of Pediatric Rheumatology, Department of Pediatrics, Children's Hospital at Montefiore/Albert Einstein College of Medicine, New York, New York, USA

KAVEH ARDALAN, MD, MS
Department of Pediatrics, Division of Pediatric Rheumatology, Duke University School of Medicine, Durham, North Carolina, USA; Departments of Pediatrics and Medical Social Sciences, Northwestern University Feinberg School of Medicine, Ann & Robert H. Lurie Children's Hospital of Chicago, Chicago, Illinois, USA

CHRISTINE M. BACHA, MD
Division of Rheumatology, Nationwide Children's Hospital, Columbus, Ohio, USA

STEPHEN J. BALEVIC, MD, MHS
Assistant Professor of Medicine and Pediatrics, Department of Pediatrics, Duke University, Duke Clinical Research Institute, Durham, North Carolina, USA

HERMINE I. BRUNNER, MD, MSc, MBA
Director, Division of Rheumatology, Department of Pediatrics, Cincinnati Children's Hospital Medical Center, University of Cincinnati College of Medicine, Cincinnati, Ohio, USA

ELLEN M. CODY, MD
Division of Pediatric Nephrology, Cincinnati Children's Hospital Medical Center, Cincinnati, Ohio, USA

MARK CONNELLY, PhD
Professor of Pediatrics, Division of Developmental and Behavioral Health, Children's Mercy Kansas City, Kansas City, Missouri, USA

COLLEEN K. CORRELL, MD, MPH
Assistant Professor, Pediatric Rheumatology, University of Minnesota, Minneapolis, Minnesota, USA

LAUREN T. COVERT, MD
Department of Pediatrics, Division of Rheumatology, Duke University Medical Center, Durham, North Carolina, USA

NATOSHIA R. CUNNINGHAM, PhD
Assistant Professor, Department of Family Medicine, Michigan State University, Michigan State University College of Human Medicine, Secchia Center, Grand Rapids, Michigan, USA

VINCENT DEL GAIZO, BS
Director of Partnerships and Patient Engagement, Childhood Arthritis and Rheumatology Research Alliance, Milwaukee, Wisconsin, USA

ASHLEY N. DANGUECAN, PhD
Department of Psychology, Division of Rheumatology, Hospital for Sick Children, Black Wing, Toronto, Ontario, Canada

CUOGHI EDENS, MD
Assistant Professor, Departments of Pediatrics and Internal Medicine, Sections of Pediatric Rheumatology and Rheumatology, University of Chicago Medicine, Chicago, Illinois, USA

INGRID GOH, PhD
Senior Research Associate, Division of Rheumatology, The Hospital for Sick Children, Child Health Evaluative Sciences, SickKids Research Institute, Toronto, Ontario, Canada

MARIA J. GUTIERREZ, MD, MHS
Division of Pediatric Allergy, Immunology and Rheumatology, Johns Hopkins University School of Medicine, Baltimore, Maryland, USA

JONATHAN S. HAUSMANN, MD
Program in Rheumatology, Division of Immunology, Boston Children's Hospital, Beth Israel Deaconess Medical Center, Division of Rheumatology and Clinical Immunology, Boston, Massachusetts, USA

ANDREA M. KNIGHT, MD, MSCE
Associate Professor, Department of Pediatrics, Division of Rheumatology, Hospital for Sick Children, University of Toronto, Toronto, Ontario, Canada

MELANIE KOHLHEIM, BS
Chair of Registry Parent/Patient Advisory Council (RPAC), Childhood Arthritis and Rheumatology Research Alliance, Milwaukee, Wisconsin, USA

JOE KOSSOWSKY, PhD, MMSc
Department of Anesthesiology, Critical Care and Pain Medicine, Boston Children's Hospital, Department of Anaesthesia, Harvard Medical School, Boston, Massachusetts, USA

SIVIA K. LAPIDUS, MD
Division of Pediatric Rheumatology, Joseph M. Sanzari Children's Hospital, Hackensack University Medical Center and Hackensack Meridian School of Medicine, Hackensack, New Jersey, USA

ERICA F. LAWSON, MD
Department of Pediatrics, Division of Rheumatology, University of California, San Francisco School of Medicine, San Francisco, California, USA

REBECCA RACHAEL LEE, PhD
Centre for Epidemiology Versus Arthritis, Centre for Musculoskeletal Research, Division of Musculoskeletal and Dermatological Sciences, Faculty of Biology, Medicine and Health, The University of Manchester, Manchester Academic Health Science Centre, Manchester, United Kingdom

TZIELAN LEE, MD
Clinical Professor of Pediatrics, Division of Allergy, Immunology and Rheumatology, Department of Pediatric Rheumatology, Stanford Children's Health, Stanford University School of Medicine, Palo Alto, California, USA

LAURA B. LEWANDOWSKI, MD, MS
Assistant Clinical Investigator, Head of Lupus Genetics and Global Health Disparities Unit, Systemic Autoimmunity Branch, National Institute of Arthritis, Musculoskeletal, and Skin Diseases, National Institutes of Health, Department of Health and Human Services, Bethesda, Maryland, USA

DONALD M. LLOYD-JONES, MD, ScM
Departments of Preventive Medicine, Medicine, and Pediatrics, Northwestern University Feinberg School of Medicine, Chicago, Illinois, USA

EYAL MUSCAL, MD, MS
Associate Professor, Section Chief, Pediatrics, Division of Rheumatology, Baylor College of Medicine, Houston, Texas, USA

MARC D. NATTER, MD
Computational Health Informatics Program, Boston Children's Hospital, Mass General Hospital for Children, Boston, Massachusetts, USA

EDWARD J. OBERLE, MD, RHMSUS
Department of Pediatrics, Division of Rheumatology, The Ohio State University, Nationwide Children's Hospital, Columbus, Ohio, USA

RAJDEEP POONI, MD, MS
Clinical Assistant Professor of Pediatrics, Division of Allergy, Immunology and Rheumatology, Department of Pediatric Rheumatology, Stanford Children's Health, Stanford University School of Medicine, Palo Alto, California, USA

LAURA PRATT, MD, RHMSUS
University of Nebraska Medical Center, Omaha, Nebraska, USA

RACHEL L. RANDELL, MD
Fellow, Division of Pediatric Rheumatology, Department of Pediatrics, Duke University School of Medicine, Durham, North Carolina, USA

BRYCE B. REEVE, PhD
Professor, Department of Population Health Sciences, Center for Health Measurement, Professor, Pediatrics, Duke University School of Medicine, Durham, North Carolina, USA

TAMAR B. RUBINSTEIN, MD, MS
Assistant Professor, Division of Pediatric Rheumatology, Department of Pediatrics Children's Hospital at Montefiore/Albert Einstein College of Medicine, New York, New York, USA

REBECCA E. SADUN, MD, PhD
Departments of Medicine and Pediatrics, Division of Rheumatology, Duke University Medical Center, Durham, North Carolina, USA

ANNA CARMELA P. SAGCAL-GIRONELLA, MD, MS
Assistant Professor, Department of Pediatrics, Hackensack Meridian School of Medicine, Nutley, New Jersey, USA; Division of Pediatric Rheumatology, Joseph M. Sanzari Children's Hospital, Hackensack, New Jersey, USA; K. Hovnanian Children's Hospital, Neptune, New Jersey, USA

SUJATA SAWHNEY, MD, MRCP, CCT
Pediatric Rheumatology Division, Institute of Child Health, Sir Ganga Ram Hospital, New Delhi, India

LAURA E. SCHANBERG, MD
Professor of Pediatrics, Division of Pediatric Rheumatology, Duke University School of Medicine, Duke Clinical Research Institute, Co-Chair, CARRA Registry and Research Oversight Committee, Co-PI, CARRA Registry, Durham, North Carolina, USA

CHRISTIAAN SCOTT, MBChB
Red Cross War Memorial Children's Hospital, University of Cape Town, Klipfontein Road, Rondebosch, Cape Town, Western Cape, South Africa

EMILY A. SMITHERMAN, MD, MSc
Assistant Professor, Division of Pediatric Rheumatology, Department of Pediatrics, The University of Alabama at Birmingham, Birmingham, Alabama, USA

ALYSHA J. TAXTER, MD, MSCE
Associate Professor, Pediatric Rheumatology, Nationwide Children's Hospital, Columbus, Ohio, USA

KATHRYN TAYLOR, DO
Pediatrics, Division of Neurology, Duke University, Durham, North Carolina, USA

TRACY V. TING, RHMSUS, MD, MSc
Department of Pediatrics, Division of Rheumatology, University of Cincinnati, Cincinnati Children's Hospital Medical Center, Cincinnati, Ohio, USA

ERIN BRENNAN TREEMARCKI, DO
Assistant Professor, Division of Pediatric Rheumatology, Department of Pediatrics, University of Utah, Salt Lake City, Utah, USA

HEATHER VAN MATER, MD, MSc
Associate Professor, Section Chief, Pediatrics, Division of Rheumatology, Duke University, Durham, North Carolina, USA

PATRICIA VEGA-FERNANDEZ, MD, MSc, RHMSUS
Department of Pediatrics, Division of Rheumatology, University of Cincinnati, Cincinnati Children's Hospital Medical Center, Cincinnati, Ohio, USA

EMILY VON SCHEVEN, MD, MAS
Professor, Division of Pediatric Rheumatology, University of California, San Francisco, San Francisco, California, USA

SHEETAL S. VORA, MD, MSc
Associate Professor, Department of Pediatrics, Atrium Health Levine Children's Hospital, Charlotte, North Carolina, USA

ELISSA R. WEITZMAN, ScD, MSc
Associate Professor, Department of Pediatrics, Harvard Medical School, Division of Adolescent/Young Adult Medicine, Boston Children's Hospital, Computational Health Informatics Program, Boston Children's Hospital, Boston, Massachusetts, USA

JENNIFER M.P. WOO, PhD, MPH
Postdoctoral Intramural Research Award Fellow, Epidemiology Branch, National Institute of Environmental Health Sciences, National Institutes of Health, Durham, North Carolina, USA

CAGRI YILDIRIM-TORUNER, MD
Assistant Professor, Department of Pediatrics, Baylor College of Medicine, Houston, Texas, USA

CHRISTINA K. ZIGLER, PhD, MSEd
Assistant Professor, Department of Population Health Sciences, Center for Health Measurement, Duke University School of Medicine, Durham, North Carolina, USA

Contents

Foreword: Pediatric Rheumatology Comes of Age: Part II xvii

Michael H. Weisman

Preface: Pediatric Rheumatology Comes of Age: Part II xix

Yukiko Kimura and Laura E. Schanberg

Patient Engagement in Pediatric Rheumatology Research 1

Vincent Del Gaizo and Melanie Kohlheim

Patient engagement in pediatric rheumatology research can ensure protocol acceptability, project relevance, facilitate a successful study, and share results with the community. Research partners can collaborate along the entire continuum of research, contributing both lived and professional experience with roles as small as a single point-in-time consultation to as large as multi-year shared leadership. Patient and caregiver partners can be found in the myriad of places-the clinic, in advocacy organizations, on social media, and through networking with existing patient partners. Patient engagement begins with relationship building and requires effective training of both researcher and patient family.

Assessing Patient-Reported Outcomes in Pediatric Rheumatic Diseases: Considerations and Future Directions 15

Christina K. Zigler, Rachel L. Randell, and Bryce B. Reeve

For children with pediatric rheumatic diseases (PRDs), the inclusion of patient-reported outcomes (PROs) is critical to inform decision making in health care delivery and research settings. PROs are direct reports from a child on their health status, without interpretation by anyone else. PROs improve understanding of the patient experience, allow clinicians to provide patient-centered care, and add value to clinical trials. When PROs cannot be collected directly from the patient, caregiver-proxy reports can provide important information on the child's more observable symptoms and functioning. In this article, we describe the current use of PROs in specific PRDs, align current research with best practice recommendations for both clinical care and research settings, highlight exciting new developments, and identify areas for future research.

Technology to Assess and Treat Pain in Pediatric Rheumatology 31

Mark Connelly and Rebecca Rachael Lee

Advancements in eHealth offer unique opportunities for assisting in and augmenting aspects of evidence-based pain evaluation and management with children and adolescents. In this article, we present an overview of some of the opportunities and challenges in pain eHealth for pediatric rheumatologists to consider while caring for children and adolescents seen in their practice.

RHEUMATIC DISEASE CLINICS OF NORTH AMERICA

FORTHCOMING ISSUES

May 2022
Cardiovascular Complications of Chronic Rheumatic Diseases
M. Elaine Husni and George A. Karpouzas, *Editors*

August 2022
Treatment Guideline Development and Implementation
Michael Ward, *Editor*

November 2022
Environmental Triggers for Rheumatic Diseases
Bryant R. England, *Editor*

RECENT ISSUES

November 2021
Pediatric Rheumatology Comes of Age: Part I
Yukiko Kimura and Laura E. Schanberg, *Editors*

August 2021
Lupus
Alfred H.J. Kim and Zahi Touma, *Editors*

May 2021
Pain in Rheumatic Diseases
Maripat Corr, *Editor*

SERIES OF RELATED INTEREST

Medical Clinics of North America
https://www.medical.theclinics.com/
Neurologic Clinics
https://www.neurologic.theclinics.com/
Dermatologic Clinics
https://www.derm.theclinics.com/
Physical Medicine and Rehabilitation Clinics of North America
https://www.pmr.theclinics.com/

THE CLINICS ARE AVAILABLE ONLINE!
Access your subscription at:
www.theclinics.com

Foreword

Pediatric Rheumatology Comes of Age: Part II

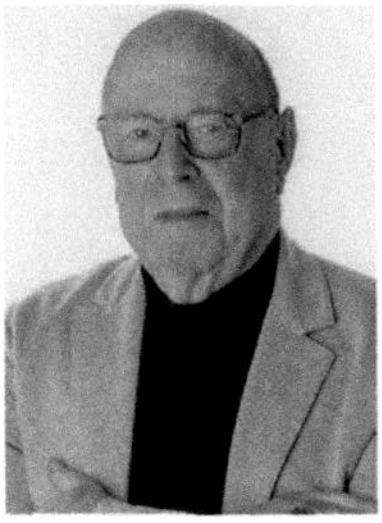

Michael H. Weisman, MD
Consulting Editor

Dr Yukiko Kimura and Dr Laura E. Schanberg have assembled two issues that reflect the remarkable changes taking place in the pediatric rheumatology community over the past 10 years. Much of this success, as reflected in the issues, is due to the strides forward in collaborative research efforts made by the various organizational care and research structures of which Laura and Yuki have played such a pivotal role and continue to do so. It is not true, however, that there has only been successes, since our editors tell us that clinical remission for childhood arthritis is not achieved in a substantial number of cases. Thus, we have these two issues, which point us on the journey just past and just ahead. The first focuses on the traditional roles of rheumatology to identify, measure, and achieve outcomes for pediatric rheumatic diseases, essentially addressing disease control as the item of primary interest. The second issue addresses our concerns for the impact of the diseases on the patient and the family, as well as the community at large. In this issue, the editors introduce us to the emerging technologies for patient-focused care and the impact of our diseases on comorbidities and other issues of personal health. They did an outstanding job and deserve much of the credit for the results.

Michael H. Weisman, MD
10800 Wilshire Blvd. #404
Los Angeles, CA 90024, USA

E-mail address:
michael.weisman@cshs.org

Rheum Dis Clin N Am 48 (2022) xvii
https://doi.org/10.1016/j.rdc.2021.10.002

Preface
Pediatric Rheumatology Comes of Age: Part II

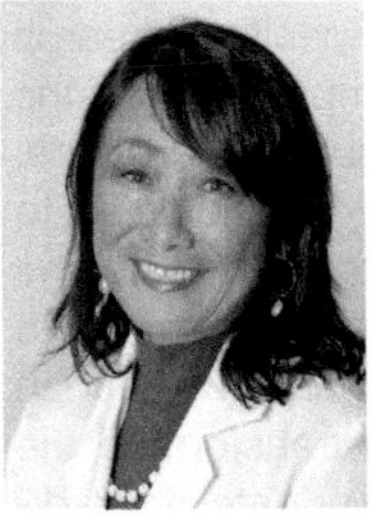
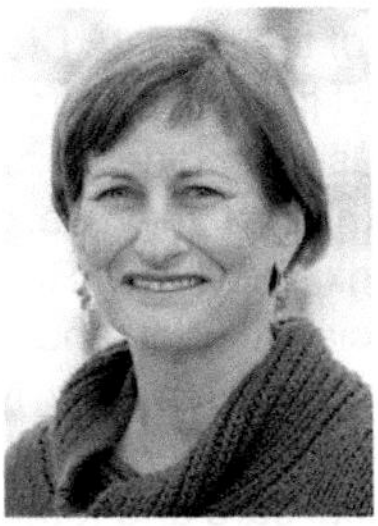

Yukiko Kimura, MD   Laura E. Schanberg, MD
Editors

The twenty-first century has been a time of enormous growth for pediatric rheumatology worldwide, spurred by the growing availability of multiple effective treatments and recognition that collaborative research is necessary to study successfully even the most common of pediatric rheumatic diseases. In North America, the incorporation and maturation of the Childhood Arthritis and Rheumatology Research Alliance (CARRA) coincide with critical progress in approaches to treatment, disease pathogenesis, and ever-expanding medication options. As treatment options expand, our understanding of autoimmunity and the recognition of the inflammatory underpinnings of disease have grown, resulting in a broadening of the definition of pediatric rheumatic diseases to include new conditions, such as autoimmune brain disease, autoinflammatory diseases, and COVID-19–related multisystem inflammatory syndrome in children (MIS-C). In addition to CARRA, the Pediatric Rheumatology Collaborative Study Group, Pediatric Rheumatology Care and Outcomes Improvement Network, Understanding Childhood Arthritis Network, the Paediatric Rheumatology European Society, and Paediatric Rheumatology International Trials Organisation have all greatly contributed to the growth of knowledge and understanding of pediatric rheumatic diseases over the last 20 years.

Despite remarkable treatment advances in the last 20 years, including the introduction of biologic disease-modifying antirheumatic drugs (bDMARDs) and targeted synthetic (ts)DMARDs, serious questions remain, including long-term safety, optimal use for individual patients, juvenile idiopathic arthritis subtypes, and other pediatric rheumatic diseases. In addition, there are significant issues concerning equity, as globally, children do not have equal access to these life-altering medications. Of note, even with access to the complete menu of bDMARDs and tsDMARDs in the United States, 30% to 50% of children in the CARRA Registry are not in clinical remission. Future research needs to focus on long-term health as well as optimal, targeted use and sequence of

Rheum Dis Clin N Am 48 (2022) xix–xx
https://doi.org/10.1016/j.rdc.2021.10.001
0889-857X/22/© 2021 Published by Elsevier Inc.

drugs, rather than simply whether drugs are efficacious in the short term. Addressing many of these concerns requires international collaborations to facilitate investigator-initiated government-sponsored large multicenter comparative effectiveness trials that incorporate translational components and patient-reported outcomes to further the understanding of disease pathogenesis and treatment impact.

It has been almost 10 years since the last pediatric-focused issue in the *Rheumatic Disease Clinics of North America*, and we are pleased to offer two issues that underscore the maturation and scope of the interests and expertise of the pediatric rheumatology community. Most topics reflect work of the CARRA Disease-Specific Research Committees and Workgroups. This issue (Part II) focuses on the life impact of pediatric rheumatic disease (mental health, cardiovascular disease, pain, substance abuse, transition to adulthood, reproductive health) and the use of new technologies to enhance care (personalized dosing of biologics and DMARDs, treatment of pain, the role of the electronic medical record, social media, and patient engagement to enhance research and patient care). Part I, published in November 2021, began with an article about the history of CARRA, which we believe has transformed the community's approach to research and clinical care and focused on updates to traditional pediatric rheumatic diseases, as well as a new condition, COVID-19–related MIS-C. We hope that these issues enhance current understanding of pediatric rheumatic disease and its treatment both within the pediatric rheumatology and, perhaps most importantly, outside of it.

Yukiko Kimura, MD
Joseph M. Sanzari Children's Hospital PC344
Hackensack University Medical Center
Hackensack Meridian School of Medicine
30 Prospect Ave
Hackensack, NJ 07601, USA

Laura E. Schanberg, MD
Duke Clinical Research Institute
Duke University School of Medicine
300 W Morgan St., Suite 800
Durham, NC 27701, USA

E-mail addresses:
yukiko.kimura@hmhn.org (Y. Kimura)
Laura.schanberg@duke.edu (L.E. Schanberg)

Patient Engagement in Pediatric Rheumatology Research

Vincent Del Gaizo, BS*, Melanie Kohlheim, BS

KEYWORDS

• Patient engagement • Stakeholder engagement • Partnering in research

KEY POINTS

- Engaging patients and caregivers in pediatric rheumatology research can assist in designing more meaningful and acceptable research projects.
- Simple steps can ensure a positive experience when engaging patients and caregivers in pediatric rheumatology research.
- "Patient engagement" has multiple interpretations. The authors define patient engagement and related terms.
- Patients and caregivers have been engaged in pediatric rheumatology research for more than 15 years.

BACKGROUND

Patient engagement has become a buzzword in health care over the past decade. Health care institutions, advocacy organizations, research networks, disease-specific registries, quality improvement (QI) networks, and the pharmaceutical industry have new-found interests in engaging patients. Patient engagement can have a significant impact on the quality of health care delivery but it must be done in the right way. Engagement that is collaborative, respectful, and promotes efficiency rather than increased workload can lead to improved outcomes. Pediatric rheumatology is one specialty that has seen tremendous success engaging patients and caregivers across numerous interfaces in research. In this article, we will define patient engagement and related terms, provide a historical overview of patient engagement in pediatric rheumatology, introduce needed perspectives, cover aspects of engagement including some pitfalls, and finally, discuss the next steps.

Childhood Arthritis and Rheumatology Research Alliance, 555 East Wells Street, Suite 1100, Milwaukee, WI 53202, USA
* Corresponding author.
E-mail address: vdelgaizo@carragroup.org

Rheum Dis Clin N Am 48 (2022) 1–13
https://doi.org/10.1016/j.rdc.2021.09.013

WHAT IS PATIENT ENGAGEMENT?

The World Health Organization[1] broadly defines patient engagement as "the facilitation and strengthening of the role of those using services as coproducers of health, and health care policy and practice." Health care providers, advocacy organizations, and institutions aim to engage patients as consumers of health care and have taken steps to ensure that the care provided meets the needs of patients and the conditions they live with. More specifically, the aim of patient engagement in research is for patients to coproduce research alongside health care professional investigators throughout the entire life cycle of any given project: from idea generation through the dissemination of results. Patients and caregivers ideally collaborate with researchers in a mutually respectful environment that encourages shared learning.

There are 2 distinct ways to engage patients and caregivers in research: one as research participants and the other as research partners. Research participants are individuals who enroll as subjects in studies in which research is being done to learn about their specific condition. Patients who come to a pediatric rheumatology clinic for care may be approached about research activities for which they may be eligible and become engaged as a patient or caregiver in those activities. They may play a passive role in the study by simply attending clinic appointments, allowing their health data to be collected, and/or have a more active role by completing additional patient-reported outcomes (PRO) surveys or become more deeply involved by being treated with an intervention, depending on the study design. In recent years, additional involvement in between study visits has become possible, with patients engaging in the study by entering interim PROs via mobile apps or other means. This has resulted in a better understanding of how patients are doing in between visits, as well as higher awareness of participation and optimally increased retention and adherence to study protocol.

A deeper level of active engagement occurs when patients and caregivers take the role of research partners in which they help design, plan, and execute studies by sitting side by side with researchers. The level of interaction between the study team and the patient partners can vary from just a few touchpoints to full integration. Patients and caregivers as research partners can include simple participation in a focus group or surveys that inform specific aims, project relevance to the community, or which assesses the acceptability of the study design. Research partners can also include patients and caregivers as fully engaged members of the study team, contributing starting with the grant application all the way through writing the article and disseminating the results. The former, more simple engagement is feasible for most of the patient families in the pediatric rheumatology community, whereas the latter higher level of engagement requires a significant investment of time and resources. The evaluation of the return on investment of engaging research partners at this level must be considered by the study team, funder, and patient or caregiver partner. Often expectations may vary from stakeholder to stakeholder, emphasizing the importance of understanding what this level of engagement will entail from all perspectives.

What patient engagement should not be is symbolic tokenization which only gives the appearance of equality and collaboration. Examples of tokenization and patronization include organizing advisory panels which do not meet and ignoring or not considering feedback provided by patients/caregivers. Patients and caregivers should not be considered for a role as a research partner simply to satisfy a requirement. Not understanding how all studies can benefit from patient engagement can result in researchers struggling to decide for which studies they should seek patient partners. A straightforward litmus test researchers should use to determine if there can be a role for patient partners is this question: Will patients be recruited to participate in this study? If the answer is yes, then there can and should be a role for patients and caregivers.

IMPACT OF PATIENT ENGAGEMENT

By involving patients and caregivers in prioritizing research questions, developing study designs, and disseminating study findings, the pediatric rheumatology research community is maximizing the impact of every dollar spent on research. To date, however, the impact of patient partners in pediatric rheumatology research has not been specifically quantified. However, feedback from researchers and patient partners has provided insightful qualitative data. Some examples can be found in **Table 1**.

HISTORY OF PATIENT ENGAGEMENT IN PEDIATRIC RHEUMATOLOGY ORGANIZATIONS

The Childhood Arthritis and Rheumatology Research Alliance (CARRA) was formed in 2002 to conduct collaborative, investigator-initiated research. During the early years, CARRA engaged with business professionals who volunteered to provide the necessary business perspective and acumen to the formation of the network. These volunteers were caregivers of pediatric rheumatology patients and therefore had a personal connection to CARRA's mission. The volunteers were invited to one early annual scientific meeting to meet the membership face to face and witness how CARRA plans research. During the meeting, the researchers formed relationships with the volunteers and began to ask questions about their opinions of the studies being planned. "Is this study important to families? Would you enroll your child in this study? Why/why not? What is important to you?" In this way, patient engagement in pediatric rheumatology was born—many years before the founding of the Patient-Centered Outcomes Research Institute (PCORI). For the next several years, the caregivers were invited back to the meeting not only to listen and learn but also to participate in discussions related to research. There were limitations in CARRA's patient engagement program in these early years because the volunteers had lived experience in only a few of the pediatric rheumatic conditions which limited the extent of patient engagement to those conditions.

The Pediatric Rheumatology Care and Outcomes Improvement Network (PR-COIN) was formed in 2011 for the pediatric rheumatology community to collaborate with patients and families on QI initiatives to improve the delivery of care and outcomes of juvenile idiopathic arthritis (JIA) treatment (PR-COIN (pr-coin.org)). PR-COIN is a learning network that aims to engage patient families in all network activities and across all participating sites. The focus of PR-COIN engagement of patients and caretakers has currently been focused solely on JIA. Geographic diversity was accomplished by bringing volunteers to the table to represent each of the sites across North America. Each site would identify an individual to engage in site-based QI initiatives and connect them with the leadership team. Those patients or caregivers would then be trained in QI, onboarded to participate as a partner, and their interest areas and skillsets assessed to identify whereby they might be able to contribute.

Advocacy organizations have also engaged pediatric rheumatology patient families as volunteers for decades. These organizations have numerous avenues by which patients, caregivers, and others can participate in organizational efforts. The Arthritis Foundation, Lupus Foundation of American, CureJM, and other organizations find that patients have powerful stories to tell to help advocate for legislation or generate

Table 1
Feedback from researchers and patient partners

Research Role	Quote
Catherine L. Young adult diagnosed with JIA as a child. Participant in Stakeholder Advisory Council for a clinical trial.	*I am very grateful for the opportunity to participate in the groundbreaking research that CARRA[1] doctors, scientists, and parents conduct. CARRA has connected me with a kind and supportive community of people who are passionate about providing great care for kids with pediatric rheumatological conditions. Additionally, CARRA has given me a cathartic and tangible way to share my personal experiences with JIA and uveitis, and to turn them into research that will positively impact the way these conditions are treated in the future. So far, my favorite opportunities with CARRA include being (on) a Stakeholder Advisory Committee member for a randomized clinical trial. It was able to use my patient perspective to guide the design of pamphlets to be provided to newly diagnosed patients and their families when they were considering joining the randomized trial. In this way, I could help provide families with all the information I wish I had known when I was diagnosed. This year, I have worked on an engagement award where I was among a few patients who brainstormed a new topic* that is, *important to us but has not yet been researched. Out of these brainstorming sessions came the framework for a new app that would both inform young patients about what medical research entails and connect researchers with patients. I think this is a fantastic way to let researchers in on the topics that are most important to patients. CARRA helps bridge the gap between providers and patients, and it makes sure that patients' voices are heard in the process of conducting research for the future.*

(*continued on next page*)

Table 1
(*continued*)

Research Role	Quote
Laura C. JIA Parent PR-COIN Steering Committee member Participant in Stakeholder Advisory Council for a clinical trial	*As a parent of a JIA young adult, I am so happy to be a part of research. My son was diagnosed in 2003 and will be 21 years old in May. Since that time, so much has changed in the world of science and research, specifically in the area of juvenile rheumatic diseases. I am committed to helping and sharing my experiences because it gives me hope that children being diagnosed today or next year will have better treatment options and ultimately better outcomes. I cannot change the experiences that my son had, but I can try my best to help future generations.*
Dr Andrea Knight PI, Engaging patients and parents to improve mental health intervention for youth with rheumatologic disease[2]	*Working with PARTNERS greatly enriched our survey project. The collaboration provided valuable input from patients and parents, all the way from the survey design phase, to recruitment, data interpretation, and disseminating the results. Involving PARTNERS resulted in a better and more meaningful study, as well as the opportunity to build productive relationships with patient and parent advocates.*
Dr Colleen Correll PI, Identifying Research Priorities among Patients and Families of Children with Rheumatic Diseases living in the United States[3]	*Working with members of PARTNERS, including parents, researchers, and administrators, helped me to create and send surveys to assess the research priorities of patients and their families. Specifically, collaborating with PARTNERS helped me to create the survey using family-friendly language, deploy the survey through affiliated patient advocacy organizations' listservs and social media sites, promote patient and family participation in the survey and focus groups, and assisted in the writing of abstracts and manuscripts.*

(*continued on next page*)

Table 1
(*continued*)

Research Role	Quote
Dr Jon Hausmann PI, Health-Related Social Media Use by Parents of Children with Rheumatic Diseases	*It was an invaluable experience to work with PARTNERS to study how parents of children with rheumatic diseases use social media to learn about their child's condition. PARTNERS connected us with parent representatives from various organizations to help us create a survey to answer questions that mattered to them. The PARTNERS network allowed us to disseminate our survey across the various patient support organizations, giving voice to families of patients with rare conditions. Our allies at PARTNERS helped us to evaluate the results and present them at national meetings. We literally could not have done this project without PARTNERS.*
Dr Stephen Balevic PI, iPERSONAL[4] study Principal Investigator	*We had a great experience working with PARTNERS. The team was very responsive and efficiently paired us with a number of great stakeholders, including patients, parents, and advisory group members. The feedback from our stakeholders and overall collaboration with PARTNERS greatly enhanced our approach and ensured a family-centered clinical trial*

Abbreviations: CARRA: Childhood Arthritis & Rheumatology Research Alliance.

funds needed to maintain organizational programming. Connecting patients and caregivers to research is another activity of these advocacy organizations, which have also facilitated conversations about drug development needs with government entities such as the Food and Drug Administration (FDA).

In Europe, the European Network for Children with Arthritis and Autoinflammatory Diseases (ENCA), a network of pediatric rheumatic disease associations (www.enca.org), formed in Paris in 2002 and represent the country-specific organizations working with children and young people with pediatric rheumatic diseases and their families throughout Europe and beyond. Their primary activities include support for children and families affected by these conditions and raising awareness. In recent years, ENCA parents who have expertise in research have been leading projects and working directly with researchers and clinicians. Members of the Board of ENCA have worked on a range of research projects and are using their skills and experiences to help build research capacity within other ENCA member organizations. These parents are mentoring other parents and patients to do the same.

The emerging trend of patient engagement in the early 2000s led to the founding of the PCORI in 2010 as part of the Affordable Care Act. In 2014, PCORI established PCORnet, a network of networks that could harness the power of large amounts of health information to facilitate patient-centered comparative effectiveness research using a common data model. Nodes of this network included Clinical Data Research

Networks (CDRNs) which included institutions and health care systems, and Patient-Powered Research Networks (PPRNs) that were disease specific and community based. One PPRN was **P**atients, **A**dvocates, **R**heumatology **T**eams **N**etwork for **R**esearch and **S**ervice (PARTNERS) a consortium consisting of 5 independent, mature entities in pediatric rheumatology and linked them with patients and caregivers: a research network (CARRA), a QI network (PR-COIN), and 3 advocacy organizations (Arthritis Foundation, Lupus Foundation of America, CureJM. PARTNERS, working with the other CDRNs and PPRNs, created the infrastructure and shared best practices to engage caregivers and patients in the research process. In addition, PCORI defined a continuum to characterize different forms of patient engagement . Caregivers and patients new to research enter as consultants. As they gain experience, they are encouraged to deepen their level of engagement to involvement and eventually shared leadership.

In pediatric rheumatology, the goal is to engage patients and caregivers at all levels. Caregivers and patients can participate at various levels over time, depending on their experience and desire.

PATIENT ENGAGEMENT PERSPECTIVES IN PEDIATRIC RHEUMATOLOGY

There are many perspectives that should be considered when engaging with caregivers and patients as research partners. One challenging dynamic in pediatric research is that primary researchers may not be working directly with the population (the patient) being enrolled in research studies. By adding the perspective of the patient family, the study team can bring in more complex needs, preferences, and dynamics. Caregivers have a different lived experience and potentially different concerns than that of a patient, so both perspectives should be included when possible. In addition, patients engaged in a study team's activities are often young adult patients who are no longer in the age group being recruited into the study. Their perspective is very valuable, especially if they can reflect back on their experiences when they were younger, but this can often be challenging to accomplish.

A good way to think about the needed perspectives of research partners is to refer to the inclusion/exclusion criteria of the proposed study. For example, a study looking to evaluate the effectiveness and tolerability of medication for newly diagnosed systemic JIA would benefit the most from partners who not only have systemic JIA, but were recently diagnosed, or have used the medication in the past. These patients and caregivers would bring their valuable lived experience to assess protocol acceptability, generalizability, and impact, while delivering key insights drawn from their own experiences. To this end, they can assist the study team in the development of recruitment and retention materials and selection of outcome measures. In addition to lived experience, caregivers and patients have wide-ranging personal and professional skills that can be useful throughout the lifecycle of the research project. Social workers, mental health professionals, graphic designers, statisticians, health literacy experts, and social media managers are just a few examples of professional roles that can add to the study team's ability to execute a research project successfully and efficiently. In addition to hard skills, patients and caregivers who have experience being engaged on a study team can effectively serve as mentors for patient families new to the role of research partner who can greatly benefit from their experiences. Finally, research teams should strive for diversity and inclusion with respect to gender, race, ethnicity, socio-economic status, geography, education level and language, to ensure the study addresses all barriers to enrollment of the target population.

BEST PRACTICES IN PATIENT ENGAGEMENT

Defining Roles

Researchers new to patient engagement often ask, "What can I have a patient partner do?" Questions like this limit the possible contributions partners can have on a project. Successful study execution relies on the completion of multiple tasks needing wide-ranging hard skills and perspectives. Instead of the question "what can we have a patient partner do?" the question should be "what tasks need to be completed to successfully execute the study?". Knowing the tasks, skills, and perspectives needed, researchers can then define the potential roles of the patient partner. Using the PCORI continuum as a guide, roles for partners can be categorized into 3 levels of engagement with increasing time commitment and varied purpose: consultation, advisory, or shared leadership (**Table 2**).

Initially, patient partners usually become involved as focus group members or survey responders. The partner time commitment is minimal and usually, the consultation is limited to a single to a few occurrences. Focus groups and surveys are valuable tools the study team can deploy quickly to measure the impact of the proposed study and acceptability of the protocol. Advisory board members have slightly deeper engagement. Although time commitment is still relatively low, the engagement lasts over several years throughout the life cycle of the project. Advisory boards enhance the study team's ability to identify barriers to recruitment and retention and create tools to address these barriers. They provide project oversight and can assist with protocol amendments needed to address recruitment and retention challenges. Advisory boards are an opportunity to engage diverse perspectives and skill sets that fill gaps in the study team.

The deepest level of engagement for a patient partner is the role of project co-leader or co-investigator. With time commitments commonly up to 0.25 FTE, the role of co-investigator should only be considered for deeply engaged, committed patient partners that can spend at least several hours per week on the project. Co-investigators can participate at multiple levels of the governance structure of the project and attend all study team calls. They can act as liaisons between the many functional groups as well as lead the Advisory Committee. Co-investigators are experienced patient partners who have often served on an Advisory Committee. In their larger role, they are an integral part of all operations-from idea generation and assisting with grant writing all the way to disseminating study results. They take an active role in recruiting, onboarding, and training all the other patient partners that will be engaged in the study.

Table 2
Possible levels of engagement

Level of Engagement	Description	Time Commitment	Purpose
Consultation	Focus group members, survey responders	Minimal, often one time	Reaching broad communities
Advisory	Stakeholder Advisory Committee members	Moderate, often for the length of the project	Patient/caregiver voice in study design
Shared Leadership	Parent/Patient Investigator, Study Team Leadership	25% FTE or sometimes more	Truly patient-centered research

TOOLS REQUIRED BEFORE ENGAGEMENT

Once the perspectives, skills, and roles needed of each patient partner are known, the principal investigator (PI) can draft a Statement of Work (SOW). The SOW is a 1–2-page tool the PI uses to advertise the engagement opportunity to the community. It clearly defines the project and the role of the patient partner in very plain language. The SOW includes project background, goals, desired perspectives, and skill sets, time commitment, and estimated start and end dates. Renumeration for the time spent should be covered but will rely on obtaining funding for the project. Guidance on the renumeration depends on the time commitment and expertise of the patient partner and can range from $25–$75 per hour. The goal of renumeration is to demonstrate that the partner's time and expertise are valued, much the same way as other researchers working on the study. Some projects do not have the budget to compensate patient partners but can still engage patients and caregivers if the SOW explains they will be volunteering their time. Partners being compensated would do so through contracts with the site or project management office.

In addition to the SOW, a Memorandum of Understanding (MOU) is prepared before engaging patient partners. The MOU is like a contract, signed and dated by the PI and the patient partner. Like the SOW, it covers the project background and goals and then provides a more granular view of the role. The MOU outlines partner responsibilities and expectations as well as the support they will receive. If renumeration is included, the MOU will explain how and when the compensation will be disbursed. Finally, the MOU should also include language that allows the partner to resign from the project or for the study team to terminate the engagement if necessary.

IDENTIFYING PATIENT PARTNERS

Many strategies can be used to find patient partners for a study:

- *Advocacy organizations* often have large lists of constituents to whom the opportunity can be advertised through email, blog posts, and events.
- *Health care providers* can approach caregivers and patients they see in the clinic.
- *The PARTNERS PPRN* maintains a database of caregivers and patients who have expressed interest in becoming engaged in research.
- *Experienced patient partners* have networks of families they know or have worked with in the past.
- *Social media groups and influencers* have large followings of caregivers and patients that can be tapped to advertise engagement opportunities.

Although a single strategy may be sufficient to meet a study's recruitment needs, using as many as possible is suggested to ensure a diverse and inclusive representation for any study.

RECRUITING, ONBOARDING, AND TRAINING

Successful patient engagement is built on respect, trust, and the development of personal relationships between the researcher and the patient/caregiver partner. Relationship building is not limited to topics related to research and should be more personal. This leads to trust while simultaneously dispelling tokenization. During the relationship-building stage, the researcher will learn the interests and skills of the patient or caregiver, which can inform potential roles for the partner in the project. Informing the research partner of their role results in a greater understanding of why they are needed in the project. The research partner will feel personally connected to the project, the investigator, and the patients who are being enrolled, which in turn deepens their engagement and commitment to the project.

New research partners often believe they are not qualified to engage in a research project. However, patient families are truly experts in the lived experience of having or caring for someone with a pediatric rheumatic disease. Explaining to the patient partner that their lived experience is a critical perspective needed on the research team empowers them to participate as a vital and engaged member of the study team. Additionally, in many circumstances, the patient or caregiver may have other useful professional or personal skillsets to add to the study team that can lead to a more efficiently run project as outlined above (see *Patient Engagement Perspectives in Pediatric Rheumatology)*.

Once the relationship is built, training of patient partners and researchers can begin. The first step of patient and caregiver training is a high-level overview explaining their role on the project, why it's needed, and some basic research terms and concepts. Partners are not trained to be researchers, but they are provided with definitions of some commonly used jargon explained in lay language. The training is done through one-on-one calls between the new partner and a mentor. Following these calls, materials can be shared to reinforce the prior conversation. Glossaries exist on the NIH and CARRA websites and terms shared with partners should be selected based on relevance to the project to avoid information overload. PCORI has an extensive library of engagement training materials from past awards, including multiple videos and materials created through a 2016 PARTNERS/Arthritis Foundation Eugene Washington Award. High-level training also includes an overview of the difference between being a research partner and "sharing your story". Research partners draw on their personal experience and apply it in a general way to speak on behalf of the community of patients, rather than simply sharing their personal story.

Researcher training includes many of the same concepts embedded in successful focus group facilitation. Respectful dialogue, active listening, and frequent knowledge checks are essential for successful patient engagement. Avoiding jargon when possible and defining terms when necessary will help families follow the discussion. Resources for researchers are available on the OMERACT[5] and PCORI[6] websites. After all members of the team are trained, onboarding can continue in a virtual group meeting whereby introductions are made and details of the project are shared.

MENTORING NEW PARENTS/PATIENTS

As more researchers seek to incorporate patient engagement in their project, there is a need for more patient and caregiver research partners. To meet the increasing demand and ensure diverse perspectives contributing to the design and execution of studies, experienced research partners have been mentoring new families. As in other mentor/mentee relationships, the mentor is a source of support and guidance for the mentee and acts as their primary point of contact for the project. Each project should consider a leadership role for experienced patient partners as well as smaller roles for new partners who can be mentored and gain valuable experience. Including these new patient partners will develop the next generation of leaders and expand opportunities across the continuum of engagement. The pediatric rheumatology community aims to build a group of highly engaged and prepared patients and caregivers who can join a study team, help to onboard and train new patients/caregivers, and continue to widen the ripple effect that has been started.

HEALTH LITERACY

A frequently overlooked aspect of patient engagement is health literacy, which goes beyond a patient or caregiver's ability to simply read health information. The definition has been expanded: for the Healthy People 2010 initiative, heath literacy was defined as "the degree to which individuals have the capacity to obtain, process, and understand basic health information and services needed to make appropriate health decisions" (Ratzen & Parker, 2000).[7] Even though most adults can read at an eighth-grade level and 20% of the population reads at or below a fifth-grade level, most health care materials are written at a 10th-grade level (https://www.aafp.org/afp/2005/0801/p463.html). To address this gap, patients and caregivers must have a seat at the table when developing study materials and dissemination plans to assist in translating to lay language. Proven techniques to lower the reading level include using short sentences, limiting the use of 3 syllable words, defining medical terms, increasing white space, and providing real-world relatable examples. Software such as Health Literacy Advisor (https://www.healthliteracyinnovations.com/products/hla) which highlights complex medical terms and suggests alternative language can also be useful in lowering the reading level. Health literate study materials facilitate participant understanding, allowing them to make an informed decision to enroll in a study and have greater understanding of the study results.

PITFALLS

The most significant pitfall in patient engagement is when an investigator engages a patient or caregiver simply to "check a box". With funding organizations pushing patient engagement as part of a grant application, an inexperienced researcher may engage a family in ways that may not offer much benefit to anyone. To avoid this, researchers in the pediatric rheumatology community new to engaging patients should be advised by experienced research partners on how to best approach, engage, train, and use the patients and caregivers in every step of the research process. In 2018, CARRA hired a Director of Patient Engagement (V.D.) for the first time, prioritizing and standardizing the concept of engaging patients in research activities at an organizational level.

Another common mistake made by study teams and experienced patient/parent partners alike is overwhelming new families with too much information. For highly engaged, knowledgeable research partners, it is easy to share too much information too soon. New families can be trained, onboarded, and empowered but if they attend meetings before they are ready and feel overwhelmed, their interest will wane and engagement will cease. When a project gets started, the pace is often rapid, and efforts to be inclusive with new parents/patient partners can backfire. There is a delicate balance between engaging enough but not overwhelming a family. This balancing point is different for individual patient participants and often hard to assess. Frequent check-ins with new families and recaps after meetings missed can reengage the new patient partner. Engaging new families in research is a slow, deliberate, stepwise process, ideally beginning with smaller roles to gain experience and self-confidence. New families can be invited to all meetings but should be told which ones are not required. They might have little to contribute initially but anyone interested in learning more about the process is likely to stay engaged and bring new skills to their next project.

Being mindful that patients and caregivers live with or care for a person with a chronic illness as well as manage full lives is critical. Pediatric rheumatic conditions flare, individuals have school, and/or work commitments, and other life events that may pull them away from research. A well-oriented and trained patient or caregiver may still need to back out to attend to life issues. Although this can be disruptive to the research process, it is an unavoidable part of working with families dealing with chronic illness. Once again, frequent check-ins and support by members of the study team can keep families up to speed on study progress, facilitating future reengagement when the time is right. Study disruption is minimized by involving several patient partners in any given research project.

Finally, identifying and recruiting patients from diverse backgrounds is a tremendous challenge. Various pediatric rheumatic conditions may preferentially affect specific races and ethnicities, so every effort must be made to recruit partners reflective of the community of patients affected by the condition. Unfortunately, access to care and trust in the health care system and research, as well as other universal diversity issues affect the populations followed by clinical care teams and may not be representative of the population at large. However, if only homogenous racial, ethnic, and sociodemographic groups are engaged, health care disparities will continue and limit the generalizability of research results.

INTEGRATING PATIENTS IN ALL ACTIVITIES

Another way to engage patients is organization (rather than project) based. Integrating patients across an entire organization increases the value of services delivered and more efficient use of resources. In CARRA, for example, a Registry Patient/Parent Advisory Committee has recently been formed to help advise CARRA Registry leadership by gathering feedback from patient communities to bring back to the Registry and its activities. Operational roles at CARRA have been developed and filled by parents as employees and subcontractors, truly bringing the voice of the patient into the day-to-day operations of this large research organization. Within the PR-COIN network, parents currently serve on every committee, including the Executive and Steering Committees that truly drive the work of this network. Within advocacy networks such as the Arthritis Foundation, patients and caregivers are taking on leadership roles in planning programs and executing events. By plugging the "consumer" into a role that helps drive the mission of an organization, patient engagement is being taken a step further to improve the patient focus and quality of the work being done.

NEXT STEPS

Patient engagement in pediatric rheumatology research has grown rapidly over the past 15 years, from a couple of caregivers in a few disease areas partnering with a few researchers, to over 100 patient partners in virtually every disease area partnering with scores of researchers. CARRA has underscored its commitment to patient engagement by hiring a full-time Director of Partnerships and Patient Engagement and setting expectations that all clinical research projects will include patients and families. However, more work is needed. Quantitatively measuring the impact of patient engagement on the research process will help sway late adopters and funders to this type of work. Newly diagnosed families have a perspective that is extremely valuable, but they are more challenging to engage as research partners because simply understanding and managing the illness is overwhelming at that stage. A patient navigator program will be piloted soon to assist newly diagnosed families and gently introduce the culture of research in pediatric rheumatology in an effort to engage them as partners. In addition, a mobile application is under development to facilitate bidirectional communication between potential patient partners and researchers. Lastly, international collaborations are a priority to ensure that best practices in North America and elsewhere can be shared and more productive patient engagement can become a global mission. Concentrated efforts must be made at organizational levels to promote more diverse, equitable, and inclusive environments to engage a more representative sample of the communities of patients served.

CLINICS CARE POINTS

- Relationship building is the first step toward patient engagement in research and leads to mutual respect and trust in the research process.
- Once the relationship is established, patients and caregivers should be approached as early in the research process as possible.
- During the idea phase of a project, experienced families can assist with the development of research aims to ensure relevance and protocol to ensure acceptability.
- Ask families interested in becoming a research partner for permission to share their contact information to introduce them to experienced research partners.

ACKNOWLEDGEMENT

The authors wish to acknowledge CARRA and the ongoing Arthritis Foundation financial support of CARRA.

REFERENCES

1. Available at: https://apps.who.int/iris/bitstream/handle/10665/252269/9789241511629-eng.pdf. Accessed February 3, 2021.
2. Available at: https://pubmed.ncbi.nlm.nih.gov/33622346/. Accessed February 25, 2021.
3. Available at: https://pubmed.ncbi.nlm.nih.gov/32062607/. Accessed February 25, 2021.
4. Available at: https://clinicaltrials.gov/ct2/show/NCT04358302?term=balevic&cond=lupus&cntry=US&draw=2&rank=1. Accessed February 25, 2021.
5. Available at: https://pubmed.ncbi.nlm.nih.gov/25877496/. Accessed February 28, 2021.
6. Available at: https://www.pcori.org/sites/default/files/PCORI-Engagement-Strategies-for-Initiating-Research-Partnerships-Info-Sheet-71917.pdf. Accessed February 28, 2021.
7. Ratzen SC, Parker RM. National Library of Medicine current bibliographies in medicine: health literacy. 2000. Introduction. Available at: https://webharvest.gov/peth04/20041105213541/http://www.nlm.nih.gov/pubs/cbm/hliteracy.pdf.

Assessing Patient-Reported Outcomes in Pediatric Rheumatic Diseases

Considerations and Future Directions

Christina K. Zigler, PhD, MSEd[a,*], Rachel L. Randell, MD[b], Bryce B. Reeve, PhD[a,c]

KEYWORDS

- Pediatric rheumatic diseases • Patient-reported outcomes
- Patient-reported outcome measures • Clinical trials • Clinical care
- Future directions

KEY POINTS

- Whenever possible, children and adolescents with PRD should report directly on their health status via PRO measures.
- When using PRO measures, researchers and clinicians should consider (1) what is important to measure, (2) who is the best source of information, (3) what is the best measure, and (4) how best to integrate the measures into the targeted setting.
- Most published research for PROs has focused on juvenile idiopathic arthritis and pediatric systemic lupus erythematosus, although there are emerging bodies of research for lesser-known conditions.
- Future directions for PROs in PRD include establishing core outcome sets, improving interpretability of scores, identifying clinically meaningful changes using a variety of methods, and identifying PROs for rare conditions.

Patient-reported outcomes (PROs) are an integral part of research and clinical care across medical specialties. Certain aspects of a patient's life, like pain, sleep quality, or daily functioning, remain unknown unless directly queried. By allowing patients to directly report on their health status, researchers and clinicians can better understand the full experiences of living with a condition or disease. Assessing PROs for children

The content is solely the responsibility of the authors and does not necessarily represent the official views of the NIH.

[a] Department of Population Health Sciences, Center for Health Measurement, Duke University School of Medicine, 215 Morris Street, Suite 235, DUMC 104023, Durham, NC 27701, USA; [b] Division of Pediatric Rheumatology, Department of Pediatrics, Duke University School of Medicine, 2301 Erwin Rd. Durham, NC 27705, USA; [c] Pediatrics, Duke University School of Medicine, 215 Morris Street, Suite 230, DUMC 104023, Durham, NC 27701, USA
* Corresponding author.
E-mail address: Christina.zigler@duke.edu

Rheum Dis Clin N Am 48 (2022) 15–29
https://doi.org/10.1016/j.rdc.2021.09.008
0889-857X/22/

and adolescents (typically 8 years or older) is an accepted practice if the measures themselves are developmentally appropriate.[1] In fact, having pediatric patients report directly on their health status is important for their autonomy and may highlight divergent perspectives compared with their parents.[2] PROs are particularly important for pediatric rheumatic diseases (PRDs), in which children may experience chronic symptoms, such as pain, and functional limitations. When children are too young or ill to self-report, caregiver-proxy measures can be used.

WHAT ARE PATIENT-REPORTED OUTCOME MEASURES?

The US Food and Drug Administration (FDA) defines PROs as "important aspects of how individuals are feeling and functioning,"[3] and PRO *measures* refer to the questionnaire the patient completes without the help of another individual. The PRO measure produces a score reflecting lower or higher levels of the PRO that may be used to inform research findings or treatment options. Many stakeholders in the health care setting recognize the importance of PROs. Both the FDA and the European Medicines Agency advocate for use of PRO measures, such as those measuring health-related quality of life (HRQOL), in clinical trials (fda.gov and ema.europa.eu). In addition to evaluating treatment efficacy and monitoring clinical symptoms, PRO measures have been used to screen patients with PRD for mental health concerns[4] and help redefine outcomes to make them more meaningful to patients (eg, redefining "clinical remission"[5]).

The potential benefits of measuring PROs in clinical care and research settings are many, but the application of rigorous standards to identify, develop, and evaluate PRO measures is relatively new (most guidance/standards published over the past 20 years). In addition, research into pediatric PROs has progressed more slowly than in adults. Although pediatric rheumatologists have proactively assessed PROs for patients with PRDs,[6] more work is needed. Thus, the goal of this article is to describe the current use of PROs in PRDs, aligning current research with best practice recommendations, and identify areas for future work.

PATIENT-REPORTED OUTCOMES IN PEDIATRIC RHEUMATIC DISEASES

Pediatric rheumatologists often focus on "disease activity" using objective measures such as laboratory and clinical biomarkers. These outcomes are important for making decisions on starting, stopping, maintaining, or escalating treatment. However, patients with rheumatic conditions often identify other priorities, including pain, fatigue, sleep quality, functioning, mental health, and medication side effects.[7] Historically, visual analog scales were used to capture this information from the family, focusing on global construct like "overall well-being" rather than specific disease or drug-related symptoms. Pediatric rheumatologists also adopted PRO measures for children and adolescents based on adult measures. For example, the Children's Health Assessment Questionnaire (CHAQ)[8] was adapted from the adult Health Assessment Questionnaire,[9] designed to capture functional status (ie, disability) for several rheumatic conditions.

As the field of health assessment has grown, rigorous methods have been applied to the design of PRO measures. Launched in 2004, the National Institutes of Health's (NIH's) Patient-Reported Outcomes Measurement Information System (PROMIS) provides researchers and clinicians access to a broad range of high-quality, universal, and freely available PRO measures.[10] PROMIS measures were rigorously developed, designed, and evaluated with state-of-the-science qualitative and quantitative methods[11,12] across a broad range of adult and pediatric populations including

PRDs.[13–15] More than 100 adult and 25 pediatric domains of symptoms, function, and well-being provide researchers and clinicians flexibility to select measures based on their needs and length of questionnaire (longer measures provide more reliable assessment). For example, a pediatric rheumatologist may choose to assess pain, fatigue, physical functioning, sleep disturbance, depression, and anxiety in clinical practice. The rheumatologist may select the PROMIS Pediatric 8-item short forms for important domains such as pain and physical functioning and select PROMIS Pediatric 4-item short forms for fatigue, sleep disturbance, depression, and anxiety. The rheumatologist may also use the PROMIS computerized adaptive testing (CAT) versions of the measures to individually tailor the assessment for each pediatric patient. Thus, PROMIS is adaptable to the needs of a care provider or researcher to yield high-quality patient-centered data for use in clinical care, research, and quality improvement.

PRO measurement greatly enhances understanding of patient's lived experience with PRD. In particular, children may experience disease impacts on life in ways not captured by biomarkers. For example, children with pediatric systemic lupus erythematosus (pSLE) reported ongoing pain and fatigue, even in the face of "normal" conventional disease activity measures.[16] In addition, some therapeutic trials that failed to meet primary disease activity end points have shown important improvement in patient symptoms (eg, hydroxycholorquine reducing pain in Sjögren syndrome[17]), but inclusion of PROs in clinical trials relies on strong measurement properties.[18] Furthermore, at an individual patient level, PROs may identify opportunities for improving patient care. Pediatric rheumatologists who screen patients for functional impairments and psychological comorbidities, which often linger after disease activity "resolves," can identify patients who might benefit from occupational therapy or counseling referrals.[4,19] There are four questions that rheumatologists should consider when identifying and implementing PROs in pediatric rheumatic disease settings (**Box 1**).

CONSIDERATION 1: STARTING AT THE BEGINNING. WHAT MATTERS TO PATIENTS?

Identifying what is meaningful to patients is a crucial first step to developing PROs. To accurately represent the voice of individuals living with disease, those individuals and their caregivers should be directly involved in deciding which HRQOL domains to assess within a specific context (eg, clinical care, research, or clinical trials; **Box 2**). The Outcome Measures in Rheumatology (OMERACT) workgroup found a strong need for patients to be involved in revising the established core domain sets (a common set of assessment variables across studies) for juvenile idiopathic arthritis (JIA)[20]; it was updated in 2018 based on input from 53 patients aged 15 to 24 years and

Box 1
Best practice: identifying and implementing patient-reported outcome measures in pediatric rheumatic disease settings

For PROs to inform decision making for pediatric rheumatic diseases, researchers and clinicians should address 4 questions:

1. What outcomes matters most to patients and is actionable for clinicians, investigators, patients, and caregivers?
2. Who is the best source for providing information on symptoms, functioning, and quality of life given the age and health condition of the child?
3. What PRO has the strongest evidence for validity and reliability to measure the targeted outcomes?
4. How do we effectively integrate PRO measures into research and health care delivery settings?

Box 2
Overview of considerations for patient-reported outcomes in pediatric rheumatic diseases

Question 1: Starting at the beginning. What matters most to patients?
- Patients and families decide what HRQOL domains to assess with PRO measures, because they are able to identify domains that are important to them and meaningfully affect their lives.
- HRQOL domains collected via PRO measures need to be relevant to the setting (eg, actionable by clinicians, related to the mechanism of action or side effects in clinical trials).
- HRQOL domains relevant to patients may differ depending on the disease or condition (eg, joint pain for patients with juvenile arthritis) or may vary by patient age (eg, body image for teenagers), whereas some domains may be more general (eg, fatigue for all pediatric rheumatic diseases).

Question 2: Who is the best source for providing information on HRQOL domains?
- Children and adolescents report directly on their health status whenever possible.
- The selection of the appropriate measure should be based on a good understanding of the target population in terms of developmental level age and abilities.
- Parental proxy report provides helpful information, but is not equivalent to child self-report.

Question 3: What is best measure of key HRQOL domains?
- Evidence supporting use of PRO measures should be specific to the target population and the purpose of the assessment.
- Recommended attributes of a PRO measure from the Scientific Advisory Committee of the Medical Outcome Trust[33] include:
  - Basis on a conceptual and measurement model
  - Reliability (including internal consistency and test-retest reliability)
  - Validity (including content validity and construct validity)
  - Responsiveness to change
  - Interpretability of scores
  - Low respondent and administrative burden
  - Availability in alternative forms
  - Cultural and language adaptations and translations
- "Legacy measures" should be evaluated on an ongoing basis to ensure their continued validity.

Question 4: How to effectively integrate PRO measures into research and health care delivery settings?
- PRO measures have been successfully integrated into pediatric clinical care and research settings.[39,40]
- Guidance documents provide specific information about integrating PRO measures into clinical research and care settings.[41,42,44]

several parents,[21] showing that (1) older children/adolescents were able to successfully participate in the process and (2) domains prioritized by patients and families were different from those of other stakeholders.[21] It cannot be overstated that asking children, adolescents, and families what is most meaningful to their lives is critical to driving patient-centered research and care. Patient and family input may be more vital in rare and less well-researched conditions like juvenile dermatomyositis (JDM), localized scleroderma(LS)/morphea, and chronic recurrent multifocal osteomyelitis/chronic nonbacterial osteomyelitis (CRMO/CNO) because of unique disease features. Furthermore, because our knowledge and understanding of these conditions is in development, incorporating patient voices has a great potential for positive impact on research and care.

Common contexts for PRO assessment are clinical care (eg, to improve patient-clinician communication, drive shared treatment decisions, provide referrals to specialists such as psychiatrists for mental health issues) and clinical trials (eg, evaluate treatment efficacy, capture medication side effects). In any context, it is important to identify outcomes important to the patients, relevant to the setting, and actionable by clinicians, caregivers, teachers, and other parties invested in the child's well-being, including themselves. Clinicians are likely to ignore outcomes less directly related to therapeutics (eg, spirituality) or that lack clear meaningfulness, which may subsequently leave patients feeling that their time completing the questionnaire was wasted.[22] Sharing PRO data with the child and family in ways that ensure the scores are meaningful helps communication with the provider and tracks health status, adding to understanding of the child's health status.

CONSIDERATION 2: WHO IS THE BEST SOURCE FOR PROVIDING OUTCOME INFORMATION?

A child's self-report is the best source for learning their feelings and function (see **Box 2**). In general, children as young as 5 years are generally capable of self-reporting aspects of HRQOL (eg, pain) with some assistance,[1] and responses become even more reliable as they get older.[23] Children at least 8 years old are often able to read and self-report independently on a broader type of outcomes such as anxiety. In particular, the PROMIS Pediatric measures were developed to be appropriate for children aged 8 to 17 years, with parent-proxy measures (when caregivers report their child's health status) available for children aged 5 to 17 years.[24,25]

When children are too young, too ill, or developmentally unable to report their own HRQOL, parent-proxy report can be a helpful method to gain information about the patient's HRQOL. However, disagreement between the child's self-report with either caregivers or clinicians' report often exists.[26] Clinicians typically have poor to fair associations with child self-report.[27] Caregiver report is more closely associated with the child's self-report, but caregivers' ratings are impacted by their own health and life experiences.[28,29] For example, as parent's own health worsens they tend to report worse health for their child.[30,31] Thus, experts recommend prioritizing child self-report unless a child is unable to complete a PRO measure, then collecting data from caregivers is appropriate. However, caregiver-reported data should not be treated as equal to child self-report, but rather an alternative helpful information source.[32]

CONSIDERATION 3: WHAT ARE ATTRIBUTES OF A HIGH-QUALITY MEASURE?

The Medical Outcomes Trust recommends 8 attributes for a quality HRQOL measure (see **Box 2**).[33] Understanding the recommended attributes can help a pediatric rheumatologist identify PRO measures that have adequate validity and reliability for the intended population in the intended context. There also are published guidance and frameworks to help clinicians and researchers evaluate existing measures for a specific purpose (eg, COSMIN methodology,[34] FDA guidance[35]).

Even PRO measures widely used in PRDs warrant critical review. There are "legacy measures" adopted early by researchers and clinicians that were never rigorously evaluated or are outdated due to changes in understanding and/or treatment of disease. Thus, it is worth revisiting legacy measures to see if they are still valid for current contexts. A recent qualitative study enrolled children and youth aged 10 to 24 years with PRDs into focus groups. When discussing psychosocial research priorities, they described the CHAQ, a widely used functional status measure in research and clinical practice, as "too long" and "did not capture their experience of their condition."[36] In a subsequent study, 52 patients aged 5 to 17 years with JIA or JDM preferred PROMIS Pediatric measures to the CHAQ. In analysis, the PROMIS pediatric measures did not show ceiling effects, although the CHAQ did.[37]

For rare conditions that lack validated PROs, generic (universal) measures like the PROMIS Pediatric measures can be useful to gather evidence on specific outcomes of interest (eg, pain, fatigue, physical functioning). Another strength of using universal measures in rare conditions is that they allow comparison of scores with more prevalent PRDs, other chronic conditions, and "healthy" populations for which there is documented normative data. In some cases, it may be useful to consider "disease-specific" measures, which are PRO measures developed and validated purposely for one population. In some cases, this can increase the likelihood that the measure is capturing information that is relevant and specific to the rare disease. The importance of reconsidering legacy measures is also critical for rarer PRDs. For example, when the Children's Dermatology Life Quality Index, a legacy measure for LS, was formally evaluated, it was found to have limited construct validity and the researchers concluded that scores were likely to underestimate the true impact of LS on patients' HRQOL.[38]

CONSIDERATION 4: HOW CAN PATIENT-REPORTED OUTCOME MEASURES INTEGRATE EFFECTIVELY INTO RESEARCH AND HEALTH CARE DELIVERY SETTINGS?

Although the use of PROs in pediatric settings lags behind adults,[39,40] there are several evidence-based guidances to help PRO implementation (see **Box 2**). The SPIRIT-PRO guidelines focus on clinical trial protocols where PRO measures are a central outcome (primary or secondary), including recommendations around intervention time points and strategies to minimize missing data.[41] Other helpful frameworks include the Consolidated Standards of Reporting Trials (CONSORT) PRO extension,[42] the Setting International Standards in Analyzing Patient-Reported Outcomes and Quality of Life Endpoints Data Consortium recommendations,[43] and the International Society for Quality of Life Research's minimum standards.[44] Despite minor differences in perspectives across the documents, recommendations are largely consistent,[45] meaning that pediatric rheumatologists can feel comfortable following any of the selected guidelines. Similar guidances are available for providers interested in implementing PRO measures in clinical practice.[46,47]

STATE OF THE FIELD

PRDs make up a group of heterogeneous, often painful, chronic conditions often affecting multiple organ systems. Specific considerations for PROs may differ between disease populations. In the following sections, we highlight research in specific disease areas. Most of the published research has focused on JIA and pSLE, although there are emerging bodies of research for lesser-known conditions like LS.

JIA: PROs have been used for several decades in JIA research across various domains, including pain intensity, pain interference, physical function, and medication side effects, and there are ongoing efforts to optimize and further incorporate PROs into research and clinical care.[48] Recently, there have been several large-scale efforts responding to the need for rigorous and patient-centric outcome measures for JIA (**Table 1**). For example, the Juvenile Arthritis Multidimensional Assessment Report (JAMAR) is a multidimensional PRO measure designed for use in standard clinical care.[49] Since its development, the JAMAR has been translated into 54 languages[50] and is currently used in a global effort of the Pediatric Rheumatology International Trials Organisation (PRINTO) to evaluate disease categories, treatment, and health status worldwide. Simultaneously, several groups are evaluating PROMIS measures in JIA.[51] Recent publications report clinically meaningful severity and minimally important differences for several PROMIS measures.[14,52] Although additional work to

Table 1
Recent, large-scale efforts to respond to the needs for rigorous and patient-centric outcome measures for juvenile idiopathic arthritis

JAMAR	A multidimensional PRO measure designed for use in standard clinical care.[49] Since development, the JAMAR has been translated into 54 languages[50] and is being used in a worldwide effort of the PRINTO to evaluate disease categories, treatment and health status worldwide[a]
International OMERACT initiative	Intended to improve outcome measurement through a data-driven, iterative consensus process, relevant stakeholders (including patients) established a JIA Working Group in 2015. Since then, the JIA Working Group has developed and updated a Core Domain Set for JIA studies[21] using OMERACT methodology, with ongoing efforts to identify and systematically evaluate the best outcome measures for the domains
The CAPTURE-JIA workgroup (United Kingdom)	Developed a core dataset to address the need for consensus PROs in JIA.[79] Because no preexisting questionnaire captured all priorities identified by patients and parents, the group developed a new questionnaire (CAPTURE-JIA PROM/PREM) using OMERACT methodology. CAPTURE-JIA PROM/PREM was recently validated and shown to be feasible for use in routine clinical care[80]
CARRA JIA Research Committee Outcomes Workgroup	With ongoing efforts endorsed by OMERACT, the working group intends to reexamine core set variables, standardize scoring of disease activity, and integrate parent assessment of overall well-being[b]

Abbreviations: CAPTURE-JIA; CARRA, The Childhood Arthritis and Rheumatology Research Alliance; JAMAR, The Juvenile Arthritis Multidimensional Assessment Report; PRINTO, Pediatric Rheumatology International Trials Organisation; PROM/PREM.
[a] https://www.printo.it/projects/past.
[b] https://carragroup.org/.

evaluate validity and reliability of PROMIS measures for JIA in specific contexts is needed, these findings and ongoing use of PROMIS underscores its usefulness in JIA.

pSLE: Several PRO measures are used to capture important domains in pSLE including pain, fatigue, physical/social functioning, and others contributing to disease burden.[53] Similar to JIA, the CHAQ has been used to assess disability in pSLE,[54] but in recent years this legacy measure has been overshadowed by several newer PROs specific to SLE, including the Lupus Quality of Life (LupusQoL), Lupus Patient Reported Outcomes, and Lupus Impact Tracker (LIT) instruments, among others. The LIT measures HRQOL in SLE across several domains including cognition, physical health, pain/fatigue impact, and medication side effects.[55] The LIT recently showed favorable psychometric properties and correlation with both patient-reported and physician-reported measures of disease activity in a pilot study of adolescents and young adults with pSLE.[55] The Simple Measure of the Impact of Lupus Erythematosus in Youngsters (SMILEY) assesses children's self-perception of quality of life[56] and has some evidence to support its validity in pSLE[57].[58] Several PROMIS Pediatric domains also have support for validity when used in pSLE.[16,52]

JDM: In general, PRO measure use in JDM is less mature than in other PRDs, but there are several ongoing efforts to advance the use of PROs. A core dataset has been developed with input from patients and parents,[59] and the Childhood Arthritis and Rheumatology Research Alliance (CARRA) JDM Research Committee Quality Measures Workgroup has partnered with patients and families in collaboration with the CureJM Foundation to evaluate the importance of various PROs and quality indicators.[60] For JDM, PROMIS measures have been evaluated for validity[61] and clinically important differences[62] and used in descriptive studies.[63]

Juvenile LS: Several different PRO measures have been used to evaluate HRQOL in this population, with largely conflicting results.[64] The disease-specific Localized Scleroderma Quality of Life Instrument (LoSQI) was designed with input from children and adolescents with LS and showed content validity using a patient-centered approach.[64,65] The LoSQI is currently used in 2 North American registries (National Registry for Childhood Onset Scleroderma and The Morphea in Adults and Children Cohort), and cross-cultural adaptation for international use is ongoing (https://www.printo.it/projects/ongoing/37).

Chronic recurrent multifocal osteomyelitis (CRMO), also known as chronic nonbacterial osteomyelitis (CNO), is a rare but increasingly recognized painful inflammatory bone disease. Recent studies highlight patient perspective on disease burden and other aspects of HRQOL.[66,67] There is a CRMO/CNO working group through OMERACT, and a prospective registry of CRMO/CNO is currently collecting PROMIS measures.

FUTURE DIRECTIONS

There are recent and ongoing efforts to develop core outcomes and core outcome assessments that incorporate PROs, including work by the Core Outcome Measures in Effectiveness Trials (COMET) initiative (https://www.cometinitiative.org/) and the International Consortium for Health Outcomes Measurement (ICHOM; https://www.ichom.org/). The FDA launched a program to develop core outcome sets as part of their patient-focused drug development (PFDD) initiative. The development of core outcome sets is typically based on a consensus-seeking process involving multiple stakeholders (including patients and patient advocates) and the published literature. Adoption of recommended core sets in research and health care delivery settings will standardize assessment of the most important HRQOL domains using high-quality measures, facilitating aggregation and comparison of results across multiple studies. We encourage similar core sets be developed for PRDs.

For any PRO measure to be clinically useful, including the PROMIS Pediatric measures, the scores have to be interpretable by end users, requiring patient and physician definitions of low versus high scores, and consensus around scores representing no/normal, mild, moderate, or severe symptom burden. One recommended approach is to conduct standard setting (also called bookmarking) studies.[68] Mann and colleagues[52] (2020) used this technique with patients with PRD, parents, and clinicians to identify severity categories for PROMIS Pediatric measures of anxiety, mobility, fatigue, and depressive symptoms.[52] Further similar studies are encouraged.

Understanding meaningful change in scores over time or difference in scores between groups also is critical to improving interpretability. There are several approaches to assess meaningful change or differences, some of which use an established clinical variable as an "anchor" for responsiveness in the PRO score.[14,69,70] For PROMIS Pediatric measures, meaningful difference estimates of 3 points were determined for most symptom and functional domains based on scale judgment methods among adolescents, caregivers, and clinicians.[71] Morgan and colleagues[14] (2017) used standard setting methods with adolescents, caregivers, and

Box 3
Recommendations for future research

- Identifying standard core outcomes sets that include both the selected health-related quality of life domain's PROs and appropriate and well-justified PRO measures for PRDs to allow for aggregation of results across studies.
- Standard setting and bookmarking studies to improve interpretability of PRO measure scores.
- Establishing meaningful change (or meaningful differences) in PRDs using clinical anchors in real-world settings.
- Increased effort to implement PRO assessment in lesser-known or rare conditions that affect children and adolescents.

clinicians for JIA and found a 5-point meaningful change for PROMIS Pediatric measures of fatigue and upper extremity function. Other domains had different meaningful change values based on the child, parent, or clinician perspectives.[14] Additional research using clinical anchors in real world settings to identify meaningful change or differences in PRD is needed.

In addition to more research in JIA and pSLE, we also recommend a stronger focus on rare PRD populations. Although there have been efforts directed at rare adult rheumatic disease populations by groups such as OMERACT to develop[72–74] disease-specific PRO measures, the lag in pediatric research is more substantial in rare PRDs. We recommend inclusion of PROs into collaborative efforts studying rare PRDs.

Finally, Internet-based technology for collecting PROs provides additional opportunities to leverage PROs to improve understanding of children's symptoms and functioning in PRD. Using technology is feasible and can improve data quality compared with paper forms.[75] Furthermore, mobile applications support more frequent assessment of symptoms and functioning, including ecological momentary assessments, which improves sensitivity and allows for dynamic assessment of outcomes in a real-world setting.[76] Other important applications for administering PROs via technology include ease of sharing data with relevant stakeholders (including back to the patient/family), although more research is needed in this area.[77] Sharing PRO data with the child and caregivers may empower them to be more knowledgeable of their condition and to changes in their conditions, resulting in better compliance with completing future PRO measures. However, the use of technology to capture PROs can exacerbate racial disparities in PRO data collection.[78] Considering health equity and access in future work is critical.

SUMMARY

Although pediatric rheumatology has been at the forefront of PRO research, knowledge gaps persist in understanding the patient experience and ensuring PRO measures are meaningful to patients, valid for a specific purpose, and useful to inform decision making for clinicians and researchers (**Box 3**).

CLINICS CARE POINTS

- Patient-reported outcome (PROs) measures can enhance improve patient-provider communication and help clinicians track outcomes over time.
- Guidances exist to support implementation of PRO measures within clinical care settings.
- Careful consideration of clinic-specific barriers and facilitators is needed when implementing PRO measures within a clinic workflow.

CONFLICTS OF INTEREST STATEMENTS

Dr C.K. Zigler reports funding via her institution from the National Institutes of Health, the U.S. Food & Drug Administration and the Childhood Arthritis and Rheumatology Research Alliance (CARRA). Dr R.L. Randell receives support from the National Institute of General Medical Sciences and the Eunice Kennedy Shriver National Institute of Child Health and Human Development (NICHD) of the National Institutes of Health (NIH) under Award Number T32GM086330. Dr R.L. Randell's spouse has current or prior employment and/or stock ownership in Merck & Co and Biogen. Dr B.B. Reeve received funding via his institution from the NIH/NIAMS grant U19AR069522.

REFERENCES

1. Varni JW, Limbers CA, Burwinkle TM. How young can children reliably and validly self-report their health-related quality of life? An analysis of 8,591 children across age subgroups with the PedsQL 4.0 Generic Core Scales. Health Qual Life Outcomes 2007;5:1.
2. Brunner HI, Klein-Gitelman MS, Miller MJ, et al. Health of children with chronic arthritis: Relationship of different measures and the quality of parent proxy reporting. Arthritis Care Res 2004;51(5):763–73.
3. Patrick DL, Burke LB, Powers JH, et al. Patient-reported outcomes to support medical product labeling claims: FDA perspective. Value Health 2007;10(Suppl 2):S125–37.
4. Yan Y, Rychlik KL, Rosenman MB, et al. Use of PROMIS® to screen for depression in children with arthritis. Pediatr Rheumatol Online J 2020;18(1):92.
5. Gul HL, Eugenio G, Rabin T, et al. Defining remission in rheumatoid arthritis: does it matter to the patient? A comparison of multi-dimensional remission criteria and patient reported outcomes. Rheumatology 2019;59(3):613–21.
6. Callahan LF. The history of patient-reported outcomes in rheumatology. Rheum Dis Clin North Am 2016;42(2):205–17.
7. Correll CK, Dave M, Paul AF, et al. Identifying research priorities among patients and families of children with rheumatic diseases living in the United States. J Rheumatol 2020;47(12):1800–6.
8. Singh G, Athreya BH, Fries JF, et al. Measurement of health status in children with juvenile rheumatoid arthritis. Arthritis Rheum 1994;37(12):1761–9.
9. Ramey D, Fries J, Singh G. Quality of life and pharmacoleconomics in clinical trials, The health assessment questionnaire 1995-status and Review. Philadelphia: Lippincott-Raven Pub; 1996. p. 227–37, 19(96).
10. Cella D, Riley W, Stone A, et al. The Patient-Reported Outcomes Measurement Information System (PROMIS) developed and tested its first wave of adult self-reported health outcome item banks: 2005-2008. J Clin Epidemiol 2010;63(11): 1179–94.
11. DeWalt DA, Rothrock N, Yount S, et al. Evaluation of item candidates: the PROMIS qualitative item review. Med Care 2007;45(5 Suppl 1):S12–21.
12. Reeve BB, Hays RD, Bjorner JB, et al. Psychometric evaluation and calibration of health-related quality of life item banks: plans for the Patient-Reported Outcomes Measurement Information System (PROMIS). Med Care 2007;45(5 Suppl 1): S22–31.
13. Bartlett SJ, Orbai AM, Duncan T, et al. Reliability and Validity of Selected PROMIS Measures in People with Rheumatoid Arthritis. PLoS One 2015;10(9):e0138543.
14. Morgan EM, Mara CA, Huang B, et al. Establishing clinical meaning and defining important differences for Patient-Reported Outcomes Measurement Information

System (PROMIS(®)) measures in juvenile idiopathic arthritis using standard setting with patients, parents, and providers. Qual Life Res 2017;26(3):565–86.
15. DeWalt DA, Gross HE, Gipson DS, et al. PROMIS(®) pediatric self-report scales distinguish subgroups of children within and across six common pediatric chronic health conditions. Qual Life Res 2015;24(9):2195–208.
16. Jones JT, Cunningham N, Kashikar-Zuck S, et al. Pain, Fatigue, and Psychological Impact on Health-Related Quality of Life in Childhood-Onset Lupus. Arthritis Care Res (Hoboken) 2016;68(1):73–80.
17. Wang SQ, Zhang LW, Wei P, et al. Is hydroxychloroquine effective in treating primary Sjogren's syndrome: a systematic review and meta-analysis. BMC Musculoskelet Disord 2017;18(1):186.
18. Izadi Z, Gandrup J, Katz PP, Yazdany J. Patient-reported outcome measures for use in clinical trials of SLE: a review. Lupus Science & Medicine 2018;5(1): e000279.
19. Azizoddin DR, Jolly M, Arora S, et al. Patient-Reported Outcomes Predict Mortality in Lupus. Arthritis Care Res (Hoboken) 2019;71(8):1028–35.
20. Morgan EM, Riebschleger MP, Horonjeff J, et al. Evidence for Updating the Core Domain Set of Outcome Measures for Juvenile Idiopathic Arthritis: Report from a Special Interest Group at OMERACT 2016. J Rheumatol 2017;44(12):1884–8.
21. Morgan EM, Munro JE, Horonjeff J, et al. Establishing an Updated Core Domain Set for Studies in Juvenile Idiopathic Arthritis: A Report from the OMERACT 2018 JIA Workshop. J Rheumatol 2019;46(8):1006–13.
22. Wilson H, Dashiell-Aje E, Anatchkova M, et al. Beyond study participants: a framework for engaging patients in the selection or development of clinical outcome assessments for evaluating the benefits of treatment in medical product development. Qual Life Res 2018;27(1):5–16.
23. Riley AW. Evidence that school-age children can self-report on their health. Ambul Pediatr 2004;4(4 Suppl):371–6.
24. Irwin DE, Gross HE, Stucky BD, et al. Development of six PROMIS pediatrics proxy-report item banks. Health Qual Life Outcomes 2012;10:22.
25. Cox ED, Dobrozsi SK, Forrest CB, et al. Considerations to Support Use of Patient-Reported Outcomes Measurement Information System Pediatric Measures in Ambulatory Clinics. J Pediatr 2021;230:198–206, e192.
26. Hinds PS, Hockenberry-Eaton M, Gilger E, et al. Comparing patient, parent, and staff descriptions of fatigue in pediatric oncology patients. Cancer Nurs 1999; 22(4):277–88.
27. Zhukovsky DS, Rozmus CL, Robert RS, et al. Symptom profiles in children with advanced cancer: Patient, family caregiver, and oncologist ratings. Cancer 2015;121(22):4080–7.
28. Roddenberry A, Renk K. Quality of life in pediatric cancer patients: the relationships among parents' characteristics, children's characteristics, and informant concordance. J Child Fam Stud 2008;17(3):402–26.
29. Addington-Hall J, Kalra L. Who should measure quality of life? Bmj 2001; 322(7299):1417–20.
30. Parsons SK, Fairclough DL, Wang J, et al. Comparing longitudinal assessments of quality of life by patient and parent in newly diagnosed children with cancer: the value of both raters' perspectives. Qual Life Res 2012;21(5):915–23.
31. Mack JW, McFatrich M, Withycombe JS, et al. Agreement between child self-report and caregiver-proxy report for symptoms and functioning of children undergoing cancer treatment. JAMA Pediatr 2020;174(11):e202861.

32. Galloway H, Newman E. Is there a difference between child self-ratings and parent proxy-ratings of the quality of life of children with a diagnosis of attention-deficit hyperactivity disorder (ADHD)? A systematic review of the literature. ADHD Attention Deficit Hyperactivity Disord 2017;9(1):11–29.
33. Aaronson N, Alonso J, Burnam A, et al. Assessing health status and quality-of-life instruments: attributes and review criteria. Qual Life Res : Int J Qual Life aspects Treat Care Rehabil 2002;11(3):193–205.
34. Terwee CB, Prinsen CAC, Chiarotto A, et al. COSMIN methodology for evaluating the content validity of patient-reported outcome measures: a Delphi study. Qual Life Res : Int J Qual Life aspects Treat Care Rehabil 2018;27(5):1159–70.
35. Guidance for industry: patient-reported outcome measures: use in medical product development to support labeling claims. In: Administration FD, Services UDoHaH, Research CfDEa, et al, eds2009.
36. Parsons S, Thomson W, Cresswell K, et al. On behalf of the Barbara Ansell National Network for Adolescent R. What do young people with rheumatic disease believe to be important to research about their condition? A UK-wide study. Pediatr Rheumatol 2017;15(1):53.
37. Craig J, Feldman BM, Spiegel L, et al. Comparing the Measurement Properties and Preferability of Patient Reported Outcome Measures in Pediatric Rheumatology: PROMIS versus CHAQ. J Rheumatol 2020;48(7):1065–72.
38. Ardalan K, Switzer GE, Zigler CK, et al. Psychometric properties of the children's dermatology life quality index in pediatric localized scleroderma 2018;3(2): 175–81.
39. Bele S, Chugh A, Mohamed B, et al. Patient-reported outcome measures in routine pediatric clinical care: a systematic review. Front Pediatr 2020;8:364.
40. Cheng L, Kang Q, Wang Y, et al. Determining the effectiveness of using patient-reported outcomes in pediatric clinical practices. J Pediatr Nurs 2020;55:100–9.
41. Calvert M, Kyte D, Mercieca-Bebber R, et al. Guidelines for inclusion of patient-reported outcomes in clinical trial protocols: the SPIRIT-PRO extension. JAMA 2018;319(5):483–94.
42. Calvert M, Blazeby J, Altman DG, et al. Reporting of patient-reported outcomes in randomized trials: the CONSORT PRO extension. Jama 2013;309(8):814–22.
43. Coens C, Pe M, Dueck AC, et al. International standards for the analysis of quality-of-life and patient-reported outcome endpoints in cancer randomised controlled trials: recommendations of the SISAQOL Consortium. Lancet Oncol 2020;21(2):e83–96.
44. Reeve BB, Wyrwich KW, Wu AW, et al. ISOQOL recommends minimum standards for patient-reported outcome measures used in patient-centered outcomes and comparative effectiveness research. Qual Life Res : Int J Qual Life aspects Treat Care Rehabil 2013;22(8):1889–905.
45. Crossnohere NL, Brundage M, Calvert MJ, et al. International guidance on the selection of patient-reported outcome measures in clinical trials: a review. Qual Life Res 2021;30(1):21–40.
46. Snyder CF, Aaronson NK, Choucair AK, et al. Implementing patient-reported outcomes assessment in clinical practice: a review of the options and considerations. Qual Life Res : Int J Qual Life aspects Treat Care Rehabil 2012;21(8): 1305–14.
47. Snyder C aW AW, editor. Users' guide to integrating patient-reported outcomes in electronic health records. Baltimore, MD: Johns Hopkins University; 2017. Funded by Patient-Centered Outcomes Research Institute (PCORI); JHU

Contract No. 10.01.14 TO2 08.01.15. Available at: http://www.pcori.org/document/users-guide-integrating-patient-reported-outcomeselectronic-health-records.
48. Hersh AO, Salimian PK, Weitzman ER. Using patient-reported outcome measures to capture the patient's voice in research and care of juvenile idiopathic arthritis. Rheum Dis Clin North Am 2016;42(2):333–46.
49. Filocamo G, Consolaro A, Schiappapietra B, et al. A new approach to clinical care of juvenile idiopathic arthritis: the Juvenile Arthritis Multidimensional Assessment Report. J Rheumatol 2011;38(5):938–53.
50. Bovis F, Consolaro A, Pistorio A, et al. Cross-cultural adaptation and psychometric evaluation of the Juvenile Arthritis Multidimensional Assessment Report (JAMAR) in 54 languages across 52 countries: review of the general methodology. Rheumatol Int 2018;38(Suppl 1):5–17.
51. Brandon TG, Becker BD, Bevans KB, et al. Patient-reported outcomes measurement information system tools for collecting patient-reported outcomes in children with juvenile arthritis. Arthritis Care Res 2017;69(3):393–402.
52. Mann CM, Schanberg LE, Wang M, et al. Identifying clinically meaningful severity categories for PROMIS pediatric measures of anxiety, mobility, fatigue, and depressive symptoms in juvenile idiopathic arthritis and childhood-onset systemic lupus erythematosus. Qual Life Res : Int J Qual Life aspects Treat Care Rehabil 2020;29(9):2573–84.
53. Holloway L, Humphrey L, Heron L, et al. Patient-reported outcome measures for systemic lupus erythematosus clinical trials: a review of content validity, face validity and psychometric performance. Health Qual Life Outcomes 2014;12:116.
54. Meiorin S, Pistorio A, Ravelli A, et al. Validation of the childhood health assessment questionnaire in active juvenile systemic lupus erythematosus. Arthritis Rheum 2008;59(8):1112–9.
55. Ganguli SK, Hui-Yuen JS, Jolly M, et al. Performance and psychometric properties of lupus impact tracker in assessing patient-reported outcomes in pediatric lupus: Report from a pilot study. Lupus 2020;29(13):1781–9.
56. Moorthy LN, Peterson MG, Baratelli M, et al. Multicenter validation of a new quality of life measure in pediatric lupus. Arthritis Rheum 2007;57(7):1165–73.
57. Moorthy LN, Peterson MG, Hassett AL, et al. Relationship between health-related quality of life and SLE activity and damage in children over time. Lupus 2009;18(7):622–9.
58. Moorthy LN, Baldino ME, Kurra V, et al. Relationship between health-related quality of life, disease activity and disease damage in a prospective international multicenter cohort of childhood onset systemic lupus erythematosus patients. Lupus 2017;26(3):255–65.
59. McCann LJ, Pilkington CA, Huber AM, et al. Development of a consensus core dataset in juvenile dermatomyositis for clinical use to inform research. Ann Rheum Dis 2018;77(2):241–50.
60. Tory HO, Carrasco R, Griffin T, et al. Comparing the importance of quality measurement themes in juvenile idiopathic inflammatory myositis between patients and families and healthcare professionals. Pediatr Rheumatol Online J 2018;16(1):28.
61. Ardalan KCD, Pachman LM, Gray EL, et al. Initial validation of patient-reported outcomes measurement information system (promis®) in children with juvenile myositis [abstract]. Arthritis Rheumatol 2017;69(suppl 10). https://acrabstracts.org/abstract/initial-validation-of-patient-reported-outcomes-measurement-information-system-promis-in-children-with-juvenile-myositis/. [Accessed 8 May 2021]. Accessed.

62. Wolfe MRA, Lai J, Coles T, et al. Estimation of clinically important differences in patient-reported outcomes measurement information system (PROMIS) measures in juvenile myositis [abstract]. Arthritis Rheumatol 2020;72(suppl 10). https://acrabstracts.org/abstract/estimation-of-clinically-important-differences-in-patient-reported-outcomes-measurement-information-system-promis-measures-in-juvenile-myositis/. [Accessed 8 May 2021]. Accessed.
63. Fahey KJGE, Chang RW, Cella D, et al. The relationship of pain, fatigue and emotional distress with quality of life in juvenile myositis [abstract]. Arthritis Rheumatol 2018; 70(suppl 10). https://acrabstracts.org/abstract/the-relationship-of-pain-fatigue-and-emotional-distress-with-quality-of-life-in-juvenile-myositis/. [Accessed 8 May 2021]. Accessed.
64. Zigler CK, Ardalan K, Lane S, et al. A novel patient-reported outcome for paediatric localized scleroderma: a qualitative assessment of content validity. The British journal of dermatology 2019;182(3):625–35. https://doi.org/10.1111/bjd.18512.
65. Zigler CK, Ardalan K, Hernandez A, et al. Exploring the impact of paediatric localized scleroderma on health-related quality of life: focus groups with youth and caregivers. Br. J. Dermatol 2020;183:692–701. https://doi.org/10.1111/bjd.18879.
66. Oliver M, Lee TC, Halpern-Felsher B, et al. Disease burden and social impact of pediatric chronic nonbacterial osteomyelitis from the patient and family perspective. Pediatr Rheumatol Online J 2018;16(1):78.
67. Silier CCG, Greschik J, Gesell S, et al. Chronic non-bacterial osteitis from the patient perspective: a health services research through data collected from patient conferences. BMJ Open 2017;7(12):e017599.
68. Cook KF, Cella D, Reeve BB. PRO-bookmarking to estimate clinical thresholds for patient-reported symptoms and function. Med Care 2019;57(Suppl 5 Suppl 1): S13–7.
69. Crosby RD, Kolotkin RL, Williams GR. Defining clinically meaningful change in health-related quality of life. J Clin Epidemiol 2003;56(5):395–407.
70. De Vet HC, Ostelo RW, Terwee CB, et al. Minimally important change determined by a visual method integrating an anchor-based and a distribution-based approach. Qual Life Res 2007;16(1):131.
71. Thissen D, Liu Y, Magnus B, et al. Estimating minimally important difference (MID) in PROMIS pediatric measures using the scale-judgment method. Qual Life Res : Int J Qual Life aspects Treat Care Rehabil 2016;25(1):13–23.
72. Robson JC, Milman N, Tomasson G, et al. Exploration, development, and validation of patient-reported outcomes in antineutrophil cytoplasmic antibody-associated vasculitis using the OMERACT process. J Rheumatol 2015;42(11): 2204–9.
73. Robson JC, Tomasson G, Milman N, et al. OMERACT endorsement of patient-reported outcome instruments in antineutrophil cytoplasmic antibody-associated vasculitis. J Rheumatol 2017;44(10):1529–35.
74. Robson JC, Dawson J, Doll H, et al. Validation of the ANCA-associated vasculitis patient-reported outcomes (AAV-PRO) questionnaire. Ann Rheum Dis 2018;77(8): 1157–64.
75. Vinney LA, Grade JD, Connor NP. Feasibility of using a handheld electronic device for the collection of patient reported outcomes data from children. J Commun Disord 2012;45(1):12–9.
76. Mofsen AM, Rodebaugh TL, Nicol GE, et al. When all else fails, listen to the patient: a viewpoint on the use of ecological momentary assessment in clinical trials. JMIR Ment Health 2019;6(5):e11845.

77. Lu DJ, Girgis M, David JM, et al. Evaluation of mobile health applications to track patient-reported outcomes for oncology patients: a systematic review. Adv Radiat Oncol 2021;6(1):100576.
78. Sisodia RC, Rodriguez JA, Sequist TD. Digital disparities: lessons learned from a patient reported outcomes program during the COVID-19 pandemic. Journal of the American Medical Informatics Association. JAMIA 2021;28(10):2265–8. https://doi.org/10.1093/jamia/ocab138.
79. McErlane F, Foster HE, Armitt G, et al. Development of a national audit tool for juvenile idiopathic arthritis: a BSPAR project funded by the Health Care Quality Improvement Partnership. Rheumatology (Oxford) 2018;57(1):140–51.
80. Lunt LE, Shoop-Worrall S, Smith N, et al. Validation of novel patient-centred juvenile idiopathic arthritis-specific patient-reported outcome and experience measures (PROMs/PREMs). Pediatr Rheumatol Online J 2020;18(1):91.

Technology to Assess and Treat Pain in Pediatric Rheumatology

Mark Connelly, PhD[a,*], Rebecca Rachael Lee, PhD[b]

KEYWORDS

• Pain • Technology • Mobile applications • Self-management • eHealth

KEY POINTS

- Assessment and management of chronic musculoskeletal pain in pediatric rheumatology are an important component of clinical care. eHealth tools hold significant potential to make these processes more accessible, efficient, engaging, and effective for children and young people.
- Despite rapid progress in the development of pain assessment and management eHealth options, the tools either are predominantly used in research studies or are in the public domain but rarely both.
- Existing eHealth assessment options incorporate a range of age-appropriate unidimensional pain assessment scales, and current eHealth management tools center on pain education principles and behavioral interventions such as relaxation training.

INTRODUCTION

Persistent musculoskeletal pain is one of the most common symptoms leading to an evaluation in pediatric rheumatology and is frequently experienced both in youth with and without established rheumatologic disease.[1–5] Optimally assessing musculoskeletal pain requires dedicated time and familiarity with and/or expertise in administering developmentally appropriate pain assessment tools. Treating musculoskeletal pain in youth similarly requires time for patient/family education and comfort with and easy access to evidence-based biopsychosocial pain management approaches. Unfortunately, neither time nor access is a luxury commonly available in contemporary rheumatology practice. Access to pediatric rheumatology is at a premium internationally.[6,7] Access

[a] Division of Developmental and Behavioral Health, Children's Mercy Kansas City, 2401 Gillham Road, Kansas City, MO 64108, USA; [b] Centre for Epidemiology Versus Arthritis, Centre for Musculoskeletal Research, Division of Musculoskeletal and Dermatological Sciences, Faculty of Biology, Medicine and Health, The University of Manchester, Manchester Academic Health Science Centre, Manchester, UK
* Corresponding author.
E-mail address: mconnelly1@cmh.edu

Rheum Dis Clin N Am 48 (2022) 31–50
https://doi.org/10.1016/j.rdc.2021.09.004
rheumatic.theclinics.com
0889-857X/22/

limitations, in turn, constrain the time spent evaluating the presence and severity of disease in pediatric rheumatology clinic visits. Pain that persists despite disease "control" may therefore be inadvertently overlooked or minimized.[8,9] Even if resource barriers are addressed, many pediatric rheumatology professionals report feeling unprepared by their medical training to assess and treat pain.[9–11]

Advancements in eHealth offer unique opportunities for assisting in and augmenting aspects of evidence-based pain evaluation and management in pediatric rheumatology practice. For the purposes of this article, we define eHealth for pain as the use of digital technologies to monitor pain, facilitate pain communication between health stakeholders, and guide pain self-management.[12] The potential benefits of eHealth for pain are numerous. Many eHealth applications are available at any time and easily integrate into the lives of today's digitally connected youth regardless of demographics.[13,14] Digital tools for supporting pain assessment and evaluation are generally viewed favorably by youth.[15,16] Features common to online and mobile software such as gamification, customizable avatars, and data-driven personalization boost engagement in a developmentally tailored way. The popularity of web platforms and smartphones in youth also help reduce the stigma associated with clinic-based behavioral pain treatments.[17] Further, empowering self-monitoring and self-management of pain through eHealth reduces in-person health care visits, which may have a beneficial downstream effect on health care costs.[18] The shift to greater reliance on digital technology-assisted pain management during the era of COVID-19 has highlighted many benefits.[19]

Digital technologies for supporting pain assessment and management in youth also are not a panacea and have important limitations. This article summarizes opportunities and challenges in pain eHealth for pediatric rheumatologists to consider when caring for children and adolescents in their practice. The intent is not to provide an exhaustive review. Rather, we present a focused review of eHealth pain applications that have specific relevance to patients seen in pediatric rheumatology clinics, are informed by contemporary pain science or have been studied empirically. We begin by reviewing evidence-based and publicly available digital tools to support pain assessment and patient–provider communication. Subsequently, we review eHealth applications intended to support pain management. We conclude by discussing challenges, gaps, and nascent aspects of eHealth for pediatric pain that likely will factor prominently in future developments.

TECHNOLOGY TO SUPPORT PAIN ASSESSMENT AND COMMUNICATION IN PEDIATRIC RHEUMATOLOGY

Pain assessment captures pain data for quantification (pain measurement) to inform diagnosis and monitor treatment response. Asking youth about their pain also is important for facilitating patient–provider conversations about pain and its impact (pain communication).[20] Technologies have several advantages over paper-based pain assessment that may facilitate improved management of chronic musculoskeletal pain. Most notably, technologies simplify multi-dimensional pain evaluation through interactive features and support automatic integration of synthesized pain data into electronic health records.[15,21] The capability of technologies to prompt children to report pain at home and automatically time-stamp entries helps empower the engagement of young patients in their care and improves the utility and credibility of captured information.[22]

Pain Assessment Using Web-Based Platforms

Web-based formats are one of the most accessible technologies to support pain assessment.[23] The Standardized Universal Pain Evaluation for Rheumatology

Providers for Children and Youth (SUPER-KIDZ) is one example of an online pain measure developed specifically for youth ages 4 to 18 years seen in pediatric rheumatology clinics.[12,24] The SUPER-KIDZ tool is a multi-dimensional online survey which has both patient and proxy pain measures. A self-report version for young children (ages 4–8 years) consists of a developmentally appropriate pain intensity scale (Faces Pain Scale-Revised[25]) and a body diagram with an anterior and posterior view for locating pain.[26,27] The self-report version for children aged 8 and above and the parent proxy-report version include items adopted from validated measures to assess pain characteristics, pain interference,[28] pain catastrophizing,[29] and emotional functioning. The SUPER-KIDZ tool has good internal consistency, responsiveness, and test–retest reliability.[24]

Another web-based pain assessment tool evaluated in pediatric rheumatology is the Iconic Pain Assessment Tool (IPAT2; **Fig. 1**). Developed by Lalloo and colleagues for evaluating adolescents with arthritis pain in clinical settings,[23] patients are able to use a range of pain quality icons to describe the type of pain experienced, assign a numerical intensity to each chosen icon (0–10 numerical rating scale) and place the icon on a body map. In usability testing of the IPAT2 with 15 adolescents (ages 14–17 years), the tool was found to be easy to use, well-liked, quick to complete (1.4 minutes), and deemed by patients to be helpful for communicating about pain with health care professionals. The IPAT2 has been recast as "PainQuILT,"[30] and licensed to a small business for eventual public deployment (C. Lalloo, personal communication, February 16th, 2021).

The PROBE system (Patient Risks, Outcomes, and Barriers Evaluation) is a web-based pain assessment tool developed using a freely available online platform (REDCap electronic data capture tool). The tool can be deployed on tablet devices for the patient (ages 3–23) and family completion while in the waiting room of pediatric

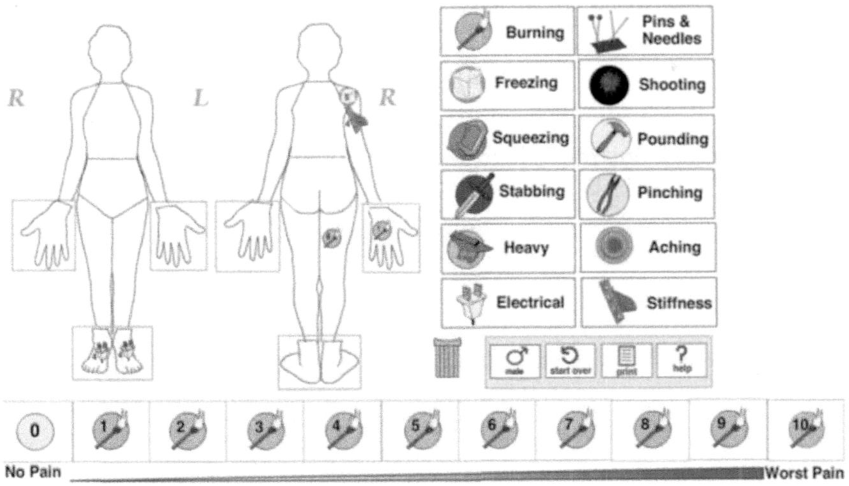

Fig. 1. *The Iconic Pain Assessment Tool Version 2.0.* The image shows a sample screen from the Iconic Pain Assessment Tool app. Pain quality and intensity icons can be dragged and dropped to the body outline. (*From* Lalloo C, Stinson J, Hochman J, Adachi J, Henry J. Adapting the Iconic Pain Assessment Tool Version 2 (IPAT2) for adults and adolescents with arthritis pain through usability testing and refinement of pain quality icons. Clin J Pain 2013;29(3):253-64; with permission.)

rheumatology clinics.[31] Information on anxiety, depression, sleep problems, family history of pain, and disease activity (eg, active joint count) are entered and automatically scored. Scores more than clinically relevant thresholds are flagged for the provider to inform clinical decision-making. The PROBE system yielded profiles that distinguished children having juvenile idiopathic arthritis (JIA) with and without chronic pain.[31] A similar but more comprehensive system for chronic pain assessment is the Pediatric Collaborative Health Outcomes Information Registry (Peds-CHOIR), a free learning health system that can be used to host tailored institution-specific chronic pain data capture.[32] Legacy and computerized adaptive testing measures for chronic pain assessment are available for use in the Peds-CHOIR system and can be completed before or at the time of clinical consultations, with data plotted graphically over time to inform clinical care.

Pain Assessment Using Mobile Devices

The first report using a mobile tool to support the assessment of pain in pediatric rheumatic disease was in 2004 by Palermo *and colleagues*.[33] They used a personal digital assistant (PDA) to compare the benefits of electronic versus paper-based pain diaries in children and young people with headaches and JIA. The randomized controlled trial analyzed the data from 60 participants who recorded pain using the device for a 7-day period. Children completed significantly more reports using the electronic diaries (mean = 6.6) than those using paper diaries (mean = 3.8), even though the pain experiences reported were similar between groups. The "e-ouch" pain diary is another early example of a mobile PDA-based pain assessment tool used in pediatric rheumatology (**Fig. 2**).[34] The e-ouch diary was designed to cue and capture pain ratings three times per day in a child's typical environment. For this tool, pain visual analog scales for measuring intensity and interference scales were adapted from the Brief Pain Inventory-Short Form.[35] In an acceptability study with participants comprised of young people (mean age 13.5 years) attending a pediatric rheumatology clinic in Canada, the tool was found to be easy, intuitive, and associated with high patient satisfaction.

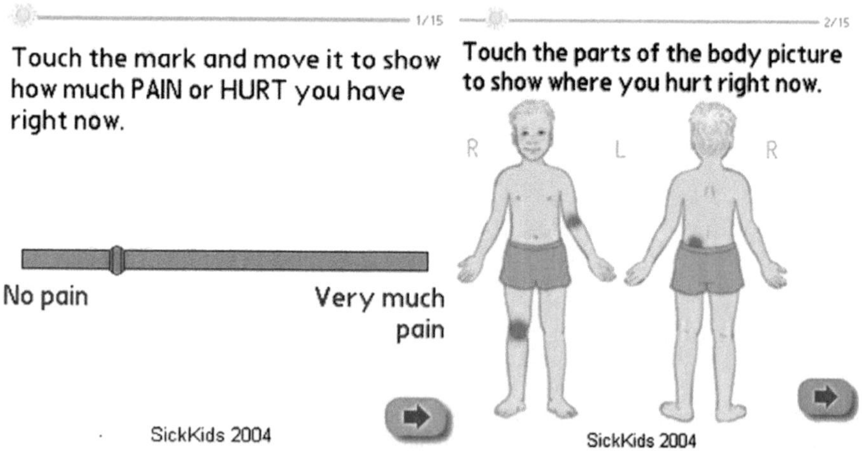

Fig. 2. *e-Ouch pain diary.* Sample images from the e-Ouch pain diary, showing screens indicating pain intensity and pain location. (*From* Stinson JN, Petroz GC, Tait G, et al. e-Ouch: Usability testing of an electronic chronic pain diary for adolescents with arthritis. Clin J Pain 2006;22:295-305 ; with permission.)

The My Pain Tracker (MPT) app is a more recent example of an evidence-based mHealth (tablet-based) pain assessment application designed specifically for use with children and young people with rheumatic disease.[36,37] MPT was found to be a useable, acceptable, and valid measure. The tool was first adapted from an interview tool used by researchers and clinicians in forensic settings.[38] MPT presents users with a digital body map on which they can "drag and drop" several different pain qualities: symbols, labels/word descriptors, size (severity), throb rate (intensity), location and emotion (**Fig. 3**). After recording pain qualities, the app then captures reports of pain interference in activities. The app has a health care professional facing interface whereby the data from the app are synthesized into visualizations that demonstrate changes in pain qualities and locations over time (see **Fig. 3**). Research exploring how pain experts and pediatric rheumatology specialists interpret pain information from patients with JIA informed the visualization design.

Mobile assessment tools discussed to this point have been used in research settings and are not publicly available. By contrast, many mobile pain assessment apps are publicly available for clinical use but have not been formally studied in a research context. Publicly available pain assessment apps typically lack patient and clinician involvement during development. A systematic review of such apps and their functions was recently published.[39] Several apps in this review are no longer available, whereas new apps have emerged. The transiency of public apps for pain assessment is a common issue. **Table 1** provides a summary of several publicly available mobile apps to consider for use in a range of ages.

TECHNOLOGY TO SUPPORT PAIN MANAGEMENT IN PEDIATRIC RHEUMATOLOGY

Many factors known to affect the sensory and emotional components of pain are potentially amenable to change through innovative and engaging applications of eHealth. For example, common modifiable targets in behavioral/self-management pain interventions that have been a focus of digital pain management tools include pain understanding and beliefs, social connectedness, health habits (eg, sleep and

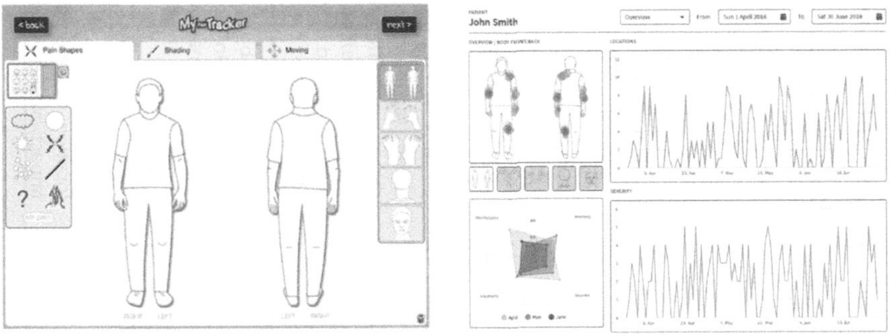

Fig. 3. *My Pain Tracker (MPT) app.* The left image shows the patient self-report screen for the My Pain Tracker app. Icons for different pain characteristics such as pain quality and intensity can be dragged and dropped to the body outline, with options to zoom in on certain body areas. The right image shows a sample image of the professional interface for monitoring data from the My Pain Tracker app. (*From* Lee RR, Shoop-Worrall S, Rashid A, Thomson W, Cordingley L "Asking Too Much?": Randomized N-of-1 Trial Exploring Patient Preferences and Measurement Reactivity to Frequent Use of Remote Multidimensional Pain Assessments in Children and Young People With Juvenile Idiopathic Arthritis J Med Internet Res 2020;22(1):e14503)

Table 1
Examples of publicly available mobile pain assessment apps for youth

App Name	Description	Compatibility	Age Group	Cost
Achy Penguin[40]	Captures information on pain intensity (selecting one of the 3 faces) and location (using an animal manikin). Following the pain-reporting interface, there also are options to choose evidence-based relaxation and distraction techniques. The app was tested in the context of postoperative pain but is suitable for other contexts to aid young children in pain reporting and coping.	iOS	Young children (aged 5–8)	Free on Apple App Store
International Children's Palliative Care Network (ICPCN) pain assessment tool[41]	Collects information on pain location (using a body manikin), quality (eg, burning, throbbing, sharp, achy), intensity (using a faces pain scale), pain movement, and use/effectiveness of pain relief techniques. Developed for palliative care but with nonspecific pain assessment features that may be useable by those with rheumatic conditions.	iOS and Android	Elementary school age and above	Free on the Apple App Store or Google Play Store
Pain Squad[42]	Assesses pain intensity (using numeric rating scale), duration, location, qualities, precipitators, impact, medications/other	iOS	Elementary school age and above	Free on the Apple App Store

	techniques tried. Initially designed for use for monitoring pain in youth with cancer. However, the app has only a few features specific to cancer and thus may still be useful in rheumatic disease. Intended to be completed twice per day and has gamification principles in-built (eg, rewards given for reporting).			
Rheumabuddy[43]	Monitors pain intensity (using a faces pain scale), duration, and location (using body manikin). Originally developed for adults with rheumatoid arthritis. The app also captures broader rheumatic disease features such as mood, fatigue, and stiffness. There is an online communities section whereby users can share experiences with other app users.	iOS and Android	Adolescents and young adults	Free on the Apple App Store or Google Play Store

Although all apps in this table are listed as free, they typically incorporate options for in-app purchases for additional features.

physical activity), mental focus, autonomic activity, and mood.[44] Offering patients' technology-assisted self-management tools as an initial approach in a stepped-care treatment model for chronic pain may be a fitting use of these emerging therapies in pediatric rheumatology clinics.[45]

Internet-Delivered Pain Interventions

eHealth developments for pediatric pain primarily have centered on internet-delivered treatment. The Teens Taking Charge Online program initially was developed for youth with JIA (**Fig. 4**).[46] This program includes online modules for teens (and parent/caregivers) pertaining to disease self-management broadly, but with evidence-based cognitive-behavioral strategies for pain management featuring prominently in the content. In particular, the "Managing Symptoms," "Coping Strategies," and "Your Lifestyle" modules comprise evidence-based psychological principles of treating pain. Iterative input from patients/families, experts in pain and rheumatology, clinicians across several disciplines, and web developers informed the development of the program. One randomized efficacy trial of the intervention demonstrated improvement in pain and pain interference in youth with JIA aged 12 to 18 years,[46] whereas another trial found the pain benefit equal to that of an online educational control.[47] The complete program is publicly available to anglophone and francophone youth with JIA in Canada and to English- and Spanish-speaking families in the US.[48–50] The Teens Taking Charge online program also was found to be acceptable and helpful for promoting and maintaining self-management skills with facilitation via video calls from trained peer mentors with JIA or chronic pain.[51,52] Usage of online peer support and mentorship in the context of pediatric chronic pain is a potentially promising area of pain eHealth but needs further evaluation.[53]

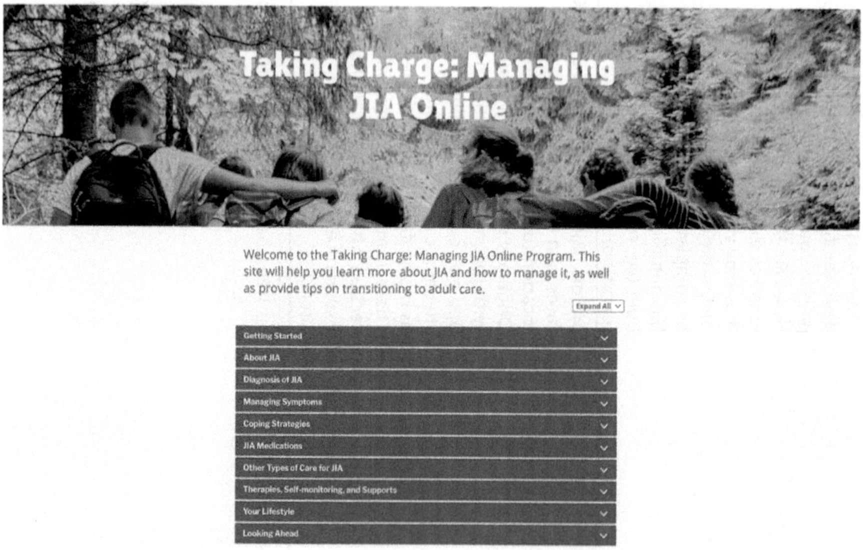

Fig. 4. *Teens Taking Charge: Managing JIA Online program.* Shown in this image is a landing page for the Teens Taking Charge program and the main program module headings. (*From* Childhood Arthritis and Rheumatology Research Alliance (CARRA, Inc.) and The Hospital for Sick Children. Taking Charge: Managing JIA. 2021. Available: https://teenstakingcharge.carragroup.org. Accessed February 28th, 2021 © The Hospital for Sick Children. All Rights Reserved.)

Other online pain interventions have focused primarily on idiopathic pain conditions. Rheumatologists providing appropriate education and resources early on for pain management in the chronic pain population helps reduce a progression of disability.[54] Web-MAP (Web-Based Management of Adolescent Pain) is an internet-delivered pain self-management program with modules comprised of education about chronic pain, training in behavioral and cognitive coping skills (eg, relaxation skills, activity pacing, sleep hygiene) and education for parents about optimal communication and pain response strategies.[55] The program uses a travel theme to engage patients and includes the aforementioned online treatment modules, daily pain diaries, audio files with relaxation instructions, progress tracker (passport), and message center to correspond with a "coach." Videos of peer models, various vignettes, illustrations, goal setting, and practice reminders are included to increase engagement and interactivity. Completing all aspects of the program requires approximately 4 hours of patient and parent/caregiver time. Results of a randomized education-controlled trial of 273 adolescents' ages 11 to 17 years (80% with musculoskeletal pain alone or in combination with abdominal pain or headaches) found that Web-MAP use predicted significantly greater reductions in activity limitations from pain than the education control condition.[55] The program has been converted for use on mobile devices and is publicly available (see the section on mobile apps).

A common component of effective behavioral interventions for pain is relaxation training.[56] There are numerous websites with the specific objective of teaching a form of relaxation usually through multimedia content (video and/or audio). The extent to which these applications are acceptable and effective for youth with pain seen in pediatric rheumatology clinics is unknown. However, if web-based resources help youth cultivate habitual relaxation practices, they are likely beneficial as long as developmentally appropriate. An example of an excellent website containing multimedia content to help with relaxation in a variety of scenarios (including acute and chronic pain) is "Imaginaction" developed by specialists at Lucile Packard Children's Hospital at Stanford.[57]

Mobile Apps for Pain Management

Of the hundreds of mobile applications purporting to teach components of pain self-management (eg, relaxation strategies, pain education), few are based on science, informed by key stakeholders, or tested for efficacy.[58] The "iCanCope" app, developed with extensive input from health care providers and youth with chronic pain, includes pain education, goal setting, training in evidence-based pain coping, and peer-based social support.[59,60] This app is undergoing testing in randomized trials and has been adapted for use in other contexts (eg, postoperative pain), but it is not yet available for clinical use. Results of a recent trial with 60 adolescents with chronic pain recruited from pediatric rheumatology centers in Canada suggested that the participants generally were adherent using the app and found it highly acceptable. By the 8-week primary study endpoint, clinically meaningful reductions in pain intensity were observed but were indistinguishable from changes observed in a condition comprised of symptom tracking only.[61]

Another mobile pain self-management app that has undergone efficacy testing in a real-world setting is WebMAP Mobile,[62] which is similar in content and features to the WebMAP Internet intervention mentioned previously but adapted for use on iOS or Android smartphone devices. In a sample of 143 youth with chronic pain aged 10 to 17 recruited from 8 clinics (5 pain clinics, 3 gastroenterology clinics) across the US, youth using the WebMAP app perceived greater global improvement than those receiving usual care.[62] However, changes in self-reported pain intensity and disability were indistinguishable between the 2 groups and only 30% of youth and parents completed treatment as intended. The WebMAP mobile app is publicly available for patient use (http://bit.do/webmapmobile).[63]

As is the case with websites, there are also numerous publicly available standalone mobile applications having the specific objective of teaching relaxation. The efficacy of these applications in improving pain typically is not tested. However, reviews of publicly available relaxation apps to consider in the context of pediatric pain have helped to delineate those that are developmentally appropriate and easy to use.[64,65] **Table 2** presents the names and description of several.

Social Media

Social media is an increasingly common means by which health researchers share clinically applicable educational content to directly engage patients and families.[66] Caution is warranted in suggesting specific social media content to patients given that much is not research-based and may be more harmful than helpful.[67–69] However, several online pain education videos have a sound scientific foundation. Pediatric rheumatologists might consider recommending one or more of these resources to patients as part of clinical care for pain. An easy to remember acronym to use when considering online videos to recommend is "CRAAP": is the video *c*urrent, *r*elevant, from a trusted *a*uthority, *a*ccurate, and without partiality or bias in *p*urpose?[70]

For chronic pain, scientifically supported "pain science education" videos that help demystify the development of chronic pain and map it to a rationale for treatment strategies can be clinically useful and potentially more palatable to patients than provider dialogue.[71] Pain science education is a common component of clinical care in pediatric pain clinics, although its unique relationship to outcomes is yet uncertain.[71–73] Animated videos can be particularly helpful for simplifying complex concepts, are generally appropriate and acceptable to adolescent patients even if not specifically developed for them, and are easy to share.[72] Examples of pain education videos that are appropriately informed by pain science and seem appropriate for youth with chronic pain include "Tame the Beast" (https://www.youtube.com/watch?v=ikUzvSph7Z4), "Mysterious Science of Pain" (https://www.youtube.com/watch?v=eakyDiXX6Uc), and "Understanding Pain in Less than 5 Minutes" (https://www.youtube.com/embed/qEWc2XtaNwg).[72,74]

For resources supporting the management of procedural pain (eg, injections), Dr Christine Chambers and colleagues in Canada have created social media campaigns on YouTube, Facebook, Twitter, and Instagram.[66] One video from their "It doesn't have to hurt" social media campaign is aimed primarily at parent/caregivers presents and provides evidence-based pain management during needle procedures in an engaging way, having reached hundreds of thousands of viewers (https://www.youtube.com/watch?v=KgBwVSYqfps).[67,75] Several other videos to support evidence-based pain management during painful procedures in children are available and are reviewed for quality in a table by Farkas and colleagues using the CRAAP test mentioned previously.[70]

Extended Reality

A promising area of digital technology for pediatric pain is the use of fully immersive or augmented reality environments.[76,77] Virtual reality, typically comprised of a computer-generated environment projected visually and auditorily on head-mounted hardware with motion tracking capability, is not new to pediatric pain, having been applied and studied in this context for more than 20 years.[78] However, costs and

Table 2
Publicly available mobile apps suitable for youth that are focused on teaching relaxation

App Name	Description	Compatibility	Age Group	Cost
Healing Buddies Comfort Kit	Provides instruction for nonpharmacological pain management strategies, including mental imagery visualization, relaxation, acupressure, aromatherapy, and positive self-talk. Can choose female or male voice. Relatively easy to use for kids and parent/caregivers to use with little guidance	iOS	Elementary school age and above	Free on the Apple App Store
Stop Breathe & Think Kids	Teaches kids how to check in with how they are feeling and how to practice mindfulness in a kid-friendly way (eg, going on "missions" to do mindful activities)	iOS	Elementary school age	Free on the Apple App Store
Breathe2Relax	Customizable breathing app that uses animated videos to demonstrate relaxed breathing techniques. Heart rate data from an Apple Watch if available can be integrated and displayed during breathing practice	iOS and Android	Elementary school age and above	Free on the Apple App Store and Google Play Store
Calm	Provided guided mindfulness meditation exercises of selectable lengths and teaches relaxed breathing strategies	iOS and Android	Elementary school age and above	Free on the Apple App Store and Google Play Store

(*continued on next page*)

Table 2
(continued)

App Name	Description	Compatibility	Age Group	Cost
Headspace	Teaches a new meditation technique each day	iOS and Android	Elementary school age and above	Free on the Apple App Store and Google Play Store
Mindful Powers	Through voice-guided stories, kids learn how to master the powers of mindfulness	iOS	Elementary school age and above	Free on the Apple App Store
Pranayama free	Uses animation to teach and pace diaphragmatic breathing, with customizable settings for beginners through advanced users	Android	Middle school age and above	Free on the Google Play Store
Simply Being	Easy customizable meditations that vary in length from 5 min to 30 min, with an option for adding music or nature sounds	iOS and Android	Middle school age and above	$1.99 on the Apple App Store and Google Play Store
Super Stretch Yoga	Pairs an animated character with real children doing yoga poses. Includes child-friendly yoga instruction with suggestions for easy breathing strategies. Quick and easy instruction; requires no knowledge or aptitude for yoga	iOS and Android	Preschool and above	Free on the Apple App Store and Google Play Store
Breathe Think Do with Sesame Street	Teaches breathing techniques (and problem-solving skills) using fun interactive games	iOS and Android	Infant, preschool	Free on the Apple App Store and Google Play Store

Although most apps are listed in this table are "free," they typically incorporate options for in-app purchases for additional features.

Data from Smith K, Iversen C, Kossowsky J, O'Dell S, Gambhir R, Coakley R. Apple apps for the management of pediatric pain and pain-related stress. Clin Pract Pediatr Psychol 2015;3(2):93-107 and Weekly T, Walker N, Beck J, Akers S, Weaver M. A review of apps for calming, relaxation, and mindfulness interventions for pediatric palliative care patients. *Children (Basel)* 2018;5(2):16.

the quality of consumer virtual reality systems have appreciably improved over time, facilitating use in clinics and at home.[76]

Virtual reality in pediatric health care has been used primarily as a means of sophisticated distraction to ease children's pain and anxiety during medical procedures. In this context, virtual reality is acceptable, generally safe for children, and associated with clinically significant reductions in pain and anxiety relative to usual care alone.[77,79] The putative neuromodulatory analgesic mechanisms of a fully immersive alternate sensory environment are common to many publicly available VR applications.[79] Thus, the choice of which types of apps to use with VR headsets during medical procedures can be informed primarily by patient preference. Some children may prefer travel apps (eg, https://vr.google.com/earth/), others may prefer games or relaxation apps. For a helpful (albeit outdated) review of commercial hardware and software virtual reality applications to consider for use in pediatric clinical practice, see the review by Won and colleagues.[80]

Extended reality applications have yet to be investigated in the context of pediatric *chronic* pain. One promising application is exploiting avatar configurations to facilitate engagement in physical therapy and cortical "remapping" of painful areas. For example, patients with fear of movement or significant guarding (eg, patients with Complex Regional Pain Syndrome) see depictions of an affected limb moving more freely in a virtual world and potentially control the movement via sensors on the non-affected limb. The perceived free movement of the painful area, in turn, helps advance gains from physical therapy.[76] The full potential of extended reality applications for the treatment of chronic pain is likely to be realized over the next decade.

DISCUSSION

Challenges and Gaps in eHealth for Pediatric Pain

There are several limitations in our current use and knowledge about technologies for the assessment and management of pediatric pain. There are a disproportionately large number of publicly available digital health applications for pain assessment and management relative to research studies evaluating their use.[58,81,82] Conversely, of the few digital pain tools evaluated for validity or efficacy, few are publicly accessible for use with young patients or providers in clinical practice.[83] Many eHealth applications for pain management were designed without comprehensive interdisciplinary input from key stakeholders such as clinicians, scientists, graphic designers, human factor experts, software engineers and most importantly, children, youth and families. This is a critical limitation because youth seen in pediatric rheumatology practices may have specific barriers to successfully using eHealth tools, such as dexterity limitations or unique emotional and support needs that should be considered during development. Challenges with data security (eg, protecting personally identifiable information entered into a technology platform) and integration of digital tools with existing data systems (eg, electronic health records) are incompletely addressed by current pain eHealth tools for youth.[84–86] Relatedly, synthesizing electronic multidimensional pain data to be meaningfully used by providers in clinical decision-making is challenging and costly.[36]

Maintaining patient engagement in digital tools over time is another key challenge for both pain assessment and treatment technologies. For digital ambulatory pain assessment, most studies in children and young people use narrow data collection windows of one to 3 weeks, with the longest sampling period of 8 weeks.[37] Having data on pain patterns over long periods of time may be especially useful in pediatric rheumatology clinical contexts, yet the extent to which children and youth will sustain engagement with assessment technologies over extended periods of time is largely unknown. By contrast, using digital technologies to repeatedly cue children to report pain over long periods of time raises concerns about promoting pain hypervigilance and reactivity, although this concern has not been substantiated in studies.[37] Digital tools to support pain self-management similarly have difficulty sustaining patient adherence. Digital self-management tools assume internal motivation to consistently engage with the technology and implement new behaviors with minimal professional oversight. Some patients may have better adherence and outcomes with face-to-face interventions.[87]

Many studies investigating the use of pain assessment and treatment technologies are conducted with children and young people aged 8 and above, with limited socio-demographic diversity in the sample. Children younger than 8 years old, those with cognitive or developmental impairments (eg, youth with autism spectrum disorder), and children with racial and ethnic diversity have been neglected in eHealth technologies for pediatric pain yet may have unique needs that are unlikely to be met with current technologies.

Emerging Areas for Pain eHealth

As technologies evolve, so does the potential to use new innovative electronic and mobile health tools to assess and monitor pain. The use of wearable devices for monitoring physiologic parameters (eg, electrodermal activity, heart rate variability, electromyography, electroencephalography), combined with advances in artificial intelligence such as machine learning, is an evolving area relatively unexplored in pediatric pain. Computers can be "taught" to identify pain occurrences or risk for pain flares with increasing accuracy by synthesizing massive volumes of data from one or more ambulatory sensors worn by a patient. These data, in turn, can cue the patient, caregiver, and/or health care professionals to implement pain prevention and management strategies in real time.[88] In the adult pain literature, wearable devices are being increasingly explored and evaluated in the context of pain assessment.[89] For pediatric pain, the feasibility of wearable sensors have been explored in the context of predicting and treating migraine and assessing pain in seriously ill hospitalized children with acute-on-chronic pain.[90–92] Specific applications in pediatric rheumatology have been mostly conceptual to date.[93] The use of wearable devices combined with artificial intelligence is an especially promising area for pediatric pain given that data collection occurs passively (overcoming adherence challenges with repeated self-report) and does not require verbal skills. Many digital companies are exploring this area. However, more data are needed to evaluate cost, feasibility, safety, validity, and efficacy.

SUMMARY

Numerous evidence-based and publicly available digital technologies currently exist to support pediatric pain assessment and management, with new applications and technologies frequently emerging. With provider awareness and discretion, current technologies have the capacity to augment the clinical evaluation and management of pain in busy rheumatology practices. However, effective pain communication and management in pediatric rheumatology requires caring and informed providers that understand pain as a sensory and emotional experience, requiring assessment and management to augment the treatment of disease activity in pediatric rheumatology clinical care.

CLINICS CARE POINTS

- There are validated digital applications for remote or in-clinic assessment of pain intensity, location, and other broader pain domains, but most of these evidence-based tools are yet to be made widely available outside of research studies.
- Public digital pain assessment tools rarely are evaluated empirically in youth or were not originally intended for rheumatology applications, but some may still be appropriate for obtaining pain self-report in the moment or over time such as the Achy Penguin mobile app (for young children 5–8 years old) and Pain Squad mobile app (ages 8 and above).
- Education about pain mechanisms can be effectively taught through publicly available digital pain websites such as the pain education module of the Teens Taking Charge Online program (originally developed for the self-management of juvenile idiopathic arthritis) and the WebMAP mobile app (originally developed for the self-management of chronic idiopathic pain). Publicly available eHealth pain management videos also enabling pain education include certain Youtube videos ("Tame the Beast," "Mysterious Science of Pain," "Understanding Pain in <5 Minutes").
- Digital tools for training in cognitive-behavioral pain coping skills have not all been evaluated for efficacy, but several that are informed by pain science may be considered for recommendation to patients seen in pediatric rheumatology: the "Imaginaction" website for teaching relaxation skills; WebMAP mobile for training in several evidence-based cognitive-behavioral pain management skills; mobile apps for teaching relaxation to cope with acute or chronic pain such as "Calm," "Mindful Powers," and "Breathe Think Do with Sesame Street" (for young children ages 5–8); and immersive virtual reality apps for managing acute pain during rheumatology procedures.

DISCLOSURE

The authors have nothing to disclose.

REFERENCES

1. Bromberg MH, Connelly M, Anthony KK, et al. Self-reported pain and disease symptoms persist in juvenile idiopathic arthritis despite treatment advances: an electronic diary study. Arthritis Rheumatol 2014;66(2):462–9.
2. Connelly M, Weiss JE, for the CARRA Registry Investigators. Pain, functional disability, and their association in juvenile fibromyalgia compared to other pediatric rheumatic diseases. Pediatr Rheumatol Online J 2019;17(1):72.
3. Khanom S, McDonagh JE, Briggs M, et al. Adolescents' experiences of fluctuating pain in musculoskeletal disorders: a qualitative systematic review and thematic synthesis. BMC Musculoskelet Disord 2020;21(1):645.
4. McGhee JL, Burks FN, Sheckels JL, et al. Identifying children with chronic arthritis based on chief complaints: absence of predictive value for musculoskeletal pain as an indicator of rheumatic disease in children. Pediatrics 2002;110(2 Pt 1):354–9.
5. Pohjankoski H, Hietanen M, Leppänen L, et al. Prolonged, widespread, disabling musculoskeletal pain of adolescents among referrals to the Pediatric Rheumatology Outpatient Clinic from the Päijät-Häme Hospital District in southern Finland. Scand J Pain 2018;18(4):621–8.
6. Correll CK, Spector LG, Zhang L, et al. Barriers and alternatives to pediatric rheumatology referrals: survey of general pediatricians in the United States. Pediatr Rheumatol Online J 2015;13:32.

7. Cox A, Piper S, Singh-Grewal D. Pediatric rheumatology consultant workforce in Australia and New Zealand: the current state of play and challenges for the future. Int J Rheum Dis 2017;20(5):647–53.
8. Defenderfer EK, Bauer K, Igler E, et al. The experience of pain dismissal in adolescence. Clin J Pain 2018;34:162–7.
9. Lee RR, Rashid A, Thomson W, et al. Reluctant to assess pain": a qualitative study of health care professionals' beliefs about the role of pain in Juvenile Idiopathic Arthritis. Arthritis Care Res (Hoboken) 2020;72(1):69–77.
10. Loeser JD, Schatman ME. Chronic pain management in medical education: a disastrous omission. Postgrad Med 2017;129:332–5.
11. Ng W, Slater H, Starcevich C, et al. Barriers and enablers influencing healthcare professionals' adoption of a biopsychosocial approach to musculoskeletal pain: a systematic review and qualitative evidence synthesis. Pain 2021. https://doi.org/10.1097/j.pain.0000000000002217.
12. Shaw T, McGregor D, Brunner M, et al. What is eHealth (6)? Development of a conceptual model for eHealth: qualitative study with key informants. J Med Internet Res 2017;19(10):e324.
13. Pew Research Center. Teens, Social media & technology 2018. Available at: https://www.pewresearch.org/internet/wp-content/uploads/sites/9/2018/05/PI_2018.05.31_TeensTech_FINAL.pdf. Accessed February 1, 2021.
14. Radovic A, Badawy SM. Technology use for adolescent health and wellness. Pediatrics 2020;145(Suppl 2):S186–94.
15. Stinson JN, Connelly M, Jibb LA, et al. Developing a standardized approach to the assessment of pain in children and youth presenting to pediatric rheumatology providers: a Delphi survey and consensus conference process followed by feasibility testing. Pediatr Rheumatol Online J 2012;10(1):7.
16. Slater H, Stinson JN, Jordan JE, et al. Evaluation of digital technologies tailored to support young people's self-management of musculoskeletal pain: mixed methods study. J Med Internet Res 2020;22(6):e18315.
17. Hunter JF, Kain ZN, Fortier MA. Pain relief in the palm of your hand: harnessing mobile health to manage pediatric pain. Paediatr Anaesth 2019;29(2):120–4.
18. Elbert NJ, van Os-Medendorp H, van Renselaar W, et al. Effectiveness and cost-effectiveness of ehealth interventions in somatic diseases: a systematic review of systematic reviews and meta-analyses. J Med Internet Res 2014;16(4):e110.
19. Eccleston C, Blyth FM, Dear BF, et al. Managing patients with chronic pain during the COVID-19 outbreak: considerations for the rapid introduction of remotely supported (eHealth) pain management services. Pain 2020;161(5):889–93.
20. Gordon DB. Acute pain assessment tools: let us move beyond simple pain ratings. Curr Opin Anaesthesiol 2015;28(5):565–9.
21. Starmer AJ, Duby JC, Slaw KM, et al. Pediatrics in the year 2020 and beyond: Preparing for plausible futures. Pediatrics 2010;126:971–81.
22. May M, Junghaenel DU, Ono M, et al. Ecological momentary assessment methodology in chronic pain research: a systematic review. J Pain 2018;19(7):699–716.
23. Lalloo C, Stinson J, Hochman J, et al. Adapting the iconic pain assessment tool version 2 (IPAT2) for adults and adolescents with arthritis pain through usability testing and refinement of pain quality icons. Clin J Pain 2013;29(3):253–64.
24. Luca NJ, Stinson JN, Feldman BM, et al. Validation of the standardized universal pain evaluations for rheumatology providers for children and youth (SUPER-KIDZ). J Orthop Sports Phys Ther 2017;47(10):731–40.

25. Hicks C, von Baeyer C, Spafford P, et al. The Faces pain scale-revised: toward a common metric in pediatric pain measurement. Pain 2001;93(2):173–83.
26. von Baeyer CL, Lin V, Seidman L, et al. Pain charts (body maps or manikins) in assessment of the location of pediatric pain. Pain Mgmt 2011;1(1):61–8.
27. Childhood Arthritis and Rheumatology Research Alliance. CARRA pain chart. 2011. Available at: https://carragroup.org/UserFiles/file/CARRA_Pain_Chart_3p_2018_v1.pdf. Accessed February 28, 2021.
28. Varni J, Stucky B, Thissen D, et al. PROMIS pediatric pain interference scale: an item response theory analysis of the pediatric pain item bank. J Pain 2010;11(11):1109–19.
29. Crombez G, Bijttebier P, Eccleston C, et al. The child version of the pain catastrophizing scale (PCS-C): a preliminary validation. Pain 2003;104:639–46.
30. Lalloo C, Stinson J, Brown S, et al. Pain-QuILT: assessing clinical feasibility of a web-based tool for the visual self-report of pain in an interdisciplianry pediatric chronic pain clinic. Clin J Pain 2014;30(11):934–43.
31. Anand V, Spalding SJ. Leveraging electronic tablets and a readily available data capture platform to assess chronic pain in children: the PROBE system. Stud Health Technol Inform 2015;216:554–8.
32. Bhandari RP, Feinstein AB, Huestis SE, et al. Pediatric-Collaborative Health Outcomes Information Registry (Peds-CHOIR): a learning health system to guide pediatric pain research and treatment. Pain 2016;157(9):2033–44.
33. Palermo T, Valenzuela D, Stork P. A randomized controlled trial of electronic versus paper pain diaries in children: Impact on compliance, accuracy, and acceptability. Pain 2004;107(3):213–9.
34. Stinson JN, Petroz GC, Tait G, et al. e-Ouch: usability testing of an electronic chronic pain diary for adolescents with arthritis. Clin J Pain 2006;22:295–305.
35. Daut RL, Cleeland CS, Flanery RC. Development of the Wisconsin Brief Pain Questionnaire to assess pain in cancer and other disease. Pain 1983;17:197–210.
36. Lee RR, Rashid A, Ghio D, et al. "Seeing pain differently": a qualitative investigation into the differences and similarities of pain and rheumatology specialists' interpretation of multidimensional mobile health pain data from children and young people with juvenile idiopathic arthritis. JMIR Mhealth Uhealth 2019;7(7):e12952.
37. Lee RR, Shoop-Worrall S, Rashid A, et al. Asking too much?": randomized n-of-1 trial exploring patient preferences and measurement reactivity to frequent use of remote multidimensional pain assessments in children and young people with juvenile idiopathic arthritis. J Med Internet Res 2020;22(1):e14503.
38. Calam RM, Jimmieson P, Cox AD, et al. Can computer-based assessment help us understand children's pain? Eur J Anaesthesiol 2000;17:284–8.
39. Zhao P, Yoo I, Lancey R, et al. Mobile applications for pain management: an app analysis for clinical usage. BMC Med Inform Decis Mak 2019;19(1):106.
40. Birmie KA, Nguyen C, Amural TD, et al. A parent–science partnership to improve postsurgical pain management in young children: co-development and usability testing of the Achy Penguin smartphone-based app. Can J Pain 2018;2(1):280–91.
41. International Children's Palliative Care Network (ICPCN). ICPCN pain assessment tool for children 2015. Available at: http://www.icpcn.org/icpcn-pain-assessment-tool-for-children/. Accessed Feburary 28, 2021.

42. Jibb LA, Stevens BJ, Nathan PC, et al. Implementation and preliminary effectiveness of a real-time pain management smartphone app for adolescents with cancer: a multicenter pilot clinical study. Pediatr Blood Cancer 2017;64(10):e26554.
43. Daman digital healthcare partners. Rheumabuddy. Available: https://www.rheumabuddy.com/english. Accessed February 28, 2021.
44. Fisher E, Law E, Dudeney J, et al. Psychological therapies for the management of chronic and recurrent pain in children and adolescents. Cochrane Database Syst Rev 2018;9(9):CD003968.
45. Stinson J, Connelly M, Kamper SJ, et al. Models of care for addressing chronic musculoskeletal pain and health in children and adolescents. Best Pract Res Clin Rheumatol 2016;30(3):468–82.
46. Stinson JN, Lalloo C, Hundert AS, et al. Teens taking charge: a randomized controlled trial of a web-based self-management program with telephone support for adolescents with juvenile idiopathic arthritis. J Med Internet Res 2020;22(7):e16234.
47. Connelly M, Schanberg LE, Ardoin S, et al. Multisite randomized clinical trial evaluating an online self-management program for adolescents with juvenile idiopathic arthritis. J Pediatr Psychol 2019;44(3):363–74.
48. Childhood Arthritis and Rheumatology Research Alliance (CARRA, Inc.) and The Hospital for Sick Children. Taking Charge: Managing JIA. 2021. Available at: https://teenstakingcharge.carragroup.org. Accessed February 28, 2021.
49. About Kids Health. Teens Taking Charge: Managing JIA Online (English version). 2017. Available: https://www.aboutkidshealth.ca/article?contentid=1087&language=english. Accessed February 28th, 2021.
50. About Kids Health. Teens Taking Charge: Managing JIA Online (French version). 2017. Available at: https://www.aboutkidshealth.ca/article?contentid=1087&language=french. Accessed February 28, 2021.
51. Stinson J, Ahola Kohut S, Forgeron P, et al. The iPeer2Peer Program: a pilot randomized controlled trial in adolescents with Juvenile Idiopathic Arthritis. Pediatr Rheumatol Online J 2016;14(1):48.
52. Ahola Kohut S, Stinson JN, Ruskin D, et al. iPeer2Peer program: a pilot feasibility study in adolescents with chronic pain. Pain 2016;157(5):1146–55.
53. Tolley JA, Michel MA, Williams AE, et al. Peer support in the treatment of chronic pain in adolescents: a review of the literature and available resources. Children (Basel) 2020;7(9):129.
54. Schechter NL, Coakley R, Nurko S. The golden half hour in chronic pediatric pain - feedback as the first intervention. JAMA Pediatr 2021;175(1):7–8.
55. Palermo TM, Law EF, Fales J, et al. Internet-delivered cognitive-behavioral treatment for adolescents with chronic pain and their parents: a randomized controlled multicenter trial. Pain 2016;157(1):174–85.
56. Brown ML, Rojas E, Gouda S. A mind-body approach to pediatric pain management. Children (Basel) 2017;4(6):50.
57. Lucile Packard Children's Hospital and Stanford Children's Health. Imaginaction 2019. Available at: http://imaginaction.stanford.edu/. Accessed February 28, 2021.
58. Lalloo C, Jibb LA, Rivera J, et al. "There's a pain app for that": review of patient-targeted smartphone applications for pain management. Clin J Pain 2015;31(6):557–63.
59. Stinson JN, Lalloo C, Harris L, et al. iCanCope with Pain™: user-centred design of a web- and mobile-based self-management program for youth with chronic pain based on identified health care needs. Pain Res Manag 2014;19(5):257–65.

60. The Hospital for Sick Children. iCanCope: living well despite pain. 2021. Available at: http://icancope.ca. Accessed February 28, 2021.
61. Lalloo C, Harris LR, Hundert AS, et al. The iCanCope pain self-management application for adolescents with juvenile idiopathic arthritis: a pilot randomized controlled trial. Rheumatology 2021;60(1):196–206.
62. Palermo TM, de la Vega R, Murray C, et al. A digital health psychological intervention (WebMAP Mobile) for children and adolescents with chronic pain: results of a hybrid effectiveness-implementation stepped-wedge cluster randomized trial. Pain 2020;161(12):2763–74.
63. Seattle Children's Pediatric Pain and Sleep Innovations Lab. WebMAP mobile app. Available at: http://bit.do/webmapmobile. Accessed February 28, 2021.
64. Smith K, Iversen C, Kossowsky J, et al. Apple apps for the management of pediatric pain and pain-related stress. Clin Pract Pediatr Psychol 2015;3(2):93–107.
65. Weekly T, Walker N, Beck J, et al. A review of apps for calming, relaxation, and mindfulness interventions for pediatric palliative care patients. Children (Basel) 2018;5(2):16.
66. Elliott SA, Dyson MP, Wilkes GV, et al. Considerations for health researchers using social media for knowledge translation: multiple case study. J Med Internet Res 2020;22(7):e15121.
67. Chambers CT, Dol J, Parker JA, et al. Implementation effectiveness of a parent-directed YouTube video ("It Doesn't Have To Hurt") on evidence-based strategies to manage needle pain: descriptive survey study. JMIR Pediatr Parent 2020;3(1):e13552.
68. Madathil KC, Rivera-Rodriguez AJ, Greenstein JS, et al. Healthcare information on YouTube: a systematic review. Health Inform J 2015;21(3):173–94.
69. Moorhead SA, Hazlett DE, Harrison L, et al. A new dimension of health care: systematic review of the uses, benefits, and limitations of social media for health communication. J Med Internet Res 2013;15(4):e85.
70. Farkas C, Solodiuk L, Taddio A, et al. Publicly available online educational videos regarding pediatric needle pain: a scoping review. Clin J Pain 2015;31(6):591–8.
71. Robins H, Perron V, Heathcote LC, et al. Pain neuroscience education: state of the art and application in pediatrics. Children 2016;3(4):43.
72. Pate JW, Heathcote LC, Simons LE, et al. Creating online animated videos to reach and engage youth: lessons learned from pain science education and a call to action. Paediatr Neonatal Pain 2020;2:131–8.
73. Heathcote LC, Pate JW, Park AL, et al. Pain neuroscience education on YouTube. PeerJ 2019;7:e6603.
74. Hunter New England Local Health District. Understanding pain and what to do about it. [Video]. Youtube. 2016. Available at: https://www.youtube.com/embed/qEWc2XtaNwg. Accessed February 17, 2021.
75. IWK Health Centre. It doesn't have to hurt. [Video]. Youtube. 2013. Available at: https://www.youtube.com/watch/KgBwVSYqfps. Accessed February 28th, 2021.
76. Won AS, Tataru CA, Cojocaru CM, et al. Two virtual reality pilot studies for the treatment of pediatric CRPS. Pain Med 2015;16(8):1644–7.
77. Eijlers R, Utens EMWJ, Staals LM, et al. Systematic review and meta-analysis of virtual reality in pediatrics: effects on pain and anxiety. Anesth Analg 2019;129(5):1344–53.
78. Hoffman HG, Doctor JN, Patterson DR, et al. Virtual reality as an adjunctive pain control during burn wound care in adolescent patients. Pain 2000;85:305–9.

79. Gold JI, Mahrer NE. Is virtual reality ready for prime time in the medical space? A randomized control trial of pediatric virtual reality for acute procedural pain management. J Pediatr Psychol 2018;43(3):266–75.
80. Won AS, Bailey J, Bailenson J, et al. Immersive virtual reality for pediatric pain. Children 2017;4(7):52.
81. Almeida AF, Rocha NP, Silva AG. Methodological quality of manuscripts reporting on the usability of mobile applications for pain assessment and management: a systematic review. Int J Environ Res Public Health 2020;17(3):785.
82. Wallace LS, Dhingra LK. A systematic review of smartphone applications for chronic pain available for download in the United States. J Opioid Manag 2014;10(1):63–8.
83. Higgins KS, Tutelman PR, Chambers CT, et al. Availability of researcher-led eHealth tools for pain assessment and management: barriers, facilitators, costs, and design. Pain Rep 2018;3(Suppl 1):e686.
84. Wu YP, Steele RG, Connelly MA, et al. Commentary: pediatric eHealth interventions: common challenges during development, implementation, and dissemination. J Pediatr Psychol 2014;39(6):612–23.
85. Hall JL, McGraw D. For telehealth to succeed, privacy and security risks must be identified and addressed. Health Aff (Millwood) 2014;33(2):216–21.
86. Butpheng C, Yeh K-H, Xiong H. Security and privacy in IoT-cloud based e-Health systems—a comprehensive review. Symmetry 2020;12(7):1191.
87. Voerman JS, Remerie S, Westendorp T, et al. Effects of a guided internet-delivered self-help intervention for adolescents with chronic pain. J Pain 2015;16(11):1115–26.
88. Nahum-Shani I, Smith SN, Spring BJ, et al. Just-in-Time Adaptive Interventions (JITAIs) in mobile health: key components and design principles for ongoing health behavior support. Ann Behav Med 2018;52(6):446–62.
89. Johnson A, Yang F, Gollarahalli S, et al. Use of mobile health apps and wearable technology to assess changes and predict pain during treatment of acute pain in sickle cell disease: Feasibility study. JMIR mHealth and uHealth 2019;7(12):e13671.
90. Connell MA, Boorigie ME. Feasibility of using "SMARTER" methodology for monitoring precipitating conditions of pediatric migraine episodes. Headache 2020;61(3):500–10.
91. Stubberud A, Tronvik E, Olsen A, et al. Biofeedback treatment app for pediatric migraine: development and usability study. Headache 2020;60(5):889–901.
92. Ajayi TA, Salongo L, Zang Y, et al. Mobile health-collected biophysical markers in children with serious illness-related pain. J Palliat Med 2020;24(4):580–8.
93. Coda A, Sculley D, Santos D, et al. Harnessing interactive technologies to improve health outcomes in juvenile idiopathic arthritis. Pediatr Rheumatol Online J 2017;15(1):40.

Instrumental Substance Use Among Youth with Rheumatic Disease—A Biopsychosocial Model

Joe Kossowsky, PhD, MMSc[a,b], Elissa R. Weitzman, ScD, MSc[c,d,e,*]

KEYWORDS

- Substance use • Self-medication • Chronic illness • Adolescents
- Instrumental substance use

KEY POINTS

- Substance use is common among youth including youth with rheumatic diseases, contributing to high levels of preventable morbidity and mortality and treatment nonadherence for youth with a chronic illness.
- Many symptoms and problems experienced by youth with a rheumatic disease, specifically pain, anxiety, stress, and sleep problems, constitute risk factors for substance use by youth.
- Some youth with rheumatic diseases report "instrumental use" of substances, that is, using to address symptoms of their disease and/or side effects of their treatments although such use has unproven benefit and poses risks for disease management.
- Screening for substance use in health care settings may help identify preventable health risks, threats to treatment management, and, for youth who report instrumental use, need for additional supportive interventions to ameliorate symptoms and disease/treatment burdens.
- Youth value screening and guidance about substance use from their specialty care providers under models that are nonjudgmental, factual, and developmentally appropriate.

INTRODUCTION

Substance use is common among adolescents and associated with myriad adverse outcomes (injury, school failure, relationship problems) and significant morbidity,

[a] Department of Anesthesiology, Critical Care and Pain Medicine, Boston Children's Hospital, Harvard Medical School, 333 Longwood Avenue, 5th Floor, Pain Treatment Service, Boston, MA 02115, USA; [b] Department of Anaesthesia, Harvard Medical School, 25 Shattuck Street, Boston, MA 02115, USA; [c] Department of Pediatrics, Harvard Medical School, 25 Shattuck Street, Boston, MA 02115, USA; [d] Division of Adolescent/Young Adult Medicine, Boston Children's Hospital, 300 Longwood Avenue, Boston, MA 02115, USA; [e] Computational Health Informatics Program, Boston Children's Hospital, Boston, MA, USA
* Corresponding authors. 300 Longwood Avenue, Boston, MA 02115.
E-mail address: elissa.weitzman@childrens.harvard.edu

Rheum Dis Clin N Am 48 (2022) 51–65
https://doi.org/10.1016/j.rdc.2021.08.003
rheumatic.theclinics.com

mortality, and economic costs annually in the United States.[1] Youth with chronic medical conditions (YCMC) including those with pediatric-onset rheumatic disease (PRD) are vulnerable to these risks and also face risks for health harms unique to their chronic illness including treatment nonadherence and poor self-care.[2,3] In addition to experiencing risks for poor outcomes and harms *because* of their substance use, for YCMC, the chronic illness experience may amplify substance use risks, *contributing to* poor outcomes. YCMC may attempt to ameliorate symptoms of disease activity and negative side effects of medications and treatments by using substances. We call substance use to alleviate symptoms and side effects of a health problem instrumental use (IU). "Self-medication" and "self-treatment" are other commonly used terms that refer to this type of substance use. This article provides a brief overview of adolescent substance use and its intersection with chronic illness and PRD including in the context of a biopsychosocial model of substance use vulnerability and emerging evidence about IU of substances. Implications for PRD clinical practice are discussed.

BRIEF OVERVIEW OF ADOLESCENT SUBSTANCE USE EPIDEMIOLOGY

Prevalence

The most common substance use behaviors among adolescents in the United States include consumption of alcohol, nicotine vapes, marijuana, and misuse of prescription medications including opioids; reports of lifetime use of these substances among adolescents in the 12th grade are 61.5%, 44.3%, 43.7%, and 14.2%, respectively.[4] Rates of use are dynamic, prevalence levels vary over time and space, in concert with social norms,[5] policies,[6] and age.[4] In nationally representative surveys from 2020, 21.3%, 37.3%, and 46.6% of 8th, 10th, and 12th graders, respectively, reported ever using an illicit substance (not including alcohol).[4] As might be expected, across substances, young age of first substance use increases the risk for development of a substance use disorder (SUD) while delayed onset is protective.[7] Details about the most commonly used substances among adolescents are reported in **Table 1**.

Intensification of Use Among Youth

Substance use behaviors are intensifying among youth for the major categories of drugs used. Over the past decade, alcohol consumption by adolescents has declined in the United States, but the percentage of youth reporting "high intensity" alcohol use (10+ drinks per occasion) has risen to about 10% of 12th graders nationally,[8] a pattern associated with a range of harms,[9] and nonmedical use of prescription drugs.[8] Marijuana is becoming the "gateway" substance that precedes and predicts other substance use.[10] Overall levels of marijuana use are mostly stable but the percentage of users reporting frequent use has risen.[11,12] Frequent and chronic marijuana use, and increased product potency are risk factors for cannabis use disorder, psychiatric problems, and other health harms.[13–15] Use of e-cigarettes or electronic vaping devices (vapes) by adolescents in high school increased nearly 1000-fold from 2011 to 2015, after which use briefly stabilized, increasing again toward the end of the decade.[16] Substantial percentages of youth (nearly 12% of high school seniors) reported daily use of nicotine vapes by 2019[17] and evidence suggests trajectories from vaping nicotine to smoking cigarettes are emerging.[16]

Polysubstance Use

Polysubstance use is common among adolescents. The most commonly reported polysubstance use pattern is the simultaneous use of alcohol and marijuana, reported

Table 1
Adolescent substance use prevalence rates and trends

							Tobacco/Nicotine										
Substances	**Alcohol**			**Marijuana**			**Cigarettes**			**Vaping**			**Prescription Opioids**		**Amphetamines**		
Typical Age of Initiation (y)	15.1[65]			13.9[66]			12.6[67]			14.1[67]			14.3[68]		16[69]		
High School Prevalence (in %), by Grade in 2019–2020																	
	8th	*10th*	*12th*	*8th*	*10th*	*12th*	*8th*	*10th*	*12th*	*8th*	*10th*	*12th*	*9/10th*	*11/12th*	*8th*	*10th*	*12th*
Lifetime Use	25.6	46.4	61.5	14.8	33.3	43.7	11.5	13.9	24.0	22.7	38.7	44.3	13.6	14.9	8.9	7.0	7.3
Annual Use	20.5	40.7	55.3	11.4	28.0	35.2	N/A			16.6	30.7	34.5	N/A		5.3	4.3	4.3
Last 30-d Use	9.9	20.3	33.6	6.5	16.6	21.1	2.2	3.2	7.5	10.5	19.3	24.5	7.0	7.3	2.2	1.9	1.7
Trends Over the Last 10 Years	Decreasing Use			No Change			Decreasing Use			Increasing Use			Insufficient years of data to assess 10-y trends. No change from 2017–2019		Decreasing Use		

Note: 2020 Prevalence rates and trends for alcohol, marijuana, tobacco/nicotine, and amphetamines were gathered from the 2020 Monitoring the Future Data.[4] 2019 Prevalence rates and trends for prescription opioid misuse was gathered from the 2019 Youth Risk Behavior Survey.[70]

Abbreviation: N/A, not assessed.

by 20% of high school seniors.[18] Both high-intensity alcohol use and daily use of marijuana predict heightened risk for concurrent use of alcohol and marijuana, whereas high-intensity alcohol use predicts recreational use of prescription drugs.[8]

Co-occurring Substance Use and Mental Health Disorders

Adolescence and young adulthood are periods of peak onset for many mental health problems.[19] Youth who experience mental health problems and substance use problems are often referred to as having a "dual-disorder" or "co-occurring problems." More than one-third (36.8%) of adolescents who met the criteria for SUD in the past year also had a major depressive episode in that time, whereas one-tenth (10.5%) of adolescents with a major depressive episode in the past year had an SUD in that time.[20] The percentage of young adults with any mental illness in the past year who have an SUD is 49.4%.[20] Depression and anxiety are common among youth with chronic illness including PRD.[21] Strong associations may be explained by the presence of predisposing factors related to both outcomes (eg, poor emotion regulation), interdependent timing (ie, experience of mental illness as a consequence of substance use, or substance use to alleviate symptoms of mental illness), or environmental exposures that increase the propensity for both mental health problems and substance use (eg, stress or trauma). Extremely few (1.3%) dually-disordered adolescents receive services for both problems,[20] and little is known about this pattern for YCMC.

SUBSTANCE USE AMONG YOUTH WITH CHRONIC ILLNESS

Prevalence and Harms

Existing research indicates that YCMC, including those with PRD, use alcohol, tobacco/nicotine, marijuana, and other drugs at levels commensurate with or above their healthy peers.[22,23] More than two-thirds of YCMC reported ever trying alcohol, of which 42.2% reported binge drinking (ie, consuming $\geq$ 4/5 drinks per occasion for women/men), 44.3% of YCMC reported ever trying tobacco, of which almost three-quarters reported regular cigarette use and 47.8% of YCMC reported lifetime use of marijuana, of which around half reported past month marijuana use.[23] Longitudinal data indicate that, compared to youth who do not have a chronic illness, YCMC may initiate substance use at younger ages and face greater risks for heavy use and associated harms later in adolescence/young adulthood, especially over transition years into early adulthood.[23]

Substance use behaviors may undermine the health status and disease management of youth with PRD. Alcohol may negatively interact with over-the-counter and prescription medications[24] and alcohol and other substance use may impact treatment adherence. The risk for medication nonadherence among YCMC who drink compared with those who do not is nearly double.[2] Moreover, substance use carries risks for poor sleep,[25] unhealthy diet,[26] and unprotected sex, heightening the risks for sexually transmitted disease and unplanned pregnancy.[27] This is especially relevant in PRD patients, given that careful planning of pregnancy, as well as the choice of medication, is critical to preventing complications, spontaneous abortions,[28] and other harms arising from unplanned pregnancy in the setting of exposure to possible teratogens.[29]

Biopsychosocial Model of Substance Use in PRD

For youth with PRD, elevated levels of sleep disturbance, stress, anxiety, depressive symptoms, and pain contribute separately and together to psychologically and neurologically mediated risks for substance use (**Fig. 1**). For teens, psychobiological risks

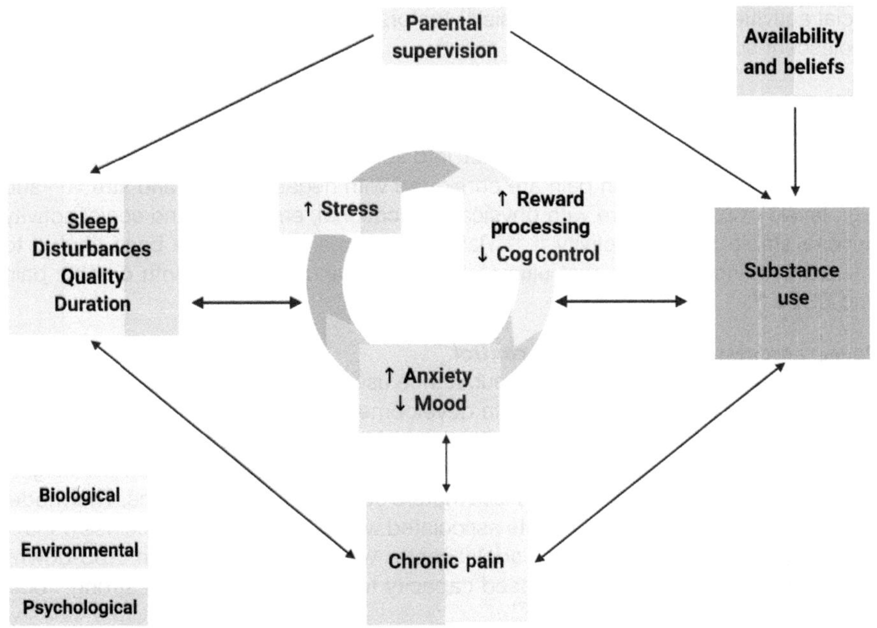

Fig. 1. Biopsychosocial model of substance use in pediatric rheumatic disease. Studies indicate bidirectional interactions among sleep disturbances, pain, and substance use. These interactions in turn are mediated via psychological and neurodevelopmental factors, including stress, anxiety, mood, cognitive control, and reward processing. Substance use is further influenced by parental supervision, availability of substances, as well as individual beliefs about the utility and risks of the substances.

are manifest during a period of rising peer influence, reduced parental monitoring,[30,31] and often, accessible and available substances.[4] Details about the specific pathways in this model and their interactions are described in the following sections.

Sleep and fatigue

PRD patients often report both sleep impairment[32] and fatigue,[33] which can lead to significant harms, including increased school absence, decreased physical functioning, and increased pain.[33] Findings suggest that pain is associated with fatigue in patients with PRD.[33] A bidirectional interaction between decreased and disturbed sleep and increased pain levels,[34] as well as higher levels of anxiety and depression,[35] has been documented, while positive emotions have been shown to act as a protective factor in the pain-sleep relationship.[32] Sleep disturbances also contribute to diminished cognitive control, making affected adolescents more likely to engage in heavy substance use during periods of worsened mood.[36]

Stress, anxiety, and depression

Children with PRD face similar psychosocial stressors as do their peers, while also confronting illness-specific challenges and negative impacts of their illness on functioning.[37] Negative body image may be caused by disease symptoms and treatment side effects, while the unpredictability of flares may be demoralizing, generating high levels of anxiety and depressive symptoms[21] and decreased quality of life.[38] Stress has been associated with increased adjustment problems, mood disorders, and disease symptoms among youth with PRD,[39,40] which in turn decrease participation in social activities on a day-to-day basis,[41] factors that may otherwise be protective of adolescent substance use.[42]

Pain

Pain is a common and clinically significant symptom of PRD, with many youths experiencing persistent pain that can continue into adulthood, even after being treated with biologics.[43–46] Increases in pain are correlated with negative mood and stress[47] and high levels of pain interfere with physical, educational, emotional, and social activity despite stable disease activity.[43,44] Pain and substance use have been shown to interact in a vicious cycle that ultimately worsens and maintains both chronic pain and SUDs.[48]

Reward processing and cognitive control

From a developmental perspective, substance use during adolescence occurs in the context of normative changes in brain development related to cognitive control and reward seeking.[49] The "dual-process" model of substance use[50] proposes that the increased propensity for substance use relies on an imbalance between the heightened activity in reward systems and less mature cognitive control systems. This model suggests that the perceived benefits associated with particular substance use behaviors are relatively overvalued by adolescents, while the limitations in "top-down" cognitive control result in a decreased capacity to regulate these often strong, "bottom-up" reward-related impulses.[51]

Instrumental Substance Use Among Youth with Rheumatic Diseases

Information is limited regarding the extent to which youth with rheumatic diseases use alcohol, marijuana, tobacco/nicotine, or other substances for relief of symptoms and side effects. In a survey of marijuana use by YCMC including youth with juvenile idiopathic arthritis and systemic lupus erythematosus, nearly one-third of adolescents who reported using marijuana did so to address symptoms and side effects of their condition, rather than for recreational purposes.[52] Among the IU group, reasons for using included to address pain (50.0%), anxiety (68.2%), nausea or upset stomach (40.9%), and appetite (45.5%). Notably, youth who reported IU were not different from those who reported recreational (noninstrumental) use in reports of overall health, mental health, or the frequency of missing activities because of their condition. However, the IU group reported younger age of onset of marijuana use, greater frequency of use, higher rates of tobacco and nicotine use, and greater intentions to use in the future—all factors that placed them at higher risk for SUD but do not support a self-medication hypothesis. A study of secondary school students throughout the province of Ontario, Canada, found nearly identical results[53]—a similar fraction of marijuana using youth reported IU, and compared to their peers who reported recreational marijuana use, the IU group reported more frequent marijuana use, higher levels of tobacco and other drug use, and were less likely to perceive marijuana as harmful. This study, with its larger sample size, found that the IU group reported worse overall health and less healthy sleep among than the youth who reported using recreationally.[53]

Qualitative research with YCMC finds that motivations for using marijuana reflect perceptions regarding use to "self-medicate" or cope. One study of adolescents with chronic illness including youth with PRD found that some youth report using marijuana to alleviate pain, and others to relieve a feeling of overall body "tightness" related to their arthritis.[3] Other youth reported perceiving that alcohol and other substance use can alleviate stress. Notably, in this study, youth with PRD taking methotrexate reported high levels of stress around the potential for alcohol use to interact with medications, which countered the desire to use. Findings echo results of other research in which youth in general report they use marijuana for relief from difficult experiences and emotions.[54]

A considerable literature exists around the use of alcohol and marijuana “to cope” with difficult experiences and emotions. Trauma, anxiety, and depression are often cited as motivating reasons for substance use by youth.[55] Youth with PRD may be at elevated risk for these problems and some youth may consider their condition and its treatment to be difficult, suggesting potential for using substances to cope with both disease and treatment burdens. Insofar as youth with PRD are at elevated risk for psychosocial problems—they may be at elevated risk for substance use as outlined in the biopsychosocial model of substance use (see **Fig. 1**).

From a psychological perspective, substance use in youth with PRD may be motivated through negative and positive reinforcement pathways as well as disruption in stress management ability. Negative reinforcement models[56] postulate that substance use is motivated by a desire to alleviate aversive states associated with PRD, such as pain, anxiety, and depression, especially if these physical and mental health symptoms are not being adequately treated. Furthermore, patients with PRD experience reduced opportunities for positive reinforcement and lower quality of life, problems they may consider to be ameliorated via the psychoactive effects of substances.[57] It is also possible that some adolescents consider substance use to be a normative and acceptable way of feeling better in contrast to taking medications, which may make them feel different, or embarrassed,[58] contributing to IU. Finally, PRD patients may also be socialized to using substances, albeit approved medications, to relieve symptoms and side effects. Notably, IU of marijuana is higher in states with more liberal marijuana laws and where marijuana use is legal for medical purposes.[59] Commercial promotion of marijuana as a healthy, benign therapeutic for anxiety, sleep, pain, and other problems may influence marijuana use among youth with PRD.

CLINICAL IMPLICATIONS: SCREENING AND SAFETY

Screening for Substance Use

Substance use, including IU by youth with PRD, jeopardizes health status and treatment adherence. As such, screening for substance use in primary and specialty care may afford opportunity to improve health behaviors and outcomes. Adolescents and young adults with chronic illnesses including PRD endorse screening for substance use in specialty care settings, which they consider to be their medical home.[3] Adolescents and young adults with PRD express strong preferences for private, direct, factual, and nonjudgmental conversations with their providers about substance use and experience providers’ questions as markers of caring and health care quality. Clear factual recommendations to avoid using substances and explanations about the negative effects of substances on health and disease including with respect to mood, medication safety/efficacy, adherence, and lifestyle risks (ie, sleep, diet, sexual, and reproductive health) are desired. When collecting behavioral health information, health care organizations can implement patient portals and electronic health records that safeguard sensitive information, for example, by restricting parental views as youth mature.[60]

Many developmentally appropriate brief screening tools to identify substance use are available along with assessment tools that will provide diagnostic information (**Table 2**). Tools can be implemented online, in advance of a visit, or at the point of care, based on provider preference and workflow. Generally speaking, youth provide

Table 2
Adolescent substance use screening tools and surveillance

Tool	Substance Use Type		Recall Period	Administration		Validated Age Range (y)	URL for More Information
	Alcohol	Drugs		Mode	Frequency		
Screening Tools							
Screening to Brief Intervention (S2BI)	X	X	Past year	Self or Clinician	Annually/As needed	11–17	https://www.drugabuse.gov/ast/s2bi/
Brief Screener for Alcohol, Tobacco, and other Drugs (BSTAD)	X	X	Past year	Self or Clinician	Annually/As needed	12–17	https://www.drugabuse.gov/ast/bstad/
Adapted NIDA Drug Use Screening Tool: Quick Screen (NMASSIST)	X	X	Past 2 wk	Self or Clinician	Annually/As needed	11–17	https://www.drugabuse.gov/nidamed-medical-health-professionals/screening-tools-resources/american-psychiatric-association-adapted-nida-modified-assist-tools
Drug Abuse Screen Test-Adolescent version (DAST-A)		X	Lifetime	Self or Clinician	Annually/As needed	13–19	http://www.socialworkerstoolbox.com/drug-abuse-screening-test-for-adolescents-dast-a/

Alcohol Screening and Brief Intervention for Youth (AUDIT)	X		Past year	Self or Clinician	Annually/ As needed	14–18	http://pubs.niaaa.nih.gov/publications/Practitioner/YouthGuide/AUDIT.pdf
CRAFFT	X	X	Past year	Self or Clinician	Annually/ As needed	12–21	https://crafft.org/
NIAAA Brief Alcohol Screening Tool	X		Past year/Lifetime	Clinician	Annually/ As needed	9–18	https://www.niaaa.nih.gov/alcohols-effects-health/professional-education-materials/alcohol-screening-and-brief-intervention-youth-practitioners-guide
Surveillance							
Monitoring the Future (MTF)[a]	X	X	Lifetime/Annual/ Past month	School, Self-administered	Yearly	High/Middle School	http://www.monitoringthefuture.org/
Youth Risk Behavior Surveillance System (YRBSS)[a]	X	X	Lifetime/Past month	School, Teacher-administered	Biennial	High/Middle School/College	https://www.cdc.gov/healthyyouth/data/yrbs/index.htm
National Survey Drug Use and Health (NSDUH)[b]	X	X	Lifetime/Annual/ Past month	Household, Interviewer-administered	Yearly	> 12 y of age	https://nsduhweb.rti.org/respweb/homepage.cfm
National Youth Tobacco Survey (NYTS)[a]		X	First use/Lifetime/ Past month	School, Self-administered	Yearly	High/Middle School	https://www.cdc.gov/tobacco/data_statistics/surveys/nyts/index.htm

[a] School based.
[b] Age based.

more detailed and reliable information when given an opportunity to report about their health behaviors online or on paper rather than verbally, and in a private setting without a parent or guardian present.[3] Studies indicate that standardized tools provided routinely generate more accurate information about patients than do clinical instincts, which can be influenced by implicit bias and moralistic assumptions.[61] Notably, both substance use and mental health screening of YCMC including those with PRD are well tolerated by youth and providers in clinical settings, with very few workflow disruptions.[62] Providers who wish to implement a screening protocol might use the S2BI which is brief, and delivers substance-specific quantity and frequency information helpful for triaging risk and assessing change. Where alcohol is a singular interest, the NIAAA Brief Screen has been validated with YCMC. Providers may additionally screen with the CRAFFT which assesses problems albeit this screen does not capture quantity/frequency information and is not substance specific hence it may not be useful for discerning change over time. In addition to implementing routine screening, providers can stay abreast of adolescent substance use patterns including by reviewing national survey programs and reports for updates on national and state trends (see **Table 1**).

Screening for Risk Factors

As indicated in **Fig. 1**, the abundance of sleep-related findings highlights the need to assess, and if needed, manage sleep problems in PRD. A detailed sleep assessment should include a thorough review of medications, including doses and timing, as many commonly used medications for PRD affect sleep staging and disturbances.[63] Similarly, screening for mental health comorbidities can provide a comprehensive picture of psychosocial wellbeing. Providers must also address patient's pain when considering the best management approach for PRD. It is important that integrated pain management strategies are used in addition to pharmacologic therapy aimed to control inflammation as soon as possible after diagnosis. Finally, psychosocial and financial burdens of having a child with chronic illness are substantial for families[64] which might contribute to both parent and child substance use. Where possible, comprehensive screening might provide insight into the family context and pinpoint adolescents at high risk for substance use and poor disease outcomes, and direct attention to the need for ameliorative interventions.

SUMMARY

In conclusion, adolescent substance use is common including among youth with PRD. Emerging evidence suggests that some youth with PRD are using substances instrumentally, to address symptoms and side effects of their conditions. A biopsychosocial model of substance use provides a coherent frame for substance use vulnerability for youth with PRD, given the high correlations among factors that are commonly reported as disease and treatment burdens by youth with PRD, and associations among these factors and substance use among youth in general. To date, studies do not show a clear picture of difference in health status between youth with PRD who are and are not using substances instrumentally. It may be that youth consider IU to be a legitimizing rationale for substance use, or a reflection of marketing and promotion of substances (especially marijuana) as effective "treatments." In either case, screening youth with PRD for substance use may identify important and potentially overlooked risk behaviors and need for psychosocial and disease management support, in line with the comprehensive attention to the whole person that all youth need and deserve.

CLINICS CARE POINTS

- Substance use is a persistent problem among adolescents with PRD, but the risk for specific substances of abuse can vary over time and place. Clinicians should stay abreast of the age-specific trends and screen for substance use using validated tools.
- Polysubstance use is common. Clinicians should pay attention to the potential that more than one substance is being used.
- Risk factors, such as sleep, pain, mood, and anxiety interact and tend to cluster together, suggesting need for a holistic assessment.
- An optimized screening approach would use validated tools that capture quantity and frequency for specific substances (ie, S2BI) coupled with a problem based screen (eg, CRAFFT).
- Social factors may provide a protective buffer or a risk environment for youth, indicating that environmental factors should be assessed as part of a high-quality assessment.
- Youth who screen positive for substance use and show signs of disordered use may need support from clinicians trained in addiction medicine.

ACKNOWLEDGMENTS

The authors thank Camila Koike and Rachele Cox for their assistance in article preparation and review.

DISCLOSURE

The authors have nothing to disclose.

REFERENCES

1. Substance Abuse and Mental Health Services Administration (US). Office of the Surgeon general (US). Facing addiction in America: the Surgeon General's report on alcohol, drugs, and health. Washington (DC): US Department of Health and Human Services; November 2016. Available at. https://www.ncbi.nlm.nih.gov/books/NBK424857/. Accessed March 9, 2021.
2. Weitzman ER, Ziemnik RE, Huang Q, et al. Alcohol and Marijuana Use and Treatment Nonadherence Among Medically Vulnerable Youth. Pediatrics 2015;136(3):450–7.
3. Weitzman ER, Salimian PK, Rabinow L, et al. Perspectives on substance use among youth with chronic medical conditions and implications for clinical guidance and prevention: A qualitative study. PLoS One 2019;14(1):e0209963.
4. Johnston LD, Miech RA, O'Malley PM, et al. Monitoring the future national survey results on drug Use, 1975-2020: overview, Key findings on adolescent drug Use. Institute for Social Research; 2021.
5. Eisenberg ME, Toumbourou JW, Catalano RF, et al. Social norms in the development of adolescent substance use: A longitudinal analysis of the International Youth Development Study. J Youth Adolesc 2014;43(9):1486–97.
6. Blevins CE, Marsh E, Banes KE, et al. The implications of cannabis policy changes in Washington on adolescent perception of risk, norms, attitudes, and substance use. Subst Abuse 2018;12. 1178221818815491.
7. DeWit DJ, Adlaf EM, Offord DR, et al. Age at first alcohol use: a risk factor for the development of alcohol disorders. Am J Psychiatry 2000;157(5):745–50.

8. McCabe SE, Veliz P, Patrick ME. High-intensity drinking and nonmedical use of prescription drugs: Results from a national survey of 12th grade students. Drug Alcohol Depend 2017;178:372–9.
9. Patrick ME, Azar B. High-intensity drinking. Alcohol Res 2018;39(1):49.
10. Copeland WE, Hill S, Costello EJ, et al. Cannabis use and disorder from childhood to adulthood in a longitudinal community sample with American Indians. J Am Acad Child Adolesc Psychiatry 2017;56(2):124–32.e2.
11. Compton WM, Han B, Jones CM, et al. Cannabis use disorders among adults in the United States during a time of increasing use of cannabis. Drug Alcohol Depend 2019;204:107468.
12. Copeland J, Rooke S, Swift W. Changes in cannabis use among young people: impact on mental health. Curr Opin Psychiatry 2013;26(4):325–9.
13. Hasin DS. US epidemiology of cannabis use and associated problems. Neuropsychopharmacology 2018;43(1):195–212.
14. Hadland SE, Harris SK. Youth marijuana use: state of the science for the practicing clinician. Curr Opin Pediatr 2014;26(4):420.
15. Keyes KM, Rutherford C, Miech R. Historical trends in the grade of onset and sequence of cigarette, alcohol, and marijuana use among adolescents from 1976–2016: Implications for "Gateway" patterns in adolescence. Drug Alcohol Depend 2019;194:51–8.
16. Walley SC, Wilson KM, Winickoff JP, et al. A public health crisis: electronic cigarettes, vape, and JUUL. Pediatrics 2019;143(6):e20182741.
17. Miech R, Johnston L, O'Malley PM, et al. Trends in adolescent vaping, 2017–2019. N Engl J Med 2019;381(15):1490–1.
18. Patrick ME, Veliz PT, Terry-McElrath YM. High-intensity and simultaneous alcohol and marijuana use among high school seniors in the United States. Subst Abus 2017;38(4):498–503.
19. Kessler RC, Amminger GP, Aguilar-Gaxiola S, et al. Age of onset of mental disorders: a review of recent literature. Curr Opin Psychiatry 2007;20(4):359–64.
20. McCance-Katz EF. The national survey on drug use and health: 2019. Substance abuse and mental health services administration. 2020. Available at: https://www.samhsa.gov/data/release/2019-national-survey-drug-use-and-health-nsduh-releases. Accessed March 9, 2021.
21. Fair DC, Rodriguez M, Knight AM, et al. Depression and anxiety in patients with juvenile idiopathic arthritis: current insights and impact on quality of life, a systematic review. Open Access Rheumatol 2019;11:237–52.
22. van Weelden M, Lourenço B, Viola GR, et al. Substance use and sexual function in juvenile idiopathic arthritis. Rev Bras Reumatol 2016;56(4):323–9.
23. Wisk LE, Weitzman ER. Substance use patterns through early adulthood: results for youth with and without chronic conditions. Am J Prev Med 2016;51(1):33–45.
24. Breslow RA, Dong C, White A. Prevalence of alcohol-interactive prescription medication use among current drinkers: United States, 1999 to 2010. Alcohol Clin Exp Res 2015;39(2):371–9.
25. Zhabenko O, Austic E, Conroy DA, et al. Substance use as a risk factor for sleep problems among adolescents presenting to the emergency department. J Addict Med 2016;10(5):331–8.
26. Naude CE, Senekal M, Laubscher R, et al. Growth and weight status in treatment-naïve 12-16 year old adolescents with alcohol use disorders in Cape Town, South Africa. Nutr J 2011;10:87.
27. Finer LB, Zolna MR. Shifts in intended and unintended pregnancies in the United States, 2001-2008. Am J Public Health 2014;104(Suppl 1):S43–8.

28. Ling N, Lawson E, von Scheven E. Adverse pregnancy outcomes in adolescents and young women with systemic lupus erythematosus: a national estimate. Pediatr Rheumatol 2018;16(1):26.
29. Ponticelli C, Moroni G. Fetal toxicity of immunosuppressive drugs in pregnancy. J Clin Med 2018;7(12):552.
30. Clark DB, Kirisci L, Mezzich A, et al. Parental supervision and alcohol use in adolescence: developmentally specific interactions. J Dev Behav Pediatr 2008; 29(4):285.
31. Kristjansson AL, James JE, Allegrante JP, et al. Adolescent substance use, parental monitoring, and leisure-time activities: 12-year outcomes of primary prevention in Iceland. Prev Med 2010;51(2):168–71.
32. Valrie CR, Bromberg MH, Palermo T, et al. A systematic review of sleep in pediatric pain populations. J Dev Behav Pediatr 2013;34(2):120–8.
33. Nijhof LN, van de Putte EM, Wulffraat NM, et al. Prevalence of severe fatigue among adolescents with pediatric rheumatic diseases. Arthritis Care Res 2016; 68(1):108–14.
34. Stinson JN, Hayden JA, Ahola Kohut S, et al. Sleep problems and associated factors in children with juvenile idiopathic arthritis: a systematic review. Pediatr Rheumatol Online J 2014;12:19.
35. Hrelic D, Rouster-Stevens K, Gewanter H, et al. Sleep problems in JIA patients: relationships with mood, pain, and functional status and health-related quality of life. J Alt Med Res 2010;2(1):97–106.
36. Hasler BP, Pedersen SL. Sleep and circadian risk factors for alcohol problems: a brief overview and proposed mechanisms. Curr Opin Psychol 2020;34:57–62.
37. Wallander JL, Varni JW. Adjustment in children with chronic physical disorders: programmatic research on a disability-stress-coping model. In: La Greca AM, Siegel LJ, Wallander JL, et al, editors. Stress and coping in child health. New York: Guilford; 1992. p. 279–98.
38. Bomba M, Meini A, Molinaro A, et al. Body experiences, emotional competence, and psychosocial functioning in juvenile idiopathic arthritis. Rheumatol Int 2013; 33(8):2045–52.
39. Timko C, Stovel KW, Baumgartner M, et al. Acute and chronic stressors, social resources, and functioning among adolescents with juvenile rheumatic disease. J Res Adolesc 1995;5(3):361–85.
40. von Weiss RT, Rapoff MA, Varni JW, et al. Daily hassles and social support as predictors of adjustment in children with pediatric rheumatic disease. J Pediatr Psychol 2002;27(2):155–65.
41. Schanberg LE, Gil KM, Anthony KK, et al. Pain, stiffness, and fatigue in juvenile polyarticular arthritis: contemporaneous stressful events and mood as predictors. Arthritis Rheum 2005;52(4):1196–204.
42. Duncan SC, Duncan TE, Strycker LA, et al. Relations between youth antisocial and prosocial activities. J Behav Med 2002;25(5):425–38.
43. Schanberg LE, Anthony KK, Gil KM, et al. Daily pain and symptoms in children with polyarticular arthritis. Arthritis Rheum 2003;48(5):1390–7.
44. Schanberg LE, Lefebvre JC, Keefe FJ, et al. Pain coping and the pain experience in children with juvenile chronic arthritis. Pain 1997;73(2):181–9.
45. Rashid A, Cordingley L, Carrasco R, et al. Patterns of pain over time among children with juvenile idiopathic arthritis. Arch Dis Child 2018;103(5):437–43.
46. Lomholt JJ, Thastum M, Herlin T. Pain experience in children with juvenile idiopathic arthritis treated with anti-TNF agents compared to non-biologic standard treatment. Pediatr Rheumatol Online J 2013;11(1):21.

47. Schanberg LE, Sandstrom MJ, Starr K, et al. The relationship of daily mood and stressful events to symptoms in juvenile rheumatic disease. Arthritis Care Res 2000;13(1):33–41.
48. Ditre JW, Zale EL, LaRowe LR. A reciprocal model of pain and substance use: transdiagnostic considerations, clinical implications, and future directions. Annu Rev Clin Psychol 2019;15:503–28.
49. Steinberg L. A social neuroscience perspective on adolescent risk-taking. Dev Rev 2008;28(1):78–106.
50. Mukherjee K. A dual system model of preferences under risk. Psychol Rev 2010; 117(1):243–55.
51. Geier CF. Adolescent cognitive control and reward processing: implications for risk taking and substance use. Horm Behav 2013;64(2):333–42.
52. Kossowsky J, Magane KM, Levy S, et al. Marijuana use to address symptoms and side effects by youth with chronic medical conditions. Pediatrics 2021; 147(3). e2020021352.
53. Wardell JD, Rueda S, Elton-Marshall T, et al. Prevalence and correlates of medicinal cannabis use among adolescents. J Adolesc Health 2021;68(1):103–9.
54. Bottorff JL, Johnson JL, Moffat BM, et al. Relief-oriented use of marijuana by teens. Subst Abuse Treat Prev Policy 2009;4(1):1–10.
55. Simpson TL, Miller WR. Concomitance between childhood sexual and physical abuse and substance use problems: A review. Clin Psychol Rev 2002;22(1): 27–77.
56. McCarthy DE, Curtin JJ, Piper ME, et al. Negative reinforcement: Possible clinical implications of an integrative model. In: Kassel JD, editor. Substance abuse and emotion. American Psychological Association; 2010. p. 15–42.
57. Boys A, Marsden J, Strang J. Understanding reasons for drug use amongst young people: a functional perspective. Health Educ Res 2001;16(4):457–69.
58. Hanghøj S, Boisen KA. Self-reported barriers to medication adherence among chronically ill adolescents: a systematic review. J Adolesc Health 2014;54(2): 121–38.
59. Sarvet AL, Wall MM, Keyes KM, et al. Self-medication of mood and anxiety disorders with marijuana: Higher in states with medical marijuana laws. Drug Alcohol Depend 2018;186:10–5.
60. Bourgeois FC, DesRoches CM, Bell SK. Ethical challenges raised by OpenNotes for pediatric and adolescent patients. Pediatrics 2018;141(6):e20172745.
61. Restrepo D, Armstrong KA, Metlay JP. Annals clinical decision making: avoiding cognitive errors in clinical decision making. Ann Intern Med 2020;172(11): 747–51.
62. Levy S, Tennermann N, Marin AC, et al. Safety protocols for adolescent substance use research in clinical settings. J Adolesc Health 2020;68(5):999–1005.
63. Wang ZJ, Zhang XQ, Cui XY, et al. Glucocorticoid receptors in the locus coeruleus mediate sleep disorders caused by repeated corticosterone treatment. Sci Rep 2015;5:9442.
64. Rayner M, Moore S. Stress and ameliorating factors among families with a seriously ill or disabled child. J Appl Psychol 2007;3:86–93.
65. Aiken A, Clare PJ, Wadolowski M, et al. Age of alcohol initiation and progression to binge drinking in adolescence: a prospective cohort study. Alcohol Clin Exp Res 2018;42(1):100–10.
66. Azagba S, Shan L, Latham K. A trend analysis of age of first marijuana use among high school students in the United States from 1991 to 2017. Health Educ Behav 2020;47(2):302–10.

67. Sharapova S, Reyes-Guzman C, Singh T, et al. Age of tobacco use initiation and association with current use and nicotine dependence among US middle and high school students, 2014–2016. Tob Control 2020;29(1):49–54.
68. Al-Tayyib A, Riggs P, Mikulich-Gilbertson S, et al. Prevalence of nonmedical use of prescription opioids and association with co-occurring substance use disorders among adolescents in substance use treatment. J Adolesc Health 2018; 62(2):241–4.
69. Austic E, McCabe SE, Stoddard S, et al. Age and cohort patterns of medical and nonmedical use of controlled medication among adolescents. J Addict Med 2015;9(5):376.
70. Jones CM, Clayton HB, Deputy NP, et al. Prescription opioid misuse and use of alcohol and other substances among high school students - youth risk behavior survey, United States, 2019. MMWR Suppl 2020;69(1):38–46.

Mental Health in Pediatric Rheumatology

An Opportunity to Improve Outcomes

Erin Brennan Treemarcki, DO[a], Ashley N. Danguecan, PhD[b], Natoshia R. Cunningham, PhD[c], Andrea M. Knight, MD, MSCE[d,*]

KEYWORDS

• Pediatric rheumatology • Mental health • Depression • Anxiety • Screening

KEY POINTS

- Mental health problems, particularly anxiety and depression, are more common in children with pediatric rheumatologic diseases (PRDs) than healthy peers.
- There are tools available to aid in tailoring mental health screening and interventions to the individual needs of the patient.
- Integration of mental health care into the pediatric rheumatology setting can improve health- and mental health-related outcomes and reduce disparities.

INTRODUCTION

The first tenet of osteopathic medicine states, "The body is a unit; the person is a unit of body, mind, and spirit."[1] Similarly, there is a clear interplay between physical health and mental health in determining overall wellness, which is particularly evident in children with pediatric rheumatologic diseases (PRDs). PRDs consist of autoimmune and autoinflammatory conditions that are often chronic, multisystem, and characterized by flares and remission including juvenile idiopathic arthritis (JIA), childhood-onset systemic lupus erythematosus (cSLE), and juvenile myositis (JM). PRDs affect physical functioning, quality of life, and mental health. In turn, mental health problems that cause significant distress or impairment can impact functioning in children with PRD. *Mental health disorders* are diagnosable psychiatric conditions categorized by distress/impairment that interferes with day-to-day functioning.[2] *Mental health*

[a] Division of Pediatric Rheumatology, Department of Pediatrics, University of Utah, 81 North Mario Capecchi Drive, 4th Floor, Salt Lake City, UT 84113, USA; [b] Department of Psychology, Division of Rheumatology, Hospital for Sick Children, 555 University Ave, Toronto, Ontario M5G 1X8, Canada; [c] Department of Family Medicine, Michigan State University, College of Human Medicine, 15 Michigan Street Northeast, Grand Rapids, MI 49503, USA; [d] Department of Pediatrics, Division of Rheumatology, Hospital for Sick Children, University of Toronto, 555 University Avenue, Toronto, Ontario M5G1X8, Canada

* Corresponding author.

E-mail address: andrea.knight@sickkids.ca

Rheum Dis Clin N Am 48 (2022) 67–90
https://doi.org/10.1016/j.rdc.2021.09.012
rheumatic.theclinics.com

symptoms, which fall on a continuum, may indicate the presence of a mental health disorder when screened with a measure that includes a clinical cut-off. Data on both mental health symptoms and mental health disorders (cumulatively referred to as mental health problems) are reviewed. This review describes the prevalence and impact of mental health problems (with a focus on anxiety and depressive symptoms) in children and young adults with rheumatologic diseases, assesses gaps in addressing mental health, and discusses opportunities to implement mental health screening into clinical practice.

PREVALENCE OF MENTAL PROBLEMS

Mental health problems impact 10% to 20% of all youth, and those with PRDs are at increased risk.[3,4] To understand the current prevalence of mental health problems in PRDs, we conducted a systematic review of the recent literature for articles published from January 2015 to January 2021. The databases MEDLINE and EMBASE were searched using strategies designed by a medical librarian and included the following MeSH terms: "pediatric," "mental health," "anxiety," "depression," "juvenile arthritis," "systemic lupus erythematosus," "myositis," and "rheumatology" (**Fig. 1**). As a methodological framework for conducting the search and reviewing articles, we used the PRISMA Scoping Review Extension reporting documentation,[5] which incorporates scoping review methods outlined by the Joanna Briggs Institute Manual of Evidence Synthesis.[6] We executed the most recent search on February 2, 2021.

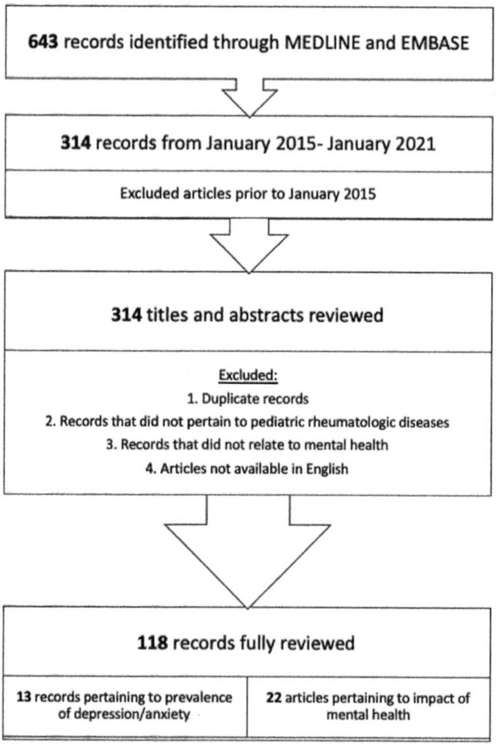

Fig. 1. Flowchart of systematic review process.

Most literature examining mental health problems in PRDs focuses on youth with JIA and cSLE. **Table 1** summarizes recent studies of the prevalence of depression and anxiety in PRDs. Our systematic review found the prevalence of anxiety ranged from 13% to 57%, and the prevalence of depression ranged from 15% to 59%. The wide variation in prevalence rates are similar to those reported in other recent systematic reviews of JIA and cSLE.[7,8] In studies of children with familial Mediterranean fever (FMF), one study did not find significant differences in the prevalence of anxiety and depression than healthy controls, but another found higher rates of anxiety, but not the depression or quality of life differences than healthy controls.[9,10] Different screening tools, sample sizes, and differences between self-report and clinician-report may contribute to the variation in prevalence rates. Disease characteristics may also play a role; a recent survey of patients with JIA, cSLE, and JM found increased rates of mental health problems in the presence of appearance-altering comorbities.[11] In addition to depression and anxiety, several studies note increased rates of adjustment disorders, social anxiety, somatic complaints, and behavioral problems.[12–14] Children with chronic nonbacterial osteomyelitis (CNO) also report problems with psychosocial wellbeing.[15] Although the literature around mental health in PRDs is largely composed of small studies, the findings consistently indicate increased the prevalence of mental health problems for these children than their peers.

The prevalence of mental health problems in patients with PRDs is similar to that from other pediatric chronic illnesses, with increased rates than healthy youth. A systematic review found an increased prevalence of anxiety ranging from 20% to 50% in youth with chronic medical conditions including asthma, type 1 diabetes, epilepsy, inflammatory bowel disease, JIA, congenital heart disease, and sickle cell disease.[16] However, a cohort of adolescents and young adults with rheumatologic diseases were found to have increased psychological distress (72%) than a cohort (42%) that included other chronic illnesses such as inflammatory bowel disease, cystic fibrosis, phenylketonuria, and craniomaxillofacial deformities.[17]

The impact of chronic disease on mental health extends beyond the affected child. In children with JM, parents and other family members endorsed emotional distress.[18] Impaired mental well-being has also been seen in caregivers of children with systemic JIA.[19] Torres-Made and colleagues identified the following areas of impact on caregivers of patients with JIA: economic impact, coping, family roles, impact of diagnosis, mental health, couple/mate relationships, impact at work, religion, and knowledge of the disease.[20] Parents of youth with JIA experience uncertainty that extends beyond medical knowledge and medical management, and these uncertainties cannot be allayed with information alone.[21] Providers should consider how to incorporate coping with uncertainty into routine care, as parental uncertainty correlates with distress in both parents and youth.[21,22] In turn, parental distress can result in increased mental health symptoms in children.[23,24] This interplay between parental and child psychological function has implications for the not just the mental health of children with PRDs but also disease-related outcomes and their overall wellbeing.

CLINICAL RELEVANCE

Mental Health Impact on Disease-Related Outcomes

Our systematic review additionally investigated the impact of mental health problems on disease-related outcomes. In youth with JIA and cSLE literature suggests an association between the symptoms of depression and anxiety and disease-related outcomes, including worse health-related quality of life (HRQOL).[25] In children with JIA

Table 1
Recent studies of depression and anxiety in youth with pediatric rheumatologic diseases

Author (Year)	Country	Study Design	Population	Sample Size		Percentage Anxiety	Percentage Depression
				Subjects	Control		
Hernandez Lember et al,[90] 2015	Colombia	Cross-sectional	cSLE	40	0	57%	37%
Jones et al,[91] 2016	USA	Cross-sectional	cSLE	60	Published norms	37%	30%
Memari et al,[92] 2016	Iran	Cross-sectional	JIA	51	75	13%	27%
Carbajal-Alonso et al,[93] 2016	Mexico	Cross-sectional	cSLE	45	0	NA	20%
Davis et al,[32] 2018	USA	Cross-sectional	cSLE	51	0	NA	58.8%
Hanns et al,[26] 2018	UK	Longitudinal	JIA	102	0	NA	15%
Kayan Okacoglu et al,[94] 2018	Turkey	Cross-sectional	JIA, PID	32 JIA 48 PID	30	25%	31%
Rubinstein et al,[95] 2018	USA	Cross-sectional	cSLE	53	0	19%	26%
Neufeld et al,[96] 2019	Canada	Cross-sectional	cSLE	51	NCS-A	36.4%	29.5%
Knight et al,[13] 2019	US, Canada	Cross-sectional	cSLE	102	0	19%	12%
Li et al,[97] 2020	Canada	Cross-sectional	JIA	80	0	22.5%	23.8%
Knight et al,[29] 2020	US	Cross-sectional	cSLE/MCTD	50	50 T1D	20%	22%
Fawole et al,[11] 2021	US, Canada	Cross-sectional	JIA, JDM, cSLE	210 JIA 173 JDM 64 cSLE	0	39%	35%

Abbreviations: cSLE, childhood-onset systemic lupus erythematosus; JDM, juvenile dermatomyositis; JIA, juvenile idiopathic arthritis; MCTD, mixed connective tissue disease; NA, not applicable; NCS-A, National Comorbidity Survey Study– Adolescent Supplement; PID, primary immunodeficiency; T1D, type 1 diabetes.

and cSLE, several studies demonstrated a relationship between depressive symptoms and increased disease activity, pain, disability, and physician global assessment.[12,26–30] Depressive symptoms in children with JIA were also associated with increased anxiety and poor peer relationships.[27] Symptoms of anxiety have been associated with increased pain, disability, and poorer physician global assessment.[31] Similar relationships between mental health symptoms and HRQOL have also been found in children with FMF, CNO, and JIA-associated uveitis.[9,15]

Mental health disorders in children with PRDs can also affect medication adherence and interactions with the health care system. In a cross-sectional sample of youth with cSLE, comorbid depression was associated with poorer medication adherence.[32] A larger study of youth in their first year after diagnosis of cSLE found that those with comorbid or newly diagnosed psychiatric disorders had increased emergency room visits and inpatient admissions than those without psychiatric disease.[33] Similar associations with increased health care utilization are also seen in adults with SLE and comorbid depression.[34] Moreover, *Chang and colleagues* found that hydroxychloroquine adherence in youth with cSLE and psychiatric comorbidity improved for those who received psychiatric treatment than those without treatment. These findings suggest that improved the recognition and treatment of mental health disorders can improve medication adherence and optimize health care utilization.[35]

There is limited literature on the long-term impacts of comorbid mental health problems in PRDs. A recent qualitative study of parents of children with JM found the diagnosis leads to particularly high levels of emotional distress early in the disease course and lingering anxiety following remission.[18] In the general population, longitudinal studies demonstrate that the consequences of mental health symptoms continue into adulthood, including increased risk for progressing to mental health disorders, suicidality, and interpersonal difficulties.[36–38]

There are also several studies assessing mental health outcomes in adults diagnosed with a PRD. In a longitudinal study of young adults with SLE, those with childhood-onset had an increased risk of a major depressive episode than those with adult-onset; depression risk was also associated with older age at assessment, lower physical function, higher disease activity, and a history of smoking.[39] Another recent study found lower HRQOL scores in the mental health domain in adults with cSLE than healthy controls.[40] Worse mental health functioning was also seen in adults with JIA than healthy peers in several studies.[41,42] However, studies have not consistently demonstrated a significant difference in mental health symptoms in adults with PRDs, even with worse HRQOL.[43–45] These contrasting findings underscore the need for additional research into the long-term effects of mental health disorders in PRDs.

Disparities in Mental Health Comorbidities in Pediatric Rheumatologic Diseases

There are known disparities in disease prevalence, severity, morbidity, and mortality within pediatric rheumatologic populations.[46–48] The disparities are most striking in youth with cSLE, which predominantly affects females from racial minority backgrounds. Than white counterparts, patients from racial or ethnic minorities with cSLE are more likely to have severe disease manifestations (eg, lupus nephritis, neuropsychiatric lupus) or die from the disease.[46] Although important strides have been made to understand mental health comorbidities in rheumatologic conditions, research findings to-date have not represented racially and socioeconomically diverse patient populations, reflecting systemic disparities in health care access and research participation.

Thus far, most mental health disparities research within pediatric rheumatology has focused on youth with cSLE. Social disadvantage is linked to poor psychosocial outcomes. For example, in one small mixed methods study of youth with cSLE or mixed connective tissue disease, there was an association between lower socioeconomic status and both poor psychosocial functioning and difficulty adapting to illness.[49] Based on a cross-sectional sample of youth with cSLE, racial and ethnic minority patients were more likely to endorse symptoms of depression.[50] Additionally, a large study of Medicaid-enrolled cSLE youth found that Black youth were less likely to receive psychiatric diagnoses and treatment.[51] One study examining race, income, and disease outcomes in JDM found racial and ethnic minority patients had worse HRQOL than White patients.[48] As per a recent systematic review on depression and anxiety in JIA, the few studies that reported on race/ethnicity had predominantly white patient samples, which precluded the analysis of race-based disparities.[7] Moving forward, it is important for investigators to intentionally recruit participants from diverse backgrounds to increase generalizability and examine potentially disparate outcomes with respect to race/ethnicity, socioeconomic status, and other social disadvantage factors.

Mental Health During COVID-19 Pandemic

The ongoing SARS-CoV-2 (COVID-19) pandemic highlights the impact of stressors on the wellbeing of children and adolescents, including those with PRDs. Stressful experiences and exposure to life stressors are associated with an increased risk of mental health problems in children and adolescents,[52–54] and the effects on physical and psychological health may persist even after the trigger has resolved.[55] Pandemic-related stressors include emotional isolation, economic loss, work and school closures, and inadequate resources for medical response.[56] The COVID-19 pandemic has been associated with increased mental health symptoms in children and adolescents including stress, anxiety, depression, and posttraumatic stress symptoms.[57–59] A national survey of US parents with children less than 18 years of age in June 2020 found the pandemic resulted in worsening mental health in both parents (27%) and children (14%) with a tandem impact in 1 in 10 families.[60] There is an increased risk for psychosocial effects of pandemics in certain populations, including those at heightened risk of COVID-19, such as the immunocompromised, and those with preexisting mental health problems.[56] These youths may be distressed about the potential health impact to themselves and/or to their loved ones. Furthermore, for those youth that has been homebound, the transition back to school or other social/recreational activities may trigger additional anxiety. Some families may be also experiencing increased stress including financial distress or increased family conflict.[60] Additionally, as reports emerge of youth with postacute sequelae of COVID-19 (PASC), also termed long COVID, these long-term health- and mental-health impacts on youth with PRD are also a consideration moving forward.[61,62]

Patients with rheumatologic conditions may be at increased risk for negative mental health outcomes related to COVID-19. A single rheumatology center explored the impact of COVID-19 on children and adults with rheumatologic diseases, noting that patient-reported flares and difficulties with access to medications were common during the pandemic peak.[63] Moreover, COVID-related distress was independently associated with worse disease activity scores and health scores. Given this already vulnerable population, it is critical to screen for and treat mental health symptoms and distress related to the pandemic.

DISCUSSION

Gaps in Knowledge

Despite evidence of the burden and impact of mental health problems on pediatric rheumatology patients, there remain many knowledge gaps. The complicated relationship between mental health and inflammatory disease, and its treatment, is not well understood. Our understanding of mental health across disease groups, as well as for patients from diverse racial and sociodemographic backgrounds is limited. Additionally, few studies address potential roles for improving mental health care through best screening practices, integration of mental health services to increase the delivery of effective treatment, and education and training opportunities for rheumatologists, despite growing evidence pointing to efficacy in general pediatrics and other pediatric chronic diseases, such as diabetes and cystic fibrosis.[64,65]

To address these gaps, a prioritized mental health research agenda was developed by the Mental Health Workgroup of the Childhood Arthritis and Rheumatology Research Alliance (CARRA), an international collaborative of greater than 550 pediatric rheumatology researchers including greater than 95% of pediatric rheumatologists in the United States and Canada, as well as allied health professionals, patients, parents, and research associates.[66] The goal of the agenda is to promote clinically relevant, important, and feasible research efforts that are likely to change clinical practice and improve care for youth with rheumatologic disease. As part of the agenda's development, a systematic review of the literature identified 5 major research domains in further need of study: (1) mental health burden and relationship to PRDs, (2) impact of mental health disorders on outcomes, (3) mental health awareness and education, (4) mental health screening, and (5) mental health treatment.[67,68] Thirty-three research topics within these domains (**Table 2**) were prioritized by importance (relevance of the topic to advancing clinical care and research), study feasibility (the ease with which research can be executed), and actionability (the ability to apply research findings toward advancing clinical care). Although the topics rated most important concern the relationship of mental health burden to rheumatologic disease and the impact of mental health on outcomes, those rated most feasible and actionable related to mental health screening. Four research topics determined to be highly important, actionable, and feasible included determining: (i) the prevalence and incidence of mental health disorders in PRDs, (ii) which mental health conditions are most important to screen, (iii) the accuracy of mental health screening tools specifically for PRDs, and (iv) the barriers and facilitators to mental health screening in the pediatric rheumatology setting.

The CARRA prioritized mental health research agenda draws attention to the need for larger scale, multi-center, longitudinal studies to investigate mental health burden, risk factors, and long-term impact on outcomes across and within disease groups. Furthermore, these studies need to include patients from diverse racial/ethnic and sociodemographic backgrounds to investigate health disparities and improve equity of mental health care as a part of comprehensive rheumatologic care. Research is also needed to determine optimal screening and proactive treatment strategies, including the validation of existing mental health screening tools, development and testing of mental health interventions (such as peer support groups and cognitive-behavioral therapy (CBT)), and investigation of implementation strategies in pediatric rheumatology settings. Additionally, research is needed to determine the best approaches to mental health education for patients, families, and clinicians.

Addressing the knowledge gaps will require enhanced multidisciplinary collaboration between rheumatology researchers and mental health professionals in psychiatry, psychology, social work, and other disciplines.[69] Consensus around routine capture of psychological data in clinical and research settings will also improve the feasibility of mental health research[70]; this could be achieved, for example, by expanding the current longitudinal CARRA disease registry to include instruments measuring mental health, as well as using newer data collection methods leveraging remote/mobile

Table 2
Topics for mental health research in pediatric rheumatology by research domain defined by the CARRA mental health workgroup[66]

Domain:	Research Topic:
1) Mental health burden and relationship to pediatric rheumatologic disease	• Determine the prevalence and incidence of mental health disorders in pediatric patients with rheumatologic disease, as well as socio-demographic and disease-specific risk factors. • Determine the relationship between mental health disorders, disease onset, and disease course. • Investigate the relationship between mental health and rheumatologic disease treatments. • Investigate the biological basis of mental health disorders. • Examine the impact of rheumatologic disease on neuropsychological development.
2) Impact of mental health disorders on outcomes	• Investigate the impact of mental health on clinical outcomes, such as disease activity. • Investigate the impact of mental health on long-term clinical outcomes, such as disease damage and mortality. • Investigate the impact of mental health on health-related behaviors, such as medication adherence. • Determine the impact of mental health on outcomes related to transition to adult care. • Investigate the impact of mental health on health care utilization and costs. • Investigate the impact of mental health on quality of life, social outcomes, education attainment, and work functioning.
3) Mental health awareness and education	• Understand the level of awareness for the importance of mental health among stakeholder groups. • Determine the impact of mental health education of patients/families on their perceived acceptability of mental health intervention. • Determine the impact of mental health education of rheumatology clinicians on their perceived feasibility/acceptability, and implementation of mental health practices/intervention. • Define gaps in knowledge for community behavioral health providers pertaining to specific mental health needs of patients with childhood-onset rheumatologic disease and their families. • Determine the impact of stakeholder education on policy change for compensation of mental health screening/intervention.

4) Mental health screening	• Determine which mental health conditions are most important to screen. • Determine the accuracy of mental health screening tools for identifying mental health conditions in specific pediatric rheumatology disease populations. • Determine the optimal timing, settings, and process for mental health screening. • Determine barriers and facilitators to mental health screening in the pediatric rheumatology setting. • Determine acceptability of mental health screening in pediatric rheumatology clinics for patients, caregivers, clinicians, and identify strategies to improve acceptability. • Determine the feasibility and sustainability of mental health screening in the pediatric rheumatology setting, including cost-effectiveness, ethical and legal aspects. • Determine the impact of mental health screening on the acceptability of mental health treatment of patients/caregivers. • Determine the efficacy of mental health screening in the pediatric rheumatology setting. • Determine the relationship between mental health screening and disease-related outcomes.
5) Mental health treatment	• Define barriers and facilitators to mental health treatment. • Determine whether adjustment/coping interventions around the time of diagnosis prevent the onset of major depression/anxiety or impact disease-related outcomes. • For different populations and different mental health disorders, determine which mental health treatment modalities are most efficacious. • Investigate the role of immunosuppressive therapy in treating mental health conditions in pediatric patients with rheumatologic disease. • Determine effective mental health treatment delivery options that differ by mode, provider, and setting. • Investigate factors contributing to socio-cultural disparities in mental health care and test interventions to reduce disparities. • Determine whether parent/caregiver-specific interventions improve mental health and disease-related outcomes. • Investigate the cost-effectiveness of mental health treatment in pediatric rheumatology setting.

Modified from Rubinstein TB, Ogbu EA, Rodriguez M, et al. Prioritized Agenda for Mental Health Research in Pediatric Rheumatology from the Childhood Arthritis and Rheumatology Research Alliance Mental Health Workgroup. J Rheumatol. Published online January 15, 2020.

and electronic health record tools.[70] Furthermore, coupling biorepositories and clinical registry data will help advance translational research examining pathophysiologic mechanisms for mental health disorders in the context of inflammatory rheumatologic diseases.

Application to Clinical Practice

Mental health screening: the eighth vital sign

Given how common and debilitating mental health problems are, Jellinek and Murphy proposed that psychosocial functioning should be considered the eighth vital sign in standard medical practice.[71] Timely assessment and treatment of mental health problems is critical for youth with PRDs given adverse impacts on medication adherence, quality of life, and health care utilization.[25,32,50] Furthermore, youth with PRDs are often on long-term medical therapies and require regular health care visits and, as such, are at risk for pediatric medical traumatic distress (PMTD), "a set of psychological and physiologic responses of children and their families to pain, injury, serious illness, medical procedures, and invasive or frightening treatment experiences."[72] Kazak and colleagues developed a model to address PMTD noting that there are different levels of care which can be offered based on patient/caregiver need.[72] The model can be applied to patients and families with PRDs, recognizing that screening and interventions for mental health disorders should be tailored to the context of the family (**Fig. 2**). All patients benefit from screening for mental health disorders, and clinical screening tools are useful to identify issues that may cause significant distress/impairment. Although it is recognized that a routine workup for a mental health condition is not feasible in a medical setting, those with increased distress may benefit from stepped, tailored care for their mental health symptoms that can be facilitated in the pediatric rheumatology setting.

Evidence supports systematic screening for mental health symptoms in chronically ill youth with implementation studies in subspecialty clinics showing that screening is both feasible and clinically meaningful.[64,73] Rheumatology patients may feel more comfortable discussing mental health issues with their pediatric rheumatologist than

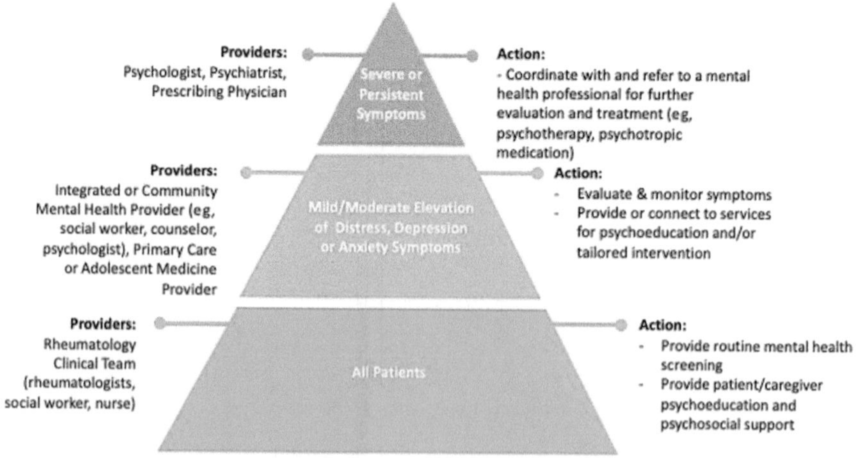

Fig. 2. Psychosocial Preventative health model.[79]. (*Adapted for* Pediatric Rheumatology from Kazak AE, Schneider S, Didonato S, Pai ALH. Family psychosocial risk screening guided by the Pediatric Psychosocial Preventative Health Model (PPPHM) using the Psychosocial Assessment Tool (PAT). Acta Oncol Stockh Swed. 2015;54(5):574 to 580.)

their general pediatrician due to more frequent visits, potentially increased availability of disease-specific mental health resources, and other differences in the patient–subspecialist relationship.[68,74] As patients with PRDs and their caregivers report that the pediatric rheumatology setting serves as their medical home, it is important for rheumatology providers to check-in, screen, monitor and address mental health problems.[75] Some patients will directly bring up mental health concerns with their medical provider and may ask for support in managing these concerns. However, patient mental health problems may not be explicitly verbalized during the medical visit, and are not always obvious to outside observers. Therefore, even when mental health problems are not explicitly communicated to the medical team, it is important to conduct regular screenings to ensure patients who need attention are identified and supported.

Screening tools used in pediatric rheumatology settings are presented in **Table 3**. In general, it is important to use consistent, psychometrically sound screening tools with known clinical cut-offs to facilitate the interpretation of results. The American Academy of Pediatrics offers freely available validated tools with cut-offs for assessing an array of mental health problems (https://www.aap.org/en-us/advocacy-and-policy/aap-health-initiatives/Mental-Health/Documents/MH_ScreeningChart.pdf). Given that COVID-19 has placed an increased burden on patients, caregivers, and medical providers, additional resources, such as validated tools to screen for COVID-19-related distress, may be helpful.

Although pediatric rheumatologists recognize the importance of assessing and treating mental health problems to promote and support overall patient wellbeing, routine screening, and intervention for mental health issues remains uncommon despite the high prevalence of anxiety and depression.[76] Access to appropriate resources is a major challenge, as a 2016 study reported that only 31% of 100 CARRA pediatric rheumatology practices had an affiliated behavioral health specialist. Even among behavioral health specialists working in pediatric rheumatology settings, inadequate follow-up and limited access to mental health services were reported, and lack of mental health protocols was an identified barrier.[74]

Established practice recommendations may help empower rheumatologists to manage mental health problems consistently and effectively. In other chronic pediatric disease communities (eg, cystic fibrosis, diabetes), specific screening, and treatment recommendations for addressing mental health symptoms have been developed, with the goal of improving psychosocial outcomes and overall disease management.[65,77,78] For pediatric rheumatology, a multi-disciplinary Task Force within the CARRA Mental Health Workgroup is currently in the process of developing recommendations to enhance mental health screening and intervention practices across rheumatology clinics with varying access to mental health resources. The goal is to enable rheumatologists to manage mental health problems using consistent, evidence-based strategies, and to provide direct guidance on all aspects of screening including who and when to screen, what to screen for, and what to do with positive screening results. Such guidance would facilitate a systematic approach for rheumatology providers to routinely identify and address mental health problems, tailored to the patient's level of need.

Mental Health Intervention

It is important to note there are no one-size-fits-all approach to mental health intervention, and treatment must be tailored based on individual patient/family needs and risk. The Psychosocial Preventative Health Model adapted for PRDs (see **Fig. 2**) provides a framework for the early identification of psychosocial distress and tiered supports to match identified levels of need and risk for patients and their families.[79] For example,

Table 3
Mental health assessments tools

Measure	Description	Age Range	Admin time (min)	Cutoffs (Yes/No)	Freely Available (Yes/No)	Available Languages
Anxiety Measures						
Beck Youth Inventories-Anxiety Inventory (BAI-Y)[98]	20 items measure anxiety symptoms to create a total raw score ranging from 0 to 60. Raw scores are converted to interpretable T-Scores: <55 = Average. 55.0–59.9 = Mildly elevated. 60.0–69.9 = Moderately Elevated. 70+ = Extremely Elevated.	7–18	5	No	No	Danish, English, French, Polish
Screen for Childhood Anxiety Related Emotional Disorders (SCARED)[25,29,88]	41 items scored on a 3-point Likert scale measure anxiety symptoms. Total scores range from 0 to 82, with a total score ≥ 25 indicating clinically significant anxiety.	8–18	10	Yes	Yes	Arabic, Chinese, Czech, English, Finnish, French, German, Hebrew, Italian, Spanish, Tamil, Thai
State-Trait Anxiety Inventory for children (STAIc)[99]	A 40-item measure querying state and trait anxiety on 4-point Likert scale. Subtest scores range from 20 to 80, with higher scores indicating greater anxiety. Scores of 39–40 and above are clinically significant.	9–12	10	Yes	No	Arabic, Cambodian, Chinese, Croatian, Czech, Danish, English, Filipino, Finnish, French, German, Greek, Hungarian, Italian, Korean, Malay, Norwegian, Persian, Polish, Portuguese, Romanian, Russian, Slovak, Spanish, Swedish, Thai, Turkish

Patient-Reported Outcomes Information Measurement System (PROMIS)[91,100,101]	8 items measure anxiety on a 5-point Likert scale to create a raw score, with higher scores indicating more symptoms. Raw scores can be interpreted as T-scores:<50 = Within normal limits. 50.0–54.9 = Mild. 55.0–64.9 = Moderate. 65+ = Severe.	8–17	5	No	Yes	Arabic, Bengali, Chinese, Czech, Dutch, English, French, German, Gujarati, Hindi, Hungarian, Italian, Japanese, Kannada, Korean, Malayalam, Marathi, Polish, Portuguese, Punjabi, Russian, Spanish, Tamil, Telugu, Ukrainian
Child Behavioral Checklist (CBCL)[92]	Frequency of problem behaviors measured through a total of 113 items from parent and youth reports. Scores in above the 97th percentile indicate a clinical range, those in the 93–97th percentile are considered borderline clinical, and those below the 93rd percentile are normal.	6–18	10	Yes	No	More than 50 translations, including Arabic, Chinese, English, French, Hindi, and Spanish
Depressive Symptom Measures						
Patient Health Questionnaire (PHQ-9)[29,32]	9 items measured on a 4-point Likert scale queries for major depression based on DSM-IV criteria. Total scores range from 0 to 27 and can be interpreted as: mild depression = 5–9, moderate depression = 10–14, moderately severe depression = 15–19, severe depression = 20–27.	12+	5	Yes	Yes	More than 50 translations, including Arabic, Chinese, English, French, Hindi, and Spanish

(*continued on next page*)

Table 3
(*continued*)

Measure	Description	Age Range	Admin time (min)	Cutoffs (Yes/No)	Freely Available (Yes/No)	Available Languages
Children's Depression Inventory (CDI)[25,88,94,99]	Measures depressive symptoms through 28 items, with each item comprised of 3 statements describing varying symptom severity. Scores between 17 and 19 and above (depending on age/gender) indicate clinical levels of depression.	7–17	5	Yes	No	English, Spanish
Mood and Feeling Questionnaire for children (MFQc)[26]	Short (13 item) and long (33 item) versions are available, and all items are measured on a 3-point Likert scale. Total scores on the short form range 0–26, with scores 12+ indicating clinical depression; total scores on the long-form range 0–66, with scores 27+ indicating clinical symptoms.	6–17	5–10	No	Yes	Arabic, English, Filipino, Finnish, German, Norwegian, Portuguese, Spanish
Patient-Reported Outcomes Measurement Information System (PROMIS)[91,100,101]	8 items measure depressive symptoms on a 5-point Likert scale to create a raw score, with higher scores indicating more symptoms. Raw scores can be interpreted as T-scores:<50 = Within normal limits. 50.0–54.9 = Mild. 55.0–64.9 = Moderate. 65+ = Severe.	8–17	5	No	Yes	Arabic, Bengali, Chinese, Czech, Dutch, French, German, Gujarati, Hebrew, Hindi, Hungarian, Italian, Japanese, Kannada, Korean, Malayalam, Marathi, Polish, Portuguese, Punjabi, Russian, Spanish, Tamil, Telugu, Ukrainian, Urdu

The Center for Epidemiologic Studies Depression Scale for children (CES-DC)[102]	20 items measure depressive symptoms, with total scores ranging from 0 to 60. Scores 15 and above indicate significant depression, whereas scores below indicate no depression symptoms.	6–17	5	Yes	Yes	English
Child Behavioral Checklist (CBCL)[92]	Frequency of problem behaviors measured through a total of 113 items from parent and youth reports. Clinical range is indicated by scores above the 97th percentile, those in the 93–97th percentile are considered borderline clinical, and those below the 93rd percentile are normal.	6–18	10	Yes	No	More than 50 translations, including Arabic, Chinese, English, French, Hindi, and Spanish

Additional Resources	**Description**	**Freely Available (Yes/No)**	**Available Languages**
American Academy of Pediatrics Mental Health Screening and Assessment Tools (https://www.aap.org/en-us/advocacy-and-policy/aap-health-initiatives/Mental-Health/Documents/MH_ScreeningChart.pdf)	List of mental health screening tools used in primary care	Yes	Resource presented in English; tools vary
COVID-19 Exposure and Family Impact Survey (https://www.healthcaretoolbox.org/tools-and-resources/covid-19-cefis.html)	COVID-19 related family distress measures for parents, adolescents, and young adults	Yes	English, Spanish

Note. Portions of this table have been adapted from Reid et al., 2021[103].

in the instance of a positive mental health screening result, follow-up recommendations are stratified based on symptom severity. Follow-up may include the monitoring of less severe symptoms and psychoeducation with mental health champion who is part of the rheumatology team. For more severe symptoms, coordinated care in communication with a primary care or adolescent medicine provider or referral to a mental health specialist, such as a counselor, psychologist, or psychiatrist is needed. Additionally, psychiatrists and trained physicians can offer pharmacologic treatment of managing mental health symptoms with more severe symptomatology (eg, severe depression, suicidal ideation).

Nonpharmacologic options are available to support pediatric rheumatology patients in managing mental health problems. Psychological treatment programs for managing pediatric chronic illnesses typically include a blend of psychoeducation, cognitive (eg, challenging maladaptive thinking, problem-solving) and behavioral (eg, relaxation training) strategies.[80] Importantly, the intervention approach can be adjusted as patient and family needs change with the disease course. Mindfulness meditation and acceptance and commitment therapies are other approaches used in treating youth with chronic illnesses, sometimes in conjunction with CBT.[81–84] Nonpharmacologic treatments for managing psychological symptoms in pediatric chronic illnesses (such as chronic pain) are available in person and virtually.[80,85] CBT is helpful for managing caregiver symptoms as well.[86] Other approaches may also be beneficial, such as engaging in peer-support programs, but further study is needed.

More virtual options are now available for youth with chronic illnesses, particularly as a result of the COVID-19 pandemic. For example, the Society for Pediatric Psychology offers patient psychoeducational tools including stress management, COVID-19 education, coping with social distancing, telehealth, and additional tools (eg, free WiFi access) for families with limited resources, https://societyofpediatricpsychology.org/content/resources-covid-19.[87] Nonpharmacologic tools to improve patient mental health can be delivered via self-management strategies (eg, web-based tools, books, apps) or with a mental health specialist embedded within or outside the medical clinic, and there is growing literature supporting their use specifically in pediatric rheumatology populations. For example, a brief tailored cognitive behavioral intervention to address mood, pain, and fatigue in youth with cSLE has been developed and a randomized controlled trial to test a remotely delivered version is currently underway.[88] Also, a self-paced app, *iCanCope,* using CBT strategies, has been shown to be feasible for users to address pain management in youth with JIA, but future work is needed to determine its effectiveness in improving health-related outcomes.[89]

Toward improving the integration of mental health care into overall care for pediatric rheumatology patients, there are tools available that can help improve patient mental health care in the scope of practice. The compendium of behavioral health integration (BHI) resources available for medical practices, https://www.ama-assn.org/delivering-care/public-health/compendium-behavioral-health-integration-resources-physician, is a practical and detailed guide about different approaches to BHI, providing strategies to initiate BHI practice (eg, increasing buy-in, assessing readiness, establishing goals), and discusses implementation (eg, designing workflow, preparing and partnering with various stakeholders, financial sustainabilities/billings, and coding information). Each step of BHI is accompanied by a companion table of resources to support medical providers with different levels of resources and practice needs that may evolve over time. In addition, patients have varying mental health needs, which may also change over time, but appropriate planning and collaboration can provide support and management to patients in the context of their medical care. For example, the rheumatologist and their team may be able to address many mild to moderate mental health concerns during the medical visit, and many states (eg, Michigan, Massachusetts) have adopted psychiatry consultation models to support the needs of patients with more complex mental health concerns.

Mental Health Education for Clinicians

Understandably, it can be challenging to address mental health issues while also caring for the patients' physical health. Pediatric rheumatology providers report multiple barriers to adequately addressing mental health care, including a lack of comfort, knowledge, or resources to effectively manage mental health concerns.[76] Potential ways to overcome barriers to addressing mental health include enhanced training for physicians and their medical team members.[67] The American Board of Pediatrics (ABP) recommends training for medical providers to accurately assess the cardinal features of depression, determine when depression is severe enough to warrant professional consultation with a specialist, and recognize the warning signs of suicide. However, in a CARRA survey of 130 pediatric rheumatologists, two-thirds reported limited mental health training (eg, only occurring in medical school) and nearly 1 in 10 reported no training at all. Most of the providers expressed interest in receiving additional mental health training.[76] Of note, providers with higher levels of training reported less barriers to engaging in mental health care. Clearly, enhanced provider education is a key component to optimizing care for rheumatology patients with mental health concerns. Recognizing the importance of mental health literacy for pediatric subspecialists, the ABP recently developed the Roadmap Project (www.abp.org/foundation/roadmap) to provide free resources to improve mental health care in subspecialty settings, as well as a framework for quality improvement efforts.

SUMMARY

Mental health problems are common in children with PRDs, impacting disease outcomes (eg, disease activity, pain), HRQOL, medication adherence, and health care utilization. There have been several significant advances in our knowledge of mental health comorbidities in youth with PRDs, although gaps remain. The prioritized mental health agenda developed by CARRA identified how these gaps may be addressed and mental health screening was rated as the most feasible and actionable area of study. In service of promoting mental health as part of general rheumatology medical care, a multi-disciplinary Task Force is developing guidance statements to empower pediatric rheumatologists in the routine and effective management of mental health issues. Moving forward, multi-center, longitudinal studies are critical for examining the impacts of mental health problems over time on disease outcomes. This work will require intentional efforts to recruit patients from diverse backgrounds to reduce known health disparities. Recognizing and addressing mental health symptoms, as an essential vital sign in the pediatric rheumatology setting, is critical to optimizing overall health and outcomes for youths with PRDs.

CLINICS CARE POINTS

- Addressing mental health problems for youth with rheumatologic disease through routine assessment and early intervention is critical to improving long-term clinical and psychosocial outcomes.
- Several mental health screening tools are freely available, and there is a spectrum of mental health interventions that can be tailored to the individualized needs of youth with rheumatologic disease.

- Integration of mental health care into the pediatric rheumatology setting is key to optimizing the accessibility of effective mental health services.
- Improving the mental health literacy of pediatric rheumatology clinicians is necessary to aid the recognition, management, and prevention of mental health disorders.
- The pediatric rheumatology community must address existing disparities in mental health care for youth with PRDs by the intentional design of intervention strategies that promote health equity.

ACKNOWLEDGMENTS

The authors would like to acknowledge medical librarian, Elizabeth Frakes, MSIS, (University of Utah), for her assistance with collecting abstracts for review, and research coordinator Samantha Ely, B.A., (Michigan State University) for her assistance in creating Figures/Tables.

DISCLOSURE

Dr E.B. Treemarcki is currently the recipient of a Research Grant from the Childhood Arthritis and Rheumatology Research Alliance and the Arthritis Foundation (CARRA-AF). Dr N.R. Cunningham is currently the recipient of a training grant from NIH/NCCIH (K23 AT009458) and a Transdisciplinary Research Grant from the Childhood Arthritis and Rheumatology Research Alliance and the Arthritis Foundation (CARRA-AF). Dr A.M Knight and Dr A.N. Danguecan have nothing to disclose.

REFERENCES

1. Tenets of Osteopathic Medicine - American Osteopathic Association. Available at: https://osteopathic.org/about/leadership/aoa-governance-documents/tenets-of-osteopathic-medicine/. Accessed March 1, 2021.
2. American Psychiatric Association. Diagnostic and statistical manual of mental disorders. 5th edition. American Psychiatric Association; 2013.
3. Avenevoli S, Swendsen J, He J-P, et al. Major depression in the national comorbidity survey-adolescent supplement: prevalence, correlates, and treatment. J Am Acad Child Adolesc Psychiatry 2015;54(1):37–44.e2.
4. Merikangas KR, He J-P, Burstein M, et al. Lifetime prevalence of mental disorders in U.S. adolescents: results from the National Comorbidity Survey Replication–Adolescent Supplement (NCS-A). J Am Acad Child Adolesc Psychiatry 2010;49(10):980–9.
5. Tricco AC, Lillie E, Zarin W, et al. PRISMA extension for scoping reviews (PRISMA-ScR): checklist and explanation. Ann Intern Med 2018;169(7):467–73.
6. Aromataris E, Munn Z, editors. JBI manual for evidence synthesis. JBI; 2020. https://doi.org/10.46658/JBIMES-20-01. Available at: https://Synthesismanual.Jbi.Global.
7. Fair DC, Rodriguez M, Knight AM, et al. Depression and anxiety in patients with juvenile idiopathic arthritis: current insights and impact on quality of life, a systematic review. Open Access Rheumatol Res Rev 2019;11:237–52.
8. Quilter MC, Hiraki LT, Korczak DJ. Depressive and anxiety symptom prevalence in childhood-onset systemic lupus erythematosus: A systematic review. Lupus 2019;28(7):878–87.

9. Durcan G, Yildiz M, Kadak MT, et al. Increased frequency of sleep problems in children and adolescents with familial Mediterranean fever: The role of anxiety and depression. Int J Rheum Dis 2020;23(10):1396–403.
10. Sönmez AÖ, Sönmez HE, Çakan M, et al. The evaluation of anxiety, depression and quality of life scores of children and adolescents with familial Mediterranean fever. Rheumatol Int 2020;40(5):757–63.
11. Fawole OA, Reed MV, Harris JG, et al. Engaging patients and parents to improve mental health intervention for youth with rheumatological disease. Pediatr Rheumatol Online J 2021;19(1):19.
12. Pascali M, Matera E, Craig F, et al. Cognitive, emotional, and behavioral profile in children and adolescents with chronic pain associated with rheumatic diseases: A case-control study. Clin Child Psychol Psychiatry 2019;24(3):433–45.
13. Knight AM, Fawole O, Reed M, et al. 92 Engaging patients and parents to improve mental health for youth with systemic lupus erythematosus [abstract]. Lupus Sci Med 2019;6(Suppl 1). https://doi.org/10.1136/lupus-2019-lsm.92.
14. Chomistek K, Johnson N, Stevenson R, et al. Patient-reported barriers at school for children with juvenile idiopathic arthritis. ACR Open Rheumatol 2019;1(3): 182–7.
15. Oliver M, Lee TC, Halpern-Felsher B, et al. Disease burden and social impact of pediatric chronic nonbacterial osteomyelitis from the patient and family perspective. Pediatr Rheumatol Online J 2018;16(1):78.
16. Cobham VE, Hickling A, Kimball H, et al. Systematic review: anxiety in children and adolescents with chronic medical conditions. J Am Acad Child Adolesc Psychiatry 2020;59(5):595–618.
17. Hamid M, Cummins L, Whitehead B, et al. Psychosocial burden of rheumatic disease in adolescents & young adults. Int J Rheum Dis 2019;22(S3):40–226.
18. Ardalan K, Adeyemi O, Wahezi DM, et al. Parent perspectives on addressing emotional health for children and young adults with juvenile myositis. Arthritis Care Res 2021;73(1):18–29.
19. Shenoi S, Horneff G, Cidon M, et al. The burden of systemic juvenile idiopathic arthritis for patients and caregivers: an international survey and retrospective chart review. Clin Exp Rheumatol 2018;36(5):920–8.
20. Torres-Made MD, Peláez-Ballestas I, García-Rodríguez F, et al. Development and validation of the CAREGIVERS questionnaire: multi-assessing the impact of juvenile idiopathic arthritis on caregivers. Pediatr Rheumatol Online J 2020; 18(1):3.
21. Pearce C, Newman S, Mulligan K. Illness uncertainty in parents of children with juvenile idiopathic arthritis. ACR Open Rheumatol 2021;3(4):250–9.
22. Fedele DA, Ramsey RR, Ryan JL, et al. The association of illness uncertainty to parent and youth adjustment in juvenile rheumatic diseases: effect of youth age. J Dev Behav Pediatr JDBP 2011;32(5):361–7.
23. Bonner MS, Ramsey RR, Ryan JL, et al. Examination of parent-child adjustment in juvenile rheumatic diseases using depression-specific indices of parent and youth functioning. J Child Health Care Prof Work Child Hosp Community 2015; 19(1):63–72.
24. Knafl K, Leeman J, Havill NL, et al. The contribution of parent and family variables to the well-being of youth with arthritis. J Fam Nurs 2015;21(4):579–616.
25. Donnelly C, Cunningham N, Jones JT, et al. Fatigue and depression predict reduced health-related quality of life in childhood-onset. Lupus 2018;27(1): 124–33.

26. Hanns L, Cordingley L, Galloway J, et al. Depressive symptoms, pain and disability for adolescent patients with juvenile idiopathic arthritis: results from the Childhood Arthritis Prospective Study. Rheumatol Oxf Engl 2018;57(8):1381–9.
27. Yan Y, Rychlik KL, Rosenman MB, et al. Use of PROMIS® to screen for depression in children with arthritis. Pediatr Rheumatol 2020;18(1):92.
28. Hoff AL, Palermo TM, Schluchter M, et al. Longitudinal relationships of depressive symptoms to pain intensity and functional disability among children with disease-related pain. J Pediatr Psychol 2006;31(10):1046–56.
29. Knight A, Weiss P, Morales K, et al. Identifying differences in risk factors for depression and anxiety in pediatric chronic disease: a matched cross-sectional study of youth with lupus/mixed connective tissue disease and their peers with diabetes. J Pediatr 2015;167(6):1397–403.e1.
30. Dimitrijevic Carlsson A, Wahlund K, Kindgren E, et al. Orofacial pain in juvenile idiopathic arthritis is associated with stress as well as psychosocial and functional limitations. Pediatr Rheumatol Online J 2019;17(1):83.
31. Hanns L, Radziszewska A, Suffield L, et al. Association of anxiety with pain and disability but not with increased measures of inflammation in adolescent patients with juvenile idiopathic arthritis. Arthritis Care Res 2020;72(9):1266–74.
32. Davis AM, Graham TB, Zhu Y, et al. Depression and medication nonadherence in childhood-onset systemic lupus erythematosus. Lupus 2018;27(9):1532–41.
33. Knight AM, Klein-Gitelman MS, Cidav Z, et al. The impact of psychiatric comorbidity on health care utilization for youth with systemic lupus erythematosus [abstract]. Arthritis Rheum 2017;69(suppl 10). Available at: https://acrabstracts.org/abstract/the-impact-of-psychiatric-comorbidity-on-health-care-utilization-for-youth-with-systemic-lupus-erythematosus/. Accessed March 1, 2021.
34. Julian LJ, Yelin E, Yazdany J, et al. Depression, medication adherence, and service utilization in systemic lupus erythematosus. Arthritis Rheum 2009;61(2):240–6.
35. Chang JC, Davis AM, Klein-Gitelman MS, et al. Impact of psychiatric diagnosis and treatment on medication adherence in youth with systemic lupus erythematosus. Arthritis Care Res 2021;73(1):30–8.
36. Harrington R, Fudge H, Rutter M, et al. Adult outcomes of childhood and adolescent depression. I. Psychiatric status. Arch Gen Psychiatry 1990;47(5):465–73.
37. Fombonne E, Wostear G, Cooper V, et al. The Maudsley long-term follow-up of child and adolescent depression. 2. Suicidality, criminality and social dysfunction in adulthood. Br J Psychiatry J Ment Sci 2001;179:218–23.
38. Kim-Cohen J, Caspi A, Moffitt TE, et al. Prior juvenile diagnoses in adults with mental disorder: developmental follow-back of a prospective-longitudinal cohort. Arch Gen Psychiatry 2003;60(7):709–17.
39. Knight AM, Trupin L, Katz P, et al. Depression risk in young adults with juvenile- and adult-onset lupus: twelve years of followup. Arthritis Care Res 2018;70(3):475–80.
40. Groot N, Shaikhani D, Teng YKO, et al. Long-term clinical outcomes in a cohort of adults with childhood-onset systemic lupus erythematosus. Arthritis Rheum Hoboken NJ 2019;71(2):290–301.
41. Foster HE, Marshall N, Myers A, et al. Outcome in adults with juvenile idiopathic arthritis: a quality of life study. Arthritis Rheum 2003;48(3):767–75.
42. Packham JC, Hall MA. Long-term follow-up of 246 adults with juvenile idiopathic arthritis: functional outcome. Rheumatol Oxf Engl 2002;41(12):1428–35.

43. Tollisen A, Selvaag AM, Aulie HA, et al. Physical functioning, pain, and health-related quality of life in adults with juvenile idiopathic arthritis: a longitudinal 30-year followup study. Arthritis Care Res 2018;70(5):741–9.
44. Paskalis G, Dimopoulou D, Trachana M, et al. AB1095 Long-term impact of juvenile idiopathic arthritis on quality of life of adult patients in greece. In: Paediatric rheumatology. vol 77. Annual European Congress of rheumatology, EULAR 2018, Amsterdam, 13–16 June 2018. BMJ Pub Group; 2018:1656.1657-1663.
45. Kearse CL, Campbell R, Oates J, et al. 154 Impact of diagnosis age on quality of life among patients with systemic lupus erythematosus. In: Abstracts. vol 6. 13th International Congress on systemic lupus erythematosus (LUPUS 2019), San Francisco, California, USA, April 5–8, 2019, Abstract Presentations. BMJ,; 2019:A111.2-A112.
46. Rubinstein TB, Knight AM. Disparities in childhood-onset lupus. Rheum Dis Clin North Am 2020;46(4):661–72.
47. Chang JC, Xiao R, Burnham JM, et al. Longitudinal assessment of racial disparities in juvenile idiopathic arthritis disease activity in a treat-to-target intervention. Pediatr Rheumatol Online J 2020;18(1):88.
48. Phillippi K, Hoeltzel M, Byun Robinson A, et al. Childhood Arthritis and Rheumatology Research Alliance (CARRA) Legacy Registry Investigators. Race, Income, and Disease Outcomes in Juvenile Dermatomyositis. J Pediatr 2017; 184:38–44.e1.
49. Knight A, Vickery M, Fiks AG, et al. The illness experience of youth with lupus/mixed connective tissue disease: a mixed methods analysis of patient and parent perspectives. Lupus 2016;25(9):1028–39.
50. Knight A, Weiss P, Morales K, et al. Depression and anxiety and their association with healthcare utilization in pediatric lupus and mixed connective tissue disease patients: a cross-sectional study. Pediatr Rheumatol Online J 2014;12:42.
51. Knight AM, Xie M, Mandell DS. Disparities in psychiatric diagnosis and treatment for youth with systemic lupus erythematosus: analysis of a national us medicaid sample. J Rheumatol 2016;43(7):1427–33.
52. Reiss F, Meyrose A-K, Otto C, et al. Socioeconomic status, stressful life situations and mental health problems in children and adolescents: Results of the German BELLA cohort-study. PLoS One 2019;14(3):e0213700.
53. Bøe T, Serlachius AS, Sivertsen B, et al. Cumulative effects of negative life events and family stress on children's mental health: the Bergen Child Study. Soc Psychiatry Psychiatr Epidemiol 2018;53(1):1–9.
54. Businelle MS, Mills BA, Chartier KG, et al. Do stressful events account for the link between socioeconomic status and mental health? J Public Health Oxf Engl 2014;36(2):205–12.
55. Yuan K, Gong Y-M, Liu L, et al. Prevalence of posttraumatic stress disorder after infectious disease pandemics in the twenty-first century, including COVID-19: a meta-analysis and systematic review. Mol Psychiatry 2021. https://doi.org/10.1038/s41380-021-01036-x.
56. Pfefferbaum B, North CS. Mental health and the covid-19 Pandemic. N Engl J Med 2020;383(6):510–2.
57. Marques de Miranda D, da Silva Athanasio B, Sena Oliveira AC, et al. How is COVID-19 pandemic impacting mental health of children and adolescents? Int J Disaster Risk Reduct IJDRR 2020;51:101845.
58. Jiao WY, Wang LN, Liu J, et al. Behavioral and emotional disorders in children during the COVID-19 Epidemic. J Pediatr 2020;221:264–6.e1.

59. Guessoum SB, Lachal J, Radjack R, et al. Adolescent psychiatric disorders during the COVID-19 pandemic and lockdown. Psychiatry Res 2020;291:113264.
60. Patrick SW, Henkhaus LE, Zickafoose JS, et al. Well-being of parents and children during the COVID-19 pandemic: a national survey. Pediatrics 2020;146(4). https://doi.org/10.1542/peds.2020-016824.
61. Ashkenazi-Hoffnung L, Shmueli E, Ehrlich S, et al. Long COVID in children: observations from a designated pediatric clinic. Pediatr Infect Dis J 2021. https://doi.org/10.1097/INF.0000000000003285.
62. Brackel CLH, Lap CR, Buddingh EP, et al. Pediatric long-COVID: An overlooked phenomenon? Pediatr Pulmonol 2021;56(8):2495–502.
63. Maldonado D, Tu E, Mahmood S, et al. Medication access difficulty and COVID-related distress are associated with disease flares in rheumatology patients during the COVID-19 pandemic. Arthritis Care Res 2020;5. https://doi.org/10.1002/acr.24531.
64. Corathers SD, Kichler J, Jones N-HY, et al. Improving depression screening for adolescents with type 1 diabetes. Pediatrics 2013;132(5):e1395–402.
65. Quittner AL, Abbott J, Georgiopoulos AM, et al. International committee on mental health in cystic fibrosis: cystic fibrosis foundation and european cystic fibrosis Society consensus statements for screening and treating depression and anxiety. Thorax 2016;71(1):26–34.
66. Rubinstein TB, Ogbu EA, Rodriguez M, et al. Prioritized agenda for mental health research in pediatric rheumatology from the childhood arthritis and rheumatology research alliance mental health workgroup. J Rheumatol 2020;15. https://doi.org/10.3899/jrheum.190361.
67. Davis AM, Rubinstein TB, Rodriguez M, et al. Mental health care for youth with rheumatologic diseases - bridging the gap. Pediatr Rheumatol Online J 2017;15(1):85.
68. Rubinstein T, Davis A, Rodriguez M, et al. Addressing mental health in pediatric rheumatology. Curr Treat Options Rheumatol 2018;4. https://doi.org/10.1007/s40674-018-0092-4.
69. Gamwell KL, Hommel KA. Comprehensive care in pediatric rheumatic diseases: a multifaceted challenge. J Rheumatol 2020;47(11):1603–5.
70. Cordingley L, Lee RR. Can we implement the new research agenda for mental health? Nat Rev Rheumatol 2020;16(4):191–2.
71. Jellinek M, Murphy JM. Screening for psychosocial functioning as the eighth vital sign. JAMA Pediatr 2021;175(1):13–4.
72. Kazak AE, Kassam-Adams N, Schneider S, et al. An integrative model of pediatric medical traumatic stress. J Pediatr Psychol 2006;31(4):343–55.
73. Iturralde E, Adams RN, Barley RC, et al. Implementation of depression screening and global health assessment in pediatric subspecialty clinics. J Adolesc Health Off Publ Soc Adolesc Med 2017;61(5):591–8.
74. Knight A, Vickery M, Faust L, et al. Gaps in mental health care for youth with rheumatologic conditions: a mixed methods study of perspectives from behavioral health providers. Arthritis Care Res 2019;71(5):591–601.
75. Knight AM, Vickery ME, Fiks AG, et al. Barriers and facilitators for mental healthcare in pediatric lupus and mixed connective tissue disease: a qualitative study of youth and parent perspectives. Pediatr Rheumatol Online J 2015;13:52.
76. Knight AM, Vickery ME, Muscal E, et al. Identifying targets for improving mental healthcare of adolescents with systemic lupus erythematosus: perspectives from pediatric rheumatology clinicians in the United States and Canada. J Rheumatol 2016;43(6):1136–45.

77. Wiener L, Kazak AE, Noll RB, et al. Standards for the psychosocial care of children with cancer and their families: an introduction to the special issue. Pediatr Blood Cancer 2015;62(Suppl 5):S419–24.
78. Delamater AM, de Wit M, McDarby V, et al. ISPAD clinical practice consensus guidelines 2018: Psychological care of children and adolescents with type 1 diabetes. Pediatr Diabetes 2018;19(Suppl 27):237–49.
79. Kazak AE, Schneider S, Didonato S, et al. Family psychosocial risk screening guided by the Pediatric Psychosocial Preventative Health Model (PPPHM) using the Psychosocial Assessment Tool (PAT). Acta Oncol Stockh Swed 2015;54(5): 574–80.
80. Eccleston C, Palermo TM, Williams AC de C, et al. Psychological therapies for the management of chronic and recurrent pain in children and adolescents. Cochrane Database Syst Rev 2014;5:CD003968.
81. Ahola Kohut S, Stinson J, Davies-Chalmers C, et al. Mindfulness-Based interventions in clinical samples of adolescents with chronic illness: a systematic Review. J Altern Complement Med N Y N 2017;23(8):581–9.
82. Ali A, Weiss TR, Dutton A, et al. Mindfulness-based stress reduction for adolescents with functional somatic syndromes: a pilot cohort study. J Pediatr 2017; 183:184–90.
83. Pielech M, Vowles KE, Wicksell R. Acceptance and commitment therapy for pediatric chronic pain: theory and application. Child Basel Switz 2017;4(2). https://doi.org/10.3390/children4020010.
84. Wicksell RK, Melin L, Lekander M, et al. Evaluating the effectiveness of exposure and acceptance strategies to improve functioning and quality of life in longstanding pediatric pain–a randomized controlled trial. Pain 2009;141(3):248–57.
85. Fisher E, Law E, Dudeney J, et al. Psychological therapies (remotely delivered) for the management of chronic and recurrent pain in children and adolescents. Cochrane Database Syst Rev 2019;4:CD011118.
86. Fisher E, Law E, Dudeney J, et al. Psychological therapies for the management of chronic and recurrent pain in children and adolescents. Cochrane Database Syst Rev 2018;2018(9). https://doi.org/10.1002/14651858.CD003968.pub5.
87. Eccleston C, Blyth FM, Dear BF, et al. Managing patients with chronic pain during the COVID-19 outbreak: considerations for the rapid introduction of remotely supported (eHealth) pain management services. Pain 2020;161(5):889–93.
88. Cunningham NR, Fussner LM, Moorman E, et al. Development and pilot testing of the treatment and education approach for childhood-onset lupus (TEACH): a cognitive behavioral treatment. Pediatr Rheumatol Online J 2019;17(1):9.
89. Lalloo C, Harris LR, Hundert AS, et al. The iCanCope pain self-management application for adolescents with juvenile idiopathic arthritis: a pilot randomized controlled trial. Rheumatol Oxf Engl 2021;60(1):196–206.
90. Hernandez Lember C, Diaz A, Vasquez R. AB0963 Anxiety and depression in pediatric systemic lupus Eritematosus. Ann Rheum Dis 2015;74(Suppl 2): 1221–4.
91. Jones JT, Cunningham N, Kashikar-Zuck S, et al. Pain, fatigue and psychological impact on health-related quality of life in childhood-onset lupus. Arthritis Care Res 2016;68(1):73–80.
92. Memari AH, Chamanara E, Ziaee V, et al. Behavioral problems in juvenile idiopathic arthritis: a controlled study to examine the risk of psychopathology in a chronic pediatric disorder. Int J Chronic Dis 2016;2016:5726236.

93. Carbajal-Alonso HL, García-Moreno NP, Rodríguez-Arreola B, et al. [Depressive disorder in Mexican pediatric patients with systemic lupus erythematosus (SLE)]. Gac Med Mex 2016;152(1):36–42.
94. Kayan Ocakoglu B, Karaca NE, Ocakoglu FT, et al. Psychological burden of pediatric primary immunodeficiency. Pediatr Int Off J Jpn Pediatr Soc 2018;60(10): 911–7.
95. Rubinstein T, Dionizovik-Dimanovski M, Smith C, et al. Screening youth with lupus for depression and anxiety in pediatric rheumatology clinics [abstract]. Arthritis Rheumatol 2018;70:1–3584.
96. Neufeld K, Silverio F, Ng L, et al. Depression and anxiety symptoms in childhood-onset systemic lupus erythematosus [abstract]. Arthritis Rheumatol 2019;71(S10):1–5420.
97. Li L, Merchant M, Gordon S, et al. Defining the prevalence of depression and anxiety symptoms in adolescents with juvenile idiopathic arthritis [abstract]. Arthritis Rheumatol 2020;72(S1):1–338.
98. Kyvsgaard N, Thastum M, Mikkelsen TS, et al. Coping strategies and anxiety in association with methotrexate-induced nausea in juvenile idiopathic arthritis. Rheumatol Int 2020;40(4):591–8.
99. Uzuner S, Sahin S, Durcan G, et al. The impact of peer victimization and psychological symptoms on quality of life in children and adolescents with systemic lupus erythematosus. Clin Rheumatol 2017;36(6):1297–304.
100. Petrongolo JL, Zelikovsky N, Keegan RM, et al. Examining uncertainty in illness in parents and children with chronic kidney disease and systemic lupus erythematosus: a mediational model of internalizing symptoms and health-related quality of life. J Clin Psychol Med Settings 2020;27(1):31–40.
101. Connelly M, Schanberg LE, Ardoin S, et al. Multisite randomized clinical trial evaluating an online self-management program for adolescents with juvenile idiopathic arthritis. J Pediatr Psychol 2019;44(3):363–74.
102. Bano S, Bosan K, Khurshid S, et al. Prevalence of depression in patients with juvenile idiopathic arthritis presenting at a tertiary care hospital. Cureus. 12(1). doi:10.7759/cureus.6807
103. Reid M, Fabricius J, Danguecan A, et al. Anxiety and depression in childhood rheumatologic conditions: a topical review. 2021. Available at:https://www.indianjrheumatol.com/preprintarticle.asp?id=309672. . Accessed March 1, 2021.

Early Sexual Health and Reproductive Implications in Pediatric Rheumatic Diseases

Cuoghi Edens, MD[a,b,*]

KEYWORDS

- Reproductive health • Pediatric rheumatology • Puberty • Menarche • Teratogens
- Human papilloma virus • Sexual orientation • Gender identity

KEY POINTS

- Reproductive health is a critical topic in pediatric rheumatology.
- Patients and parents have a keen interest in how their diagnosis and medications affect their reproductive health.
- Rheumatologists, primary care providers, endocrinologists, women's health care providers, urologists, and fertility specialists are needed to meet the reproductive health care needs of patients with pediatric-onset rheumatic diseases.
- Pediatric-onset rheumatic diseases influence multiple milestones along the progression from childhood to adolescence.

"What will happen when my child grows up?" is a common question posed in the pediatric rheumatologist's office. This prompt usually leads to an explanation of the chronicity of most rheumatic diseases. However, growing up isn't just about a child's physical wellbeing and health in regard to their rheumatic disease; conceptually, it includes a child's ability to obtain higher education, have gainful employment, contribute to society, form long-term romantic relationships, and have offspring of their own.

Sexual and reproductive health is defined by the United Nations and World Health Organization as a "state of physical, mental, and social well-being and not merely the absence of disease, dysfunction, or infirmity, in all matters relating to the reproductive system, its functions, and its processes."[1] The definition clarifies that sexual health requires a positive, respectful approach to sexuality and sexual relationships that are free of coercion, discrimination, or violence. The topic of sexual and reproductive health may seem out of place in pediatric rheumatology, but as medical providers

[a] Department of Pediatrics, Section Pediatric Rheumatology, University of Chicago Medicine, 5841 South Maryland Avenue, C104-A, MC5044, Chicago, IL 60637, USA; [b] Department of Internal Medicine, Section of Rheumatology, University of Chicago Medicine, 5841 South Maryland Avenue, C104-A, MC5044, Chicago, IL 60637, USA
* Corresponding author.
E-mail address: cedens@peds.bsd.uchicago.edu
Twitter: @CuoghiE (C.E.)

Rheum Dis Clin N Am 48 (2022) 91–112
https://doi.org/10.1016/j.rdc.2021.09.015

to those with life-long diseases, we are fortunate to help our patients and families navigate the progression from childhood to adulthood; although as subspecialists, we may lack knowledge or expertise to be proficient in the topic.

There is a multitude of reasons this topic deserves examination in pediatric rheumatology. In a subspecialty without cures, most of the rheumatic conditions diagnosed in childhood persist into adulthood with approximately 20% of systemic lupus (SLE) patients diagnosed in childhood[2] and 50% of juvenile idiopathic arthritis (JIA) patients continuing rheumatology care as adults.[3] Adolescent and young adult (AYA) rheumatic disease patients and their families have identified medication safety, sexual activity, family planning, peer relations, and dating as topics of interest in reproductive health.[4] AYA prefer to receive this information from health care providers, particularly their rheumatologists.[5]

Pediatric rheumatologists admit discomfort with reproductive issues[6] and assume their patient's primary care provider is addressing the topic. Unfortunately, this assumption is false; pediatricians also lack comfort and time to discuss these sensitive subjects.[7] Subspecialists engage with their patients more often than their primary care provider, whom patients may see only once a year for well-child visits. Even when these visits are attended, only 70% of adolescents receive information or counseling on sexuality[8] with a mere 40 seconds being the average time a provider spends when they do address sexual and reproductive health.[9] Paradoxically, some of the most ill and complex rheumatic disease patients do not have primary care providers.[10] The close bond a rheumatology provider forms with patients and families is a key reason pediatric rheumatology clinic is an ideal place to discuss sexual and reproductive health issues with their patients. As one parent stated, "Subspecialists may feel it isn't their 'area of expertise', but they are often the ones we trust most."[11] Like their parents, patients also trust the information their medical providers impart.[12]

PUBERTY

Transitioning from childhood into adulthood is a natural progression most often defined by physical growth. Changes in height and hair distribution, breasts, and genitalia are the hallmark signs, measured by sexual maturity rating, also known as Tanner staging. Many external forces can affect puberty and pubertal delay in an otherwise healthy child can indicate a potential inflammatory process. Delayed puberty is defined as the absence of testis enlargement or breast development at an age that is 2 to 2.5 SD later than the population mean, typically age 14 for boys and age 13 for girls.[13]

Puberty delay is prevalent in pediatric rheumatic diseases. In childhood-onset SLE (cSLE), delayed pubertal onset is present in 15% and 24% of the females and males, respectively.[14] Due to this prevalence, it has been suggested that pubertal delay be included in the assessment of cumulative damage in cSLE.[15] JIA can also contribute to puberty delay, which occurs in approximately 15% of children with this diagnosis.[16,17] A patient's JIA subtype may impact puberty onset with systemic JIA patients less delayed than others, although for unclear reasons.[18] It is uncertain if disease duration and activity impact puberty timing; most recent evidence suggests it does not rather it is the diagnosis of JIA itself.[19] Recommendations support the assessment of pubertal stage every 6 months starting at 9 years of age in children with JIA due to associated delays.[20] Routine evaluation of pubertal progress and discussion of risks contributing to pubertal delay has also been proposed.[21]

Corticosteroid use appears to play a role in the pubertal delay. Corticosteroids alter the gonadotropin-releasing hormone (GnRH)–gonadotropin-gonadic (GGG) axis resulting in downstream gonadal dysfunction likely from circulating inflammatory cytokines like interleukin-1, interleukin-6, and tumor necrosis factor-alpha, which impact insulin growth factor-1 (IGF-1).[22–24] Even after stopping corticosteroids, puberty onset remains delayed in patients with JIA.[25] This delay may be dose-dependent and cumulative over the course of corticosteroid use.[14,18]

Juvenile dermatomyositis (JDM) patients analyzed by the Pediatric *Rheumatology* International Trials Organisation (PRINTO) experienced delayed puberty in over one-third of subjects, independent of gender.[26] Although other more rare diseases in pediatric rheumatology have not been studied, exposure to corticosteroids and associated delayed puberty seen in other inflammatory diseases such as inflammatory bowel disease (IBD) illustrate the importance of evaluating sexual development in rheumatic disease care.[27]

Little is written about puberty causing stable JIA to flare although anecdotal evidence exists. Theoretically, alterations in sex hormones with resultant cytokine changes could affect disease activity but remains to be evaluated.[28,29] As uveitis activity has a biphasic course with a quiescent phase around the age of 9 years and increased activity during early puberty, diligent uveitis screening is required as patients mature.[30] Evidence suggests that cSLE flares with pubertal changes. Prospective evaluation of prepubertal SLE patients found that Tanner stages 2 and 3 were associated with disease flares, raising the postulation that sex hormones and adipokines may play a role in disease activity.[31]

The effects of delayed puberty are not just lag in sexual maturation, but associated reduction in one's peak bone mass, increasing the possibility of current or future bone fragility. For a population already at risk for growth delay from corticosteroids, further impaired bone growth from delayed puberty may contribute to short stature and merits treatment.[32,33] Depression, oppositional behavior, psychosomatic complaints, change in school performance, bullying, and general social immaturity can be rooted in pubertal delay in addition to low self-esteem.[34]

Puberty is also important developmentally outside of physical attributes. Beginning in early adolescence, preteens may seek more privacy as well as explore ways to seek independence.[35] Egocentric preteens may push boundaries and react strongly if parents or guardians reinforce limits, translating clinically to the rejection of rheumatic disease medications and other therapies. Evolving peer interactions also have repercussions by creating anxiety about peer knowledge of their diagnosis, issues with self-esteem rooted in having a chronic illness, and the desire to be a "normal" teen. As children continue to age, it is developmentally appropriate for them to seek increasing levels of independence from their families. This, coupled with their brain's immature ability to coordinate complex decisions, maintain impulse control, and consider multiple options and consequences potentially creates a conflict over their medical care. In adolescence, medication ownership often transfers from parent to the patient with subsequent adherence declines. Acknowledging this with patients before it occurs and implementing compliance monitoring strategies may improve patient outcomes.[36] Medication compliance hovers between 50% and 60% in pediatric rheumatic diseases, likely impacted by the developmental changes of adolescence.[37,38]

As children progress into middle adolescence around age 14, romantic interests and sexual relationships in addition to the exploration of sexual identity expand as do experimentation and risky behaviors; both must be taken into consideration in rheumatic disease care. The beginning of late adolescence (18–21) coincides with other life transitions like higher education, military participation, full-time employment, living separate from one's family, and committed romantic relationships. Late adolescence is often when patients with chronic medical conditions transfer their medical care from pediatric to adult providers, a critical time in the lives of those with rheumatic conditions.[39–41]

Coined the "review of symptoms for adolescents", the HEADSSS assessment is recommended by the American Academy of Pediatrics (AAP) as well as EULAR (European League Against Rheumatism)/PReS (Pediatric Rheumatology European Society) in their transition care guidelines for those with juvenile-onset rheumatic diseases.[42] This brief interview focuses on the assessment of the Home environment, Education and Employment, Eating, peer-related Activities, Drugs, Sexuality, Suicide/depression, and Safety from injury and violence and is recommended at least annually (**Table 1**).[43] Of note, pediatric rheumatologists do not commonly perform the HEADSS assessment.[44]

Puberty is also a time for changes in clinical practice, again highlighting why its acknowledgment is important. As outlined in the AAP Bright Futures initiative, the office confidentiality policy should be explained to the adolescent and parent, establishing that the adolescent will spend time alone with the provider beginning between ages 11 and 14.[45,46] The clinician should now acknowledge the adolescent as the

Table 1
Sexuality-specific HEADSSS assessment suggested questioning

	First-Line Questions	Follow-up Questions
Sexuality	• Have you ever been in a romantic relationship? • Tell me about the people who have dated • Have any of your relationships been sexual, like involving kissing or touching or sex? • Are you attracted to anyone now? • Are you interested in boys or girls? Both? Neither? Maybe not sure right now?	• Ask about Menarche, last menstrual period (LMP), and menstrual cycles • Have any of your relationship been violent? • What does the term "safe sex" mean to you? • Have you ever sent unclothes photos of your on email or text? • Have you ever been forced or pressured into doing something sexual you didn't want to do? • Have you ever been touched sexually in a way that you didn't want? • Have you ever been raped, on a date or any other time? • How many sexual partners have you had altogether? • Have you ever been pregnant or worried you might be pregnant? • Have you ever gotten someone pregnant or worried that might have happened? • What are you using for birth control? Are you satisfied with this method? • Do you use condoms every time you have intercourse? • Have you ever had a sexually transmitted infection or worried you had one? • Are your sexual activities enjoyable

primary history provider, not the parent. This includes the provider introducing themselves to the patient before the parent, making eye contact with the adolescent, and having the adolescent seated (in clothing) next to the seated provider, rather than on the examination table, for the interview. Implemented at routine clinic visits in early adolescence, this becomes routine and helps the adolescent take responsibility for their health care and lay the foundation for eventual transfer to adult care. The process is also aided by a clinic or institutional transition policy.[47]

MENARCHE AND MENSTRUAL CYCLES

Menarche, the start of one's menstrual cycle, is an important personal, social, and medical milestone. Median age of menarche in the developed world remains between 12 and 13 years of age, typically occurring 2 to 3 years after thelarche.[48] Akin to puberty, the timing of menarche is affected by several variables.

JIA has been associated with a delay in menarche.[19,49,50] Time to menarche lags 1 to 2 years in JIA patients compared to the general population.[51] Corticosteroid use, JIA subtype, disease duration, and severity are hypothesized as possible factors contributing to the delay.[50,52] It is imperative to determine if biological therapies and pursuit of medicated remission alter the timing of menarche in JIA patients; however, these investigations have not yet been undertaken.

Onset of menses is similarly delayed in patients with cSLE by 1 to 2 years.[53–55] Disease activity plays an independent role with higher SLEDAI and SLICC scores found in AYA who develop oligomenorrhea or amenorrhea.[54,56] Duration of disease and corticosteroid use also correlate with menarchal delay.[55] Beyond delay, studies find menstrual irregularities in as high as 50% of cSLE patients.[57] Females diagnosed with cSLE prepubertally have significantly worst disease severity across all disease aspects than those diagnosed later in adolescence, impacting puberty timing.[58] In subanalyses, cyclophosphamide is an independent factor affecting menarche timing and causing secondary amenorrhea.[59] JDM patients too are noted to have delayed menarche.[60] Women with menarche onset before age 11 are more likely to develop SLE and rheumatoid arthritis (RA) over their lifetime.[61]

Across ages, inflammatory diseases contribute to secondary amenorrhea if diagnosed after menarche.[14,62] Patients with rheumatic diseases experiencing secondary amenorrhea have abnormal follicular stimulating hormone (FSH), luteinizing hormone (LH), and low progesterone levels. Medications aside, delayed menarche and disruption of established cycles, like puberty, is the downstream effect of inflammation on the GGG axis, decreasing pituitary function resulting in inappropriate progesterone levels.[53,57] Delayed menarche is associated with low bone density and increased cardiovascular disease, amplifying existing risk in rheumatic disease patients.[63]

Absence of menarche by age 15 or within 3 years of thelarche, cycles less than 21 days or greater than 45 days, heavy menses, or menses lasting longer than 7 days should be evaluated by a specialist.[64] Once menarche has occurred, the date of last menses should be routinely obtained across medical settings. Secondary amenorrhea, defined as the cessation of menses for 3 months or 6 months if prior menses was irregular, requires evaluation including testing for pregnancy as well as endocrinopathies.[65]

Aside from the effect of one's rheumatic disease on menarche and menses, other aspects of one's menstrual cycle can greatly contribute to overall health. AYA with active rheumatic diseases may already have significant school absenteeism due to disease activity and medical appointments. Menorrhagia and dysmenorrhea can add to missed school, occupation, athletics, extracurricular activities, and social events, amplifying a lack of peer normalcy, and contributing to decreased quality of life.[66–68] Anemia, a presenting symptom in more than 50% of pediatric patients with cSLE and JIA,[69] can be worsened by anemia from one's menstrual cycle. Fatigue is a common symptom of rheumatic diseases that waxes and wanes over the menstrual cycle,[70] compounded by other factors like medication side effects and anemia. Lastly, self-care during one's menstrual cycle can be difficult due to one's rheumatic disease, for example, changing a tampon during a JIA flare or with significant joint damage or contractures.[4,52]

Hormonal changes accompanying one's menstrual cycle have been associated with disease flares and increased disease activity in adults with RA and SLE,[71] but is undocumented in AYA with rheumatic diseases. The timing of menstrual cycle-related flares varies in SLE compared with RA; however, all subjects noted changes in pain, fatigue, and disease activity with cyclic hormonal changes.[72,73] Rheumatic disease activity and its relation to menstrual cycles likely occurs in the pediatric population and is an area warranting investigation.

Extremely painful or irregular menses are another reason for pause in any adolescent. Generally not diagnosed until their mid-to-late 20s, 60% of women with endometriosis report having symptoms before age 15.[74] Though silent forms exist, symptoms include pelvic pain, dyspareunia, dysmenorrhea and menorrhagia.[75] Women with endometriosis have an increased frequency of SLE, Sjögren's syndrome, IBD, and RA.[76–78]

Polycystic ovarian syndrome (PCOS) has a prevalence of at least 7% in the general population.[79] Typically presenting early in one's reproductive life as oligo- or amenorrhea, hirsutism, and other signs of androgen excess, a formal PCOS diagnosis is typically not made until when this endocrinopathy complicates conception.[80] Confounding the diagnosis of PCOS in patients with rheumatic diseases is the use of exogenous corticosteroids which contribute to acne, weight gain, hirsutism, hypertension, insulin resistance, and medication or inflammatory state-induced oligomenorrhea, mimicking the diagnosis.[81] Although PCOS pathogenesis is unclear, research examining the relationship between PCOS and rheumatic diseases suggests increased incidence.[82]

SEXUAL ORIENTATION AND GENDER IDENTITY

More often thought of as sexual orientation and a person's identity in relation to the gender or genders to which they are typically attracted, one's sexuality is an important part of maturation. Formation of healthy sexuality is a notable developmental milestone for all young people, dependent on information acquisition and developing attitudes, beliefs, and values about consent, sexual orientation, gender identity, relationships, and intimacy. Assessing sexual orientation and gender identity in subspecialty clinics is easily accomplished through the aforementioned HEADSSS assessment.

Nomenclature used in discussing gender and sexual orientation is evolving to extend inclusivity. LGBTQIA+ is the newest umbrella term that includes those who identify as intersex and asexual (or ally) in addition to previously included lesbian, gay, bisexual, transgender, and questioning.[83] Transgender and gender nonconforming (TGNC) is a term used to cover the spectrum of nonbinary gender identities and sexual orientations. In a 2016 survey of over 80,000 teenagers, almost 3% identified as TGNC, an increase from prior.[84]

An alarming 20% of those surveyed had been refused medical care because of their TGNC status, which may equate to a delay or lack of rheumatic disease diagnosis in this population.[85] When seeking medical care, LGBTQAI+ patients may be concerned about a perceived lack of confidentiality, the reaction of the health care provider up on disclosure, or the provider's assumption of heterosexuality or cisgender. In forming an open, therapeutic relationship with patients, which is often the crux of medication compliance, recognition and acceptance of a patient's sexual orientation and gender identity conveys inclusivity, competence, and most of all, caring. Noncisgender persons have increased mental health needs and bear the burden of bullying, discrimination, and stigmatization, issues more common in patients with pediatric rheumatic diseases, which can have a cumulative effect when patients face both.[86,87]

Simple steps are taken in the clinical setting including inquiry and acknowledgment of a patient's gender identification and sexual orientation facilitate care. This includes not assuming cisgender, asking about and then addressing patients with their preferred pronouns, and not assuming heterosexual relationships when inquiring. Patient areas can be made TGNC friendly with symbols establishing the clinic as welcoming to those across the gender identity spectrum with nondiscrimination policies displayed. Providers may consider wearing lapel pins, name badge accessories, or other insignia as an outward sign of acceptance and inclusivity. In addition to medical care providers, clinic staff, and other health care workers that interact with patients should be included in educational efforts focused on inclusive practices to increase the comfort and trust of TGNC patients and improve their interaction with the health care system. Electronic health care records can also be modified to include preferred name, gender identity, and pronouns.[88]

HUMAN PAPILLOMA VIRUS AND GYNECOLOGIC CANCERS

The most notable sexually transmitted infection (STI) facing pediatric patients is human papilloma virus (HPV), with peak time for obtaining HPV after the first sexual encounter for any gender.[89] Transmitted through the skin to skin contact during oral, vaginal, or anal sex, HPV infects 14 million persons a year.[90] When analyzed by age, 33% of 14 to 19-year-old and 54% of 20 to 24-year-old females are infected with a strain of HPV. At least 14% of college students are infected with HPV yearly.[91,92] These age ranges are important to note as prior health care transition research revealed most pediatric rheumatologists care for patients well into their 20s.[41]

Typically symptomless, HPV follows an indolent course and is the causative agent of more than 90% of cervical cancer diagnoses,[93] in addition to anogenital warts, vaginal, oropharyngeal, and penile cancers. HPV vaccination is efficacious in lowering these diagnoses.[94–96] The CDC's Advisory Committee on Immunization Practices recommends vaccination for girls and boys well in advance of sexarche. All children age 11 to 12 years are recommended to receive the 2-shot series; however, those with "immunocompromising conditions" which includes the use of immunosuppressive agents are recommended the 3-shot series.[97] Intended for adults, the American College of Rheumatology (ACR) also recommends HPV vaccination before or during treatment with DMARDs and biologics.[98] Unfortunately, there is very low uptake of HPV vaccines in the general population and those with rheumatic diseases.[99,100]

The lack of vaccination in those with rheumatic diseases is concerning, as multiple studies have demonstrated increased precancerous and cancerous lesions in women across the spectrum of rheumatic diseases.[101–105] Increased risk of precancerous lesions and cancer is likely multifactorial with immunosuppression playing a role as well as the lack of routine screening in addition to low vaccination rates.

HPV vaccination is safe as well as immunogenic in pediatric patients with both JIA and cSLE.[106–108] Vaccination should be strongly encouraged in both men and women with rheumatic diseases confidently as the development of rheumatic diseases or disease flare does not correlate with vaccine administration.[109,110]

Cervical and Other Gynecologic Cancers

The American Cancer Society recommendations for cervical cancer screening have greatly changed in the past 20 years. Although controversial, age 25 is now the preferred age to initiate cervical cancer screening, no matter age of sexarche or sexual orientation, although other organizations continue to recommend age 21.[111] Preferred screening now consists of HPV testing alone.[112] However, these recommendations are not applicable to all populations. Due to the increased risk of cervical abnormalities and lack of HPV clearance in patients with rheumatic diseases, additional guidelines exist for patients on immunosuppressive medications. All women with SLE and women with RA on immunosuppressive therapy should follow cervical cancer screening guidelines for HIV-infected women. This includes testing beginning at sexarche or age 21 with subsequent yearly evaluations. Women with RA not on immunosuppressant therapy should follow screening guidelines for the general population. There is no delineation for patients with pediatric-onset rheumatic diseases or other rheumatic diseases presumably at equal risk.[113] While young women with JIA do not have statistically significant increased infection rates or cervical abnormalities than the general public,[114] this is difficult data to interpret given the lack of longitudinal evaluation.

Additional considerations for cervical cancer screening in young women with rheumatic diseases include the ability to maintain dorsal lithotomy position despite arthritic disease in the hip, pelvis, or spine, avascular necrosis, or joint replacement. Vaginal dryness from sicca symptoms can also complicate testing.

The risk of other gynecologic cancers in patients with rheumatic diseases varies. Women with RA have decreased risk of breast, uterine, and ovarian cancer with no consensus found in SLE, although disease duration correlated with increased risk.[115–117]

Testicular Cancer

Although there is no increased incidence in patients with rheumatic diseases, testicular cancer is the most common cancer among men aged 15 to 34 years and therefore may present in the rheumatology clinic. Testicular cancer is comparatively rare and there are no screening recommendations for adolescent or adult males by clinician examination or patient self-examination.[118]

REPRODUCTIVE HEALTH IMPLICATIONS OF RHEUMATIC MEDICATIONS

Parents of children across the age and rheumatic diseases spectrum have concerns about medications and their effect on their child's reproductive potential, as do rheumatologists and patients. Thankfully, out of the growing list of medications used to treat pediatric rheumatic diseases, very few have implications on fertility or pregnancy. However, it is critical to recognize that medications do not undergo testing in pregnant women; rather this information comes from postmarketing analysis and case reports. In lieu of human clinical trial data, animal Developmental and Reproductive Toxicology (DART) studies are used to assess: (1) *reproductive toxicity* including alterations of the reproductive cycle, sexual behavior, sperm or egg production (quality and quantity), pregnancy outcomes, labor and delivery, and, lactation and (2) *developmental toxicity* referring to adverse effects on the developing fetus that result from exposure before conception, pre and postnatal, and up to the time of sexual maturity.

Teratogenic medications may cause birth defects via a toxic effect on an embryo or fetus. A subcategory of teratogens, called abortogens, induce abortion. Multiple organizations including the ACR have published evidence-based expert opinion statements addressing medication safety in pregnancy to clarify the confusing and now defunct ordinal system implemented in the United States and other countries.[119,120] Although details of these statements may differ as well as become outdated as research that is more robust is completed, currently recognized teratogens commonly used in rheumatology include *cyclophosphamide, leflunomide, methotrexate, and mycophenolate.* Recommendations surrounding medication management concerning pregnancy planning are shown in **Table 2**; however, unplanned pregnancy, a more likely scenario in AYA using these medications, lacks standardized guidance. Inappropriately in this situation, a common default is to recommend termination due to teratogenic concern even though congenital malformation risk is ~25% or less for these medications.

Cyclophosphamide is an alkylating agent that induces cellular apoptosis. Cyclophosphamide's beneficial immunomodulatory effects include elimination of T regulatory cells and induction of T cell growth factors. Infertility is dose dependent in both genders but also age dependent in females, with those less than 25 years of age faring better.[59,121–123] For men, a cumulative dosing limit of less than 7.5 g/m^2 has been established in oncology based on results showing sperm count recovery within that range.[124] 30% of cSLE patients who received high cumulative doses of cyclophosphamide have decreased ovarian reserve, which is not recoverable.[125]

An important consideration with cyclophosphamide use in rheumatic diseases is disease chronicity. Lower cyclophosphamide dosing used in rheumatic disease protocols benefit AYA with cSLE and ANCA-associated vasculitis (AAV), but cumulative dosing over the reproductive lifetime of the patient with a chronic illness including potential redosing for flare impacts long-term fertility impact. Sadly, AYA with cSLE or AAV treated with cyclophosphamide receive little counseling concerning effects on reproductive potential nor are they referred to a fertility specialist for preservation strategies.[126]

Cyclophosphamide is highly teratogenic when administered during pregnancy. Malformations of skeleton, palate, limbs, and eyes are common when administered early in pregnancy. Fetal growth retardation and severe bone marrow hypoplasia occur when administered later in pregnancy. Contraception use should be ensured in childbearing aged patients while receiving cyclophosphamide. ACR guidelines recommend screening for pregnancy before administration to prevent fetal exposure.[127] Due to its effect on spermatogenesis, recommendations suggest that those desiring to father a child, 3 months should lapse from last cyclophosphamide dose to conception.[128]

Methotrexate Outside of rheumatology, large doses of methotrexate are used as an abortive agent. Therefore the prescribing provider should counsel women prescribed methotrexate and their families on reliable contraception and subsequently follow-up to verify contraceptive use due to this risk, although the rheumatology dose is relatively small. Methotrexate carries a 10% risk of congenital malformations but a miscarriage rate nearing 50%.[129] Notably, the risk of spontaneous abortion and congenital malformation are *not* present after stopping. With its use as a chemotherapy agent in higher doses than used in rheumatic diseases, infertility is a concern. Although women who use methotrexate for RA have demonstrated subfertility, this was not associated with methotrexate use itself but rather felt to be disease-related.[130] Most studies have looked at methotrexate use in adulthood; rare is the pediatric study that has evaluated the effect of cumulative methotrexate use in children.[131,132] Studies show no long-term effect on spermatogenesis and methotrexate does not need to be stopped in men for conception.[128] ACR guidelines recommend women stop methotrexate 1 to 3 months before conception, allowing for medication depletion, disease stabilization, and transition to pregnancy-compatible medication.[120]

Table 2
Pregnancy compatibility of rheumatic medications[a]

	Compatible		Caution/Conditional		Not Compatible
Pre-Conception	Adalimumab	Golimumab	Abatacept	Discontinue at conception[b]	Cyclophosphamide+
	Anakinra	Hydroxychloroquine	Anakinra	Discontinue at conception	Leflunomide
	Azathioprine/6-MP	Infliximab	Belimumab	Discontinue at conception	Lenalidomide
	Belimumab	NSAIDs +	Cyclosporine	Monitor for HTN	Methotrexate
	Certolizumab	Prednisone+ (<20mg/day)	NSAIDs+	Discontinue if conception delay	Mycophenolate
	Colchicine	Rituximab	Prednisone+ >20mg/day	Discontinue at conception	Mycophenolic Acid
	Etanercept	Sulfasalazine+	Rituximab	Discontinue at conception	Thalidomide
			Secukinumab/IL-17 agents	Discontinue at conception	
			Ustekinumab/IL-23 agents	Discontinue at conception	
			Tacrolimus	Monitor for HTN	
			Tocilizumab/IL-6 agents	Discontinue at conception	
			Tofacitinib/other JAKi	Discontinue at conception	
Pregnancy	Adalimumab[c]	Prednisone	Abatacept	Limited data	Cyclophosphamide
	Azathioprine/6-MP	Sulfasalazine	Anakinra	Limited data	Leflunomide
	Certolizumab	Tacrolimus	Belimumab	Limited data	Lenalidomide
	Colchicine		NSAIDs	Stop at 20 weeks	Methotrexate
	Cyclosporine		Rituximab	Life/organ threatening disease	Mycophenolate

	Etanercept[c]		Secukinumab/IL-17 agents	Limited data	Mycophenolic Acid
	Golimumab[c]		Ustekinumab/IL-23 agents	Limited data	Thalidomide
	Hydroxychloroquine		Tocilizumab/IL-6 agents	Limited data	
	Infliximab[c]		Tofacitinib/other JAKi	Limited data	
Breastfeeding[d]	Abatacept	Etanercept	Tofacitinib/other JAKi	Limited data, small molecules	Cyclophosphamide
	Adalimumab	Golimumab			Leflunomide
	Anakinra	Hydroxychloroquine			Lenalidomide
	Azathioprine/6-MP	Infliximab			Methotrexate
	Belimumab	NSAIDs			Mycophenolate
	Certolizumab	Prednisone			Mycophenolic Acid
	Colchicine	Rituximab			Thalidomide
	Cyclosporine	Sulfasalazine			
	Tacrolimus				
	Secukinumab/IL-17 agents				
	Tocilizumab/IL-6 agents				
	Ustekinumab/IL-23 agents				

[a] Adapted from Sammaritano L et al. 2020 American College of Rheumatology Guideline for the Management of Reproductive Health in Rheumatic and Musculoskeletal Diseases. Arthritis Rheumatol. 2020 Apr;72(4):529-556.
[b] Decision to discontinue any medication at conception should be had in discussion with patient, subspecialist, women's health provider, and after review of most up to date literature.
[c] If well controlled rheumatic disease, consider discontinuation in 3rd trimester due to increased placental transfer, if flares can restart. Do not discontinue if patient has IBD.
[d] Monoclonal antibodies are large molecules with low passage rate into breast milk, if any does pass, likely destroyed in the infant's gastrointestinal tract. +Medications that may affect fertility, sulfasalazine only impacts men.

Mycophenolate Studies of mycophenolate have not demonstrated an effect on male or female fertility when used in the treatment of rheumatic diseases or organ transplants.[128] However, substantial evidence exists that mycophenolate causes congenital malformations and contributes to miscarriage, leading the FDA to create a risk evaluation and mitigation strategy (REMS) program to educate providers and patients of these risks as well as contraception needs while on the medication. Based on solid organ transplant data, 45% of pregnant patients taking mycophenolate experienced a spontaneous abortion and 22% of live births resulted in congenital malformations involving the jaw and ear.[133] Dual contraceptives are recommended for sexually active women of childbearing age unless the patient has an intrauterine device (IUD) in place or if they/their partner has undergone sterilization surgery.[134] Recommendations to stop mycophenolate 3 months before attempting conception allows for transition to pregnancy-compatible medications and monitoring for increased disease activity.[120]

Leflunomide While controversial, leflunomide continues to be categorized as a teratogenic medication.[135] Animal studies using supratherapeutic doses of leflunomide demonstrate increased fetal loss and malformations; however, human studies have been less conclusive.[136] Existing recommendations include stopping the medication before conceiving and, due to enterohepatic recycling, proceeding with a cholestyramine or charcoal washout followed by serum level assessment. If conception occurs while on leflunomide, washout is recommended. Due to disease chronicity, pediatric patients may have been on leflunomide previously but not while trying to conceive. In such cases, if a serum level is still elevated, washout should be pursued. Pregnancies occurring after the washout procedure, including those conceived on leflunomide, have had positive outcomes.[137]

Sulfasalazine Male-specific concerns exist with the use of sulfasalazine, which can cause reversible azoospermia. However, no teratogenic and female fertility concerns have been found, and sulfasalazine is recommended for use in pregnant females with inflammatory arthritis.[120] If a male on sulfasalazine is having difficulty conceiving, recommendations are to hold it for 3 months and perform a semen analysis. Routine discontinuation of sulfasalazine before conception is not necessary.[128]

Nonsteroidal anti-inflammatory drugs (NSAIDs) The most common medication class used in rheumatic diseases has significant reproductive health ramifications. Due to prostaglandin effects, women can experience a reduction in ovulation, which appears to reverse once the NSAID is stopped.[138,139] Men using high doses of aspirin or NSAIDs may have decreased spermatogenesis that also appears reversible with cessation. If having difficulty conceiving, NSAIDs should be held for men or women

NSAIDs also have repercussions during pregnancy. Much debate exists between obstetricians and rheumatologists over the safety of NSAIDs in early pregnancy with questionable effects on embryo implantation and miscarriage. Evidence-based guidelines from the ACR establish compatibility in the 1st and 2nd trimester for patients with rheumatic diseases.[120] However, the ACR guidelines were created before the FDA warning regarding NSAIDs as contributory to oligohydramnios and related fetal renal disorders and advised avoidance after 20 weeks gestation.[140] Third trimester NSAID use is associated with premature closure of the ductus arteriosus, leading to fetal pulmonary hypertension.[141]

Corticosteroids High levels of corticosteroids stimulate the release of somatostatin, inhibit the release of growth hormone, IGF-1, and IGF binding protein, decrease the expression of receptors for growth hormone and IGF-1, and reduce the level of IGF binding protein. High levels of corticosteroids can also reduce proliferation in growth plate chondrocytes by inhibiting the expression of receptors for growth hormone and

IGF-1. Furthermore, corticosteroids interfere with normal bone development by increasing the level of proteolysis in nearby muscle tissue.[142]

Prednisone and other corticosteroids affect fertility in several ways; however, it is difficult to differentiate their side effects from that of an assumingly active rheumatic disease. Suppressing the GGG axis, prednisone can lead to gonadal dysfunction. Corticosteroids can affect menses regularity, duration, and heaviness.[143] Notably, doses greater than 7.5 mg/d of prednisone increases time to conceive.[144]

Controversy exists as to the safety of corticosteroids in pregnancy, however, recent studies do not suggest an increased risk of congenital malformation such as cleft lip/palate as formerly reported.[145] The risks and benefits of corticosteroids in pregnancy must be weighed with the mother's health paramount as disease activity correlates with poor outcomes for both mother and baby. Preterm delivery and premature rupture of membranes have been associated with cortico steroid use, but here too it is impossible to remove rheumatic or other autoimmune disease activity from this equation.[146] Prednisone doses of 20 mg or less (or other steroid equivalents) are safer in pregnancy.[120] Corticosteroid use in pregnancy may increase the incidence of gestational diabetes and hypertension. Prednisone and other nonfluorinated corticosteroids do not offer fetal lung maturation benefits, so mothers with impending premature delivery need the recommended fluorinated steroid treatment.[147]

Additional medications concerns There are other medications commonly used in rheumatic disease patients that are teratogenic including angiotensin-converting enzyme inhibitors (ACEis), angiotensin II receptor blockers (ARBs), warfarin, lenalidomide, and thalidomide. The latter 2 have mandatory REMS programs required to regulate prescription. ACEis and ARBs can cause congenital malformations in all trimesters resulting in oligohydramnios[148] and should be stopped before conception or at a positive pregnancy test. Fetal warfarin syndrome affects about 10% of pregnancies. Pregnant patients on warfarin should be transitioned to heparin products at therapeutic dosing.[149]

Patient education regarding medication risks is key to protecting future fertility and pregnancy. Reassurance of long-term medication safety pertaining to fertility is also important, as this worry is a cause of medication noncompliance.[150] Clinical implementation of procedures to increase patient education and pregnancy testing is easy and effective.[151]

SUMMARY

Reproductive health is closely intertwined with rheumatic diseases in children. Provision of reproductive health care is essential to well-rounded rheumatic disease care. Collaboration with a patient's primary care providers, various women's health specialists, adolescent medicine, endocrinologists, and urologists helps address the spectrum of reproductive health needs of patients with pediatric rheumatic diseases through coordinated clinical care and explorative research to fill the gaps that exist while improving the quality of life and outcomes. Pediatric rheumatologists may lack time, desire, knowledge, and training on reproductive health topics; however, opening the conversation, assessing for concerning behaviors, acknowledging concerns, providing a confidential outlet, and helping a patient seek care with a provider who can address their needs and concerns is well within their scope. These conversations should be open, free of judgment, and without the assumption of binary gender or sexual orientation to adequately provide care to all patients. Patient and provider discomfort surrounding these topics can be lessened, particularly regarding medication safety, by routinely presenting this information to patients and families often and early in their care.

CLINICS CARE POINTS

- Routinely assess puberty stage and menarche status.
- Routinely perform HEADSSS assessment to obtain a thorough social history.
- Establish confidentiality with patients at age 11 to 14 and begin talking to them without family members present.
- Create an accepting, inclusive environment for all gender identities and sexual orientations in the pediatric rheumatology clinic.
- Recommend HPV vaccine to all patients (3 dose series for cSLE patients and those on immunosuppressive medications).
- Encourage age/gender-appropriate cancer screenings.
- Discuss potential rheumatic disease and medication implications on reproductive health with patients of all ages and their families.

DISCLOSURE

The author has nothing to disclose.

REFERENCES

1. WHO. Reproductive Health. 2021. Available at: https://www.who.int/westernpacific/health-topics/reproductive-health. Accessed June 5, 2021.
2. Duarte C, CM, Ines L, Liang M, et al. In: Lahita RG, editor. Systemic lupus erythematosus. 5th edition. Academic Press; 2011.
3. Oen K, Malleson PN, Cabral DA, et al. Disease course and outcome of juvenile rheumatoid arthritis in a multicenter cohort. J Rheumatol 2002;29(9):1989–99.
4. Carandang K, Mruk V, Ardoin SP, et al. Reproductive health needs of adolescent and young adult women with pediatric rheumatic diseases. Pediatr Rheumatol Online J 2020;18(1):66.
5. Ronis T, Frankovich J, Yen S, et al. Pilot study of reproductive health counseling in a pediatric rheumatology clinic. Arthritis Care Res (Hoboken) 2014;66(4):631–5.
6. De Ranieri D, Onel K, Wagner-Weiner L, and Tesher MS. Pregnancy and Contraception in Adolescents and Teens with SLE: Are pediatric rheumatologists adequately Screening and Educating Their Patients? [Abstract]. 2012 ACR/ARHP Annual Meeting. Washington, DC. November 9-14, 2012.
7. Grubb LK, Powers M. Committee On A. Emerging Issues in Male Adolescent Sexual and Reproductive Health Care. Pediatrics 2020;145(5):e20200627.
8. Boekeloo BO. Will you ask? Will they tell you? Are you ready to hear and respond?: barriers to physician-adolescent discussion about sexuality. JAMA Pediatr 2014;168(2):111–3.
9. Alexander SC, Fortenberry JD, Pollak KI, et al. Sexuality talk during adolescent health maintenance visits. JAMA Pediatr 2014;168(2):163–9.
10. Yazdany J, Tonner C, Trupin L, et al. Provision of preventive health care in systemic lupus erythematosus: data from a large observational cohort study. Arthritis Res Ther 2010;12(3):R84.
11. Pickles DM, Lihn SL, Boat TF, et al. A roadmap to emotional health for children and families with chronic pediatric conditions. Pediatrics 2020;145(2):e20191324.

12. Ott MA, Rosenberger JG, McBride KR, et al. How do adolescents view health? Implications for state health policy. J Adolesc Health 2011;48(4):398–403.
13. Palmert MR, Dunkel L. Clinical practice. Delayed puberty. N Engl J Med 2012; 366(5):443–53.
14. Rygg M, Pistorio A, Ravelli A, et al. A longitudinal PRINTO study on growth and puberty in juvenile systemic lupus erythematosus. Ann Rheum Dis 2012;71(4): 511–7.
15. Gutierrez-Suarez R, Ruperto N, Gastaldi R, et al. A proposal for a pediatric version of the Systemic Lupus International Collaborating Clinics/American College of Rheumatology Damage Index based on the analysis of 1,015 patients with juvenile-onset systemic lupus erythematosus. Arthritis Rheum 2006;54(9): 2989–96.
16. El Badri D, Rostom S, Bouaddi I, et al. Sexual maturation in Moroccan patients with juvenile idiopathic arthritis. Rheumatol Int 2014;34(5):665–8.
17. Aggarwal B, Bhalla AK, Singh S. Sexual maturation in boys with juvenile rheumatoid arthritis. Rheumatol Int 2011;31(11):1419–21.
18. Maher SE, Ali FI. Sexual maturation in Egyptian boys and girls with juvenile rheumatoid arthritis. Rheumatol Int 2013;33(8):2123–6.
19. Van Pelt P, Hokken-Koelega A, Dolhain R, et al. Puberty and disease activity in JIA. Pediatr Rheumatol 2014;12, P151.
20. Kao KT, Denker M, Zacharin M, et al. Pubertal abnormalities in adolescents with chronic disease. Best Pract Res Clin Endocrinol Metab 2019;33(3):101275.
21. de Gruijter NM, Naja M, Peckham H, et al. A systematic review exploring the bidirectional relationship between puberty and autoimmune rheumatic diseases. Pediatr Rheumatol Online J 2021;19(1):47.
22. Gore AC, Attardi B, DeFranco DB. Glucocorticoid repression of the reproductive axis: effects on GnRH and gonadotropin subunit mRNA levels. Mol Cell Endocrinol 2006;256(1–2):40–8.
23. Wong SC, Dobie R, Altowati MA, et al. Growth and the Growth Hormone-Insulin Like Growth Factor 1 Axis in Children With Chronic Inflammation: Current Evidence, Gaps in Knowledge, and Future Directions. Endocr Rev 2016;37(1): 62–110.
24. d'Angelo DM, Di Donato G, Breda L, et al. Growth and puberty in children with juvenile idiopathic arthritis. Pediatr Rheumatol Online J 2021;19(1):28.
25. Machado SH, Xavier RM, Lora PS, et al. Height and sexual maturation in girls with juvenile idiopathic arthritis. J Pediatr (Rio J) 2020;96(1):100–7.
26. Nordal E, Pistorio A, Rygg M, et al. Growth and puberty in juvenile dermatomyositis: a longitudinal cohort study. Arthritis Care Res (Hoboken) 2020;72(2): 265–73.
27. Ballinger AB, Savage MO, Sanderson IR. Delayed puberty associated with inflammatory bowel disease. Pediatr Res 2003;53(2):205–10.
28. Fisher C, Ciurtin C, Leandro M, et al. Similarities and differences between juvenile and adult spondyloarthropathies. Front Med (Lausanne) 2021;8:681621.
29. Webb K, Peckham H, Radziszewska A, et al. Sex and Pubertal Differences in the Type 1 Interferon Pathway Associate With Both X Chromosome Number and Serum Sex Hormone Concentration. Front Immunol 2018;9:3167.
30. Hoeve M, Kalinina Ayuso V, Schalij-Delfos NE, et al. The clinical course of juvenile idiopathic arthritis-associated uveitis in childhood and puberty. Br J Ophthalmol 2012;96(6):852–6.
31. O'Neil K and Rakestra A. Hormone and Adipokine Effects on cSLE Disease Activity During Puberty. Proceedings of the 2019 Childhood Arthritis and

Rheumatology Research Alliance (CARRA) Annual Scientific Meeting Pediatric Rheumatology 2019;17(73) Louisville, KY April 10-14, 2019.
32. Simon D, Lucidarme N, Prieur AM, et al. Treatment of growth failure in juvenile chronic arthritis. Horm Res 2002;58(Suppl 1):28–32.
33. Bechtold S, Ripperger P, Hafner R, et al. Growth hormone improves height in patients with juvenile idiopathic arthritis: 4-year data of a controlled study. J Pediatr 2003;143(4):512–9.
34. Kulin HE. Delayed puberty. J Clin Endocrinol Metab 1996;81(10):3460–4.
35. Allen B and Waterman H. Stages of adolescence. American Academy of Pediatrics; 2019. Available at: https://www.healthychildren.org/English/ages-stages/teen/Pages/Stages-of-Adolescence.aspx. Accessed July 10, 2021.
36. Taddeo D, Egedy M, Frappier JY. Adherence to treatment in adolescents. Paediatr Child Health 2008;13(1):19–24.
37. Favier LA, Taylor J, Loiselle Rich K, et al. Barriers to adherence in juvenile idiopathic arthritis: a multicenter collaborative experience and preliminary results. J Rheumatol 2018;45(5):690–6.
38. Scalzi LV, Hollenbeak CS, Mascuilli E, et al. Improvement of medication adherence in adolescents and young adults with SLE using web-based education with and without a social media intervention, a pilot study. Pediatr Rheumatol Online J 2018;16(1):18.
39. Ardoin S. Transitions in Rheumatic Disease: Pediatric to Adult Care. Pediatr Clin North Am 2018;65(4):867–83.
40. Lawrence S, Neinstein CEI. Young Adults Remain Worse Off Than Adolescents. J Adolesc Health 2013;55(5):559–61.
41. Johnson KR, Edens C, Sadun RE, et al. Differences in Healthcare Transition Views, Practices, and Barriers Among North American Pediatric Rheumatology Clinicians From 2010 to 2018. J Rheumatol 2021;48(9):1442–9.
42. Foster HE, Minden K, Clemente D, et al. EULAR/PReS standards and recommendations for the transitional care of young people with juvenile-onset rheumatic diseases. Ann Rheum Dis 2017;76(4):639–46.
43. Goldenring J, Rosen D. Getting into adolescent heads: An essential update. Contemporary Pediatrics 2004;21:64.
44. Spitznagle JBN, Adams A, Onel K, et al. Identifying Targets to Improve the Assessment of Psychosocial Risk Factors in Adolescent Patients: Perspectives from Pediatric Rheumatology Fellows in the United States and Canada [abstract]. Arthritis Rheumatol 2020;72.
45. Hagan JF, Shaw JS. Bright futures: guidelines for health supervision of infants, children, and adolescents. 4th edition. Elk Grove Village (IL): American Academy of Pediatrics; 2017.
46. White PH, Cooley WC. Transitions Clinical Report Authoring G, American Academy Of P, American Academy Of Family P, American College Of P. Supporting the Health Care Transition From Adolescence to Adulthood in the Medical Home. Pediatrics 2018;142(5):e20182587.
47. Marcell AV, Burstein GR. Committee On A. Sexual and Reproductive Health Care Services in the Pediatric Setting. Pediatrics 2017;140(5):e20172858.
48. Chumlea WC, Schubert CM, Roche AF, et al. Age at menarche and racial comparisons in US girls. Pediatrics 2003;111(1):110–3.
49. Lurati A, Salmaso A, Teruzzi B, et al. Relationship between delayed menarche and bone density in patients affected by juvenile idiopathic arthritis. Pediatr Rheumatol 2008;6:P45.

50. Fraser PA, Hoch S, Erlandson D, et al. The timing of menarche in juvenile rheumatoid arthritis. J Adolesc Health Care 1988;9(6):483–7.
51. Woźniak S. Rheumatoid arthritis – peculiarity in children. Ped Prakt. 1998;6:13–6.
52. Rusconi R, Corona F, Grassi A, et al. Age at menarche in juvenile rheumatoid arthritis. J Pediatr Endocrinol Metab 2003;16(Suppl 2):285–8.
53. Medeiros PB, Febronio MV, Bonfa E, et al. Menstrual and hormonal alterations in juvenile systemic lupus erythematosus. Lupus 2009;18(1):38–43.
54. Pasoto SG, Mendonca BB, Bonfa E. Menstrual disturbances in patients with systemic lupus erythematosus without alkylating therapy: clinical, hormonal and therapeutic associations. Lupus 2002;11(3):175–80.
55. Silva CA, Leal MM, Leone C, et al. Gonadal function in adolescents and young women with juvenile systemic lupus erythematosus. Lupus 2002;11(7):419–25.
56. Shabanova SS, Ananieva LP, Alekberova ZS, et al. Ovarian function and disease activity in patients with systemic lupus erythematosus. Clin Exp Rheumatol 2008;26(3):436–41.
57. Silva CA, Hilario MO, Febronio MV, et al. Risk factors for amenorrhea in juvenile systemic lupus erythematosus (JSLE): a Brazilian multicentre cohort study. Lupus 2007;16(7):531–6.
58. Hui-Yuen JS, Imundo LF, Avitabile C, et al. Early versus later onset childhood-onset systemic lupus erythematosus: Clinical features, treatment and outcome. Lupus 2011;20(9):952–9.
59. Ioannidis JP, Katsifis GE, Tzioufas AG, et al. Predictors of sustained amenorrhea from pulsed intravenous cyclophosphamide in premenopausal women with systemic lupus erythematosus. J Rheumatol 2002;29(10):2129–35.
60. Aikawa NE, Sallum AM, Leal MM, et al. Menstrual and hormonal alterations in juvenile dermatomyositis. Clin Exp Rheumatol 2010;28(4):571–5.
61. Costenbader KH, Feskanich D, Stampfer MJ, et al. Reproductive and menopausal factors and risk of systemic lupus erythematosus in women. Arthritis Rheum 2007;56(4):1251–62.
62. Nonato DR, Barbosa VS, Rodrigues DL, et al. Menstrual disturbances in systemic lupus erythematosus patients using immunossuppressants. Rev Bras Reumatol 2010;50(5):501–15.
63. Zhu J, Chan YM. Adult consequences of self-limited delayed puberty. Pediatrics 2017;139(6):e20163177.
64. American Academy of Pediatrics Committee on A, American College of O, Gynecologists Committee on Adolescent Health Care, Diaz A, Laufer MR, Breech LL. Menstruation in girls and adolescents: using the menstrual cycle as a vital sign. Pediatrics 2006;118(5):2245–50.
65. Practice Committee of the American Society for Reproductive Medicine. Current evaluation of amenorrhea. Fertil Steril 2006;86(5 Suppl 1):S148–55.
66. Knox B, Azurah AG, Grover SR. Quality of life and menstruation in adolescents. Curr Opin Obstet Gynecol 2015;27(5):309–14.
67. Bruinvels G, Goldsmith E, Blagrove R, et al. Prevalence and frequency of menstrual cycle symptoms are associated with availability to train and compete: a study of 6812 exercising women recruited using the Strava exercise app. Br J Sports Med 2021;55(8):438–43.
68. De Sanctis V, Soliman A, Bernasconi S, et al. Primary dysmenorrhea in adolescents: prevalence, impact and recent knowledge. Pediatr Endocrinol Rev 2015; 13(2):512–20.

69. Al-Hemairi MH, Albokhari SM, Muzaffer MA. The Pattern of Juvenile Idiopathic Arthritis in a Single Tertiary Center in Saudi Arabia. Int J Inflam 2016;2016: 7802957.
70. Li SH, Lloyd AR, Graham BM. Physical and mental fatigue across the menstrual cycle in women with and without generalised anxiety disorder. Horm Behav 2020;118:104667.
71. Latman NS. Relation of menstrual cycle phase to symptoms of rheumatoid arthritis. Am J Med 1983;74(6):957–60.
72. Colangelo K, Haig S, Bonner A, et al. Self-reported flaring varies during the menstrual cycle in systemic lupus erythematosus compared with rheumatoid arthritis and fibromyalgia. Rheumatology (Oxford) 2011;50(4):703–8.
73. Birru Talabi M, Eudy AM, Jayasundara M, et al. Pregnancy, periods, and "The Pill": exploring the reproductive experiences of women with inflammatory arthritis. ACR Open Rheumatol 2019;1(2):125–32.
74. Greene R, Stratton P, Cleary SD, et al. Diagnostic experience among 4,334 women reporting surgically diagnosed endometriosis. Fertil Steril 2009; 91(1):32–9.
75. Agarwal SK, Chapron C, Giudice LC, et al. Clinical diagnosis of endometriosis: a call to action. Am J Obstet Gynecol 2019;220(4):354.e1–12.
76. Harris HR, Costenbader KH, Mu F, et al. Endometriosis and the risks of systemic lupus erythematosus and rheumatoid arthritis in the Nurses' Health Study II. Ann Rheum Dis 2016;75(7):1279–84.
77. Xue YH, You LT, Ting HF, et al. Increased risk of rheumatoid arthritis among patients with endometriosis: a nationwide population-based cohort study. Rheumatology (Oxford) 2021;60(7):3326–33.
78. Shigesi N, Kvaskoff M, Kirtley S, et al. The association between endometriosis and autoimmune diseases: a systematic review and meta-analysis. Hum Reprod Update 2019;25(4):486–503.
79. Azziz R, Woods KS, Reyna R, et al. The prevalence and features of the polycystic ovary syndrome in an unselected population. J Clin Endocrinol Metab 2004; 89(6):2745–9.
80. Bremer AA. Polycystic ovary syndrome in the pediatric population. Metab Syndr Relat Disord 2010;8(5):375–94.
81. Oray M, Abu Samra K, Ebrahimiadib N, et al. Long-term side effects of glucocorticoids. Expert Opin Drug Saf 2016;15(4):457–65.
82. Edens C, Antonelli M. Polycystic Ovarian Syndrome in Rheumatic Disease [abstract]. Arthritis Rheumatol 2017;69(suppl 10).
83. Gold M. The ABCs of L.G.B.T.Q.I.A.+. New York Times. 2018. Available at: https://www.nytimes.com/2018/06/21/style/lgbtq-gender-language.html. Accessed May 5, 2021.
84. Rider GN, McMorris BJ, Gower AL, et al. Health and Care Utilization of Transgender and Gender Nonconforming Youth: A Population-Based Study. Pediatrics 2018;141(3):e20171683.
85. Grant J, Mottet L, Tanis L, et al. Injustice at every turn: a report of the national transgender discrimination survey. Washington: National Center for Transgender Equality and National Gay and Lesbian Task Force; 2011.
86. Eisenberg ME, Gower AL, Nic Rider G, et al. At the Intersection of Sexual Orientation and Gender Identity: Variations in Emotional Distress and Bullying Experience in a Large Population-based Sample of U.S. Adolescents. J LGBT Youth 2019;16(3):235–54.

87. Becerra-Culqui TA, Liu Y, Nash R, et al. Mental Health of Transgender and Gender Nonconforming Youth Compared With Their Peers. Pediatrics 2018; 141(5).
88. Lemelman M. Transformation of gender care: where we are and next steps. University of Chicago, Comer Children's Hospital;April 8, 2021.
89. Kreisel KM, Spicknall IH, Gargano JW, et al. Sexually Transmitted Infections Among US Women and Men: Prevalence and Incidence Estimates, 2018. Sex Transm Dis 2021;48(4):208–14.
90. CDC. Genital HPV Infection – Fact Sheet. Human Papillomavirus (HPV). 2016. Available at: https://www.cdc.gov/std/hpv/HPV-FS-print.pdf.
91. Dunne EF, Unger ER, Sternberg M, et al. Prevalence of HPV infection among females in the United States. JAMA 2007;297(8):813–9.
92. Steinau M, Hariri S, Gillison ML, et al. Prevalence of cervical and oral human papillomavirus infections among US women. J Infect Dis 2014;209(11):1739–43.
93. Hopenhayn C, Christian A, Christian WJ, et al. Prevalence of human papillomavirus types in invasive cervical cancers from 7 US cancer registries before vaccine introduction. J Low Genit Tract Dis 2014;18(2):182–9.
94. Mix JM, Van Dyne EA, Saraiya M, et al. Assessing Impact of HPV Vaccination on Cervical Cancer Incidence among Women Aged 15-29 Years in the United States, 1999-2017: An Ecologic Study. Cancer Epidemiol Biomarkers Prev 2021;30(1):30–7.
95. Liao C, Caesar M, Chan C, et al. HPV associated cancers in the United States over the last 15 years: Has screening or vaccination made any difference? Journal of Clinical Oncology 2021;39(15_suppl).
96. Drolet M, Benard E, Perez N, et al. Group HPVVIS. Population-level impact and herd effects following the introduction of human papillomavirus vaccination programmes: updated systematic review and meta-analysis. Lancet 2019; 394(10197):497–509.
97. Wodi AP, Ault K, Hunter P, et al. Advisory Committee on Immunization Practices Recommended Immunization Schedule for Children and Adolescents Aged 18 Years or Younger — United States, 2021. MMWR Morb Mortal Wkly Rep 2021; 70:189–92.
98. Singh JA, Furst DE, Bharat A, et al. 2012 update of the 2008 American College of Rheumatology recommendations for the use of disease-modifying antirheumatic drugs and biologic agents in the treatment of rheumatoid arthritis. Arthritis Care Res (Hoboken) 2012;64(5):625–39.
99. Feldman CH, Hiraki L, Lii J, et al. Human Papillomavirus vaccine uptake among children and young adults with autoimmune diseases. Arthritis Rheum 2013; 65(suppl 10).
100. Bizjak M, Blazina S, Zajc Avramovic M, et al. Vaccination coverage in children with rheumatic diseases. Clin Exp Rheumatol 2020;38(1):164–70.
101. Kim SC, Feldman S, Moscicki AB. Risk of human papillomavirus infection in women with rheumatic disease: cervical cancer screening and prevention. Rheumatology (Oxford) 2018;57(suppl_5):v26–33.
102. Corbitt K, Lopez I, Culpepper S. Sjogren's syndrome and its risk of cervical lesions [abstract]. Arthritis Rheumatol 2020;72.
103. Feldman CH, Liu J, Feldman S, et al. Risk of high-grade cervical dysplasia and cervical cancer in women with systemic lupus erythematosus receiving immunosuppressive drugs. Lupus 2017;26(7):682–9.

104. Kim SC, Glynn RJ, Giovannucci E, et al. Risk of high-grade cervical dysplasia and cervical cancer in women with systemic inflammatory diseases: a population-based cohort study. Ann Rheum Dis 2015;74(7):1360–7.
105. Wadstrom H, Arkema EV, Sjowall C, et al. Cervical neoplasia in systemic lupus erythematosus: a nationwide study. Rheumatology (Oxford) 2017;56(4):613–9.
106. Heijstek MW, Scherpenisse M, Groot N, et al. Immunogenicity and safety of the bivalent HPV vaccine in female patients with juvenile idiopathic arthritis: a prospective controlled observational cohort study. Ann Rheum Dis 2014;73(8): 1500–7.
107. Esposito S, Corona F, Barzon L, et al. Immunogenicity, safety and tolerability of a bivalent human papillomavirus vaccine in adolescents with juvenile idiopathic arthritis. Expert Rev Vaccines 2014;13(11):1387–93.
108. Soybilgic A, Onel KB, Utset T, et al. Safety and immunogenicity of the quadrivalent HPV vaccine in female Systemic Lupus Erythematosus patients aged 12 to 26 years. Pediatr Rheumatol Online J 2013;11:29.
109. Liu EY, Smith LM, Ellis AK, et al. Quadrivalent human papillomavirus vaccination in girls and the risk of autoimmune disorders: the Ontario Grade 8 HPV Vaccine Cohort Study. CMAJ 2018;190(21):E648–55.
110. Grimaldi-Bensouda L, Guillemot D, Godeau B, et al. Autoimmune disorders and quadrivalent human papillomavirus vaccination of young female subjects. J Intern Med 2014;275(4):398–408.
111. American College of Obstetricians and Gynecologists. Updated Cervical Cancer Screening Guidelines. 2021. Available at: https://www.acog.org/clinical/clinical-guidance/practice-advisory/articles/2021/04/updated-cervical-cancer-screening-guidelines. Accessed May 25, 2021.
112. Fontham ETH, Wolf AMD, Church TR, et al. Cervical cancer screening for individuals at average risk: 2020 guideline update from the American Cancer Society. CA Cancer J Clin 2020;70(5):321–46.
113. Moscicki AB, Flowers L, Huchko MJ, et al. Guidelines for cervical cancer screening in immunosuppressed women without HIV infection. J Low Genit Tract Dis 2019;23(2):87–101.
114. Ferreira GRV, Tomioka RB, Queiroz LB, et al. Lower genital tract infections in young female juvenile idiopathic arthritis patients. Adv Rheumatol 2019; 59(1):50.
115. Parikh-Patel A, White RH, Allen M, et al. Risk of cancer among rheumatoid arthritis patients in California. Cancer Causes Control 2009;20(6):1001–10.
116. Cobo-Ibanez T, Urruticoechea-Arana A, Rua-Figueroa I, et al. Hormonal dependence and cancer in systemic lupus erythematosus. Arthritis Care Res (Hoboken) 2020;72(2):216–24.
117. Nordstrom BL, Mines D, Gu Y, et al. Risk of malignancy in children with juvenile idiopathic arthritis not treated with biologic agents. Arthritis Care Res (Hoboken) 2012;64(9):1357–64.
118. United States Preventative Service Task Force (USPSTF). Screening for testicular cancer: brief evidence update. Rockville (MD): Agency for Healthcare Research and Quality; 2004.
119. Gotestam Skorpen C, Hoeltzenbein M, Tincani A, et al. The EULAR points to consider for use of antirheumatic drugs before pregnancy, and during pregnancy and lactation. Ann Rheum Dis 2016;75(5):795–810.
120. Sammaritano LR, Bermas BL, Chakravarty EE, et al. 2020 American College of Rheumatology Guideline for the Management of Reproductive Health in

Rheumatic and Musculoskeletal Diseases. Arthritis Care Res (Hoboken) 2020; 72(4):461–88.
121. Boumpas DT, Austin HA 3rd, Vaughan EM, et al. Risk for sustained amenorrhea in patients with systemic lupus erythematosus receiving intermittent pulse cyclophosphamide therapy. Ann Intern Med 1993;119(5):366–9.
122. Meistrich ML, Wilson G, Brown BW, et al. Impact of cyclophosphamide on long-term reduction in sperm count in men treated with combination chemotherapy for Ewing and soft tissue sarcomas. Cancer 1992;70(11):2703–12.
123. Aikawa NE, Sallum AM, Pereira RM, et al. Subclinical impairment of ovarian reserve in juvenile systemic lupus erythematosus after cyclophosphamide therapy. Clin Exp Rheumatol 2012;30(3):445–9.
124. Gajjar R, Miller SD, Meyers KE, et al. Fertility preservation in patients receiving cyclophosphamide therapy for renal disease. Pediatr Nephrol 2015;30(7): 1099–106.
125. Brunner HI, Bishnoi A, Barron AC, et al. Disease outcomes and ovarian function of childhood-onset systemic lupus erythematosus. Lupus 2006;15(4):198–206.
126. Nahata L, Sivaraman V, Quinn GP. Fertility counseling and preservation practices in youth with lupus and vasculitis undergoing gonadotoxic therapy. Fertil Steril 2016;106(6):1470–4.
127. Yazdany J, Panopalis P, Gillis JZ, et al. A quality indicator set for systemic lupus erythematosus. Arthritis Rheum 2009;61(3):370–7.
128. Bermas BL. Paternal safety of anti-rheumatic medications. Best Pract Res Clin Obstet Gynaecol 2020;64:77–84.
129. Weber-Schoendorfer C, Chambers C, Wacker E, et al. Pregnancy outcome after methotrexate treatment for rheumatic disease prior to or during early pregnancy: a prospective multicenter cohort study. Arthritis Rheumatol 2014;66(5):1101–10.
130. Martinez Lopez JA, Loza E, Carmona L. Systematic review on the safety of methotrexate in rheumatoid arthritis regarding the reproductive system (fertility, pregnancy, and breastfeeding). Clin Exp Rheumatol 2009;27(4):678–84.
131. Ferreira GRV, Tomioka RB, Aikawa NE, et al. Ovarian reserve in young juvenile idiopathic arthritis patients. Mod Rheumatol 2019;29(3):447–51.
132. de Araujo DB, Yamakami LY, Aikawa NE, et al. Ovarian reserve in adult patients with childhood-onset lupus: a possible deleterious effect of methotrexate? Scand J Rheumatol 2014;43(6):503–11.
133. Sifontis NM, Coscia LA, Constantinescu S, et al. Pregnancy outcomes in solid organ transplant recipients with exposure to mycophenolate mofetil or sirolimus. Transplantation 2006;82(12):1698–702.
134. Mycophenolate REMS. Available at: https://www.mycophenolaterems.com/. Accessed Sept 5, 2021.
135. Andreoli L, Bertsias GK, Agmon-Levin N, et al. EULAR recommendations for women's health and the management of family planning, assisted reproduction, pregnancy and menopause in patients with systemic lupus erythematosus and/ or antiphospholipid syndrome. Ann Rheum Dis 2017;76(3):476–85.
136. Fukushima R, Kanamori S, Hirashiba M, et al. Teratogenicity study of the dihydroorotate-dehydrogenase inhibitor and protein tyrosine kinase inhibitor Leflunomide in mice. Reprod Toxicol 2007;24(3–4):310–6.
137. Chambers CD, Johnson DL, Robinson LK, et al. Birth outcomes in women who have taken leflunomide during pregnancy. Arthritis Rheum 2010;62(5): 1494–503.

138. Uhler ML, Hsu JW, Fisher SG, et al. The effect of nonsteroidal anti-inflammatory drugs on ovulation: a prospective, randomized clinical trial. Fertil Steril 2001; 76(5):957–61.
139. Mendonca LL, Khamashta MA, Nelson-Piercy C, et al. Non-steroidal anti-inflammatory drugs as a possible cause for reversible infertility. Rheumatology (Oxford) 2000;39(8):880–2.
140. Food and Drug Administration. FDA recommends avoiding use of NSAIDs in pregnancy at 20 weeks or later because they can result in low amniotic fluid. October 15, 2020. Available at: https://www.fda.gov/media/142967/download.
141. Koren G, Florescu A, Costei AM, et al. Nonsteroidal antiinflammatory drugs during third trimester and the risk of premature closure of the ductus arteriosus: a meta-analysis. Ann Pharmacother 2006;40(5):824–9.
142. Klaus G, Jux C, Fernandez P, et al. Suppression of growth plate chondrocyte proliferation by corticosteroids. Pediatr Nephrol 2000;14(7):612–5.
143. Perloff WH, Channick BJ. Effect of prednisone on abnormal menstrual function. Am J Obstet Gynecol 1959;77(1):138–43.
144. Brouwer J, Hazes JM, Laven JS, et al. Fertility in women with rheumatoid arthritis: influence of disease activity and medication. Ann Rheum Dis 2015; 74(10):1836–41.
145. Park-Wyllie L, Mazzotta P, Pastuszak A, et al. Birth defects after maternal exposure to corticosteroids: prospective cohort study and meta-analysis of epidemiological studies. Teratology 2000;62(6):385–92.
146. Palmsten K, Bandoli G, Watkins J, et al. Oral corticosteroids and risk of preterm birth in the california medicaid program. J Allergy Clin Immunol Pract 2021;9(1): 375–84.e5.
147. ACOG Committee Opinion No. 475: antenatal corticosteroid therapy for fetal maturation. Obstet Gynecol 2011;117(2 Pt 1):422–4.
148. Friedman JM. ACE inhibitors and congenital anomalies. N Engl J Med 2006; 354(23):2498–500.
149. Starling LD, Sinha A, Boyd D, et al. Fetal warfarin syndrome. BMJ Case Rep 2012;2012. bcr2012007344.
150. Harry O, Crosby LE, Smith AW, et al. Self-management and adherence in childhood-onset systemic lupus erythematosus: what are we missing? Lupus 2019;28(5):642–50.
151. Cooper AM, Horwitz M, Becker ML. Improving the safety of teratogen prescribing practices in a pediatric rheumatology clinic. Pediatrics 2019;143(4): e20180803.

The Impact of Pediatric Rheumatic Diseases on Sexual Health, Family Planning, and Pregnancy

Cuoghi Edens, MD[a,b,*]

KEYWORDS

- Reproductive health • Pediatric rheumatology • Pregnancy • Contraception
- Infertility • Sexual transmitted infections • Marriage • Dating

KEY POINTS

- Reproductive health is an integral topic in pediatric rheumatology.
- Having a pediatric-onset rheumatic disease greatly impacts romantic relationships and sexual intercourse.
- Patients with pediatric rheumatic disease need multi-disciplinary care to meet their family planning needs and desires.
- Successful pregnancies are possible in patients with rheumatic diseases diagnosed in childhood.

INTRODUCTION

As a child progresses through adolescence and matures into a young adult, they face new challenges in regard to their rheumatic disease and potential implications on their reproductive and sexual health. Rheumatology care providers must address the expanding potential for social activity changes that may affect a patient's disease or treatment. As most pediatric-onset rheumatic diseases continue well into late adolescence and young adulthood,[1,2] an age group still cared for by pediatric rheumatologists,[3] these specialists must address pertinent reproductive health topics such as contraception, sex, and pregnancy.[4] As they become active participants in their health care, patients begin to ask questions about their rheumatic disease and its impact on their reproductive future and desire to take part in these conversations.[5]

[a] Department of Pediatrics, Section of Pediatric Rheumatology, University of Chicago Medicine, 5841 South Maryland Avenue, C104-A, MC5044, Chicago, IL 60637, USA; [b] Department of Internal Medicine, Section of Rheumatology, University of Chicago Medicine, 5841 South Maryland Avenue, C104-A, MC5044, Chicago, IL 60637, USA
* Corresponding author.
E-mail address: cedens@peds.bsd.uchicago.edu
Twitter: @CuoghiE (C.E.)

Rheum Dis Clin N Am 48 (2022) 113–140
https://doi.org/10.1016/j.rdc.2021.09.016
rheumatic.theclinics.com

As a young adults likely engaging in sexual intercourse, increased adverse events can occur unless appropriately counseled, which is unlikely to be happening in the primary care setting due to avoidance, time constraints, and lack of primary care altogether.[6–8] Although pediatric providers may feel a patient engaging in "adult" activities may be better served by rheumatologists trained to see older patients inquiry into sexual health is also lacking in the adult care environment.[9,10] The close and frequent-contact relationship adolescent and young adult (AYA) patients have with their pediatric rheumatology provider can be leveraged to address reproductive and sexual health.

Most rheumatic diseases have a female predilection; therefore, more greatly impacting childbearing and its prevention, while raising questions about fertility. Medical and social lore also exist regarding rheumatic diseases and multiple facets of reproductive health, particularly pregnancy, and rheumatologists are called on to dispel these myths. Men also benefit from addressing these topics as they too have concerns about the impact of their disease on reproductive health. Although pediatric rheumatologists' knowledge may be modest, patients desire their involvement in their sexual and reproductive health, particularly around topics such as pregnancy.[11]

SEX

Sex is an innate behavior on the biological ascent to adulthood. Almost one-half of the US high school students have had sex, roughly 7% before the age of 13. Three percent and 11% of men and women, respectively, ages 15 to 19, report a sexual experience with the same-sex partner.[12] Although presumed to be sexually inactive or disinterested, neither chronic illness nor physical disability hampers one's sexual activity; adolescent and young adult (AYA) patients are as sexually active as their peers.[13,14] This bias, however, limits the sexual education this population receives from medical providers.[15] Data show that a comparable number of patients with juvenile idiopathic arthritis (JIA) are as sexually active as the general population.[16]

Pediatric rheumatologists do not routinely screen for sexual activity, with only 12% inquiring and only one-third comfortable doing so.[17] Primary care providers are also deficient in this investigation.[18] Embarrassment around sex exists in the patient–provider relationship, making it a difficult topic for either party to bring up.[19] AYA with rheumatic diseases revealed altered discussions around sex and intimacy, with the discussions being less private and not just with their partner but including family and care team.[5]

Rheumatic diseases complicate sexual intercourse physically and contribute to sexual dysfunction. In adults, inflammatory arthritis and systemic lupus erythematosus (SLE) affect intercourse and intimacy due to pain or fear of pain, fatigue, erectile dysfunction, diminished sexual desire, and sexual function fluctuations with disease flares.[20–22] In the limited, dated pediatric data that exists, a large proportion of patients with JIA expressed disease-related sexual dysfunction.[16,23] Arthritis involving the hip, a joint commonly afflicted by JIA, contributes the most to sexual dysfunction in adults.[24] One could postulate that temporomandibular joint involvement, also commonly affected by JIA, could contribute to pain or impairment during kissing or oral sex in addition to self-esteem issues and worry over appearance due to micrognathia. Rheumatic diseases that affect the hand whether muscle, joint, skin, or vasculature can also contribute to sexual dysfunction. Cardiopulmonary involvement may also physically hamper sexual activity.

Vaginal and oral dryness from primary or secondary Sjögren's syndrome in SLE, rheumatoid arthritis (RA), and systemic sclerosis and can lead to significant sexual dysfunction as well as pain.[25,26] Specifically in patients with systemic sclerosis, genital skin tightening causes physical sexual dysfunction.[27] Chronic noninflammatory musculoskeletal pain and fibromyalgia, common comorbidities in patients with rheumatic diseases, may also contribute to sexual dysfunction.[26,28] Concomitant anxiety and depression, prevalent across rheumatic diseases, also affect sexual interest and libido as can negative body image whether from disease or medications.[29,30]

Sexual health and satisfaction with one's sex life contribute highly to the overall quality of life, even for those in poor health. Those in poorer health report lower sexual satisfaction. Accordingly, sexual health should be a routine part of patient assessments.[31] Psychological dimensions of a sexual relationship including being there for another person, psychological closeness, feeling loved, and caring for someone are often reported lacking in patients with rheumatic disease.[32,33] Literature that specifically looks at pediatric sexual dysfunction is sparse, what exists shows AYA across genders fare better than adults sexually, suggesting that a diagnosis earlier in life allows for more adept compensation and adaptation.[34,35]

Medications used to treat rheumatic diseases may contribute to sexual dysfunction. Those that cause hirsutism, hair loss, acne, or weight gain, affect self-esteem. Corticosteroids are known to decrease sexual drive.[36]

Sadly sexual violence is increased in those with chronic diseases.[14,37] Those 12 to 34 years of age have the highest rates of rape and sexual assault with unwanted first sexual encounters reported among 11% of both female and male subjects 18 to 24.[38,39] As the medical provider a patient may trust most, this uncomfortable topic may arise and pediatric rheumatologists need to be able to provide resource information and care for the patient.

CONTRACEPTIVES AND EMERGENCY CONTRACEPTION

Although identified as a top concern of pediatric rheumatologists, at this time there are no guidelines specifically addressing contraception in those with pediatric rheumatic diseases. Guidelines do exist from the American College of Obstetrics and Gynecology (ACOG) and American Academy of Pediatrics (AAP) on contraception appropriateness in those less than 18 years of age, regardless of medical history.[40] The United States Medical Eligibility Criteria provides contraception guidance based on diagnosis or medical history and denotes contraception compatibility through evidence-based (often limited) categorization.[41] In 2020, the American College of Rheumatology (ACR) published *Guideline for the Management of Reproductive Health in Rheumatic and Musculoskeletal Diseases* outlining recommendations to enhance the care of adults with rheumatic diseases.[42] Although some of the recommendations are ill-suited for the pediatric population, the evidence-based contraception guidelines can be used in the pediatric rheumatic community, as age is not an exclusion to any contraceptive.[43] Contraception recommendations are based on antiphospholipid antibody (aPL) status, rheumatic disease, disease activity, and reliability. Aligning with ACR guidelines, both the AAP and ACOG support the use of long-acting reversible contraceptives (LARCs) in the pediatric population due to their efficacy, increased compliance, and decreased risk of thrombosis than other contraceptives. Neither sexual activity nor prior pregnancy is prerequisites for LARCs, which include hormonal and copper intrauterine devices (IUDs) as well hormonal implants.[43,44] Condoms should be advised in all patients due to their unique ability to prevent sexually transmitted infections (STIs).

Contraception plays an important role in the care of patients with rheumatic diseases of all ages, although decreased contraceptive utilization has been found than their peers.[45] Preventing unwanted pregnancy is a health care aim among teens and young adults including those with rheumatic diseases. Teratogenic medication use and disease processes that could be made worse by pregnancy or cause a negative fetal outcome, coupled with the socioeconomic impacts of teen pregnancy that disproportionately affect patients of color who also more often have systemic rheumatic diseases, highlight contraception needs in pediatric rheumatology. Research has also shown that pregnancy outcomes for those with rheumatic diseases improve if conception is planned, allowing for the transition to pregnancy-compatible medications, optimal disease control, and appropriate prenatal care.[46,47] In the United States, approximately 50% of all pregnancies are unplanned, but in the 15 to 19 age range, this escalates to over 80%,[48] the age range coinciding with a peak onset of many rheumatic diseases. In view of this statistical, it is not surprising that over 50% of female adolescents report using the withdrawal method or condoms alone for contraception, which have only 50% and 80% efficacy, respectively.[38]

Table 1 provides evidence-based contraception guidance specific to patients with rheumatic disease. Gynecologic and rheumatic tradition exist that combined hormone contraceptives, or even more conservatively, progestin-only methods are not suitable for patients with rheumatic disease, particularly those with SLE, irrespective of aPL status, due to the risk of thrombosis or disease flare; *however, this has been disproven*.[49,50] APL status is an important determinant of contraceptive appropriateness across diseases, with positivity seen not only in SLE but also upwards of one-fourth of patients with JIA, RA, Sjögren's, and mixed connective tissue disease (MCTD).[51–55] Screening for these coagulation risk factors is prudent in all rheumatology patients seeking contraception. Other rheumatology-specific concerns arise when evaluating specific contraceptives. Most of the pediatric rheumatology patients are on immunosuppressive agents so LARCs potentially could increase postinsertion infections; however, this has not been documented in rheumatology patients nor seen in other immunocompromised populations.[56,57] Thrombocytopenia and the use of anticoagulants are also a procedural concern; however, this is theoretic as no published literature demonstrates poor outcomes in this population.

Table 1
Contraception in patients with rheumatic diseases[a]

(Arrows: Compliance − to +; Effectiveness − to +)

	Positive aPL testing in any rheumatic disease	Negative aPL testing		Special considerations in AYA
		SLE	Other rheumatic disease	
Progestin Implant[b]	✓	✓	✓	Discrete once healed, high cost if not using insurance/rec'ing at low-cost clinic. Irregular bleeding
IUD[b] (hormonal or copper)	✓	✓	✓	Discrete, invasive procedure, high cost if not using insurance/rec'ing at low-cost clinic. Cramping/heavier menses w/copper IUD
DMPA Injection	—	✓	✓	Discrete but needs to be administered q3months. Loss of bone mass. Weight gain & irregular bleeding
Progesterone Only Pill	✓	✓	✓	Daily consistency to be effective. Prescription needed
Contraceptive Patch	✗	✗	✓	Discrete, weekly self-placement. Prescription needed
Contraceptive Ring	✗	—	✓	Discrete, monthly self-insertion. Prescription needed
Combined Hormone Contraceptive Pill	✗	—	✓	Discrete, daily. Prescription needed. Best for Acne, PMS
Barrier Protection	✓	✓	✓	No prescription needed for some forms, STI protection

Key
✓ Strongly recommend
- Conditionally recommend
✗ Recommend against

[a]Adapted from Sammaritano L et al . 2020 American College of Rheumatology Guideline for the Management of Reproductive Health in Rheumatic and Musculoskeletal Diseases. Arthritis Rheumatol. 2020 Apr;72(4):529-556.
[b]Long-acting reversible contraception (LARC)

Although contraception in adult patients is most often used for pregnancy-prevention, pediatric patients use contraceptives to manage acne, premenstrual syndrome (PMS), premenstrual dysphoric disorder (PMDD), dysmenorrhea, metrorrhagia, menorrhagia, hirsutism, polycystic ovarian syndrome (PCOS), endometriosis, menstruation-related iron deficiency anemia, and menstrual headaches. Contraceptives are also used to regulate cycles allowing for the ease of participation in sports, work, travel, and educational pursuits.[58] Patients with rheumatic diseases may also welcome the contraceptive side effects of oligomenorrhea or amenorrhea as a significant upper extremity or hip arthritis, sclerodactyly, or other rheumatic disease manifestation can make menstrual care difficult.

Noncontraceptive benefits of contraception specific for rheumatic disease patients include disease improvement with fewer flares reported in adult SLE and RA contraception users.[9,59–61] Menorrhagia for those on anticoagulants may improve as most contraceptive modalities decrease uterine lining thickness as its pregnancy-prevention mechanism.[62] The detrimental sequelae of systemic inflammation and corticosteroids use on bone health is abated by certain contraceptives. Medroxyprogesterone acetate (DMPA) injections, however, can negatively impact bone mass, specifically of concern in female teenagers, as girls accrue at least a third of their bone mass during adolescence. Multiple organizations have suggested a 2-year limit on the use of DMPA due to this finding, which may be potentiated in those with rheumatic diseases.[63]

Pediatric rheumatologists do not often discuss contraception with patients on teratogenic medications and unplanned pregnancies are a consequence.[17,64,65] Although no formal program exists, the use of known teratogens commonly used to treat rheumatic diseases such as cyclophosphamide, methotrexate, leflunomide, and angiotensin enzyme inhibitors merit at minimum a discussion of contraception need due to their teratogenic effects. Medications with teratogenic risk, such as mycophenolate mofetil, thalidomide, and lenalidomide, have recommendations for dual contraception from the FDA risk evaluation and mitigation strategy (REMS) program.[66–68] Rheumatologists may not have the training or time to have effective in-depth contraception conversations, however, should be able to refer a patient to such resources, collaborate with appropriate providers, and be aware of state-specific laws in regards to access.[69–71]

Barriers to contraception use in AYA include stigma, cost, confidentiality, provider misconceptions or beliefs of appropriateness, religious concerns, peer pressure, partner influence, and misconceptions about fertility. Few AYA acknowledges that the unawareness of contraception itself is a barrier to use.[72] Even the most counseled and prepared patient can have contraception failures, choose not to take contraceptives, or be the victim of sexual violence. Emergency contraception is available and recommended for all ages. Gynecologic societies are clear that there is no restriction to emergency contraception, including in those with increased risk of thrombosis or autoimmune diseases. **Table 2** reviews emergency contraception options that should be made available to patients with pediatric rheumatic disease.

Although contraception most often focuses on those with childbearing capabilities, discussing barrier contraception with male patients to prevent STIs as well as undesired fatherhood is also prudent. Men play a significant role in contraception choice and pregnancy prevention of women partners and want to be involved in this decision making although may have little knowledge.[73,74]

Abortion

The rate of induced abortion in those with rheumatic diseases is unclear. Although increased incidence might be expected in this population specifically due to

Table 2
Emergency contraception for adolescents and young adults with rheumatic diseases

Type	Timing after Sex	Restrictions	Advantages	Access
Copper IUD	Within 120 h	Wilson's Disease Copper allergy *Ok in SLE and aPL+* Expensive w/o insurance or low-cost clinic	Can remain in place long-term Discrete after placement	Requires appointment and procedure
Hormonal IUD[a]	Within 120 h	Breast cancer history *Ok in SLE and aPL+* Expensive w/o insurance or low-cost clinic	Can remain in place long-term Discrete after placement	Requires appointment and procedure
Ulipristal	Within 120 h	Less effective >88 kg *Ok in SLE and aPL+*	Discreet One time dose	Prescription needed
Levonorgestrel	Best <72 h, up to 120 h	Less effective >70 kg *Ok in SLE and aPL+*	Discreet One time dose	No prescription needed Available at pharmacies and online
Combined Hormonal Contraceptives "Yuzpe Method"	Best <72 h	**Avoid** if aPL + or other thrombophilia **Avoid** if the history of thrombosis *Ok in SLE*	Can be continued for ongoing prevention	Prescription needed

[a] Mirena® and Liletta® are the hormonal IUDs studied for emergency contraception.

conception while on teratogenic medications and disease activity or organ involvement that may contribute to an unsafe pregnancy, limited studies have not shown a significant increase compared to the general population.[75,76] Termination should be offered to patients with rheumatic diseases who do not desire to continue their pregnancy. Patients who conceive on teratogenic medications should be counseled on risks and pregnancy options, but due to the relatively low rates of teratogenicity, termination should not be the rule. Evaluation of patients after an abortion should be attempted due to potential disease flare which can occur akin to spontaneous abortion and in the postpartum period.[77]

SEXUALLY TRANSMITTED INFECTIONS

Significant health consequences including pregnancy complications, infertility, enhanced HIV transmission, and psychosocial sequelae can be traced to STIs. The most prevalent STIs in the United States include *Treponema pallidum* (syphilis),

Neisseria gonorrhoeae, Chlamydia trachomatis, Trichomonas vaginalis, hepatitis B, herpes simplex virus (HSV), human immunodeficiency virus (HIV), and human papillomavirus (HPV). STIs are spread predominantly by any mode of sexual contact in addition to blood or placental transfer. Although most rheumatic diseases do not go unnoticed for long, people can have an STI without overt symptoms for years contributing to the asymptomatic spread.

In the United States, whereby teen pregnancy rates have declined over recent years due to increased contraceptive availability, STIs rates have paradoxically increased.[78] Youth aged 15 to 24 years comprise 27% of the sexually active population but account for more than 50% of new STI cases each year.[79] As the provider seeing AYA more often than their primary care providers, rheumatologists play an important role in STI testing as well as diagnosis, particularly due to overlapping symptoms with rheumatic diseases. Having one STI increases the risk of contracting another, so STI screening needs to be broad. Clinically, STIs can cause rheumatic disease flares, mimic active disease, or cause symptoms unresponsive to immunosuppression.[80,81] It is unclear if being immunocompromised increases STI acquisition or symptoms, theoretically could contribute to severity. Notably, all 50 states allow minors to consent for STI testing and treatment and[71] a majority allow the prescription of STI treatment to partners in an effort to deter spread.[82]

Gonorrhea, Chlamydia, Trichomoniasis

Sixty-five percent of chlamydia cases and 50% of gonorrhea cases are found in 15 to 24 years old, making it a diagnosis likely to show up in the rheumatology clinic.[79] Women, as they are more often symptomatic, have increased incidence.[83] Although pelvic inflammatory disease (PID) is synonymous with gonorrhea and chlamydia, infection with either pathogen is a significant cause of infertility in both women and men.[84,85]

Evaluating for these STIs is important diagnostically as reactive and gonococcal arthritis can manifest as seronegative RA arthritis, spondyloarthritis, tenosynovitis as well as enthesitis-related arthritis. Onset typically occurs within 3 months of the sexual contraction. Both gonococcal and chlamydia-related arthritides are associated with HLA-B27 positivity.[86] Sexually acquired reactive arthritis is self-limited with resolution within 6 months on average, although a small percentage of patients may experience recurrent episodes or have a chronic course. Disseminated gonococcal infection can include fever, migratory arthritis, skin lesions, erythema nodosum, endocarditis, perihepatitis, osteomyelitis, pericarditis, and meningitis, overlapping with many rheumatic processes.[87] Screening for gonorrhea and chlamydia is recommended by the US Prevention Task Force (USPTF), AAP, ACOG for sexually active women age $\leq$24. Male screening is not recommended, but testing should be performed if symptomatic or having a known contact.

Often tested in unison with gonorrhea and chlamydia, trichomoniasis also causes PID and reactive arthritis. It is the most prevalent nonviral STI in the United States.[88] Screening recommendations do not exist.

Human Immunodeficiency Virus

Rash, myalgia, fatigue, fevers, oral sores, leukopenia, anemia, and thrombocytopenia can all be presenting symptoms of acute HIV, easily mistaken as SLE, inflammatory bowel disease (IBD), or Behcet's disease if a careful infectious investigation is not undertaken. Antinuclear antibody (ANA), as well as other antibody positivity, is often present in HIV-infected patients.[89,90] HIV can manifest with sicca symptoms due to diffuse idiopathic lymphocytic syndrome, easily misdiagnosed as parotitis presumed secondary to Sjögren's syndrome. HIV is part of the differential in a high-risk patient, particularly of the male gender with generalized lymphadenopathy with negative autoimmune serologies.[91] Arthritis and arthralgias have been described in patients with HIV and associated diagnoses include HIV-associated arthropathy, seronegative spondyloarthropathies, reactive arthritis, psoriatic arthritis, and RA. Osteonecrosis, vasculitis, and myositis are rare manifestations of HIV.[92] HIV screening is recommended once between ages 15 and 18 by the USPTF and is part of AAP recommendations, with annual screening for those high-risk.

Herpes Simplex Virus

HSV is among the most prevalent STIs. Usually subclinical, symptoms include recurrent, painful genital and or anal lesions, easily confused with Behcet's disease or IBD.[93] Patients with SLE with active disease are at increased risk of new and reactivated HSV.[94–96] Immunosuppression from medications including those used in rheumatology can resurrect quiescent oral or urogenital lesions, often resulting in medication noncompliance and discontinuation. Severe disseminated HSV also occurs in patients with rheumatic disease who are significantly immunocompromised. HSV screening is not recommended.

Syphilis

Teens and young adults are increasingly diagnosed with syphilis as its prevalence is growing in the general population.[97] Known as the "great imitator," syphilis should be part of the differential diagnosis for many patients with complex or multisystem a rheumatologist may be asked to provide consultation. Vasculitis of all vessel sizes, uveitis, SLE, sarcoidosis, Behcet's, and inflammatory arthritis have all been subsequently diagnosed as syphilis, this is complicated by ANA, anticardiolipin antibody, and rheumatoid factor positivity often found with this STI.[98–103] Syphilis screening is recommended only in high-risk groups, however, with increasing rates of this STI, practice change may be on the horizon.

Hepatitis B

Contacted through bodily fluids, hepatitis B is 50 to 100 times more infectious than HIV. Although infection most commonly causes hepatic inflammation both acute and chronic, there is an association with RA, polyarteritis nodosa, and mixed cryoglobulinemia and can present early on as serum sickness.[104,105] Screening recommendations exist before starting biologic therapy. Hepatitis B is part of the routine vaccinations recommended by the CDC for children and adults.[106] HPV is discussed in detail elsewhere (Early Sexual Health and Reproductive Implications in Pediatric Rheumatic Diseases).

ROMANTIC RELATIONSHIPS AND MARRIAGE

The impact of rheumatic disease on platonic relationships in pediatric rheumatology is complex. Likely multifactorial with unique attributes for each rheumatic disease, the range of physical and emotional challenges a rheumatic disease proposes may make romantic relationships difficult, particularly those that are long-term. As pediatric diseases are often more aggressive than their adult counterparts,[2,107] those diagnosed in childhood may be particularly affected due to potentially more severe health complications, distressing physical symptoms caused by the disease or treatment, overlapping mental health diagnoses, and other socialization factors facing those with chronic illnesses. If fertility is affected, this can negatively influence one's desire to pursue companionship. AYA with JIA note challenges in dating such as when to disclose their rheumatic diagnosis and worry that their partner will not understand their disease.[5,108]

Chronic illnesses strain relationships, whether new or well established, particularly if dealing with pain and physical limitations, not to mention medication side effects and disease-associated fatigue or body changes. Long-term physical and psychosocial impairment may hamper an AYA's relationship status and sexual activity.[109,110] In rheumatic diseases, relationships with sexual partners may take longer to establish, possibly because the relationship is not just a romantic partner but also potentially a caregiver.[111] Self-esteem, low in pediatric patients with chronic illnesses,[30] correlates closely with the quality of romantic relationships.[112] Age of diagnosis may impact relationship outcomes, whether resilience, adaptation, or disease remission is the reason, patients diagnosed younger have better psychosocial outcomes.[113]

Age at marriage as well as overall marriage rate are affected by a JIA diagnosis, patients with JIA being older and less likely to get married, even when compared with adult-onset arthritis counterparts.[16,114,115] More recent studies continue to demonstrate similar themes including worry regarding finding a partner and concern over partner disease comprehension and insight expressed by both patients and parents,[5] although rates of marriage in the biologic treatment era are now comparable to the general public.[116] The trend of remaining unpartnered is also present in patients with juvenile dermatomyositis (JDM) and childhood-onset SLE (cSLE).[117,118] Gender may play a role as males with JIA have greater difficulties than non-JIA men and JIA women establishing platonic relationships, although in SLE the opposite was found.[115] Marriage and marriage-like partnerships can positively influence both mental and physical quality of life in patients with rheumatic diseases, despite barriers to their formation.[119,120]

FERTILITY, OVARIAN INSUFFICIENCY, AND FERTILITY PRESERVATION

Most parents hope their child will eventually have children of their own, but when your child has a chronic illness, these aspirations may be curtailed.[121] Patients and parents of those with rheumatic diseases have expressed concern over the effect of their diagnosis on future fertility.[5,122] Infertility by definition is the failure to achieve a clinical pregnancy after 12 months of regular unprotected intercourse, whereas subfertility is a delay to achieve pregnancy.[123] The potential effects of pediatric rheumatic diseases on a child's future childbearing or fathering abilities are multifactorial with both disease and treatment-related contributors.

Inflammation itself likely impacts fertility in both men and women across rheumatic diseases. Plausibly, illness duration, with cumulative periods of disease flare, could itself contribute to infertility.[124] As pediatric-onset diseases can be more severe, and by the definition are of longer duration, infertility repercussions may be a reflection of uncontrollable variables such as disease severity at the onset and duration of disease. Alterations in the gonadotropin-releasing hormone (GnRH)–gonadotropin–gonadic (GGG) axis from physical stressors, illness, or medications such as corticosteroids have downstream effects on the hormones, which directly influence fertility, such as GnRH, prolactin, luteinizing hormone (LH), and follicle-stimulating hormone (FSH).[125] The resultant effect of systemic inflammation, therefore, causes gonadal dysfunction. This is best assessed through biochemical and ultrasonographic markers, as menses and testosterone formation can continue although infertility is present.

Antisperm, anticorpus luteum, and antiovary antibodies have been found in increasing numbers of patients with rheumatic diseases, although is it unclear if they contribute to difficulty conceiving.[126–128] Men of all ages with SLE have sperm abnormalities, decreased testicular volume, and impaired spermatogenesis, exclusive of treatment.[129,130] Testicular Sertoli cells, essential for sperm maturation, are diminished in testes of male lupians.[131] Gonadal function in women with SLE is abnormal with notable hormonal derangements. Antral follicle count, an estimation of ovarian reserve, is low in cSLE.[132,133]

Although some studies have found fertility unaffected in patients with JIA, as determined by live births, hormonal, and ultrasound parameters more specific to fertility potential have told a different story.[124] Serum markers reveal a decreased ovarian reserve independent of age, disease duration, medications, inflammatory markers, or disease activity scores.[134] Studies of patients with inflammatory arthropathy demonstrate lower anti-Müllerian hormone (AMH) levels than controls, AMH being a surrogate marker for ovarian reserve.[74,135] Following suit, women with RA pursue in vitro fertilization and intrauterine insemination more often than their peers.

Other inflammatory diseases diagnosed in childhood seem to have a causal relationship with a decreased ovarian reserve and therefore the possibility of fertility including Behcet's disease and periodic fever syndromes, likely due to ongoing systemic inflammation; however, sperm quality seems to be preserved.[136–138] Male JDM patients have abnormal sperm morphology.[138,139] Ovarian reserve is decreased in adults with Sjögren's patients and inflammatory myopathies, so infertility potentially exists in children diagnosed with these as well.[140]

Premature ovarian insufficiency (POI), defined as clinical end-stage ovarian function in women less than 40 years old, has replaced the former term premature ovarian failure. Thought to affect about 1% of the population, those affected are more likely to have associated autoimmunity with studies showing up to a 40% prevalence.[141,142] Increased POI is found in SLE, Sjögren's syndrome, RA, MCTD, systemic sclerosis, and antiphospholipid antibody syndrome (APS), although not well characterized in pediatric-onset disease.[143] POI may be due to abnormal self-recognition by the immune system, similar to other rheumatic disease pathogenesis, as oocyte antibodies, and lymphocytic oophoritis can also be present.[144] Determining the true cause of POI in patients with rheumatic diseases is challenging due to the concomitant use of cytotoxic agents obscuring causation.[145] Contradictory research exists as to whether SLE on its own, outside of cyclophosphamide use, contributes to POI, but evidence is accumulating toward a negative association.[132,146–148] Patients with long-standing and more severe JIA have increased incidence of POI.[16] POI has not been found in patients with JDM and young adults across inflammatory myopathies.[149]

Fertility preservation for AYA comes in many forms; however, most are not appropriate for the urgency and acuity of those with rheumatic diseases. Oocyte stimulation and ovarian tissue preservation, while effective, are often unsafe, costly, and timely in what are often critically ill patients with numerous risk factors for significant side effects.[150] Gaining popularity with hopes of becoming standard of care, GnRH agonists bring the ovaries to a prepubertal "resting" state, whereas receiving cytotoxic treatment and have been used with promising results, even long-term.[151–155] Challenges exist in using GnRH agonists due to insurance coverage as well as timing, but should be considered in menarchal patients in consultation with women's health specialists.

Cryopreservation, colloquially termed "sperm banking," should be offered to male patients Tanner III and beyond due to undergoing long-term cytotoxic therapy likely to result in gonadal dysfunction.[156] In studies of both pediatric nephrologists and rheumatologists, men with cSLE and ANCA-associated vasculitis (AAV) receiving cyclophosphamide are rarely offered this procedure despite the ease of collection and long term success.[157,158] Male fertility preservation is also fraught with hurdles to implementation. Fertility preservation guidelines exist from the ACR, the American Society of Reproductive Medicine, and multiple oncologic societies.[159,160] Inability to bear children has long-lasting psychological implications and efforts should be made to prevent this.[161]

PCOS, endometriosis, and STIs are also significant contributors to infertility in those with rheumatic diseases.[162,163]

PREGNANCY

A sentinel topic in the growing body of reproductive health and rheumatology knowledge, pregnancy is an area of interest for those with pediatric rheumatic diseases as well as their families. Most patients with AYA and their families focus more on future childbearing potential than pregnancy success, disease activity, or medication use during pregnancy.[5]

Teen pregnancy is a public health concern. Each year, approximately 750,000 15 to 19 year olds become pregnant, at least 80% of these pregnancies are unplanned.[164] Teen pregnancy has decreased over the past decade; however, racial and ethnic disparities exist, with higher rates of birth and abortion among Black and Hispanic adolescents, notably those with more severe, systemic rheumatic diseases.[165] Socioeconomic disadvantage exists for pregnant teens, of whom 20% will have a repeat teen birth.[166] 60% of teen parents do not graduate high school and only 2% graduate college.[167,168] Children born to teens are more likely to be placed in foster care, not finish high school, be incarcerated, and become teen parents themselves.[169] These sobering statistics highlight the personal and societal benefits of contraception.[170]

Pregnancies that occur when patients are still under the care of a pediatric rheumatologist often trigger an abrupt, uncoordinated transfer to adult rheumatic care out of provider anxiety and inexperience.[171] Complicated by delays and hurdles inherent in the current health care environment and a shortage of rheumatologists, a sudden change in rheumatic care due to a most-often unexpected pregnancy lacks the recommended transition preparation and assessment that increases the likelihood of success.[172] The transition period is one of the well-recognized health care vulnerability and medical treatment interruptions which can result in significant and even life-threatening disease flares, amplified by a high-risk pregnant AYA patient abruptly advised to transfer their rheumatic care.[173]

How does one help patients avoid an unplanned pregnancy? The HEADSSS assessment is a convenient, validated instrument to determine sexual activity.[174] The validated, patient-focused One Key Question "Would you like to become pregnant in the next year?"[175] easily identifies at-risk patients—those that are sexually active and answer "No" but are not using effective contraception as revealed on further questioning. It can also identify patients actively trying to become pregnant and aid in preconception counseling, medication changes, and disease optimization. This question, while geared to those able to carry children, can also be used for those able to father children with minor alterations.

Decreased number of children, increased age at first pregnancy, fear of passing their disease on to their children, fear of inability to care for a child or pregnant self, or deciding whether to conceive at all are concerns raised by AYA with pediatric rheumatic diseases.[16,115,176,177] Rheumatic disease activity and disability correlate negatively with these future childbearing concerns. Although treatment has improved dramatically, worries about disease implications on future childbearing remain the same and are similar to adults.[5] Future studies are needed to determine if improved medical management alters childbearing trends in those with pediatric-onset rheumatic diseases.

Few studies have specifically analyzed pregnancy outcomes in patients with cSLE while still under pediatric care. Unfortunately, studies evaluating pregnancies in adult patients rarely include disease duration as a variable, so it is unclear if cSLE is an additional pregnancy risk above and beyond the well-established risk factors of lupus nephritis, hypertension, antiphospholipid antibodies, active disease at conception or during pregnancy, and an unplanned pregnancy.[178–181] The only study to compare cSLE versus SLE did not find disease duration contributory.[182]

Adult-onset lupus pregnancies are more likely to be complicated by preeclampsia, preterm delivery, intrauterine growth restriction, low birth weight, stillbirth, and cesarean section than the general public. These poor outcomes are directly related to the prior list of risk factors. Maternal and infant death are also increased significantly than the general population.[183] Although progress has been made to reduce these statistics, lupus pregnancy outcomes continue to be worse than the public.[184] AYA SLE pregnancies have been specifically examined. Brazilian AYA with cSLE demonstrated significantly elevated spontaneous abortion rates (21%), correlating with elevated SLEDAI scores; however, study results were confounded by teratogenic medication use. Premature birth was increased and associated with glomerulonephritis, proteinuria, and hypertension if present early in pregnancy.[185] A review of AYA lupians in the United States had significantly increased incidence of pre-eclampsia/eclampsia, maternal death, preterm birth, spontaneous abortion, and induced abortion than age-matched controls.[186] As in adult studies, lower disease activity leading to improved pregnancy outcomes can be inferred.[187]

Studies regarding JIA pregnancy outcomes exist. The collection of studies, however, is small in subject number, span decades of JIA treatment advancements as well as the globe, making generalizations challenging. Further complicating the understanding of pregnancy outcomes in JIA, most of the studies only examine pregnancies in patients with a current diagnosis of JIA, so a patient with a prior diagnosis now in remission off medication are excluded as are patients whose diagnosis is changed on entering adult care, limiting data applicability. Like patients with adult-onset inflammatory arthritis, patients with JIA are more likely to have spontaneous abortions, preeclampsia, cesarean section delivery, premature delivery, postpartum hemorrhage, low birth weight infants, increased neonatal intensive care unit admissions, and increased neonatal mortality. For unclear reasons, increased cardiovascular comorbidities, including hypertension, have been reported in pregnant JIA patients.[16,187–194] It is promising that studies evaluating more modern cohorts show improved outcomes.[195] Corticosteroids and active disease preconception and during pregnancy are associated with poorer outcomes, particularly preterm delivery.[196] Biologic treatments either prior or during pregnancy and male use of DMARDs do not contribute to negative pregnancy outcomes.[197,198] Rheumatology medication compatibility preconception, during pregnancy, and in lactation can be found in **Table 3**; however, as a rapidly changing field, review of most recent research is encouraged, particularly for newer medications.

Noninfectious uveitis stays active early in pregnancy, and then, like inflammatory arthritis, improves in the 2nd trimester with the lowest activity in the 3rd trimester.[199] Unfortunately, like joint symptoms, uveitis also flares postpartum. In the case of JDM and autoinflammatory diseases, flares happen during pregnancy as well as after, increasing the risk of poor outcomes.[200–204] Pregnant women with any rheumatic disease should have maternal–fetal medicine as part of their pregnancy care team in

Table 3
Pregnancy compatibility of rheumatic medications[a]

	Compatible		Caution/Conditional		Not Compatible
Pre-Conception	Adalimumab	Golimumab	Abatacept	Discontinue at conception[b]	Cyclophosphamide+
	Anakinra	Hydroxychloroquine	Anakinra	Discontinue at conception	Leflunomide
	Azathioprine/6-MP	Infliximab	Belimumab	Discontinue at conception	Lenalidomide
	Belimumab	NSAIDs +	Cyclosporine	Monitor for HTN	Methotrexate
	Certolizumab	Prednisone+ (<20mg/day)	NSAIDs+	Discontinue if conception delay	Mycophenolate
	Colchicine	Rituximab	Prednisone+ >20mg/day	Discontinue at conception	Mycophenolic Acid
	Etanercept	Sulfasalazine+	Rituximab	Discontinue at conception	Thalidomide
			Secukinumab/IL-17 agents	Discontinue at conception	
			Ustekinumab/IL-23 agents	Discontinue at conception	
			Tacrolimus	Monitor for HTN	
			Tocilizumab/IL-6 agents	Discontinue at conception	
			Tofacitinib/other JAKi	Discontinue at conception	
Pregnancy	Adalimumab[c]	Prednisone	Abatacept	Limited data	Cyclophosphamide
	Azathioprine/6-MP	Sulfasalazine	Anakinra	Limited data	Leflunomide
	Certolizumab	Tacrolimus	Belimumab	Limited data	Lenalidomide
	Colchicine		NSAIDs	Stop at 20 weeks	Methotrexate
	Cyclosporine		Rituximab	Life/organ threatening disease	Mycophenolate

(*continued on next page*)

Table 3
(continued)

	Etanercept[c]		Secukinumab/IL-17 agents	Limited data	Mycophenolic Acid
	Golimumab[c]		Ustekinumab/IL-23 agents	Limited data	Thalidomide
	Hydroxychloroquine		Tocilizumab/IL-6 agents	Limited data	
	Infliximab[c]		Tofacitinib/other JAKi	Limited data	
Breastfeeding[d]	Abatacept	Etanercept	Tofacitinib/other JAKi	Limited data, small molecules	Cyclophosphamide
	Adalimumab	Golimumab			Leflunomide
	Anakinra	Hydroxychloroquine			Lenalidomide
	Azathioprine/6-MP	Infliximab			Methotrexate
	Belimumab	NSAIDs			Mycophenolate
	Certolizumab	Prednisone			Mycophenolic Acid
	Colchicine	Rituximab			Thalidomide
	Cyclosporine	Sulfasalazine			
	Tacrolimus				
	Secukinumab/IL-17 agents				
	Tocilizumab/IL-6 agents				
	Ustekinumab/IL-23 agents				

[a] Adapted from Sammaritano L et al. 2020 American College of Rheumatology Guideline for the Management of Reproductive Health in Rheumatic and Musculoskeletal Diseases. Arthritis Rheumatol. 2020 Apr;72(4):529 to 556.

[b] Decision to discontinue any medication at conception should be had in discussion with patient, subspecialist, women's health provider, and after the review of most up to date literature.

[c] If well controlled rheumatic disease, consider discontinuation in 3rd trimester due to increased placental transfer, if flares can restart. Do not discontinue if the patient has IBD.

[d] Monoclonal antibodies are large molecules with a low passage rate into breast milk, if any does pass, likely destroyed in the infant's gastrointestinal tract. +Medications that may affect fertility, sulfasalazine only impacts men.

addition to rheumatology, obstetrics, and other subspecialists based on disease manifestations.

Aside from the risks inherent to pregnancy itself or medications, there are disease-specific topics that merit mention. Due to the increased risk of pre-eclampsia in women with SLE and APS, low-dose aspirin is recommended to reduce the development of this serious pregnancy complication.[205] This recommendation may spread to other rheumatic diseases in the future. Patients with positive aPLs and thrombotic APS with or without SLE, face additional pregnancy challenges including maternal thrombosis as well as miscarriage, stillbirth, and preeclampsia.[206] Guidelines exist for perinatal anticoagulation to decrease negative outcomes.[207] Low dose aspirin is also recommended by ACR for patients with positive aPLs to aid in the reduction of preeclampsia. Increasingly seen across rheumatic diseases, patients should, therefore, be tested for aPLs if pregnant, considering, or multiple miscarriages.

While most often not contemplating pregnancy while receiving pediatric rheumatology care, patients with anti-SSA and anti-SSB antibody positivity need counseling due to their antibody status and its associated risk of future pregnancy complications, regardless of their diagnosis. Anti-SSA, and less so anti-SSB, antibodies cross the placenta with possible dermatologic, hepatic, hematopoietic, and, most concerning, cardiac sequelae, collectively coined neonatal lupus. High-risk obstetric care, provided by maternal fetal medicine, including fetal cardiac monitoring is recommended and hydroxychloroquine is considered to decrease the risk of congenital heart block.[42] Anti-SSA and anti-SSB antibody screening should occur in all rheumatic disease pregnancies due to its presence in SLE, MCTD, systemic sclerosis, and inflammatory arthritis.[208] Lastly, the pediatric rheumatologist needs to be aware of the relative contraindications to pregnancy in patients with rheumatic disease and share this information with patients and families (**Box 1**). Screening pulmonary function testing and echocardiogram should be considered in patients with multi-organ system diseases when trying to conceive.

Box 1
Relative contraindications to pregnancy in rheumatic diseases[a]

Pulmonary hypertension

Severe restrictive lung disease (FVC < 1 L)

Severe valvular heart disease or advanced heart failure

Significant renal disease (Creatinine >2.8 mg/dL)

Cerebral vascular event in the past 6 mo

Severe preeclampsia or HELLP on aspirin and heparin

Teratogenic medications

[a]European Society of Gynecology (ESG); Association for European Pediatric Cardiology (AEPC); German Society for Gender Medicine (DGesGM), Regitz-Zagrosek V, et al. ESC Committee for Practice Guidelines. ESC Guidelines on the management of cardiovascular diseases during pregnancy: the Task Force on the Management of Cardiovascular Diseases during Pregnancy of the European Society of Cardiology (ESC). Eur Heart J. 2011 Dec;32(24):3147 to 97.

Data from Moroni, Gabriella et al. Pregnancy in lupus nephritis American Journal of Kidney Diseases, Volume 40, Issue 4, 713 to 720. de Jesus GR, Mendoza-Pinto C, de Jesus NR, Dos Santos FC, Klumb EM, Carrasco MG, Levy RA. Understanding and Managing Pregnancy in Patients with Lupus. Autoimmune Dis. 2015

Disease flares postpartum, theoretically due to rapid cytokine changes[209] and prolactin elevation,[210] are seen across the spectrum of rheumatic diseases. Adult literature across rheumatic diseases support the importance of well-controlled disease preconception and during pregnancy to lessen the likelihood of flare and optimize outcomes.[76,211] Pediatric postpartum data are limited to JIA whereby postpartum flares occur in upwards of 75% of pregnancies.[177,212,213] Postpartum disease activity has significant repercussions on a mother's ability to care for herself and her child, not to mention associated mental health concerns and accrued joint and organ damage.[214]

Assisted reproductive technologies (ARTs) such as in vitro fertilization should be offered to those with rheumatic diseases.[42] Stable autoimmune diseases without major organ damage do not affect ART outcomes. Successful pregnancy rates are similar to those of the general public. ART does not seem harmful to patients with preexisting autoimmune diseases, although precautions are indicated in those with a thrombotic history, APS, or positive aPLs.[215]

SUMMARY

As patients age, pediatric rheumatologists can play an important role in promoting their reproductive and sexual health. STIs and unintended pregnancies in AYA are preventable health outcomes with potentially serious, permanent sequelae. Rheumatology care presents unique opportunities to provide comprehensive education and reproductive health care services to adolescents and young adults. Patients with pediatric onset-rheumatic diseases require multi-disciplinary care throughout their lifetime to address their family planning needs and attain personal goals. Successful pregnancies are achievable, the best outcomes are associated with appropriate planning. Despite the progress of diagnostics and therapeutics across pediatric rheumatology over the last 20 years, questions remain about the impact of rheumatic diseases and their treatment on the many facets of reproductive health particularly relationships, infertility, pregnancy, and postpartum care.

CLINICS CARE POINTS

- Conduct pregnancy testing before the prescription/administration of teratogenic medications.
- Evaluate for STIs as they are common and mimic rheumatic diseases.
- Pursue fertility preservation for males Tanner stage III or greater as well as postmenarchal females undergoing cyclophosphamide treatment.
- Safe and effective contraceptives exist for all rheumatology patients, including those with antiphospholipid antibodies and a history of thrombosis.
- Emergency contraceptives are appropriate for patients with rheumatic diseases.
- Ask the One Key Question "Would you like to become pregnant in the next year?" to assess pregnancy intentions.
- Planned pregnancies have better maternal and fetal outcomes in patients with rheumatic diseases.

DISCLOSURE

The authors have nothing to disclose.

REFERENCES

1. Duarte CCM, Ines L, Liang M. In: Lahita Robert G, editor. Systemic lupus erythematosus. 5th Edition. Academic Press; 2011.
2. Oen K, Malleson PN, Cabral DA, Rosenberg AM, Petty RE, Cheang M. Disease course and outcome of juvenile rheumatoid arthritis in a multicenter cohort. J Rheumatol 2002;29(9):1989–99.
3. Johnson KR, Edens C, Sadun RE, et al. Differences in Healthcare Transition Views, Practices, and Barriers Among North American Pediatric Rheumatology Clinicians From 2010 to 2018. J Rheumatol 2021;48(9):1442–9.
4. Hays KLC, Huynh B, Ronis T, Edelheit B, Cook K, Mruk V, Edens C. Reproductive Health Knowledge Gaps, Needs, and Barriers Identified by Pediatric Rheumatology Providers [abstract]. Arthritis Rheumatol 2021;73.
5. Carandang K, Mruk V, Ardoin SP, et al. Reproductive health needs of adolescent and young adult women with pediatric rheumatic diseases. Pediatr Rheumatol Online J 2020;18(1):66.
6. Boekeloo BO. Will you ask? Will they tell you? Are you ready to hear and respond?: barriers to physician-adolescent discussion about sexuality. JAMA Pediatr 2014;168(2):111–3.
7. Alexander SC, Fortenberry JD, Pollak KI, et al. Sexuality talk during adolescent health maintenance visits. JAMA Pediatr 2014;168(2):163–9.
8. Yazdany J, Tonner C, Trupin L, et al. Provision of preventive health care in systemic lupus erythematosus: data from a large observational cohort study. Arthritis Res Ther 2010;12(3):R84.
9. Birru Talabi M, Eudy AM, Jayasundara M, et al. Pregnancy, Periods, and "The Pill": Exploring the Reproductive Experiences of Women with Inflammatory Arthritis. ACR Open Rheumatol 2019;1(2):125–32.
10. Birru Talabi M, Clowse MEB, Blalock SJ, Hamm M, Borrero S. Perspectives of Adult Rheumatologists Regarding Family Planning Counseling and Care: A Qualitative Study. Arthritis Care Res (Hoboken) 2020;72(3):452–8.
11. Wolgemuth T, Stransky OM, Chodoff A, Kazmerski TM, Clowse MEB, Birru Talabi M. Exploring the Preferences of Women Regarding Sexual and Reproductive Health Care in the Context of Rheumatology: A Qualitative Study. Arthritis Care Res (Hoboken) 2021;73(8):1194–200.
12. Chandra A, Mosher WD, Copen C, Sionean C. Sexual behavior, sexual attraction, and sexual identity in the United States: data from the 2006-2008 National Survey of Family Growth. Natl Health Stat Rep 2011;(36):1–36.
13. Alvin P, de Tournemire R, Anjot MN, Vuillemin L. [Chronic illness in adolescence: ten pertinent questions]. Arch Pediatr 2003;10(4):360–6.
14. Suris JC, Resnick MD, Cassuto N, Blum RW. Sexual behavior of adolescents with chronic disease and disability. J Adolesc Health 1996;19(2):124–31.
15. Holland-Hall C, Quint EH. Sexuality and Disability in Adolescents. Pediatr Clin North Am 2017;64(2):435–49.
16. Packham JC, Hall MA. Long-term follow-up of 246 adults with juvenile idiopathic arthritis: social function, relationships and sexual activity. Rheumatology (Oxford) 2002;41(12):1440–3.
17. De Ranieri D, Onel K, Wagner-Weiner L, and Tesher MS. Pregnancy and Contraception in Adolescents and Teens with SLE: Are pediatric rheumatologists adequately Screening and Educating Their Patients?. 2012 ACR/ARHP Annual Meeting. Washington, DC. November 9-14, 2012.

18. Britto MT, Rosenthal SL, Taylor J, Passo MH. Improving rheumatologists' screening for alcohol use and sexual activity. Arch Pediatr Adolesc Med 2000;154(5):478–83.
19. Ryan KL, Arbuckle-Bernstein V, Smith G, Phillips J. Let's Talk About Sex: A Survey of Patients' Preferences When Addressing Sexual Health Concerns in a Family Medicine Residency Program Office. PRiMER 2018;2:23.
20. Restoux LJ, Dasariraju SR, Ackerman IN, Van Doornum S, Romero L, Briggs AM. Systematic Review of the Impact of Inflammatory Arthritis on Intimate Relationships and Sexual Function. Arthritis Care Res (Hoboken) 2020; 72(1):41–62.
21. Bourg M, Ruyssen-Witrand A, Bettiol C, Parinaud J. Fertility and sexuality of women with inflammatory arthritis. Eur J Obstet Gynecol Reprod Biol 2020; 251:199–205.
22. Garcia Morales M, Callejas Rubio JI, Peralta-Ramirez MI, et al. Impaired sexual function in women with systemic lupus erythematosus: a cross-sectional study. Lupus 2013;22(10):987–95.
23. Moghadam ZB, Rezaei E, Faezi ST, Zareian A, Ibrahim FM, Ibrahim MM. Prevalence of sexual dysfunction in women with systemic lupus erythematosus and its related factors. Reumatologia 2019;57(1):19–26.
24. Abdel-Nasser AM, Ali EI. Determinants of sexual disability and dissatisfaction in female patients with rheumatoid arthritis. Clin Rheumatol 2006;25(6):822–30.
25. Maddali Bongi S, Del Rosso A, Orlandi M, Matucci-Cerinic M. Gynaecological symptoms and sexual disability in women with primary Sjogren's syndrome and sicca syndrome. Clin Exp Rheumatol 2013;31(5):683–90.
26. Tristano AG. The impact of rheumatic diseases on sexual function. Rheumatol Int 2009;29(8):853–60.
27. Bhadauria S, Moser DK, Clements PJ, et al. Genital tract abnormalities and female sexual function impairment in systemic sclerosis. Am J Obstet Gynecol 1995;172(2 Pt 1):580–7.
28. Briggs AM, Slater H, Van Doornum S, et al. Chronic primary or secondary non-inflammatory musculoskeletal pain is associated with disrupted sexual function and relationships: a systematic review. Arthritis Care Res (Hoboken) 2021.
29. Gutweniger S, Kopp M, Mur E, Gunther V. Body image of women with rheumatoid arthritis. Clin Exp Rheumatol 1999;17(4):413–7.
30. Fair DC, Rodriguez M, Knight AM, Rubinstein TB. Depression And Anxiety In Patients With Juvenile Idiopathic Arthritis: Current Insights And Impact On Quality Of Life, A Systematic Review. Open Access Rheumatol 2019;11:237–52.
31. Flynn KE, Lin L, Bruner DW, et al. Sexual Satisfaction and the Importance of Sexual Health to Quality of Life Throughout the Life Course of U.S. Adults. J Sex Med 2016;13(11):1642–50.
32. Josefsson KA, Gard G. Women's experiences of sexual health when living with rheumatoid arthritis–an explorative qualitative study. BMC Musculoskelet Disord 2010;11:240.
33. Kvien TK, Uhlig T. Quality of life in rheumatoid arthritis. Scand J Rheumatol 2005; 34(5):333–41.
34. de Avila Lima Souza L, Gallinaro AL, Abdo CH, et al. Effect of musculoskeletal pain on sexuality of male adolescents and adults with juvenile idiopathic arthritis. J Rheumatol 2009;36(6):1337–42.
35. Pitta AC, Ferreira GRV, Tomioka RB, et al. Sexual function in female juvenile idiopathic arthritis patients. Adv Rheumatol 2019;59(1):13.

36. Tristano AG. Impact of rheumatoid arthritis on sexual function. World J Orthop 2014;5(2):107–11.
37. Alriksson-Schmidt AI, Armour BS, Thibadeau JK. Are adolescent girls with a physical disability at increased risk for sexual violence? J Sch Health 2010; 80(7):361–7.
38. Martinez G, Copen CE, Abma JC. Teenagers in the United States: sexual activity, contraceptive use, and childbearing, 2006-2010 national survey of family growth. Vital Health Stat 2011;23(31):1–35.
39. MC B. The National intimate partner and sexual violence Survey (NISVS): 2010 summary report. Atlanta, GA: National Center for Injury Prevention and Control, Centers for Disease Control and Prevention; 2011.
40. Ott MA, Sucato GS, Committee on A. Contraception for adolescents. Pediatrics 2014;134(4):e1257–81.
41. Curtis KM, Tepper NK, Jatlaoui TC, et al. U.S. Medical Eligibility Criteria for Contraceptive Use, 2016. MMWR Recomm Rep 2016;65(3):1–103.
42. Sammaritano LR, Bermas BL, Chakravarty EE, et al. 2020 American College of Rheumatology Guideline for the Management of Reproductive Health in Rheumatic and Musculoskeletal Diseases. Arthritis Care Res (Hoboken) 2020; 72(4):461–88.
43. Medical Eligibility Criteria for Contraceptive Use. 5th edition. Geneva: World Health Organization; 2015.
44. Committee on Adolescent Health Care Long-Acting Reversible Contraception Working Group, The American College of Obstetricians and Gynecologists. Committee opinion no. 539: adolescents and long-acting reversible contraception: implants and intrauterine devices. Obstet Gynecol 2012;120(4):983–8.
45. Dalkilic E, Tufan AN, Oksuz MF, et al. Comparing female-based contraceptive methods in patients with systemic lupus erythematosus, rheumatoid arthritis and a healthy population. Int J Rheum Dis 2014;17(6):653–7.
46. Clowse ME, Magder LS, Witter F, Petri M. The impact of increased lupus activity on obstetric outcomes. Arthritis Rheum 2005;52(2):514–21.
47. Bortoluzzi A, Andreoli L, Carrara G, et al. Improved Pregnancy Outcome in Patients With Rheumatoid Arthritis Who Followed an Ideal Clinical Pathway. Arthritis Care Res (Hoboken) 2021;73(2):166–72.
48. Guttmacher Institute. Adolescent sexual and reproductive health in the United States 2019. https://www.guttmacher.org/united-states/teens. Accessed September 2, 2021.
49. Petri M, Kim MY, Kalunian KC, et al. Combined oral contraceptives in women with systemic lupus erythematosus. N Engl J Med 2005;353(24):2550–8.
50. Sanchez-Guerrero J, Uribe AG, Jimenez-Santana L, et al. A trial of contraceptive methods in women with systemic lupus erythematosus. N Engl J Med 2005; 353(24):2539–49.
51. Gladd DA, Olech E. Antiphospholipid antibodies in rheumatoid arthritis: identifying the dominoes. Curr Rheumatol Rep 2009;11(1):43–51.
52. Avcin T, Ambrozic A, Bozic B, Accetto M, Kveder T, Rozman B. Estimation of anticardiolipin antibodies, anti-beta2 glycoprotein I antibodies and lupus anticoagulant in a prospective longitudinal study of children with juvenile idiopathic arthritis. Clin Exp Rheumatol 2002;20(1):101–8.
53. Rai R, Swetha T. Association of anti-phospholipid antibodies with connective tissue diseases. Indian Dermatol Online J 2015;6(2):89–91.

54. Fauchais AL, Lambert M, Launay D, et al. Antiphospholipid antibodies in primary Sjogren's syndrome: prevalence and clinical significance in a series of 74 patients. Lupus 2004;13(4):245–8.
55. Serra CR, Rodrigues SH, Silva NP, Sztajnbok FR, Andrade LE. Clinical significance of anticardiolipin antibodies in juvenile idiopathic arthritis. Clin Exp Rheumatol 1999;17(3):375–80.
56. Stringer EM, Kaseba C, Levy J, et al. A randomized trial of the intrauterine contraceptive device vs hormonal contraception in women who are infected with the human immunodeficiency virus. Am J Obstet Gynecol 2007;197(2):144 e141–148.
57. WHO. Intrauterine Devices. In: Medical Eligibility Criteria for Contraceptive Use. 3 ed. Reproductive health and research World health Organizaiton. 2004.
58. Bailey MJ, Hershbein B, Miller AR. The opt-in revolution? Contraception and the gender gap in wages, 2012 wages. Am Econ J Appl Econ 2012;4(3):225–54.
59. Petri M, Robinson C. Oral contraceptives and systemic lupus erythematosus. Arthritis Rheum 1997;40(5):797–803.
60. Birru Talabi M, Clowse MEB, Blalock SJ, Moreland L, Siripong N, Borrero S. Contraception Use Among Reproductive-Age Women With Rheumatic Diseases. Arthritis Care Res (Hoboken) 2019;71(8):1132–40.
61. Amini L, Kalhor M, Haghighi A, Seyedfatemi N, Hosseini F. Effect of oral contraceptive pills on rheumatoid arthritis disease activity in women: A randomized clinical trial. Med J Islam Repub Iran 2018;32:61.
62. Pisoni CN, Cuadrado MJ, Khamashta MA, Hunt BJ. Treatment of menorrhagia associated with oral anticoagulation: efficacy and safety of the levonorgestrel releasing intrauterine device (Mirena coil). Lupus 2006;15(12):877–80.
63. Quint EH, O'Brien RF, Committee On A, North American Society for P, Adolescent G. Menstrual Management for Adolescents With Disabilities. Pediatrics 2016;138(1).
64. Hays KSK, Bundy D, Wallis E, Ruth NM. Rates of Contraceptive Use and Unintended Pregnancy in Teen Girls Prescribed Teratogenic Medications [abstract]. Arthritis Rheumatol 2017;69.
65. Stancil SL, Miller M, Briggs H, Lynch D, Goggin K, Kearns G. Contraceptive Provision to Adolescent Females Prescribed Teratogenic Medications. Pediatrics 2016;137(1).
66. Mycophenolate REMS. Available at: https://www.mycophenolaterems.com/. Accessed September 2, 2021.
67. Lenolidomide REMS. Available at: https://revlimidhcp.com/mds/rems. Accessed September 2, 2021.
68. Thalidomide REMS. Available at: https://www.thalomidrems.com. Accessed September 2, 2021.
69. Marcell AV, Burstein GR, Committee On A. Sexual and Reproductive Health Care Services in the Pediatric Setting. Pediatrics 2017;140(5).
70. Kaye KSK, Sloup C. The fog zone: how misperceptions, magical thinking, and ambivalence put young adults at risk for unplanned pregnancy. Washington, DC: National Campaign to Prevent Teen and Unplanned Pregnancy; 2009.
71. Guttmacher Institute. State policies in brief. An overview of minors' consent law. 2021. Available at: https://www.guttmacher.org/state-policy/explore/overview-minors-consent-law. Accessed May 15, 2021.
72. Brown S, Guthrie K. Why don't teenagers use contraception? A qualitative interview study. Eur J Contracept Reprod Health Care 2010;15(3):197–204.

73. Richards MJ, Peters M, Sheeder J, Kaul P. Contraception and Adolescent Males: An Opportunity for Providers. J Adolesc Health 2016;58(3):366–8.
74. Brown S. They think it's all up to the girls': gender, risk and responsibility for contraception. Cult Health Sex 2015;17(3):312–25.
75. Vinet E, Kuriya B, Pineau CA, Clarke AE, Bernatsky S. Induced abortions in women with rheumatoid arthritis receiving methotrexate. Arthritis Care Res (Hoboken) 2013;65(8):1365–9.
76. Dissanayake TD, Maksymowych WP, Keeling SO. Peripartum issues in the inflammatory arthritis patient: A survey of the RAPPORT registry. Sci Rep 2020; 10(1):3733.
77. Brouwer J, Laven JS, Hazes JM, Dolhain RJ. Brief Report: Miscarriages in Female Rheumatoid Arthritis Patients: Associations With Serologic Findings, Disease Activity, and Antirheumatic Drug Treatment. Arthritis Rheumatol 2015; 67(7):1738–43.
78. National Academies of Sciences E, Medicine. Sexually transmitted infections: Adopting a sexual health paradigm. Washington, DC: The National Academies Press; 2021.
79. Division of STD Prevention NCfHA. Viral Hepatitis, STD, and TB Prevention, Centers for Disease Control and Prevention Sexually Transmitted Diseases: Adolescents and Young Adults. 2021. Available at: https://www.cdc.gov/std/life-stages-populations/adolescents-youngadults.htm. Accessed June 10, 2021.
80. To U, Kim J, Chia D. Lupus flare: an uncommon presentation of disseminated gonorrhea. Case Rep Med 2014;2014:626095.
81. Tikly M, Diese M, Zannettou N, Essop R. Gonococcal endocarditis in a patient with systemic lupus erythematosus. Br J Rheumatol 1997;36(2):270–2.
82. CDC. Legal Status of Expedited Partner Therapy (EPT). 2021. Available at:https://www.cdc.gov/std/ept/legal/default.htm. . Accessed September 25, 2021.
83. CDC Surveillance and Data Management Branch, Division of STD Prevention. Sexually transmitted disease Surveillance 2015. Atlanta, GA: US Department of Health and Human Services; 2016.
84. Ochsendorf FR. Sexually transmitted infections: impact on male fertility. Andrologia 2008;40(2):72–5.
85. Tsevat DG, Wiesenfeld HC, Parks C, Peipert JF. Sexually transmitted diseases and infertility. Am J Obstet Gynecol 2017;216(1):1–9.
86. Carlin E, Flew S. Sexually acquired reactive arthritis. Clin Med (Lond) 2016; 16(2):193–6.
87. Devine PA. Extrapelvic manifestations of gonorrhea. Prim Care Update OB/GYNS 1998;5:233–7.
88. Kreisel KM, Spicknall IH, Gargano JW, et al. Sexually Transmitted Infections Among US Women and Men: Prevalence and Incidence Estimates, 2018. Sex Transm Dis 2021;48(4):208–14.
89. Kulthanan K, Jiamton S, Omcharoen V, Linpiyawan R, Ruangpeerakul J, Sivayathorn A. Autoimmune and rheumatic manifestations and antinuclear antibody study in HIV-infected Thai patients. Int J Dermatol 2002;41(7):417–22.
90. Iordache L, Bengoufa D, Taulera O, et al. Nonorgan-specific autoantibodies in HIV-infected patients in the HAART era. Medicine (Baltimore) 2017;96(10): e6230.
91. N L. HIV InSite: Rheumatologic and musculoskeletal manifestations of HIV 1998. Available at: http://hivinsite.ucsf.edu/InSite?page=kb-04-01-15. Accessed May 14, 2021.

92. Adizie T, Moots RJ, Hodkinson B, French N, Adebajo AO. Inflammatory arthritis in HIV positive patients: A practical guide. BMC Infect Dis 2016;16:100.
93. McQuillan G, Kruszon-Moran D, Flagg EW, Paulose-Ram R. Prevalence of Herpes Simplex Virus Type 1 and Type 2 in Persons Aged 14-49: United States, 2015-2016. NCHS Data Brief 2018;(304):1–8.
94. Reis AD, Mudinutti C, de Freitas Peigo M, et al. Active human herpesvirus infections in adults with systemic lupus erythematosus and correlation with the SLEDAI score. Adv Rheumatol 2020;60(1):42.
95. Kapoor TMP, Bhandari B, Li J, Bathon J, Nguyen S, Askanase AD. Herpetic Viruses in Lupus [abstract]. Arthritis Rheumatol 2016;68.
96. Sunzini F, McInnes I, Siebert S. JAK inhibitors and infections risk: focus on herpes zoster. Ther Adv Musculoskelet Dis 2020;12. 1759720X20936059.
97. Barrow RYAF, Bolan GA, Workowski KA. Recommendations for Providing Quality Sexually Transmitted Diseases Clinical Services, 2020. MMWR Recomm Rep 2020;68:1–20.
98. Cerny EH, Farshy CE, Hunter EF, Larsen SA. Rheumatoid factor in syphilis. J Clin Microbiol 1985;22(1):89–94.
99. Duarte JA, Henriques CC, Sousa C, Alves JD. Lupus or syphilis? That is the question! BMJ Case Rep 2015;2015.
100. Im JH, Chung MH, Park YK, et al. Antinuclear antibodies in infectious diseases. Infect Dis (Lond) 2020;52(3):177–85.
101. Qureshi SMK, Ezeonyeji A, et al. aIFRI0448FOURCASES OF SYPHILIS MIMICKING RHEUMATOLOGICAL CONDITIONS PRESENTING TO THE GENERAL RHEUMATOLOGY SERVICE AT ST GEORGES HOSPITAL ,LONDON ,UK IN 2018 -2019. Ann Rheum Dis 2020;79:821.
102. Wang Y, Yang L, Zhang ZL. [Panuveitis with oral and genital ulcer misdiagnosed as Behcet's disease: two cases report and literature review]. Beijing Da Xue Xue Bao Yi Xue Ban 2016;48(5):910–4.
103. Lao SMP. REACTIVE ARTHRITIS IN SYPHILIS MIMICKING RHEUMATOID ARTHRITIS: A CASE REPORT. Ann Rheum Dis 2021;80:1357.
104. Fernandes B, Dias E, Mascarenhas-Saraiva M, et al. Rheumatologic manifestations of hepatic diseases. Ann Gastroenterol 2019;32(4):352–60.
105. Koutsianas C, Thomas K, Vassilopoulos D. Reactivation of hepatitis B virus infection in rheumatic diseases: risk and management considerations. Ther Adv Musculoskelet Dis 2020;12.
106. Hagan JFSJ. In: Bright futures: guidelines for health Supervision of infants, children, and adolescents. 4th ed. Elk Grove Village, IL: American Academy of Pediatrics; 2017.
107. Aggarwal A, Srivastava P. Childhood onset systemic lupus erythematosus: how is it different from adult SLE? Int J Rheum Dis 2015;18(2):182–91.
108. Secor-Turner M, Scal P, Garwick A, Horvath K, Wells CK. Living with juvenile arthritis: adolescents' challenges and experiences. J Pediatr Health Care 2011;25(5):302–7.
109. Oliveira S, Ravelli A, Pistorio A, et al. Proxy-reported health-related quality of life of patients with juvenile idiopathic arthritis: the Pediatric Rheumatology International Trials Organization multinational quality of life cohort study. Arthritis Rheum 2007;57(1):35–43.
110. Peterson LS, Mason T, Nelson AM, O'Fallon WM, Gabriel SE. Psychosocial outcomes and health status of adults who have had juvenile rheumatoid arthritis: a controlled, population-based study. Arthritis Rheum 1997;40(12):2235–40.

111. Hamilton A. Sexual problems in arthritis and allied conditions. Int Rehabil Med 1981;3(1):38–42.
112. Pinquart M. Self-esteem of children and adolescents with chronic illness: a meta-analysis. Child Care Health Dev 2013;39(2):153–61.
113. April KT, Cavallo S, Feldman DE. Children with juvenile idiopathic arthritis: are health outcomes better for those diagnosed younger? Child Care Health Dev 2013;39(3):442–8.
114. Guan M, Wang J, Zhu Z, et al. Comparison in clinical features and life impact between juvenile-onset and adult-onset ankylosing spondylitis. Turk J Med Sci 2014;44(4):601–5.
115. Ostensen M, Almberg K, Koksvik HS. Sex, reproduction, and gynecological disease in young adults with a history of juvenile chronic arthritis. J Rheumatol 2000;27(7):1783–7.
116. Bruze G, Askling J, Horne A, et al. Juvenile idiopathic arthritis, marriage and parenthood: a Nationwide matched cohort study. Oxford): Rheumatology; 2021.
117. Chalmers A, Sayson R, Walters K. Juvenile dermatomyositis: medical, social and economic status in adulthood. Can Med Assoc J 1982;126(1):31–3.
118. Brailovski E, Vinet E, Pineau CA, et al. Marital status and age of systemic lupus erythematous diagnosis: the potential for differences related to sex and gender. Lupus Sci Med 2019;6(1):e000325.
119. Tamayo T, Fischer-Betz R, Beer S, Winkler-Rohlfing B, Schneider M. Factors influencing the health related quality of life in patients with systemic lupus erythematosus: long-term results (2001–2005) of patients in the German Lupus Erythematosus Self-Help Organization (LULA Study). Lupus 2010;19(14):1606–13.
120. Reese JB, Somers TJ, Keefe FJ, Mosley-Williams A, Lumley MA. Pain and functioning of rheumatoid arthritis patients based on marital status: is a distressed marriage preferable to no marriage? J Pain 2010;11(10):958–64.
121. Illum NO, Bonderup M, Gradel KO. Parents' Expressions of Concerns and Hopes for the Future and Their Concomitant Assessments of Disability in Their Children. Clin Med Insights Pediatr 2018;12.
122. Favier LA, Taylor J, Loiselle Rich K, et al. Barriers to Adherence in Juvenile Idiopathic Arthritis: A Multicenter Collaborative Experience and Preliminary Results. J Rheumatol 2018;45(5):690–6.
123. Khizroeva J, Nalli C, Bitsadze V, et al. Infertility in women with systemic autoimmune diseases. Best Pract Res Clin Endocrinol Metab 2019;33(6):101369.
124. Sarkar O, Bahrainwala J, Chandrasekaran S, et al. A. Agarwal Impact of inflammation on male fertility. Front Biosci (Elite Ed) 2011;3:89–95.
125. Silverman MN, Sternberg EM. Glucocorticoid regulation of inflammation and its functional correlates: from HPA axis to glucocorticoid receptor dysfunction. Ann N Y Acad Sci 2012;1261:55–63.
126. Tsaliki M, Koelsch KA, Chambers A, Talsania M, Scofield RH, Chakravarty EF. Ovarian antibodies among SLE women with premature menopause after cyclophosphamide. Int J Rheum Dis 2021;24(1):120–4.
127. Pasoto SG, Viana VS, Mendonca BB, Yoshinari NH, Bonfa E. Anti-corpus luteum antibody: a novel serological marker for ovarian dysfunction in systemic lupus erythematosus? J Rheumatol 1999;26(5):1087–93.
128. Marcus ZH, Hess EV. Antisperm antibodies in patients with systemic lupus erythematosus. Arthritis Rheum 1981;24(3):569–70.
129. Soares PM, Borba EF, Bonfa E, Hallak J, Correa AL, Silva CA. Gonad evaluation in male systemic lupus erythematosus. Arthritis Rheum 2007;56(7):2352–61.

130. Silva CA, Hallak J, Pasqualotto FF, Barba MF, Saito MI, Kiss MH. Gonadal function in male adolescents and young males with juvenile onset systemic lupus erythematosus. J Rheumatol 2002;29(9):2000–5.
131. Suehiro RM, Borba EF, Bonfa E, et al. Testicular Sertoli cell function in male systemic lupus erythematosus. Rheumatology (Oxford) 2008;47(11):1692–7.
132. Medeiros PB, Febronio MV, Bonfa E, Borba EF, Takiuti AD, Silva CA. Menstrual and hormonal alterations in juvenile systemic lupus erythematosus. Lupus 2009; 18(1):38–43.
133. Aikawa NE, Sallum AM, Pereira RM, et al. Subclinical impairment of ovarian reserve in juvenile systemic lupus erythematosus after cyclophosphamide therapy. Clin Exp Rheumatol 2012;30(3):445–9.
134. Ferreira GRV, Tomioka RB, Aikawa NE, et al. Ovarian reserve in young juvenile idiopathic arthritis patients. Mod Rheumatol 2019;29(3):447–51.
135. Henes M, Froeschlin J, Taran FA, et al. Ovarian reserve alterations in premenopausal women with chronic inflammatory rheumatic diseases: impact of rheumatoid arthritis, Behcet's disease and spondyloarthritis on anti-Mullerian hormone levels. Rheumatology (Oxford) 2015;54(9):1709–12.
136. Mont'Alverne AR, Yamakami LY, Goncalves CR, Baracat EC, Bonfa E, Silva CA. Diminished ovarian reserve in Behcet's disease patients. Clin Rheumatol 2015; 34(1):179–83.
137. Oner G, Muderris II. Assessment of ovarian reserve based on hormonal parameters, ovarian volume, and antral follicle count in women with familial Mediterranean fever. Eur J Obstet Gynecol Reprod Biol 2013;170(2):449–51.
138. Tiseo BC, Cocuzza M, Bonfa E, Srougi M, Silva CA. Male fertility potential alteration in rheumatic diseases: a systematic review. Int Braz J Urol 2016;42(1): 11–21.
139. Moraes AJ, Pereira RM, Cocuzza M, Casemiro R, Saito O, Silva CA. Minor sperm abnormalities in young male post-pubertal patients with juvenile dermatomyositis. Braz J Med Biol Res 2008;41(12):1142–7.
140. Karakus S, Sahin A, Durmaz Y, et al. Evaluation of ovarian reserve using anti-mullerian hormone and antral follicle count in Sjogren's syndrome: Preliminary study. J Obstet Gynaecol Res 2017;43(2):303–7.
141. Ayesha Jha V, Goswami D. Premature Ovarian Failure: An Association with Autoimmune Diseases. J Clin Diagn Res 2016;10(10):QC10–2.
142. Grossmann B, Saur S, Rall K, et al. Prevalence of autoimmune disease in women with premature ovarian failure. Eur J Contracept Reprod Health Care 2020; 25(1):72–5.
143. Betterle C, Dal Pra C, Mantero F, Zanchetta R. Autoimmune adrenal insufficiency and autoimmune polyendocrine syndromes: autoantibodies, autoantigens, and their applicability in diagnosis and disease prediction. Endocr Rev 2002;23(3): 327–64.
144. Ebrahimi M, Akbari Asbagh F. Pathogenesis and causes of premature ovarian failure: an update. Int J Fertil Steril 2011;5(2):54–65.
145. Ceccarelli F, Orefice V, Perrone G, et al. Premature ovarian failure in patients affected by systemic lupus erythematosus: a cross-sectional study. Clin Exp Rheumatol 2020;38(3):450–4.
146. Mayorga J, Alpizar-Rodriguez D, Prieto-Padilla J, Romero-Diaz J, Cravioto MC. Prevalence of premature ovarian failure in patients with systemic lupus erythematosus. Lupus 2016;25(7):675–83.

147. Oktem O, Guzel Y, Aksoy S, Aydin E, Urman B. Ovarian function and reproductive outcomes of female patients with systemic lupus erythematosus and the strategies to preserve their fertility. Obstet Gynecol Surv 2015;70(3):196–210.
148. Lawrenz B, Henes J, Henes M, et al. Impact of systemic lupus erythematosus on ovarian reserve in premenopausal women: evaluation by using anti-Muellerian hormone. Lupus 2011;20(11):1193–7.
149. Aikawa NE, Sallum AM, Leal MM, Bonfa E, Pereira RM, Silva CA. Menstrual and hormonal alterations in juvenile dermatomyositis. Clin Exp Rheumatol 2010; 28(4):571–5.
150. Dooley MA, Nair R. Therapy Insight: preserving fertility in cyclophosphamide-treated patients with rheumatic disease. Nat Clin Pract Rheumatol 2008;4(5): 250–7.
151. Clowse ME, Behera MA, Anders CK, et al. Ovarian preservation by GnRH agonists during chemotherapy: a meta-analysis. J Womens Health (Larchmt) 2009; 18(3):311–9.
152. Blumenfeld Z, Haim N. Prevention of gonadal damage during cytotoxic therapy. Ann Med 1997;29(3):199–206.
153. Somers EC, Marder W, Christman GM, Ognenovski V, McCune WJ. Use of a gonadotropin-releasing hormone analog for protection against premature ovarian failure during cyclophosphamide therapy in women with severe lupus. Arthritis Rheum 2005;52(9):2761–7.
154. Orefice V, Ceccarelli F, Perrone G, et al. Treatment with Gonadotropin Releasing Hormone Agonists in Systemic Lupus Erythematosus Patients Receiving Cyclophosphamide: A Long-term Follow-up Study. Isr Med Assoc J 2020;22(6): 343–7.
155. Brunner HI, Silva CA, Reiff A, et al. Randomized, double-blind, dose-escalation trial of triptorelin for ovary protection in childhood-onset systemic lupus erythematosus. Arthritis Rheumatol 2015;67(5):1377–85.
156. Ranganathan P, Mahran AM, Hallak J, Agarwal A. Sperm cryopreservation for men with nonmalignant, systemic diseases: a descriptive study. J Androl 2002;23(1):71–5.
157. Nahata L, Sivaraman V, Quinn GP. Fertility counseling and preservation practices in youth with lupus and vasculitis undergoing gonadotoxic therapy. Fertil Steril 2016;106(6):1470–4.
158. Miller SD, Li Y, Meyers KE, Caplan A, Miller VA, Ginsberg JP. Fertility preservation in paediatric nephrology: results of a physician survey. J Ren Care 2014; 40(4):257–62.
159. Practice Committee of the American Society for Reproductive Medicine. Electronic address aao. Fertility preservation in patients undergoing gonadotoxic therapy or gonadectomy: a committee opinion. Fertil Steril 2019;112(6): 1022–33.
160. Font-Gonzalez A, Mulder RL, Loeffen EA, et al. Fertility preservation in children, adolescents, and young adults with cancer: Quality of clinical practice guidelines and variations in recommendations. Cancer 2016;122(14):2216–23.
161. Canada AL, Schover LR. The psychosocial impact of interrupted childbearing in long-term female cancer survivors. Psychooncology 2012;21(2):134–43.
162. Practice Committee of the American Society for Reproductive Medicine. Definitions of infertility and recurrent pregnancy loss: a committee opinion. Fertil Steril 2020;113(3):533–5.
163. Bulletti C, Coccia ME, Battistoni S, Borini A. Endometriosis and infertility. J Assist Reprod Genet 2010;27(8):441–7.

164. Randeva HS, Tan BK, Weickert MO, et al. Cardiometabolic aspects of the polycystic ovary syndrome. Endocr Rev 2012;33(5):812–41.
165. Kost K, Isaac M-Z. U.S. Teenage pregnancies, births and abortions, 2011: state trends by age, race and ethnicity. New York: Guttmacher Institute; 2016.
166. CDC. Preventing Repeat Teen Births. 2013. Available at: https://www.cdc.gov/vitalsigns/teenpregnancy/index.html. Accessed September 25, 2021.
167. Meade CS, Kershaw TS, Ickovics JR. The intergenerational cycle of teenage motherhood: an ecological approach. Health Psychol 2008;27(4):419–29.
168. Hoffman SD. By the numbers: the public costs of adolescent childbearing. Washington, D.C.: The National Campaign to Prevent Teen Pregnancy; 2006.
169. Committee on Adolescent Health C. Committee Opinion No 699: Adolescent Pregnancy, Contraception, and Sexual Activity. Obstet Gynecol 2017;129(5):e142–9.
170. Committee JE. The Economic Benefits of birth control and access to family planning. United States Congress2020. Available at: https://www.jec.senate.gov/public/_cache/files/d0a67745-74ff-439c-a75a-aacc47e0abc1/jec-fact-sheet—economic-benefits-of-access-to-family-planning.pdf.
171. Sadun RE, Chung RJ, Maslow GR. Transition to Adult Health Care and the Need for a Pregnant Pause. Pediatrics 2019;143(5).
172. White PH, Cooley WC. Transitions Clinical Report Authoring Group; American Academy of Pediatrics; American Academy of Family Physicians; American College of Physicians. Supporting the Health Care Transition From Adolescence to Adulthood in the Medical Home. Pediatrics 2018;142(5). CWTCRAGAAOPAAOFPACOP.
173. Betz CL, Smith K. Measuring health care transition planning outcomes: Challenges and issues. Int J Child Adolesc Health 2010;3:463–72.
174. Goldenring JMRD. Getting into adolescent heads: an essential update. Contemp Pediatr 2004;21.
175. Bellanca HK, Hunter MS. ONE KEY QUESTION(R): Preventive reproductive health is part of high quality primary care. Contraception 2013;88(1):3–6.
176. Wallenius M, Skomsvoll JF, Irgens LM, et al. Parity in patients with chronic inflammatory arthritides childless at time of diagnosis. Scand J Rheumatol 2012;41(3):202–7.
177. Ostensen M. Pregnancy in patients with a history of juvenile rheumatoid arthritis. Arthritis Rheum 1991;34(7):881–7.
178. Ko HS, Ahn HY, Jang DG, et al. Pregnancy outcomes and appropriate timing of pregnancy in 183 pregnancies in Korean patients with SLE. Int J Med Sci 2011;8(7):577–83.
179. Wagner SJ, Craici I, Reed D, et al. Maternal and foetal outcomes in pregnant patients with active lupus nephritis. Lupus 2009;18(4):342–7.
180. Madazli R, Yuksel MA, Oncul M, Imamoglu M, Yilmaz H. Obstetric outcomes and prognostic factors of lupus pregnancies. Arch Gynecol Obstet 2014;289(1):49–53.
181. Chakravarty EF, Colon I, Langen ES, et al. Factors that predict prematurity and preeclampsia in pregnancies that are complicated by systemic lupus erythematosus. Am J Obstet Gynecol 2005;192(6):1897–904.
182. Saavedra MA, Miranda-Hernandez D, Sanchez A, et al. Pregnancy outcomes in women with childhood-onset and adult-onset systemic lupus erythematosus: a comparative study. Rheumatol Int 2016;36(10):1431–7.
183. Lateef A, Petri M. Managing lupus patients during pregnancy. Best Pract Res Clin Rheumatol 2013;27(3):435–47.

184. Mehta B, Luo Y, Xu J, et al. Trends in Maternal and Fetal Outcomes Among Pregnant Women With Systemic Lupus Erythematosus in the United States: A Cross-sectional Analysis. Ann Intern Med 2019;171(3):164–71.
185. Silva CA, Hilario MO, Febronio MV, et al. Pregnancy outcome in juvenile systemic lupus erythematosus: a Brazilian multicenter cohort study. J Rheumatol 2008;35(7):1414–8.
186. Ling N, Lawson E, von Scheven E. Adverse pregnancy outcomes in adolescents and young women with systemic lupus erythematosus: a national estimate. Pediatr Rheumatol Online J 2018;16(1):26.
187. Chen D, Lao M, Zhang J, et al. Fetal and Maternal Outcomes of Planned Pregnancy in Patients with Systemic Lupus Erythematosus: A Retrospective Multicenter Study. J Immunol Res 2018;2018:2413637.
188. Feldman DE, Vinet E, Berard A, et al. Heart Disease, Hypertension, Gestational Diabetes Mellitus, and Preeclampsia/Eclampsia in Mothers With Juvenile Arthritis: A Nested Case-Control Study. Arthritis Care Res (Hoboken) 2017;69(2):306–9.
189. Ehrmann Feldman D, Vinet E, Bernatsky S, et al. Birth Outcomes in Women with a History of Juvenile Idiopathic Arthritis. J Rheumatol 2016;43(4):804–9.
190. Ostensen M. Problems related to pregnancy in patients with juvenile chronic arthritis. Rev Rhum Engl Ed 1997;64(10 Suppl):196S–7S.
191. Mohamed MA, Goldman C, El-Dib M, Aly H. Maternal juvenile rheumatoid arthritis may be associated with preterm birth but not poor fetal growth. J Perinatol 2016;36(4):268–71.
192. Remaeus K, Johansson K, Askling J, Stephansson O. Juvenile onset arthritis and pregnancy outcome: a population-based cohort study. Ann Rheum Dis 2017;76(11):1809–14.
193. Al-Hemairi MH, Albokhari SM, Muzaffer MA. The Pattern of Juvenile Idiopathic Arthritis in a Single Tertiary Center in Saudi Arabia. Int J Inflam 2016;2016:7802957.
194. Alpigiani MGSP, Callegari S, Lorini R. Pregnancy outcomes in women affected by juvenile idiopathic arthritis. Pediatr Rheumatol Online J 2014;12.
195. Zhang-Jian SJ, Yang HY, Chiu MJ, et al. Pregnancy outcomes and perinatal complications of Asian mothers with juvenile idiopathic arthritis - a case-control registry study. Pediatr Rheumatol Online J 2020;18(1):9.
196. Smith CJF, Forger F, Bandoli G, Chambers CD. Factors Associated With Preterm Delivery Among Women With Rheumatoid Arthritis and Women With Juvenile Idiopathic Arthritis. Arthritis Care Res (Hoboken) 2019;71(8):1019–27.
197. Drechsel P, Studemann K, Niewerth M, et al. Pregnancy outcomes in DMARD-exposed patients with juvenile idiopathic arthritis-results from a JIA biologic registry. Rheumatology (Oxford) 2020;59(3):603–12.
198. Pontikaki IGM, Argolini L, et al. Pregnancy Outcome in Patients Affected by Juvenile Idiopathic Arthritis (JIA) Exposed To Biological Agents: A Monocentric Experience in A Tertiary Centre of Milan. Ann Rheum Dis 2016;75.
199. Chiam NP, Lim LL. Uveitis and gender: the course of uveitis in pregnancy. J Ophthalmol 2014;2014:401915.
200. Madu AE, Omih E, Baguley E, Lindow SW. Juvenile dermatomyositis in pregnancy. Case Rep Obstet Gynecol 2013;2013:890107.
201. Gerfaud-Valentin M, Hot A, Huissoud C, Durieu I, Broussolle C, Seve P. Adult-onset Still's disease and pregnancy: about ten cases and review of the literature. Rheumatol Int 2014;34(6):867–71.

202. Abdulkarim S, Otieno F, Ali SK. Adult-onset Still's disease triggered by pregnancy. Proc (Bayl Univ Med Cent). 2019;32(2):229–30.
203. Ben-Chetrit E, Levy M. Reproductive system in familial Mediterranean fever: an overview. Ann Rheum Dis 2003;62(10):916–9.
204. Ota K, Kwak-Kim J, Takahashi T, Mizunuma H. Pregnancy complicated with PFAPA (periodic fever, aphthous stomatitis, pharyngitis and cervical adenitis) syndrome: a case report. BMC Pregnancy Childbirth 2018;18(1):207.
205. ACOG Committee Opinion No. 743. Low-Dose Aspirin Use During Pregnancy. Obstet Gynecol 2018;132(1):e44–52.
206. Bramham K, Hunt BJ, Germain S, et al. Pregnancy outcome in different clinical phenotypes of antiphospholipid syndrome. Lupus 2010;19(1):58–64.
207. Committee on Practice Bulletins-Obstetrics ACoO. Gynecologists. Practice Bulletin No. 132: Antiphospholipid syndrome. Obstet Gynecol 2012;120(6): 1514–21.
208. Martinez-Sanchez N, Perez-Pinto S, Robles-Marhuenda A, et al. Obstetric and perinatal outcome in anti-Ro/SSA-positive pregnant women: a prospective cohort study. Immunol Res 2017;65(2):487–94.
209. Ostensen M, Forger F, Nelson JL, Schuhmacher A, Hebisch G, Villiger PM. Pregnancy in patients with rheumatic disease: anti-inflammatory cytokines increase in pregnancy and decrease post partum. Ann Rheum Dis 2005;64(6):839–44.
210. Vieira Borba V, Shoenfeld Y. Prolactin, autoimmunity, and motherhood: when should women avoid breastfeeding? Clin Rheumatol 2019;38(5):1263–70.
211. Davis-Porada J, Kim MY, Guerra MM, et al. Low frequency of flares during pregnancy and post-partum in stable lupus patients. Arthritis Res Ther 2020; 22(1):52.
212. Garcia-Fernandez A, Gerardi MC, Crisafulli F, et al. Disease course and obstetric outcomes of pregnancies in juvenile idiopathic arthritis: are there any differences among disease subtypes? A single-centre retrospective study of prospectively followed pregnancies in a dedicated pregnancy clinic. Clin Rheumatol 2021;40(1):239–44.
213. Musiej-Nowakowska E, Ploski R. Pregnancy and early onset pauciarticular juvenile chronic arthritis. Ann Rheum Dis 1999;58(8):475–80.
214. Ostensen M, Rugelsjoen A. Problem areas of the rheumatic mother. Am J Reprod Immunol 1992;28(3–4):254–5.
215. Lockshin MD. Autoimmunity, infertility and assisted reproductive technologies. Lupus 2004;13(9):669–72.

Transitioning to Adulthood with a Rheumatic Disease

A Case-Based Approach for Rheumatology Care Teams

Rebecca E. Sadun, MD, PhD[a,b,*], Lauren T. Covert, MD[b],
Erica F. Lawson, MD[c]

KEYWORDS

• Adolescent and young adult • Youth with special health care needs
• Health care transition and transfer • Pediatric rheumatology

KEY POINTS

- Pediatric rheumatology patients experience increased morbidity and mortality at the time of transfer.
- Pediatric rheumatologists ought to orient families to transition and transfer by early adolescence, coach families on the shared management model so that teens learn self-management skills, practice an adult model of care that includes time alone with the teen at most visits, and inform families about what to expect posttransfer.
- Transfer is most likely to succeed when patients are medically and socially stable and when there is direct communication between the pediatric and adult rheumatology teams.
- The adult rheumatologist can help retain transferring patients by attending to families' specific needs during the first clinic visit.
- Got Transition's Six Core Elements of Health Care Transition 3.0 offers evidence-based tools to assist with transition and transfer.

INTRODUCTION

Health care transition, or the gradual shift from a child- and family-centered system to an adult-oriented health care model, represents an important part of the journey to adulthood for youth with rheumatic diseases. The goals of health care transition are

[a] Department of Medicine, Division of Rheumatology, Duke University Medical Center, Durham, NC, USA; [b] Department of Pediatrics, Division of Rheumatology, Duke University Medical Center, Durham, NC, USA; [c] Department of Pediatrics, Division of Rheumatology, University of California San Francisco School of Medicine, San Francisco, CA, USA
* Corresponding author. Division of Rheumatology, Duke University Medical Center, Durham, NC, USA.
E-mail address: rebecca.sadun@duke.edu

Rheum Dis Clin N Am 48 (2022) 141–156
https://doi.org/10.1016/j.rdc.2021.09.011 rheumatic.theclinics.com
0889-857X/22/

to (1) prepare young people to independently manage their condition and effectively access health care and (2) ensure an organized process that facilitates the movement from pediatric to adult care systems.[1]

The concept of health care transition should be introduced to families during early adolescence.[2] The medical team can support patients and families in the gradual turnover of day-to-day health-related responsibilities to the maturing patient.[3] This transition to self-sufficiency, including medication management and appointment making, is like a dance: when the patient is developmentally ready to take a step forward, the parent follows his or her lead and steps back, while keeping watch for signs that the adolescent may not be meeting their responsibilities, requiring the parent to step back in. The health care team serves as a coach, providing guidance and support, helping to keep the dance both fluid and purposeful. In contrast to the more longitudinal and holistic process of health care transition, *transfer* to adult care represents the switch from pediatric to adult health care providers.[2]

Patients with serious health conditions are at high risk for poor outcomes during the transition period. National data demonstrate that young people aged 18 to 25 years experience worse health status than those aged 12 to 17 years or 26 to 34 years[4] and that for youth with chronic conditions, morbidity and mortality rates worsen following transfer.[5] Furthermore, about half of patients fail to establish care in adult rheumatology after leaving pediatric care.[6,7] Loss of health insurance coverage, difficulty accessing adult care, and competing personal priorities can lead to poor adherence to routine care and medications, increasing the risk of disease flare and hospitalization.[8,9]

Evidence demonstrates that a structured transition process decreases gaps in care during transition.[10,11] Since health care transition recommendations were first introduced in *Pediatrics* in 1996,[12] guidelines and best practices have continued to evolve.[2,13] The Six Core Elements of Healthcare Transition were developed to provide a structured framework for the practical implementation of health care transition processes, beginning with the dissemination of a practice-wide transition policy and concluding with the completion of transfer and successful integration into adult care.[14]

The cases that follow illustrate the complexity and challenges of transition and transfer, while highlighting best practices.

CASE #1: STARTING THE TRANSITION PROCESS (AGE 12–16 YEARS)

A 14-year-old girl, diagnosed at age 18 months with oligoarticular juvenile idiopathic arthritis (JIA) complicated by bilateral uveitis, is currently being managed with adalimumab and weekly oral methotrexate. At her routine pediatric rheumatology appointment, she spends most of the visit looking at her phone, while her mother provides an update on how she is doing and asks thoughtful questions. Interested in assessing the patient's disease knowledge, the pediatric rheumatologist asks the parent to leave the room briefly. The patient knows that she has arthritis, including "in my eyes," and states, "I take a bunch of pills every Friday, and I get a shot every other Friday." She does not know the names of her medications, which her mother administers. On further questioning, the patient reveals that she has been sexually active for the past 6 months and is "using condoms sometimes," despite being on methotrexate.

Introduce Health Care Transition Early

Introducing health care transition to families during early adolescence (age 12–14 years) provides time for young patients to develop self-care skills and adjust to the idea of transferring from a pediatric specialist to adult specialist. Transfer commonly occurs between the ages of 18 and 23 years, with timing often influenced by institutional and health insurance policies, patient preference, and geographic mobility. Transfer is a stressful event for many patients and families, both in concept and execution.[15] A written *transition policy*, which describes the practice-wide approach to health care transition, can serve as a tool to introduce the concept to families.[16] Transition policies outline the age range at which patients are expected to transfer to adult providers, as well as changes in privacy and consent laws that occur when patients turn 18 years.

Provide Disease Education

Children diagnosed in early childhood who are entering adolescence may be ready for additional disease education, having "outgrown" the rudimentary explanation provided to them at diagnosis. Although it is challenging for a busy clinician to find time to assess and address gaps in disease knowledge, patients across multiple studies have expressed a preference for receiving health information from their health care team.[17–19] Colleagues in nursing and social work can play vital roles in providing this education, either one-on-one or via group sessions. Group sessions additionally provide the opportunity for patients to meet peers living with rheumatic conditions and allow parents to develop relationships with and learn from each other. Video communication platforms may provide an efficient and feasible approach to group transition preparation, reducing the travel burden for families and the time burden for providers.[20] Community-based organizations, such as the Arthritis Foundation and the Lupus Foundation of America, also provide important opportunities for age-appropriate education outside the clinic visit, including educational events, support groups, and summer camps.[21]

Assess Transition Readiness and Set Self-Management Goals

Early adolescence is a critical period to support patient engagement and self-management. The process can be initiated with a *transition readiness assessment*, performed in clinic or before the visit. A variety of transition readiness assessment instruments exist, most applicable across chronic conditions. One of the most commonly used and best-validated tools is the Transition Readiness Assessment Questionnaire, which assesses self-management and self-advocacy skills.[22] Other validated transition readiness assessment measures include the TRANSITION-Q[23] and the STARx.[24] Providers can administer the measures at multiple time points to track the ongoing development of self-management skills. However, even a single assessment may be useful as a jumping-off point to discuss goals for self-management. For example, if a patient seems to be independent in medication management but has difficulty asking questions during the medical visit, a goal could be for the patient to ask 2 questions at the next visit. Motivational interviewing[25] and shared decision-making[26] are helpful techniques in setting goals for self-management.

Spend Time without Parents in the Room

Spending time alone with their health care provider helps adolescents develop self-advocacy skills, ask and answer questions independently, and address confidential health concerns. Time alone with the physician is a metric used in a variety of transition studies and patient-reported transition measures.[27] In rheumatology clinic, where we regularly prescribe teratogenic medications to young female patients, time speaking with the patient alone gives providers a chance to confidentially assess and address high-risk behaviors, including unprotected sex and substance use, and ask about anxiety and depression, which occur at high rates in young adults with rheumatic diseases.[28,29] With a parent out of the room, a young adult may have the courage to request contraception or reveal confidential and important social history details that are relevant to care. Providers often feel uncomfortable asking parents to leave the room, but research demonstrates that most parents believe time alone with the physician is appropriate and important for adolescents.[30]

Track and Monitor Transition

Transition tracking and monitoring ensures that all patients with chronic rheumatic conditions receive transition preparation, as outlined in a practice's transition policy. Tracking and monitoring is often accomplished through the creation of a transition registry. Although data can be entered into transition registries manually, integration with the electronic medical record (EMR) makes it easier to identify transition-age patients and track receipt of transition interventions. The health care team can generate reports on a recurring basis to identify patients who are ready to begin transition preparation or are approaching transfer. More complex EMR infrastructure may be used to track transition milestones over time or send documents and questionnaires directly to patients (such as a transition policy or a transition readiness assessment) via the EMR's patient portal.[31,32]

CASE #2: PREPARING FOR TRANSFER (AGE 17–21 YEARS)

An 18-year-old young woman with systemic lupus erythematosus (SLE) diagnosed at age 14 years presents to her pediatric rheumatologist for routine follow-up with new complaints of malar rash and morning knee stiffness. She admits to missing a few doses of her medications (mycophenolate mofetil and hydroxychloroquine) in recent weeks due to preoccupation with studying. She will be starting at an out-of-state college next fall. Laboratories are consistent with mild SLE flare. In addition to suggesting a plan for the current flare, you discuss that once she starts college, she is likely to continue to grapple with significant academic stress and will benefit from having a plan in place to support her health. She should establish rheumatology care locally and register with the Office of Disability Services at her university, so she can receive accommodations as needed.

Create a Transfer Plan

Although readiness for an adult model of care, disease control, and patient or family preference ideally guide the timing of transfer, a geographic move or insurance requirements may also dictate transfer timing. Transfer preparation beginning at least 18 months before the anticipated date of transfer provides time to address health insurance changes, set self-management goals, and schedule an appointment with a new adult rheumatology provider. Moreover, the time allows young adult patients and their parents to prepare for transfer, avoiding the sense of abandonment associated with an abrupt and unanticipated departure from the pediatric clinic. Recent single-center data demonstrated that receiving a referral from the pediatric rheumatologist to an adult rheumatologist, continuous insurance coverage, and younger age at referral correlate with a shorter time between last pediatric and first adult rheumatology visits.[9]

In addition to transferring during a time of medical stability, transferring during a time of social stability increases the chances of a young adult attending a scheduled appointment, adhering to medical management, and pursuing referrals. In cases where a pediatric rheumatologist is uncomfortable caring for a patient—as with a pregnant teen[33,34]—we recommend a period of co-management, during which time an adult rheumatologist can see the patient and offer management recommendations, whereas the pediatric rheumatologist can continue to see the patient and be a source of stability for the family. Young women often feel vulnerable during pregnancy and when abruptly transferred, may feel abandoned by the medical team.[35] The same can be true for young adults transferred amid acute struggles with mental health, including substance abuse. For some pediatricians, the aforementioned challenges are viewed as a ticket out of pediatrics, but young adults faced with such challenges often benefit from the continuity of a longstanding relationship with a trusted physician.

Address Privacy and Consent at Age 18 Years

Before age 18 years, consent for medical care is generally obtained from a parent or guardian, and most medical information can be shared with caregivers.[36] After age 18 years, patients must provide their own consent for medical care. Their health information is legally protected under the Health Insurance Portability and Accountability Act Privacy Rule.[37] In order to legally share information with parents and caregivers, the patient must sign a consent form, which is kept in the medical record.[38]

Rheumatology Care at College

A variety of models can be applied to care for patients with rheumatic diseases who travel far from home to attend college. Patients may be ready for transfer to a local adult provider at age 18 years. Alternatively, patients may prefer to continue care close to home with their existing pediatric rheumatology provider, attending routine medical visits between semesters and leveraging telehealth for acute care visits, as needed. Of note, there may be restrictions on out-of-state telehealth care, which needs investigation before implementing a care plan that relies on this approach. Finally, a hybrid model works well for many patients, with a local adult rheumatology provider at college in addition to ongoing pediatric rheumatology care at home. In this scenario, we encourage patients to establish with the local adult provider as soon as they arrive at college, ensuring timely access whenever a flare arises. A recent US-based insurance claims study of young adult patients with SLE found that greater than 30% of patients had a period of overlapping care, with visits to both adult and pediatric providers.[39] The success of this model depends on close communication between providers to ensure a coherent plan of care. Regardless of which strategy a young adult chooses, he or she should be encouraged to perform *all* aspects of care—from filling the pill box to requesting refills—independently for several months before leaving home, affording the opportunity to identify challenges and even make mistakes while still under the supervision of a parent.

Colleges are not required to provide personalized support on par with an individualized education plan; nevertheless, Section 504 of the Rehabilitation Act of 1973 and the Americans with Disabilities Act require equal access for people with disabilities and protection against discrimination.[40] To qualify for accommodations, patients with chronic rheumatic conditions must register with the college's Office of Disability Services (which sometimes bears an alternate name), even if their disease is well controlled. In the event of a flare, being registered will facilitate immediate access to needed accommodations, such as extensions on deadlines for assignments or postponing examinations.

CASE #3: SETTING THE PATIENT UP FOR A SUCCESSFUL TRANSFER (AGE 18–23 YEARS)

A 19-year-old young woman was diagnosed at age 14 years with SLE presenting as rash and arthritis, now well controlled on hydroxychloroquine monotherapy. She attends community college classes and works part-time. She calls with complaints of a new malar rash and sets up an appointment with her pediatric rheumatologist for the following week. When the patient arrives to check in, her Medicaid is expired, as she turned 19 years the month prior and is therefore newly uninsured. She leaves without seeing a provider to avoid liability for the cost of the clinic visit. Her pediatric rheumatologist places an urgent referral to adult rheumatology at the same academic medical center and prescribes a month of low-dose steroids as a temporizing measure. The patient accepts the "next available new appointment" with the adult rheumatologist, which is in 6 months. At the patient's first adult rheumatology appointment, she has 2+ bilateral lower extremity edema. Her urinalysis demonstrates 2 g of proteinuria, and creatinine is elevated at 2.9. She is admitted to the hospital for new-onset lupus nephritis, with kidney biopsy showing moderate chronicity.

Prepare for Predictable Lapses in Insurance

For young adults on their parents' private insurance, a common time to lose insurance is at age 26 years, as parental insurance options currently extend through age 25 years. However, patients with Medicaid may lose insurance sooner, typically on their 18th, 19th, or 21st birthday, depending on the state. Planning for alternate insurance coverage before insurance is lost is crucial. For patients with significant chronic medical illnesses, such as SLE, it is often possible for the patient to qualify for an extension of Medicaid coverage. However, the process requires an application, takes time to receive approval, and is not guaranteed. Full-time student status or full-time employment will likely provide insurance options, whereas part time status with either rarely does. A handful of national companies offer insurance to part-time employees, and patients with chronic medical diagnoses can be advised to consider employment options with these companies.[41]

If a patient unexpectedly loses insurance, the pediatric rheumatology team can counsel the patient and family as to how to reenroll. The pediatric provider who knows the patient well may be able to provide documentation that assists the young adult in extending his/her Medicaid coverage based on chronic illness or disability. The process is likely to be faster and more effective if initiated through the system in which the patient is already receiving care, as opposed to waiting for the patient to establish care with an adult provider.

Ensure Communication between Pediatric and Adult Rheumatologists

The adult rheumatologist in the aforementioned case was not aware of the medical urgency to see the flaring patient, and the pediatric rheumatologist was not aware how far in the future the patient was scheduled in the adult clinic. To prevent such scenarios, EULAR/PReS rheumatology transition guidelines recommend both a written medical summary and direct contact between the transferring pediatric rheumatologist and the accepting adult rheumatologist.[13] For written communication, Got Transition offers multiple disease-agnostic tools, including a Transfer of Care Checklist,[42] a Transfer of Care Letter,[43] and a Transfer of Care Medical Summary.[44] In addition The American College of Rheumatology Transition Toolkit includes medical summary templates specifically for JIA and SLE.[45,46] Although transfer documentation is sent directly to the accepting provider whenever possible, a medical summary should

Box 1
TRANSFERS mnemonic for pretransfer communication between pediatric and adult teams

Treatment history

Recent complications, Recent medication changes, and so forth

Adherence challenges (including suspected root causes)

Needs (eg, other subspecialists to transition or mental health needs)

Social history, Social challenges

Financial/insurance challenges

Emotional or intellectual challenges

Reasons that this is a good (or precarious) time for transfer

Summary of patient characteristics (eg, a favorite activity, academic interests, or personal goals)

Modified from Sadun RE, Schanberg LE. Transition and transfer of the patient with paediatric-onset lupus: a practical approach for pediatric and adult rheumatology practices. Lupus Sci Med. 2018;5(1):e000282.

also be given to all transferring patients with instructions to bring it to their first adult rheumatology visit, in case the transfer summary is not received by the adult practice.

When a pediatric provider is communicating with an adult provider, the mnemonic TRANSFERS (**Box 1**) offers a model for clinical practice.[47]

In addition to treatment history and next steps in care, it is helpful for the pediatric provider to offer insight into the patient's social history. For example, the pediatric rheumatologist might know that the patient is not averse to immunomodulatory medications but lives with a grandmother who opposes allopathic medications. It is also important to young adult patients that providers discuss "important aspects of (their) life" during visits.[17] Pediatric rheumatologists can use transfer documentation to help adult providers get to know their patients (eg, "Johnny loves animals and wants to become a vet tech"), facilitating adult rheumatology providers developing a strong connection with new young adult patients.

Ensure Care Continuity at the Time of Transfer

New appointments with an adult rheumatologist may be scheduled 6 months or longer out, with the workforce shortage predicted to make it harder to get new patient appointments in the future.[48] For a complex or active patient, it may not be safe to go 6 months without follow-up. It is therefore important for the pediatric provider to maintain ownership of the patient until he or she has established with an adult rheumatologist. It is also important to know the date of the first adult appointment to ensure that sufficient medication refills are provided.[49] For patients on infusion medications, it may be necessary to contact the adult rheumatologist's office before the first visit to facilitate prompt initiation of prior authorization and infusion center scheduling.

CASE #4: INTEGRATION INTO ADULT CARE (AGE 18–26 YEARS)

A 21-year-old young woman with JIA pages through the hospital operator to talk to the on-call pediatric rheumatologist. She has run out of methotrexate and needs refills. The pediatric rheumatologist has not seen her in 9 months. At her last visit, transfer to adult rheumatology was discussed. The patient relays that she went to a new adult rheumatologist several months prior but then decided not to follow-up, explaining that she did not like the doctor who saw her. Her mother, who also was present for the adult rheumatology visit, wants her daughter "to stay with pediatrics" because the adult rheumatologist wanted to change her daughter's medications "without knowing her medical history" and because the adult visit felt rushed.

Prepare for Differences between Adult and Pediatric Rheumatology Practice

The employment of several best practices could have prevented this typical patient "bounce back" scenario. Much of a successful transfer centers on educating young adult patients and their families about what to expect in adult care. Explaining

Table 1
Common differences between pediatric and adult rheumatology practice

Pediatric Rheumatology Practice	Adult Rheumatology Practice
Family-centered interaction	Patient-centered interaction
Parent present for most or all of clinic visit	Patients often interviewed and examined without parent
Multidisciplinary care including physical therapy, social work, and nurse-led medication teaching available	Multidisciplinary care may not be available
Multispecialty clinics to optimize care coordination and reduce clinic appointments, for example, Lupus Clinic with pediatric rheumatology and nephrology	Clinic appointments for individual subspecialties are distinct
Longer clinic visits at more frequent intervals	Shorter clinic visits with less frequent follow-up
More availability for urgent visits	Less availability for urgent visits
Leniency with late arrival to clinic appointments	Strict no-show policies
Comprehensive physical examination at every visit	Focused physical examination at follow-up visits
Care addresses psychosocial needs and mental health	Psychosocial needs and mental health care may be addressed via referrals
Care may address primary care needs such as routine vaccinations and contraception	Routine health maintenance may be deferred to primary care physician
More frequent screening for rare complications of disease, for example, interstitial lung disease or pulmonary hypertension	More frequent screening for common adult comorbidities, for example, osteoporosis or dyslipidemia
Antirheumatic medications prescribed more frequently and/or at higher doses	Fewer or lower dose antirheumatic medications may be prescribed
Goal is often to achieve complete remission without evidence of disease activity	Low disease activity without functional impairments sometimes tolerated
Infusion medications may be used to overcome medication non-adherence	Responsibility rests with the patient to adhere to medications
Child-friendly clinic environment with bright colors and games available	More stark clinic environment

Adapted from Sadun RE, Schanberg LE. Transition and transfer of the patient with paediatric-onset lupus: a practical approach for pediatric and adult rheumatology practices. *Lupus Sci Med.* 2018;5(1):e000282.

differences between adult and pediatric rheumatology practice enables patients to feel more confident and less apprehensive about transfer and prevents feelings of being "pushed" into adult care.[50] Patients and their families can anticipate cultural and logistic differences and will be less taken aback by the first adult visit. Some of these differences are outlined in **Table 1**.

Address the Needs of Young Adult Patients and Parents

The process of transition does not end the day a young adult transfers. As such, the adult rheumatologist needs to work with patient-parent dyads. For adult rheumatologists, it is important to recognize that parents may feel excluded and resentful toward a provider who asks them to leave the room for the bulk of a clinic visit, especially for a first visit. Although the adult rheumatologist appropriately encourages patient autonomy by speaking directly to the patient and reserving at least a few minutes to interview the young adult alone, this must be balanced with parental engagement by inviting parents to add details to the patient's history, hear the rationale for treatment options, and provide feedback at the patient's discretion.[51] The goal is to give the young adult increasingly more voice in the visit without alienating parents.

When working with young adults, it is important to keep in mind that the prefrontal cortex does not fully mature until the mid-to-late 20s, and as a result, young adult patients tend to concentrate on current symptoms and their impact on daily life rather than the long-term trajectory of disease, including possible late complications from deferred care. In qualitative interviews with young adult patients with JIA, for example, patients emphasized the need for health care to "fit in" with their daily lives.[52] Thus, focusing on the "here and now" as opposed to long-term prognosis may lead to better medication adherence and more reliable follow-up. In addition, young adult patients report high levels of pain intensity and functional disability, while having high rates of depression, anxiety, and other mental health disorders,[17] all of which interfere with adherence. In contrast to reprimanding patients or using scare tactics, motivational interviewing techniques are a more effective way to encourage behavior change in young adults.[53]

Finally, it is important for adult rheumatologists to incorporate best practices from adolescent medicine, a field that focuses on the care of patients ages 12 to 26 years.[54] The HEADSS mnemonic for social history[55] (**Box 2**) was designed to identify targets

Box 2
HEADSS mnemonic for taking a thorough psychosocial history of a young adult patient

Home (Where do you live and who lives with you?)

Education and employment (What are you good at in school/work? What is hard for you? What kinds of grades do you get? What kind of work do you do?)

Activities (What do you do for fun? What do you do with friends?)

Drugs (Many young people experiment with drugs and alcohol. Have you or your friends ever tried them?)

Sexuality (Have you ever had a sexual relationship with anyone? If so, was it with boys, girls, or both?)

Suicidality (Have you ever had thoughts of hurting yourself or others?)

Adapted from Getting into adolescent heads. Accessed March 5, 2021. https://www.contemporarypediatrics.com/view/getting-adolescent-heads

for a harms-reduction approach—for example, the need to address contraception to avoid unplanned pregnancies, especially in women on teratogenic medications—and to identify what is important to the healthy growth and development of the patient, such as educational and vocational goals.

Build Rapport at the Introductory Adult Rheumatology Clinic Visit

The initial focus of the first adult rheumatology visit is orienting the patient to adult practice. This involves discussing the preferred methods of communication, clinic policies, expectations, and guidance on what to do in urgent and emergent situations. After a brief welcome and orientation to the adult practice, the focus of the visit shifts to fostering good rapport with the patient to build a strong foundation of trust.

Among adolescents with rheumatic conditions, adult providers are often perceived as not having enough time and not being empathic toward them as a person and only focusing on their disease.[17,51] By dedicating time to discuss the patient's daily life outside of his/her disease, the adult rheumatologist is much more likely to develop an effective relationship and be able to align care and messaging with the young adult's priorities.

Contributing to alignment is minimizing treatment changes at the first visit.[47] Young adult patients often fear that clinicians in the adult setting will change their care plan, leading to medical instability and increased risk of disease flare.[17] If changes are crucial, adult providers should speak directly to the young adult in jargon-free terminology and allow ample opportunity for the patient to express his/her opinions. As discussed in Case 3, although it is appropriate to invite parents to ask questions and offer feedback during initial visits, speaking with young adult patients alone bolsters trust and allows for confidentiality.[56]

A helpful mnemonic for how to orient a young adult patient to adult care is WELCOME (**Box 3**).[47]

Communicate after Transfer

Ideally at least 2 direct communications between pediatric and adult rheumatologists take place—one before and one after transfer—either in person during a combined

Box 3
WELCOME mnemonic for key elements of the first adult rheumatology visit after transfer

Welcome and congratulate the patient on graduating to adult care

Explain key similarities and differences between pediatric and adult care (outlined in **Table 1**)

Let the patient and parents know their respective roles (eg, the patient answers questions first, after which input from the parent is appreciated)

Communication with the pediatric provider: reassure the patient you are in touch as needed

Opportunity for the patient and parents to ask questions about the new clinic (before beginning medical aspects of the visit)

Minimize medical changes during the first adult clinic visit

Expectations: supportively convey expectations of the patient and parents (eg, be sure to arrive 15 minutes before your appointment, as patients who are more than 5 minutes late will be rescheduled)

Modified from Sadun RE, Schanberg LE. Transition and transfer of the patient with paediatric-onset lupus: a practical approach for pediatric and adult rheumatology practices. Lupus Sci Med. 2018;5(1):e000282.

transition clinic or via telephone or electronic communication.[13] The posttransfer communication, 3 to 6 months after the last pediatric rheumatology visit, helps establish that the patient showed up to the adult clinic and has ongoing follow-up scheduled. It also offers opportunities for consultation to ensure the best outcome for the patient and builds collaborative partnerships between pediatric and adult rheumatologists. It is optimal to have a transition coordinator within the pediatric rheumatology clinic to support the communication between health care professionals within a multidisciplinary team, such as the primary rheumatologists, physical therapists, social workers, and other subspecialists. Transition coordinators can also obtain anonymous feedback from patients and families to drive improvements with the transition process.

Although it is desirable to have seamless communication between providers following transfer, this often is difficult to execute—clinics often lack a transition coordinator, and identifying and communicating with the correct provider can be time-consuming. Although it may not be feasible to close the loop between rheumatologists with every young adult patient who transfers care, it is of paramount importance to make sure adequate communication occurs for patients at high risk of medical instability or of being lost to follow-up. Proactively communicating with the adult rheumatologist for these high-risk patients can have a life-changing impact on patient outcomes.

SUMMARY

Transition is a process best started in early adolescence and continued even after transfer to adult care.[2,47] The pediatric team can equip patients with disease knowledge, self-management skills, and awareness of what to expect in the adult rheumatology health care system. Although the presence of a transition coordinator or transition clinic[57–59] facilitates a structured transition process, these resources do not exist at many institutions. Time constraints inherent in rheumatology practice require addressing transition practically, in a way that is feasible and efficient for both families and care teams. Pragmatic best practices include introducing the concept of transition early, developing and distributing a transition policy, using quick readiness assessment tools to guide conversations around self-management goals, leveraging EMR reports to identify patients approaching transfer age, and providing a medical summary to share with the adult rheumatologist.

With tools, templates, and resources from Got Transition[14,60] and the ACR transition toolkit,[61] the key elements of transition can be incorporated into busy pediatric rheumatology clinic settings. Particularly when patients are at high risk for poor outcomes, pediatric and adult rheumatologists ought to communicate about the patient before and after transfer to ensure care continuity and promote the adult rheumatologist's understanding of key medical and social issues. Communication using the TRANSFER mnemonic[47] can take as few as 5 minutes and may help avoid downstream consequences such as flares due to care delays. To improve patient integration into adult care, the adult rheumatologist can focus on management of the patient-parent-physician triad, recognizing the challenge of transfer for families and using the WELCOME mnemonic to guide the initial visit.[47] The adult rheumatology team may need to support the young adult in the continual development of self-management skills over the next several years.

Most young adults with childhood-onset rheumatic conditions carry the burden of disease throughout their lifetime. As rheumatology providers, we are responsible for delivering care that grows with our patients. By embracing the role of "transition coaches," pediatric and adult rheumatology care teams can help our young patients thrive in adulthood.

CLINICS CARE POINTS

- The website https://gottransition.org/ and the ACR's online Transition Toolkit provide free, evidence-based transition tools, such as a Transition Policy, Transfer of Care Checklist, Transfer of Care Letter, Transfer of Care Medical Summary, and Transition Readiness Assessment Tools.
- Pediatric rheumatologists should discuss transition early and often, gradually implementing an adult model of care while the adolescent patient is still in pediatric care. This should include spending time alone with the patient without the parent in the room and familiarizing patients and families with differences between pediatric and adult care (**Table 1**).
- When a patient reaches the age of 18, the rheumatology team should explain the implications of the Health Insurance Portability and Accountability Act (HIPAA) on communication between providers and parents.
- The mnemonic TRANSFERS (**Box 1**) guides the pre-transfer handoff conversation between pediatric and adult rheumatology providers. EULAR/PReS guidelines recommend pre-transfer and post-transfer communication between pediatric and adult rheumatologists.
- Only 50% of transferring rheumatology patients return to see the adult rheumatologist after the first visit. The mnemonic WELCOME (**Box 3**) guides adult providers in steps to help young adult rheumatology patients feel comfortable during their first visit so as to encourage their integration into adult rheumatology care.
- Adult rheumatologists should familiarize themselves with readiness assessment tools, recognizing that the work of transition does not end with transfer and that many young adult patients will continue to need guidance as they develop self-management skills.
- Pediatric and adult rheumatology providers serve as coaches for young adult patients and their families - before, during, and after transfer.

DISCLOSURE

Dr R.E. Sadun is the recipient of a Clinician Scholar Educator Award from the Rheumatology Research Foundation to complete a project that entails developing a transition curriculum for rheumatology fellows.

REFERENCES

1. Sabbagh S, Ronis T, White PH. Pediatric rheumatology: addressing the transition to adult-orientated health care. Open Access Rheumatol 2018;10:83–95.
2. White PH, Cooley WC. Transitions Clinical Report Authoring Group, American Academy of Pediatrics, American Academy of Family Physicians, American College of Physicians. Supporting the Health Care Transition From Adolescence to Adulthood in the Medical Home. Pediatrics 2018;142(5). https://doi.org/10.1542/peds.2018-2587.
3. Ardoin SP. Transitions in rheumatic disease. Pediatr Clin North Am 2018;65(4):867–83.
4. Neinstein LS, Irwin CE. Young adults remain worse off than adolescents. J Adolesc Health 2013;53(5):559–61.
5. Betz CL. Approaches to transition in other chronic illnesses and conditions. Pediatr Clin North Am 2010;57(4):983–96.

6. Jensen PT, Paul GV, LaCount S, et al. Assessment of transition readiness in adolescents and young adults with chronic health conditions. Pediatr Rheumatol Online J 2017;15(1):70.
7. Hart LC, Pollock M, Hill S, et al. Association of transition readiness to intentional self-regulation and hopeful future expectations in youth with illness. Acad Pediatr 2017;17(4):450–5.
8. Bitencourt N, Kramer J, Bermas BL, et al. Clinical team perspectives on the psychosocial aspects of transition to adult care for patients with childhood-onset systemic lupus erythematosus. Arthritis Care Res (Hoboken) 2021;73(1):39–47.
9. Bitencourt N, Bermas BL, Makris UE, et al. Time to completed visit and healthcare utilization among young adults transferring from pediatric to adult rheumatologic care in a safety-net hospital. Arthritis Care Res (Hoboken) 2020. https://doi.org/10.1002/acr.24409.
10. Schmidt A, Ilango SM, McManus MA, et al. Outcomes of pediatric to adult health care transition interventions: an updated systematic review. J Pediatr Nurs 2020;51:92–107.
11. Weissberg-Benchell J, Shapiro JB. A review of interventions aimed at facilitating successful transition planning and transfer to adult care among youth with chronic illness. Pediatr Ann 2017;46(5):e182–7.
12. Transition of care provided for adolescents with special health care needs. American Academy of Pediatrics Committee on Children with Disabilities and Committee on Adolescence. Pediatrics 1996;98(6 Pt 1):1203–6. Available at: https://pediatrics.aappublications.org/content/pediatrics/98/6/1203.full.pdf.
13. Foster HE, Minden K, Clemente D, et al. EULAR/PReS standards and recommendations for the transitional care of young people with juvenile-onset rheumatic diseases. Ann Rheum Dis 2017;76(4):639–46.
14. McManus M, White P, Pirtle R, et al. Incorporating the six core elements of health care transition into a medicaid managed care plan: lessons learned from a pilot project. J Pediatr Nurs 2015;30(5):700–13.
15. Johnson K, Edens C, Sadun RE, et al. Differences in health care transition views, practices, and barriers amongst north american pediatric rheumatology clinicians from 2010 to 2018. J Rheumatol 2021. https://doi.org/10.3899/jrheum.200196.
16. McManus M, White P, Barbour A, et al. Pediatric to adult transition: a quality improvement model for primary care. J Adolesc Health 2015;56(1):73–8.
17. Jiang I, Major G, Singh-Grewal D, et al. Patient and parent perspectives on transition from paediatric to adult healthcare in rheumatic diseases: an interview study. BMJ Open 2021;11(1):e039670.
18. Frederick NN, Bober SL, Berwick L, et al. Preparing childhood cancer survivors for transition to adult care: The young adult perspective. Pediatr Blood Cancer 2017;64(10). https://doi.org/10.1002/pbc.26544.
19. Applebaum MA, Lawson EF, von Scheven E. Perception of transition readiness and preferences for use of technology in transition programs: teens' ideas for the future. Int J Adolesc Med Health 2013;25(2):119–25.
20. Gray WN, Wagoner ST, Schaefer MR, et al. Transition to Adult IBD Care: A Pilot Multi-Site, Telehealth Hybrid Intervention. J Pediatr Psychol 2021;46(1):1–11.
21. Faith MA, Mayes S, Pratt CD, et al. Improvements in hope and beliefs about illness following a summer camp for youth with chronic illnesses. J Pediatr Nurs 2019;44:56–62.

22. Wood DL, Sawicki GS, Miller MD, et al. The Transition Readiness Assessment Questionnaire (TRAQ): its factor structure, reliability, and validity. Acad Pediatr 2014;14(4):415–22.
23. Klassen AF, Grant C, Barr R, et al. Development and validation of a generic scale for use in transition programmes to measure self-management skills in adolescents with chronic health conditions: the TRANSITION-Q. Child Care Health Dev 2015;41(4):547–58.
24. Nazareth M, Hart L, Ferris M, et al. A parental report of youth transition readiness: the Parent STARx Questionnaire (STARx-P) and Re-evaluation of the STARx Child Report. J Pediatr Nurs 2018;38:122–6.
25. Apodaca TR, Tsai SL, Miller MK, et al. Implementing motivational interviewing in a pediatric hospital. Mo Med 2014;111(3):212–6.
26. McKenzie RB, Sanders L, Bhattacharya J, et al. Health care system factors associated with transition preparation in youth with special health care needs. Popul Health Manag 2019;22(1):63–73.
27. Sawicki GS, Garvey KC, Toomey SL, et al. Preparation for transition to adult care among medicaid-insured adolescents. Pediatrics 2017;140(1). https://doi.org/10.1542/peds.2016-2768.
28. Fair DC, Rodriguez M, Knight AM, et al. Depression and anxiety in patients with juvenile idiopathic arthritis: current insights and impact on quality of life, a systematic review. Open Access Rheumatol 2019;11:237–52.
29. Ardalan K, Adeyemi O, Wahezi DM, et al. Parent perspectives on addressing emotional health for children and young adults with juvenile myositis. Arthritis Care Res (Hoboken) 2021;73(1):18–29.
30. Miller VA, Friedrich E, García-España JF, et al. Adolescents spending time alone with pediatricians during routine visits: perspectives of parents in a primary care clinic. J Adolesc Health 2018;63(3):280–5.
31. Volertas SD, Rossi-Foulkes R. Using quality improvement in resident education to improve transition care. Pediatr Ann 2017;46(5):e203–6.
32. Szalda D, Steinway C, Greenberg A, et al. Developing a hospital-wide transition program for young adults with medical complexity. J Adolesc Health 2019;65(4):476–82.
33. Maddux MH, Ricks S, Bass J. Preparing patients for transfer of care: practices of primary care pediatricians. J Community Health 2015;40(4):750–5.
34. Nabbout R, Teng T, Chemaly N, et al. Transition of patients with childhood onset epilepsy: Perspectives from pediatric and adult neurologists. Epilepsy Behav 2020;104(Pt A):106889.
35. Sadun RE, Chung RJ, Maslow GR. Transition to adult health care and the need for a pregnant pause. Pediatrics 2019;143(5):e20190541.
36. Pfister HR, Ingargiola SR. Privacy please: health consent laws for minors in the information age. Available at: https://www.chcf.org/wp-content/uploads/2017/12/PDF-PrivacyPleaseHealthConsentMinors.pdf.
37. Health information privacy law and policy. Available at: https://www.healthit.gov/topic/health-information-privacy-law-and-policy.
38. Turning 18: What it means for your health. Available at: https://www.gottransition.org/resource/?turning-18-english.
39. Chang JC, Knight AM, Lawson EF. Patterns of Healthcare Use and Medication Adherence among Youth with Systemic Lupus Erythematosus during Transfer from Pediatric to Adult Care. J Rheumatol 2021;48(1):105–13.
40. Cory RC. Disability services offices for students with disabilities: a campus resource. New Dir High Educ 2011;154:27–36.

41. 10 Companies that offer part-time jobs with benefits. Available at: https://www.indeed.com/career-advice/finding-a-job/companies-that-offer-part-time-jobs-with-benefits. Accessed March 5, 2021.
42. Sample transfer of care checklist. Available at: https://gottransition.org/6ce/?leaving-transfer-checklist. Accessed March 5, 2021.
43. Sample transfer letter. Available at: https://gottransition.org/6ce/?leaving-transfer-letter.
44. Transfer of care medical summary and emergency care plan. Available at: https://gottransition.org/6ce/?leaving-medical-summary-emergency-plan. Accessed March 5, 2021.
45. Medical summary: juvenile idiopathic arthritis. Available at: https://www.rheumatology.org/Portals/0/Files/Medical-Summary-JIA.pdf. Accessed March 5, 2021.
46. Medical summary: systemic lupus erythematosus. Available at: https://www.rheumatology.org/Portals/0/Files/Medical-Summary-SLE.pdf. Accessed March 5, 2021.
47. Sadun RE, Schanberg LE. Transition and transfer of the patient with paediatric-onset lupus: a practical approach for paediatric and adult rheumatology practices. Lupus Sci Med 2018;5(1):e000282.
48. Battafarano DF, Ditmyer M, Bolster MB, et al. 2015 American College of Rheumatology Workforce Study: supply and demand projections of adult rheumatology workforce, 2015-2030. Arthritis Care Res 2018;70(4):617–26.
49. Mannion ML, Xie F, Baddley J, et al. Analysis of health care claims during the peri-transfer stage of transition from pediatric to adult care among juvenile idiopathic arthritis patients. Pediatr Rheumatol 2016;14(1):49.
50. Zhou H, Roberts P, Dhaliwal S, et al. Transitioning adolescent and young adults with chronic disease and/or disabilities from paediatric to adult care services – an integrative review. J Clin Nurs 2016;25(21–22):3113–30.
51. Shaw KL, Southwood TR, McDonagh JE. User perspectives of transitional care for adolescents with juvenile idiopathic arthritis. Rheumatology 2004;43(6):770–8.
52. Howland S, Fisher K. Looking through the patient lens – Improving best practice for young people with juvenile idiopathic arthritis transitioning into adult care. SpringerPlus 2015;4(1):111.
53. Carcone AI, Naar S, Clark J, et al. Provider behaviors that predict motivational statements in adolescents and young adults with HIV: a study of clinical communication using the Motivational Interviewing framework. AIDS Care 2020;32(9):1069–77.
54. Moreno M, Thompson L. What is adolescent and young adult medicine? JAMA Pediatr 2020;174(5):512.
55. Getting into adolescent heads. Available at: https://www.contemporarypediatrics.com/view/getting-adolescent-heads. Accessed March 5, 2021.
56. Shaw KL. Transitional care for adolescents with juvenile idiopathic arthritis: a Delphi study. Rheumatology 2004;43(8):1000–6.
57. Chu PY, Maslow GR, von Isenburg M, et al. Systematic review of the impact of transition interventions for adolescents with chronic illness on transfer from pediatric to adult healthcare. J Pediatr Nurs 2015;30(5):e19–27.
58. Clemente D, Leon L, Foster H, et al. Systematic review and critical appraisal of transitional care programmes in rheumatology. Semin Arthritis Rheum 2016;46(3):372–9.

59. Annunziato RA, Baisley MC, Arrato N, et al. Strangers headed to a strange land? A pilot study of using a transition coordinator to improve transfer from pediatric to adult services. J Pediatr 2013;163(6):1628–33.
60. Six core elements of health care transition. Available at: https://gottransition.org/six-core-elements/. Accessed March 3, 2021.
61. Pediatric to adult rheumatology care transition. Available at: https://www.rheumatology.org/Practice-Quality/Pediatric-to-Adult-Rheumatology-Care-Transition. Accessed March 5, 2021.

Cardiovascular Health in Pediatric Rheumatologic Diseases

Kaveh Ardalan, MD, MS[a,b,c,*], Donald M. Lloyd-Jones, MD, ScM[d,e,f], Laura E. Schanberg, MD[g]

KEYWORDS

- Cardiovascular health • Cardiovascular disease • Pediatric rheumatology
- Systemic lupus erythematosus • Juvenile dermatomyositis
- Juvenile idiopathic arthritis

KEY POINTS

- The American Heart Association defines cardiovascular health as the sum of protective factors against later life cardiovascular disease.
- Patients with juvenile systemic lupus erythematosus, juvenile dermatomyositis, and juvenile idiopathic arthritis experience early loss of cardiovascular health and high long-term cardiovascular disease risk.
- Rheumatologic disease–related factors such as chronic inflammation and endothelial dysfunction interact bidirectionally with traditional cardiovascular health factors such as obesity, potentiating the long-term risk of cardiovascular disease in patients with pediatric rheumatologic diseases.
- Pharmacologic interventions may mitigate cardiovascular risk by controlling underlying rheumatic disease activity, decreasing chronic inflammation, and improving cardiovascular health factors such as lipid profile.

Continued

[a] Department of Pediatrics, Division of Pediatric Rheumatology, Duke University School of Medicine, T909 Children's Health Center, DUMC Box 3212, Durham, NC 27710, USA; [b] Department of Pediatrics, Northwestern University Feinberg School of Medicine, Ann & Robert H. Lurie Children's Hospital of Chicago; [c] Department of Medical Social Sciences, Northwestern University Feinberg School of Medicine, Ann & Robert H. Lurie Children's Hospital of Chicago; [d] Department of Preventive Medicine, Northwestern University Feinberg School of Medicine, Suite 1400, 680 North Lake Shore Drive, Chicago, IL 60611, USA; [e] Department of Medicine, Northwestern University Feinberg School of Medicine, Suite 1400, 680 North Lake Shore Drive, Chicago, IL 60611, USA; [f] Department of Pediatrics, Northwestern University Feinberg School of Medicine, Suite 1400, 680 North Lake Shore Drive, Chicago, IL 60611, USA; [g] Department of Pediatrics, Division of Pediatric Rheumatology, Duke Clinical Research Institute, Duke University School of Medicine, T909 Children's Health Center, DUMC Box 3212, Durham, NC 27710, USA

* Corresponding author. T909 Children's Health Center, DUMC Box 3212, Durham, NC 27710.
E-mail address: kaveh.ardalan@duke.edu

Rheum Dis Clin N Am 48 (2022) 157–181
https://doi.org/10.1016/j.rdc.2021.09.006 rheumatic.theclinics.com

Continued

- Nonpharmacologic interventions that address health behaviors, psychosocial factors, and health disparities may further decrease cardiovascular disease risk in patients with pediatric rheumatologic disease.

INTRODUCTION

Although most rheumatic disease outcomes are improving, cardiovascular disease (CVD) remains a leading cause of mortality in adults with systemic lupus erythematosus, dermatomyositis, and rheumatoid arthritis.[1,2] Myocardial infarction and stroke are more common in adults with rheumatologic diseases, occur at younger ages than the general population, and are associated with higher mortality and morbidity.[3–7] Rheumatologic disease independently predicts incident CVD, whereas traditional cardiovascular risk scores underestimate the magnitude of risk.[8] Traditional and disease-related CVD risk factors are evident in children with juvenile systemic lupus erythematosus (JSLE), juvenile dermatomyositis (JDM), and juvenile idiopathic arthritis (JIA). JSLE is associated with premature atherosclerosis beginning in childhood as well as early myocardial infarction and stroke.[9,10] The Atherosclerosis Prevention in Pediatric Lupus Erythematosus (APPLE) trial found that the rate of carotid intima media thickness (cIMT) progression is greater in patients with JSLE than in familial dyslipidemia.[11] Patients with JDM have higher rates of most cardiovascular risk factors and comorbidities than the general pediatric population.[12] By early adulthood, patients with JIA frequently demonstrate unfavorable cardiometabolic profiles.[13–18] Although the increased risk of CVD in JSLE, JDM, and JIA is evident, effective interventions remain elusive. This review (1) introduces the American Heart Association's (AHA) definition of cardiovascular health (CVH) and its relevance in pediatric rheumatologic diseases; (2) describes the "perfect storm" arising from the interplay of traditional and disease-related cardiovascular risk factors in pediatric rheumatologic diseases; and (3) highlights potential interventions to mitigate CVD risk in youth with pediatric rheumatologic diseases.

DEFINING CARDIOVASCULAR HEALTH AND ITS RELEVANCE TO PEDIATRIC RHEUMATOLOGIC DISEASES

What is Cardiovascular Health?

The AHA published Strategic Impact Goals in 2010 with a pediatric follow-up in 2016 outlining the novel construct of CVH.[19,20] The AHA's 2010 statement describes CVH as a measure for tracking progress in *primordial prevention* of CVD, defined as population-wide efforts to prevent individual-level development of risk factors for CVD, as opposed to primary or secondary prevention (ie, for individuals with established risk factors or CVD events).[19] CVH is a positive health construct, not only indicating absence of disease but also identifying health factors and behaviors associated with favorable long-term prognosis. CVH is composed of individual components that are (1) rigorously supported by epidemiologic, clinical, and mechanistic data; (2) simple to measure; (3) understandable to patients and other stakeholders; and (4) actionable for all patients including children.[19,20] An ideal CVH phenotype defined by AHA includes optimal levels of 7 health behaviors and factors (ie, healthy diet; high physical activity; nonsmoking; lean body mass index [BMI]; and optimal values for blood total cholesterol, fasting blood glucose, and blood pressure). Ideal CVH is associated with dramatically lower long-term risks of CVD events, premature mortality, other chronic diseases of aging, and lower health care costs (**Box 1**).[19,20]

CVH is operationalized by categorizing individual metrics as "poor," "intermediate," or "ideal," assigning a corresponding score ranging from 0 to 2 to each metric, and then summing individual item scores to generate a CVH summary score (range: 0–14) that can be categorized as "low," "moderate," or "high."[19–21]

Poor Cardiovascular Health Leads to Higher Cardiovascular Disease Risk

Ideal CVH is rare in adults, and poorer CVH is associated with incident CVD events and risk indicators such as arterial stiffness.[21–25] Ideal CVH is also uncommon in childhood, and the prevalence of high childhood CVH may be decreasing.[26–33] CVH is highest at birth and declines by adulthood, but dramatically worsening CVH is often evident even in early childhood. Ideal BMI rates decline from 77% at 2 to 5 years old to 67% by 6 to 11 years old. Ideal diet is rare in early childhood, and poor diet and higher BMI correlate with hypercholesterolemia and hypertension in the first 11 years of life.[33] Overweight and obese children are at especially high risk of early CVH loss.[29] By young adulthood, ideal CVH occurs in as little as 1% of the population, and poorer CVH is associated with higher cIMT.[30] Cross-sectional CVH assessments in childhood predict subclinical cardiovascular measures in adulthood more than 20 years later, including cIMT/arterial elasticity,[34] cardiac structure/function,[35] hypertension, lipids, and metabolic syndrome.[36] Patients who regain a degree of CVH later in life have a lower risk of subclinical atherosclerosis in middle adulthood, suggesting a critical period in early life for promoting CVH.[37] Differing trajectories of CVH decline also independently predict adult CVD outcomes. Individuals with rapidly declining

Box 1
Contributors to cardiovascular disease risk in pediatric rheumatologic diseases

Cardiovascular Health Factors:
- Smoking status
- Physical activity
- Diet quality
- Blood pressure
- Body mass index
- Total cholesterol
- Fasting blood glucose

Disease-Related Risk Factors:
- Chronic inflammation and immune dysregulation
  - Persistent disease activity
  - Elevated hsCRP
  - Cytokines (eg, TNF-α, interleukin-6, interferons)
  - Neutrophil extracellular traps
- Endothelial dysfunction
- Lupus nephritis and/or proteinuria (JSLE)
- Neuropsychiatric lupus manifestations (JSLE)
- Antiphospholipid antibodies
- Lipodystrophy (JDM)
- Homocysteine

Additional Factors:
- Corticosteroids and immunosuppressive treatment
- Depression and psychological stress
- Adverse childhood experiences
- Health disparities (eg, race/ethnicity, socioeconomic status)

CVH trajectories during childhood have greater cIMT by middle age, independent of cross-sectional assessments of CVH.[28] Favorable CVH in late adolescence predicts lower rates of CVD events/death at 32 years follow-up across demographic groups (ie, race/ethnicity, sex).[38] Social determinants of health, including lower family income and minority race, also predict poorer CVH.[26,27,39–42]

Relevance of Cardiovascular Health in Pediatric Rheumatologic Diseases

With increasing awareness of CVD risks in pediatric rheumatologic diseases, routine screening and intervention, particularly for patients with JSLE, are considered indicators of high-quality care.[43,44] However, cardiovascular screening in routine rheumatology practice lags behind recommendations.[45,46] CVH is feasible to measure in adult and pediatric practice,[47,48] and the inverse correlation of CVH scores with inflammatory markers[48–50] supports adoption of CVH monitoring in pediatric rheumatology clinical and research settings where existing data in JSLE, JDM, and JIA suggest poorer CVH than the general pediatric population.

Cardiovascular health indicators in juvenile systemic lupus erythematosus

Dyslipidemia occurs in up to 63% of patients with JSLE overall and more frequently with higher disease activity or nephritis.[51–53] Dyslipidemia is prominent at JSLE diagnosis but improves during treatment.[54]The APPLE trial and other studies demonstrated that lipid profiles fluctuate throughout JSLE disease course with specific lipid subtypes differentially affected by complex interactions between disease activity, steroid dosage, nephritis, and proteinuria.[11,54–57] Even in the absence of active disease, steroid use, and nephritis, JSLE confers a high risk of dyslipidemia.[58]

In addition to dyslipidemia, other CVH metrics are frequently unfavorable in JSLE. Hypertension occurs in up to two-thirds of patients with JSLE.[59,60] At least one-third of participants in the APPLE trial had been diagnosed with hypertension and/or reported a history of antihypertensive medication use[11,61] and uncontrolled hypertension often persists years after diagnosis.[62] Hypertension in JSLE is associated with disease activity, inflammation, nephritis, obesity, and measures of subclinical CVD including cIMT, pulse wave velocity, and left ventricular mass index.[60,62,63] In addition to hypertension, roughly 25% of patients with JSLE are obese, and they demonstrate higher adiposity associated with corticosteroid use, lower aerobic fitness, less physical activity, poorer quality of life, and worse functional outcomes.[60,64–67] Metabolic syndrome is prevalent in JSLE and is associated with both disease activity and steroid use.[68] Although there are limited data on diet quality and smoking status among patients with JSLE, up to 80% of patients with JSLE report poor diets,[69] and although tobacco use may not be prevalent in patients with JSLE, rates of smoking and e-cigarette use have not been monitored longitudinally.[60]

Cardiovascular health indicators in juvenile dermatomyositis

Although less attention has been paid to CVH factors in JDM compared with JSLE, patients with JDM experience poor CVH in childhood that declines through adulthood. Analyses of greater than 10 years of National Inpatient Sample data demonstrated that patients hospitalized with JDM had higher rates of hypertension, obesity, diabetes, lipid abnormalities, atherosclerosis, and other cardiovascular/cerebrovascular risk factors and comorbidities than other hospitalized pediatric patients.[12] Overweight/obesity occurs in nearly half of patients with JDM alongside hypertriglyceridemia (47%), elevated fasting insulin (41%), metabolic syndrome (25%), and hypertension (23.5%).[70] Unfavorable CVH factors, particularly dyslipidemia and hyperinsulinemia, are especially common in patients with JDM with lipodystrophy.[71,72] Kozu and colleagues found higher rates of hypertriglyceridemia, hypercholesterolemia, and low high-density lipoprotein (HDL) in patients with JDM versus controls.[73] Sedentary behavior is common in JDM, with 95% of patients falling short of recommended physical activity levels.[74] Poor CVH in JDM persists into adulthood. Compared with healthy controls, adults with JDM have more proatherogenic lipid profiles (eg, higher proinflammatory oxidized HDL levels) and higher blood pressure.[75] Nearly 10% of adults with JDM had documented hypertension despite low disease activity at long-term follow-up.[76] Although data on CVH factors in adults with JDM remain scarce, data from patients with adult-onset dermatomyositis corroborate concern for poor CVH, given high rates of metabolic syndrome (34%–40%), diabetes mellitus (18%–29%), and hypertension (up to 62%).[77–79] Although diet quality and smoking are understudied in JDM, a study of adults with dermatomyositis found that despite similar rates of smoking compared with control patients (~11%), dermatomyositis was associated with far higher rates of metabolic syndrome, diabetes, and stroke.[77]

Cardiovascular health indicators in juvenile idiopathic arthritis

Adults with rheumatoid arthritis have significantly higher risks of CVD, comparable with adult lupus and dermatomyositis.[2] Patients with JIA frequently experience poor CVH, leading to concern about adverse long-term cardiovascular outcomes.[80] Obesity is prevalent in JIA and associated with early deleterious cardiovascular changes, dyslipidemia, and insulin resistance.[81] Dyslipidemia is most common in systemic-onset JIA, as compared with other JIA subtypes, and among patients with JIA with active disease, whereas adequate treatment response predicts improvement in dyslipidemia.[82,83] Girls with JIA have higher BMI and fat mass than controls.[84] Rates of overweight/obesity vary by JIA subtype. Patients with refractory polyarticular JIA and juvenile psoriatic arthritis are more likely to be overweight/obese than other JIA subtypes and the general pediatric population.[85,86] Steroid use and low physical activity predict elevated BMI in children with JIA.[87] Overweight/obesity may be more prevalent in patients with JIA, even patients with inactive disease, compared with controls,[88] but this is not consistent across studies.[89] Among patients with enthesitis-related arthritis, higher BMI is associated with difficulty achieving clinically inactive disease, a worrisome finding given uncontrolled inflammation may contribute to long-term cardiovascular risk.[90] Inadequate physical activity is prevalent in JIA, even during low disease activity, and may contribute to subclinical atherosclerosis.[80,91–94] Poor CVH, exemplified by high rates of metabolic syndrome, is common in adults with JIA.[13] Increased fat mass and low lean body mass have been noted in adults with active JIA.[14] Long-term follow-up of adults with JIA reveals higher rates of hypertension, tobacco smoking, insulin resistance, and family history of CVD.[15,16] First-time mothers with JIA have higher rates of heart disease, prepregnancy hypertension, and preeclampsia/eclampsia.[17]

PERFECT STORM: INTERPLAY OF DISEASE-RELATED RISKS AND POOR CARDIOVASCULAR HEALTH IN PEDIATRIC RHEUMATOLOGIC DISEASE

Children with rheumatologic disease are recognized by the AHA for higher CVD risk due to both poor CVH and disease-related factors (see **Box 1**).[95] A systematic review in adults with SLE demonstrated higher rates of premature coronary heart disease due to the presence of poor CVH, disease-related inflammation, and nephritis, leading to greater CVD risk than calculated by traditional cardiovascular risk scoring systems.[96] The bidirectional interplay of poor CVH and disease-related factors such as chronic inflammation, endothelial dysfunction, and medication effects (eg, corticosteroids) creates a “perfect storm” for poor long-term cardiovascular outcomes in patients with JSLE, JDM, and JIA (**Fig. 1**).[43,57,78,97]

Chronic Inflammation and Cardiovascular Health Factors in Pediatric Rheumatologic Diseases

JSLE, JDM, and JIA are marked by chronic inflammation, which contributes to worse long-term cardiovascular outcomes. Patients with JSLE with higher disease activity are more likely to have subclinical atherosclerosis, even after adjusting for creatinine clearance, proteinuria, and steroid use.[69] Measures of inflammation associated with CVD, including tumor necrosis factor-alpha (TNFα) and high-sensitivity C-reactive protein (hsCRP), are higher in JSLE versus control patients, with similar findings emerging in JDM and JIA regarding variable levels of TNFα and associated CVD risk.[81,98,99] Increased inflammation is associated with decreased heart rate variability and systolic/diastolic dysfunction in JSLE, JDM, and JIA.[100–104] Subclinical systolic/diastolic dysfunction in JDM is predicted by persistent skin disease activity, inflammatory biomarkers, and dyslipidemia.[100,101] In addition to cytokines, abnormal levels of adipokines have been noted in JSLE, JDM, and JIA.[18,75,105] Aberrant neutrophil function also contributes to atherosclerotic plaque formation/rupture and heightened cardiovascular risk in JSLE and JDM.[106–109] Platelet-derived S100A8/A9, a biomarker associated with inflammation, is elevated even among patients with inactive lupus and is strongly associated with CVD, particularly myocardial infarction.[110,111] Patients with JSLE, JDM, and JIA thus face elevated cardiovascular disease risk due to the confluence of multiple proinflammatory pathways.

Chronic inflammation in pediatric rheumatologic diseases contributes to dyslipidemia, hypertension, and hyperinsulinemia, leading to early loss of CVH. JSLE disease activity is strongly associated with dyslipidemia, higher low-density lipoprotein (LDL) particle

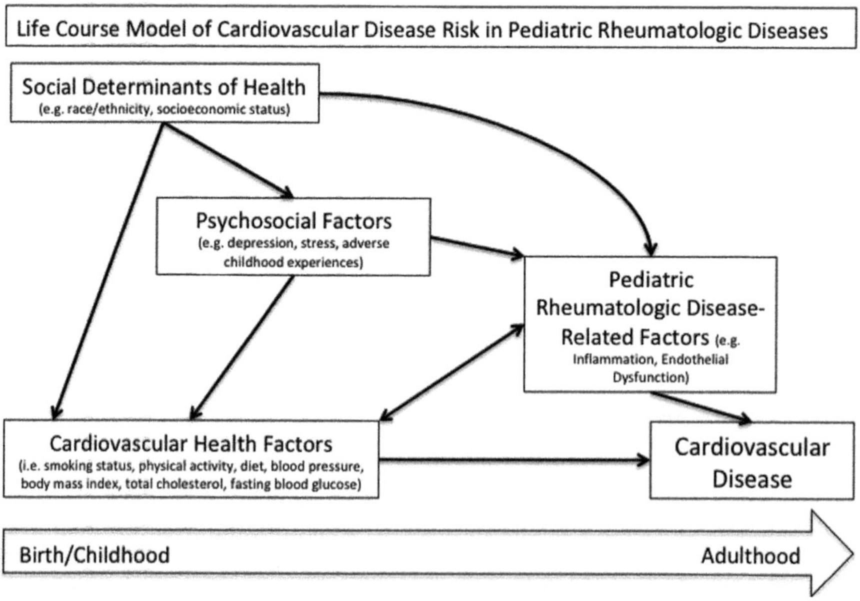

Fig. 1. Conceptual schema of relationships between cardiovascular health (protective factors), pediatric rheumatologic disease–related risk factors, psychosocial factors, and cardiovascular disease over the life course.

oxidizability, and insulin resistance.[51,54,112] Post hoc analyses of APPLE trial data found measures of disease activity and inflammation are associated with dyslipidemia, hypertension, and atorvastatin response.[61,113–115] Even in patients with well-controlled JSLE, lipid profiles remain proatherogenic and correlate with subclinical inflammation.[58,116] In JDM, proinflammatory cytokines, abnormal neutrophil function, and clinical disease activity correlate with dyslipidemia and hyperinsulinemia.[70,73,75,101,108,117] Higher disease activity and inflammation also predict dyslipidemia and proatherogenic inflammatory lipid profiles in patients with JIA, with improvement on achieving inactive disease especially in the setting of TNF inhibitor use.[83,118–120]

Just as chronic inflammation may worsen CVH, poor CVH can in turn exacerbate disease activity and chronic inflammation. Obesity in JSLE and JIA are associated with elevated cytokines, such as TNFα, that are associated with increased CVD risk.[118,121,122] Tobacco smoke exposure is proinflammatory[123] and may contribute to rheumatologic disease activity.[124–129] Finally, poor diet is associated with higher inflammation, although further study in pediatric rheumatologic diseases is needed to identify optimal diet composition.[130–134]

Endothelial dysfunction contributes to cardiovascular risk in pediatric rheumatologic diseases

Structural and functional endothelial abnormalities occur commonly in JSLE, JDM, and JIA and are associated with higher lifetime cardiovascular risk.[135,136] Nondipping blood pressure is prevalent in lupus, including JSLE, and associated with endothelial dysfunction, atherosclerotic changes, and abnormal myocardial deformation even when overt hypertension is absent.[137–139] Increased carotid arterial stiffness index is common in patients with JSLE, especially during active disease, compared with matched controls.[140,141] Detection of endothelial dysfunction varies based on the modality used, with increased cIMT noted most often in up to 60% of patients with JSLE, but lower rates of abnormal reactive hyperemia index, pulse wave velocity, and brachial artery reactivity.[60,116,139] Serum biomarkers of endothelial dysfunction are elevated during active JSLE.[142] Endothelial progenitor cells (EPC), which participate in vascular repair, are decreased in number and function in JSLE, and inhibition of type I Interferon reverses impairment of EPC differentiation.[143] The vasculitis component of the SLE disease activity index and abnormal nailfold capillaroscopy are both associated with diastolic dysfunction.[144,145] Endothelial dysfunction is thus a hallmark feature of JSLE and represents an important pathophysiologic mechanism for elevated CVD risk in this population.

Endothelial dysfunction in the setting of vasculopathy is a hallmark of JDM.[146] Adults with JDM demonstrate worse cIMT, brachial artery reactivity, and carotid-radial pulse wave velocity than healthy controls, and serum biomarkers of vasculopathy correlate with cIMT.[75,147] Circulating endothelial cells and microparticles, which measure endothelial cell injury, are high in JDM and correlate with disease activity, cytokine levels, and thrombotic tendency.[147] A subset of patients with JDM with inactive disease demonstrate persistent elevation in endothelial injury biomarkers.[136] A pilot study did not identify decreased EPC numbers in JDM, although EPC function was not assessed and the study may have been limited by small sample size.[148] In another study, abnormal reactive hyperemia index was noted in 50% of the participants with JDM.[149] The relationship of endothelial dysfunction with myocardial function remains understudied, with one study finding no association between nailfold capillary abnormalities and cardiac parameters.[150]

Endothelial dysfunction has received less attention in JIA, although it may be a concern particularly by adulthood. No differences in pulse wave velocity were found between JIA and control patients, although the study excluded patients with cardiovascular risk factors and predominantly enrolled oligoarticular patients who may experience less systemic inflammation than other JIA subtypes.[151] In another study, cIMT did not differ between adults with JIA and controls, although endothelial activation and oxidative stress were higher in patients with JIA.[18] Adults with JIA demonstrate higher pulse wave velocity in association with elevated diastolic blood pressure.[16] EPC responses to exercise were blunted in patients with JIA, suggesting less effective vascular repair potentially worsening endothelial dysfunction.[152]

Other disease-related cardiovascular risk factors

Corticosteroids and other disease-related factors (eg, nephritis, lipodystrophy) contribute to poor CVH and higher CVD risk in children with rheumatologic diseases. Studies on the impact of corticosteroids on CVH in pediatric rheumatologic diseases demonstrate mixed findings, with most focusing on JSLE. Corticosteroids cause BMI to rapidly increase in children with rheumatic diseases and half do not return to their premorbid BMI particularly if high doses are administered.[153] Higher cumulative corticosteroid dosage predicts higher LDL-cholesterol and metabolic syndrome in JSLE, and prednisone dose reduction is associated with improved lipid profiles after controlling for disease activity.[55,58,68] However, corticosteroids may also protect against dyslipidemia in patients with JSLE by decreasing disease activity, suggesting mixed impacts on CVH.[54] The APPLE trial and another smaller study demonstrated a nonlinear relationship of corticosteroid dosage with cIMT, with protective effects at lowest and highest dosages and deleterious impact at intermediate dosages,[11,60,154] reflecting the shifting balance of corticosteroids' effects on inflammation, endothelial function, and CVH factors. The impact of corticosteroids on CVH in JDM and JIA has not been studied in detail, although nonlinear relationships similar to those seen in JSLE are likely in these populations as well.

Renal involvement in JSLE is also an independent cardiovascular risk factor that can worsen CVH (eg, dyslipidemia) and worsen endothelial dysfunction.[56,142,155,156] Nephrotic-range proteinuria in JSLE is associated with dyslipidemia, hypertension, increased cIMT, and worse ventricular function.[51,55,58,60,144,157] Lupus nephritis, neuropsychiatric manifestations of JSLE, and antiphospholipid antibodies also predict late-onset heart failure and right ventricular dysfunction.[158,159] Elevated homocysteine levels in patients with JSLE, particularly those with nephritis, are associated with higher total and LDL-cholesterol levels, endothelial dysfunction, atherosclerosis, and cardiovascular events.[53,56,160–162]

Finally, lipodystrophy is prevalent in JDM and is associated with dyslipidemia, especially hypertriglyceridemia, insulin resistance, and abnormal adipokine levels in JDM.[71,72,75] More generalized forms of lipodystrophy in JDM are associated with more severe disease features and higher rates of insulin resistance and steatohepatitis.[163]

POTENTIAL INTERVENTIONS AND FUTURE DIRECTIONS

Pharmacologic Interventions

Given the contribution of inflammation to cardiovascular risk, controlling rheumatologic disease activity is likely important for risk reduction (**Box 2**). Studies suggest some immunosuppressive agents (eg, methotrexate,[164] TNFα inhibitors[119,120]) may be protective, whereas others (eg, cyclosporine[73]) are less favorable for long-term cardiovascular outcomes. Hydroxychloroquine is associated with improved lipid profile,[165] decreased incidence of atrial fibrillation,[166] and lower rates of coronary artery disease in adults with lupus,[167] although validation of these findings in JSLE and

Box 2
Potential interventions and targets for cardiovascular health promotion in pediatric rheumatologic diseases

Pharmacologic:
- Immunosuppression and control of disease activity (eg, TNF inhibitors)
- Hydroxychloroquine
- Low-dose aspirin
- Novel antiinflammatory agents (eg, colchicine)
- Lipid-lowering agents (eg, statins)
- Antihypertensive agents (eg, ACE inhibitors)
- Hyperinsulinemia
- Vitamin D

Nonpharmacological:
- Cardiovascular risk factor screening programs
- Physical activity interventions (eg, wearable devices, structured exercise regimens)
- Dietary interventions (eg, nutritional education, Mediterranean diet)
- Smoking cessation
- Emotional distress (eg, stress, depression, anxiety)
- Positive psychological well-being and coping
- Trauma-informed care/resiliency interventions for childhood adversity
- Health equity interventions to address disparities

JDM is required. Low-dose aspirin alone[168] or in combination with hydroxychloroquine[169] may decrease the risk of cardiovascular events in adults through antithrombotic and antiinflammatory mechanisms, although further study in pediatric populations is needed. Novel uses of antiinflammatory agents, such as colchicine, for cardiovascular risk reduction may warrant further study in pediatric rheumatologic diseases.[170]

In addition to controlling inflammation, pharmacologic strategies can bolster CVH by addressing dyslipidemia, hypertension, and insulin resistance (see **Box 2**). In adults with lupus, statins are associated with lower rates of CVD[171] with protective effects on endothelial function independent of effects on lipid profile,[172] but they remain underutilized even in "at-risk" lupus patients.[173] The APPLE study is the largest randomized controlled trial in JSLE to date and assessed the use of atorvastatin for slowing cIMT progression. Although primary endpoints were not met, post hoc analyses suggest that postpubertal status, hypovitaminosis D, elevated hsCRP, and C4 genetic variants may identify patients who could benefit from atorvastatin, although prospective confirmatory studies are needed.[11,61,113,115] The impact of vitamin D on CVH and cardiovascular risk in pediatric rheumatologic diseases deserves further study given that higher vitamin D levels are associated with decreased inflammation, improved endothelial function, lower disease activity, and lower rates of metabolic syndrome.[114,174–179] Adults with lupus reaching lower blood pressure targets were found to have fewer cardiovascular events[180]; identification of optimal blood pressure targets in children with rheumatologic diseases deserves further study. Pharmacologic management of insulin resistance may improve cardiometabolic profile and decrease inflammation,[181,182] but studies in children with rheumatologic diseases are needed to better understand the impact of disease- and treatment-related factors on beta cell function[183] and the role of pharmacotherapy in managing hyperinsulinemia.

Nonpharmacological Interventions

Nonpharmacological interventions can also promote CVH and reduce cardiovascular risk in JSLE, JDM, and JIA (see **Box 2**). Although international guidelines recommend routine assessment of cardiovascular risk factors in adults and children with lupus, multiple studies demonstrate lack of patient awareness and inadequate screening.[45,46,184,185] Quality improvement methods have been used to increase rates of lipid screening in patients with JSLE by increasing awareness and protocolizing risk assessments.[44]

Behavioral interventions promoting healthy lifestyles may improve CVH in patients with pediatric rheumatologic diseases. Increased physical activity may decrease chronic inflammation and endothelial dysfunction, addressing both traditional and disease-related cardiovascular risk factors.[186–191] Pilot studies of internet-based physical activity promotion, wearable physical activity trackers, and resistance exercise interventions have demonstrated feasibility in patients with JIA.[192–195] Although structured exercise therapy is safe and effective in lupus and dermatomyositis, future studies should assess interventions that minimize sedentary behavior and increase motivation for physical activity.[196–199] Higher quality diets (eg, Mediterranean diet, higher fiber intake) are associated with favorable body composition, lower triglycerides, and decreased homocysteine, whereas nutritional education interventions in JSLE demonstrate favorable effects on adiposity and lipid profile.[130,200–202] Finally, the authors recommend that future studies assess smoking rates and identify prevention and cessation programs that are feasible, acceptable, and effective in pediatric rheumatologic disease populations.[184,203]

Psychosocial contributors to CVH and CVD are important targets for intervention (see **Box 1**). The AHA has recognized CVD risks associated with depression as well as protective effects of positive psychological well-being (see **Fig. 1**).[204,205] Children with rheumatologic diseases frequently experience psychological stress, anxiety, and depression, and their mental health needs often go unmet.[206–208] Depression in adults with lupus is associated with more rapid cIMT progression, coronary artery calcification, and carotid plaques, likely mediated by systemic inflammation that is also triggered by emotional distress, although pediatric studies are lacking.[188,209–212] Psychological interventions that address anxiety, depression, and coping skills in children with rheumatologic diseases could exert beneficial effects on cytokine balance and CVH, but further study is required.[42,213–216]

Adverse childhood experiences (ACEs) are intense early life stressors (eg, abuse, parental loss) that are associated with worse cardiovascular outcomes in adulthood.[217] The impact of ACEs on cardiovascular risk and CVH is likely mediated by a combination of maladaptive health behaviors (eg, medication nonadherence), psychosocial factors (eg, depression), and biological factors (eg, chronic inflammation, endothelial dysfunction), but trauma-informed care models may buffer negative health impacts (see **Fig. 1**).[218–221] Emerging evidence suggests that ACEs such as child abuse are associated with incident lupus, worse functional outcomes in adults with lupus, and a dose-dependent association with childhood-onset forms of arthritis, but ACEs' impact on CVH has not been studied in pediatric rheumatologic disease populations.[222–224] The contribution of ACEs to CVD risk in pediatric rheumatology patients, as well as resilience factors that could buffer the deleterious effects of ACEs, deserve further study.

Finally, the authors recommend studying interventions that address health disparities in CVH and CVD risk in pediatric rheumatologic diseases, given that other disparate health outcomes have been noted in JSLE, JDM, and JIA (see **Fig. 1**).[225–229] Studies demonstrate significantly worse cardiovascular outcomes in Black, Hispanic, and economically disadvantaged adults with lupus,[230–234] but there is currently scant data on CVH disparities in children with rheumatologic diseases.[56,59]

SUMMARY

Patients with JSLE, JDM, and JIA face higher lifetime CVD risk than unaffected children. CVH, defined as the sum of protective factors against CVD, declines in childhood and is lost prematurely in children with rheumatologic diseases. Chronic inflammation and endothelial dysfunction potentiate the lifetime risk of CVD in JSLE, JDM, and JIA. Pharmacologic management of disease activity, inflammation, and CVH factors may reduce long-term CVD risk. In addition, interventions addressing healthy behaviors, psychological well-being, and social determinants of health can improve CVH in children with rheumatologic diseases. Further studies are needed to determine the effectiveness of specific interventions and the mediators and moderators of these effects.

CLINICS CARE POINTS

- CVH is composed of 7 protective factors that can be feasibly measured in pediatric practice.
- Routine assessment of CVH factors in patients with JSLE, JDM, and JIA is warranted.
- Disease-related cardiovascular risk factors such as chronic inflammation and endothelial dysfunction should be monitored.
- Controlling underlying disease activity may help reduce cardiovascular risk in pediatric rheumatologic diseases.
- Pharmacologic and nonpharmacologic interventions for CVH promotion in pediatric rheumatologic diseases are warranted.

DISCLOSURE

Dr K. Ardalan receives salary support from Cure JM Foundation to assist with clinical trial design with ReveraGen BioPharma but does not receive any funding or compensation from ReveraGen BioPharma; he also receives salary/grant support from the Childhood Arthritis and Rheumatology Research Alliance (CARRA) and Rheumatology Research Foundation. Dr D.M. Lloyd-Jones has no commercial or financial conflicts to disclose. Dr L.E. Schanberg receives salary support from CARRA, Inc; DSMB member for Sanofi and UCB; grant support from PCORI and BMS.

REFERENCES

1. Tektonidou MG, Lewandowski LB, Hu J, et al. Survival in adults and children with systemic lupus erythematosus: a systematic review and Bayesian meta-analysis of studies from 1950 to 2016. Ann Rheum Dis 2017;76(12):2009–16.
2. Ferguson LD, Sattar N, McInnes IB. Managing cardiovascular risk in patients with rheumatic disease. Med Clin North Am 2021;105(2):247–62.
3. Yazdany J, Pooley N, Langham J, et al. Systemic lupus erythematosus; stroke and myocardial infarction risk: a systematic review and meta-analysis. RMD Open 2020;6(2):e001247.
4. Rai SK, Choi HK, Sayre EC, et al. Risk of myocardial infarction and ischaemic stroke in adults with polymyositis and dermatomyositis: a general population-based study. Rheumatology 2016;55(3):461–9.
5. Barbhaiya M, Feldman CH, Chen SK, et al. Comparative risks of cardiovascular disease in patients with systemic lupus erythematosus, diabetes mellitus, and in general Medicaid recipients. Arthritis Care Res 2020;72(10):1431–9.

6. Ramos-Rodriguez AJ, Cancel-Artau KJ, Lemor A, et al. The in-hospital burden of dermatomyositis on patients with acute myocardial infarction: a nationwide cross-sectional analysis from 2004 to 2015. J Am Acad Dermatol 2021;85(4):1006–8.
7. Ke S-R, Liu C-W, Wu Y-W, et al. Systemic lupus erythematosus is associated with poor outcome after acute myocardial infarction. Nutr Metab Cardiovasc Dis 2019;29(12):1400–7.
8. Colaco K, Ocampo V, Ayala AP, et al. Predictive utility of cardiovascular risk prediction algorithms in inflammatory rheumatic diseases: a systematic review. J Rheumatol 2020;47(6):928–38.
9. Groot N, Shaikhani D, Teng YKO, et al. Long-term clinical outcomes in a cohort of adults with childhood-onset systemic lupus erythematosus. Arthritis Rheumatol 2019;71(2):290–301.
10. Sozeri B, Deveci M, Dincel N, et al. The early cardiovascular changes in pediatric patients with systemic lupus erythematosus. Pediatr Nephrol 2013;28(3):471–6.
11. Schanberg LE, Sandborg C, Barnhart HX, et al. Use of atorvastatin in systemic lupus erythematosus in children and adolescents. Arthritis Rheum 2012;64(1):285–96.
12. Silverberg JI, Kwa L, Kwa MC, et al. Cardiovascular and cerebrovascular comorbidities of juvenile dermatomyositis in US children: an analysis of the National Inpatient Sample. Rheumatology 2018;57(4):694–702.
13. Sule S, Fontaine K. Metabolic syndrome in adults with a history of juvenile arthritis. Open Access Rheumatol 2018;10:67–72.
14. Brabnikova Maresova K, Jarosova K, Pavelka K, et al. The association between lean mass and bone mineral content in the high disease activity group of adult patients with juvenile idiopathic arthritis. BMC Musculoskelet Disord 2014;15(1):51.
15. Anderson JH, Anderson KR, Aulie HA, et al. Juvenile idiopathic arthritis and future risk for cardiovascular disease: a multicenter study. Scand J Rheumatol 2016;45(4):299–303.
16. Aulie HA, Selvaag AM, Günther A, et al. Arterial haemodynamics and coronary artery calcification in adult patients with juvenile idiopathic arthritis. Ann Rheum Dis 2015;74(8):1515–21.
17. Feldman DE, Vinet É, Bérard A, et al. Heart disease, hypertension, gestational diabetes mellitus, and preeclampsia/eclampsia in mothers with juvenile arthritis: a nested case-control study. Arthritis Care Res 2017;69(2):306–9.
18. Aranda-Valera IC, Arias de la Rosa I, Roldán-Molina R, et al. Subclinical cardiovascular risk signs in adults with juvenile idiopathic arthritis in sustained remission. Pediatr Rheumatol 2020;18(1):59.
19. Lloyd-Jones DM, Hong Y, Labarthe D, et al. Defining and setting national goals for cardiovascular health promotion and disease reduction: the American Heart Association's Strategic Impact Goal through 2020 and beyond. Circulation 2010;121(4):586–613.
20. Steinberger J, Daniels SR, Hagberg N, et al. Cardiovascular health promotion in children: challenges and opportunities for 2020 and beyond: a scientific statement from the American Heart Association. Circulation 2016;134(12):e236–55.
21. Folsom AR, Yatsuya H, Nettleton JA, et al. Community prevalence of ideal cardiovascular health, by the American Heart Association definition, and relationship with cardiovascular disease incidence. J Am Coll Cardiol 2011;57(16):1690–6.

22. Huffman MD, Capewell S, Ning H, et al. Cardiovascular health behavior and health factor changes (1988–2008) and projections to 2020: results from the National Health and Nutrition Examination Surveys. Circulation 2012;125(21): 2595–602.
23. Oyenuga AO, Folsom AR, Cheng S, et al. Greater adherence to Life's Simple 7 Is associated with less arterial stiffness: the Atherosclerosis Risk in Communities (ARIC) Study. Am J Hypertens 2019;32(8):769–76.
24. Ramírez-Vélez R, Saavedra JM, Lobelo F, et al. Ideal cardiovascular health and incident cardiovascular disease among adults: a systematic review and meta-analysis. Mayo Clinic Proc 2018;93(11):1589–99.
25. Dong C, Rundek T, Wright CB, et al. Ideal cardiovascular health predicts lower risks of myocardial infarction, stroke, and vascular death across whites, blacks, and hispanics: the Northern Manhattan Study. Circulation 2012;125(24): 2975–84.
26. Dong H, Yan Y, Liu J, et al. Alarming trends in ideal cardiovascular health among children and adolescents in Beijing, China, 2004 to 2014. Int J Cardiol 2017;231: 264–70.
27. Gooding HC, Ning H, Perak AM, et al. Cardiovascular health decline in adolescent girls in the NGHS cohort, 1987–1997. Prev Med Rep 2020;20:101276.
28. Allen NB, Krefman AE, Labarthe D, et al. Cardiovascular health trajectories from childhood through middle age and their association with subclinical atherosclerosis. JAMA Cardiol 2020;5(5):557–66.
29. Fyfe-Johnson AL, Ryder JR, Alonso A, et al. Ideal cardiovascular health and adiposity: implications in youth. J Am Heart Assoc 2018;7(8):e007467.
30. Oikonen M, Laitinen TT, Magnussen CG, et al. Ideal cardiovascular health in young adult populations from the United States, Finland, and Australia and its association with cIMT: the International Childhood Cardiovascular Cohort Consortium. J Am Heart Assoc 2013;2(3):e000244.
31. Henriksson P, Henriksson H, Gracia-Marco L, et al. Prevalence of ideal cardiovascular health in European adolescents: the HELENA study. Int J Cardiol 2017; 240:428–32.
32. Shay CM, Ning H, Daniels SR, et al. Status of cardiovascular health in US adolescents: prevalence estimates from the National Health and Nutrition Examination Surveys (NHANES) 2005–2010. Circulation 2013;127(13):1369–76.
33. Ning H, Labarthe DR, Shay CM, et al. Status of cardiovascular health in US children up to 11 years of age: the National Health and Nutrition Examination Surveys 2003–2010. Circ Cardiovasc Qual Outcomes 2015;8(2):164–71.
34. Pahkala K, Hietalampi H, Laitinen TT, et al. Ideal cardiovascular health in adolescence: effect of lifestyle intervention and association with vascular intima-media thickness and elasticity (The Special Turku Coronary Risk Factor Intervention Project for Children [STRIP] Study). Circulation 2013;127(21):2088–96.
35. Laitinen TT, Ruohonen S, Juonala M, et al. Ideal cardiovascular health in childhood—Longitudinal associations with cardiac structure and function: The Special Turku Coronary Risk Factor Intervention Project (STRIP) and the Cardiovascular Risk in Young Finns Study (YFS). Int J Cardiol 2017;230:304–9.
36. Laitinen TT, Pahkala K, Magnussen CG, et al. Ideal cardiovascular health in childhood and cardiometabolic outcomes in adulthood: the cardiovascular risk in young finns study. Circulation 2012;125(16):1971–8.
37. Laitinen TT, Pahkala K, Magnussen CG, et al. Lifetime measures of ideal cardiovascular health and their association with subclinical atherosclerosis: the Cardiovascular Risk in Young Finns Study. Int J Cardiol 2015;185:186–91.

38. Perak AM, Ning H, Khan SS, et al. Associations of late adolescent or young adult cardiovascular health with premature cardiovascular disease and mortality. J Am Coll Cardiol 2020;76(23):2695–707.
39. Islam SJ, Kim JH, Baltrus P, et al. Neighborhood characteristics and ideal cardiovascular health among black adults: results from the Morehouse-Emory Cardiovascular (MECA) Center for Health Equity. Ann Epidemiol 2020. https://doi.org/10.1016/j.annepidem.2020.11.009.
40. Henriksson P, Henriksson H, Labayen I, et al. Correlates of ideal cardiovascular health in European adolescents: the HELENA study. Nutr Metab Cardiovasc Dis 2018;28(2):187–94.
41. Unger E, Diez-Roux AV, Lloyd-Jones DM, et al. Association of neighborhood characteristics with cardiovascular health in the Multi-Ethnic Study of Atherosclerosis. Circ Cardiovasc Qual Outcomes 2014;7(4):524–31.
42. Pulkki-Råback L, Elovainio M, Hakulinen C, et al. Cumulative effect of psychosocial factors in youth on ideal cardiovascular health in adulthood: the Cardiovascular Risk in Young Finns Study. Circulation 2015;131(3):245–53.
43. Fanouriakis A, Kostopoulou M, Alunno A, et al. 2019 update of the EULAR recommendations for the management of systemic lupus erythematosus. Ann Rheum Dis 2019;78(6):736–45.
44. Smitherman EA, Huang B, Furnier A, et al. Quality of care in childhood-onset systemic lupus erythematosus: report of an intervention to improve cardiovascular and bone health screening. J Rheumatol 2020;47(10):1506–13.
45. Costenbader KH, Wright E, Liang MH, et al. Cardiac risk factor awareness and management in patients with systemic lupus erythematosus: cardiac risk factors in SLE. Arthritis Rheum 2004;51(6):983–8.
46. Scalzi LV, Ballou SP, Park JY, et al. Cardiovascular disease risk awareness in systemic lupus erythematosus patients. Arthritis Rheum 2008;58(5):1458–64.
47. Blackett P, Farrell K, Truong M, et al. Feasibility of ideal cardiovascular health evaluation in a pediatric clinic setting. Adv Prev Med 2018;2018:1–7.
48. Hernández-Martínez A, Gavilán-Carrera B, Vargas-Hitos JA, et al. Ideal cardiovascular health in women with systemic lupus erythematosus: association with arterial stiffness, inflammation, and fitness. Int J Cardiol 2021;330:2017–213.
49. Gaye B, Tafflet M, Arveiler D, et al. Ideal cardiovascular health and incident cardiovascular disease: heterogeneity across event subtypes and mediating effect of blood biomarkers: the PRIME study. J Am Heart Assoc 2017;6(10):e006389.
50. González-Gil EM, Santabárbara J, Ruiz JR, et al. Ideal cardiovascular health and inflammation in European adolescents: the HELENA study. Nutr Metab Cardiovasc Dis 2017;27(5):447–55.
51. Tyrrell PN, Beyene J, Benseler SM, et al. Predictors of lipid abnormalities in children with new-onset systemic lupus erythematosus. J Rheumatol 2007;34(10):2112–9.
52. El-Gamasy M, Abd Elsalam M, Abd-El Latif A, et al. Predictive values of dyslipidemia and B-type natriuretic peptide levels in juvenile systemic lupus erythematosus: a two center-experience. Saudi J Kidney Dis Transpl 2019;30(4):863.
53. Ortiz TT, Terreri MT, Caetano M, et al. Dyslipidemia in pediatric systemic lupus erythematosus: the relationship with disease activity and plasma homocysteine and cysteine concentrations. Ann Nutr Metab 2013;63(1–2):77–82.
54. Sarkissian T, Beyenne J, Feldman B, et al. The complex nature of the interaction between disease activity and therapy on the lipid profile in patients with pediatric systemic lupus erythematosus. Arthritis Rheum 2006;54(4):1283–90.

55. Sarkissian T, Beyene J, Feldman B, et al. Longitudinal examination of lipid profiles in pediatric systemic lupus erythematosus. Arthritis Rheum 2007;56(2):631–8.
56. Ardoin S, Schanberg L, Sandborg C, et al. Laboratory markers of cardiovascular risk in pediatric SLE: the APPLE baseline cohort. Lupus 2010;19(11):1315–25.
57. Ilowite NT, Samuel P, Ginzler E, et al. Dyslipoproteinemia in pediatric systemic lupus erythematosus. Arthritis Rheum 1988;31(7):859–63.
58. Machado D, Sarni ROS, Abad TTO, et al. Lipid profile among girls with systemic lupus erythematosus. Rheumatol Int 2017;37(1):43–8.
59. Ostrov BE, Min W, Eichenfield AH, et al. Hypertension in children with systemic lupus erythematosus. Semin Arthritis Rheum 1989;19(2):90–8.
60. Quinlan C, Kari J, Pilkington C, et al. The vascular phenotype of children with systemic lupus erythematosus. Pediatr Nephrol 2015;30(8):1307–16.
61. Mulvihill E, Ardoin S, Thompson SD, et al. Elevated serum complement levels and higher gene copy number of complement *C4B* are associated with hypertension and effective response to statin therapy in childhood-onset systemic lupus erythematosus (SLE). Lupus Sci Med 2019;6(1):e000333.
62. Avar Aydin PO, Shan J, Brunner HI, et al. Blood pressure control over time in childhood-onset systemic lupus erythematous. Lupus 2018;27(4):657–64.
63. Canpolat N, Kasapcopur O, Caliskan S, et al. Ambulatory blood pressure and subclinical cardiovascular disease in patients with juvenile-onset systemic lupus erythematosus. Pediatr Nephrol 2013;28(2):305–13.
64. Sule S, Fontaine K. Abnormal body composition, cardiovascular endurance, and muscle strength in pediatric SLE. Pediatr Rheumatol 2016;14(1):50.
65. Houghton KM, Tucker LB, Potts JE, et al. Fitness, fatigue, disease activity, and quality of life in pediatric lupus. Arthritis Rheum 2008;59(4):537–45.
66. Mina R, Klein-Gitelman MS, Nelson S, et al. Effects of obesity on health-related quality of life in juvenile-onset systemic lupus erythematosus. Lupus 2015;24(2):191–7.
67. Lilleby V, Haugen M, Mørkrid L, et al. Body composition, lipid and lipoprotein levels in childhood-onset systemic lupus erythematosus. Scand J Rheumatol 2007;36(1):40–7.
68. Sinicato NA, Postal M, de Oliveira Peliçari K, et al. Prevalence and features of metabolic syndrome in childhood-onset systemic lupus erythematosus. Clin Rheumatol 2017;36(7):1527–35.
69. Medeiros PBS, Salomão RG, Teixeira SR, et al. Disease activity index is associated with subclinical atherosclerosis in childhood-onset systemic lupus erythematosus. Pediatr Rheumatol 2021;19(1):35.
70. Coyle K, Rother KI, Weise M, et al. Metabolic abnormalities and cardiovascular risk factors in children with myositis. J Pediatr 2009;155(6):882–7.
71. Verma S, Singh S, Bhalla AK, et al. Study of subcutaneous fat in children with juvenile dermatomyositis. Arthritis Rheum 2006;55(4):564–8.
72. Huemer C, Kitson H, Malleson PN, et al. Lipodystrophy in patients with juvenile dermatomyositis — evaluation of clinical and metabolic abnormalities. J Rheumatol 2001;28(3):610–5.
73. Kozu KT, Silva CA, Bonfa E, et al. Dyslipidaemia in juvenile dermatomyositis: the role of disease activity. Clin Exp Rheumatol 2013;31(4):638–44.
74. Pinto AJ, Yazigi Solis M, de Sá Pinto AL, et al. Physical (in)activity and its influence on disease-related features, physical capacity, and health-related quality of life in a cohort of chronic juvenile dermatomyositis patients. Semin Arthritis Rheum 2016;46(1):64–70.

75. Eimer MJ, Brickman WJ, Seshadri R, et al. Clinical status and cardiovascular risk profile of adults with a history of juvenile dermatomyositis. J Pediatr 2011; 159(5):795–801.
76. Tsaltskan V, Aldous A, Serafi S, et al. Long-term outcomes in juvenile myositis patients. Semin Arthritis Rheum 2020;50(1):149–55.
77. de Moraes MT, de Souza FHC, de Barros TBM, et al. Analysis of metabolic syndrome in adult dermatomyositis with a focus on cardiovascular disease: metabolic syndrome and CVD in DM. Arthritis Care Res 2013;65(5):793–9.
78. Silva M, Borba E, Mello S, et al. Serum adipocytokine profile and metabolic syndrome in young adult female dermatomyositis patients. Clinics 2016;71(12): 709–14.
79. Limaye VS, Lester S, Blumbergs P, et al. Idiopathic inflammatory myositis is associated with a high incidence of hypertension and diabetes mellitus: clinical associations of inflammatory myositis. Int J Rheum Dis 2010;13(2):132–7.
80. Bohr A-H, Fuhlbrigge RC, Pedersen FK, et al. Premature subclinical atherosclerosis in children and young adults with juvenile idiopathic arthritis. A review considering preventive measures. Pediatr Rheumatol 2016;14(1):3.
81. Głowińska-Olszewska B, Bossowski A, Dobreńko E, et al. Subclinical cardiovascular system changes in obese patients with juvenile idiopathic arthritis. Mediators Inflamm 2013;2013:436702.
82. Ilowite NT, Samuel P, Beseler L, et al. Dyslipoproteinemia in juvenile rheumatoid arthritis. J Pediatr 1989;114(5):823–6.
83. Shen C-C, Yao T-C, Yeh K-W, et al. Association of disease activity and antirheumatic treatment in juvenile idiopathic arthritis with serum lipid profiles: a prospective study. Semin Arthritis Rheum 2013;42(6):590–6.
84. Caetano MC, Sarni ROS, Terreri MTL, et al. Excess of adiposity in female children and adolescents with juvenile idiopathic arthritis. Clin Rheumatol 2012; 31(6):967–71.
85. Markula-Patjas KP, Ivaska KK, Pekkinen M, et al. High adiposity and serum leptin accompanied by altered bone turnover markers in severe juvenile idiopathic arthritis. J Rheumatol 2014;41(12):2474–81.
86. Samad A, Stoll ML, Lavi I, et al. Adiposity in juvenile psoriatic arthritis. J Rheumatol 2018;45(3):411–8.
87. Schenck S, Niewerth M, Sengler C, et al. Prevalence of overweight in children and adolescents with juvenile idiopathic arthritis. Scand J Rheumatol 2015; 44(4):288–95.
88. Grönlund M-M, Kaartoaho M, Putto-Laurila A, et al. Juvenile idiopathic arthritis patients with low inflammatory activity have increased adiposity. Scand J Rheumatol 2014;43(6):488–92.
89. Markula-Patjas K, Valta H, Pekkinen M, et al. Body composition and adipokines in patients with juvenile idiopathic arthritis and systemic glucocorticoids. Clin Exp Rheumatol 2015;33(6):924–30.
90. Makay B, Gücenmez ÖA, Ünsal E. Inactive disease in enthesitis-related arthritis: association of increased body mass index. J Rheumatol 2016;43(5):937–43.
91. Nørgaard M, Herlin T. Specific sports habits, leisure-time physical activity, and school-educational physical activity in children with juvenile idiopathic arthritis: patterns and barriers. Arthritis Care Res 2019;71(2):271–80.
92. Bohr A-H, Nielsen S, Müller K, et al. Reduced physical activity in children and adolescents with juvenile idiopathic arthritis despite satisfactory control of inflammation. Pediatr Rheumatol 2015;13(1):57.

93. Risum K, Hansen BH, Selvaag AM, et al. Physical activity in patients with oligo- and polyarticular juvenile idiopathic arthritis diagnosed in the era of biologics: a controlled cross-sectional study. Pediatr Rheumatol 2018;16(1):64.
94. Bos GJFJ, Lelieveld OTHM, Armbrust W, et al. Physical activity in children with juvenile idiopathic arthritis compared to controls. Pediatr Rheumatol 2016; 14(1):42.
95. Kavey RE, Allada V, Daniels SR, et al. Cardiovascular risk reduction in high-risk pediatric patients: a scientific statement from the American Heart Association Expert Panel on Population and Prevention Science; the Councils on Cardiovascular Disease in the Young, Epidemiology and Prevention, Nutrition, Physical Activity and Metabolism, High Blood Pressure Research, Cardiovascular Nursing, and the Kidney in Heart Disease; and the Interdisciplinary Working Group on Quality of Care and Outcomes Research: Endorsed by the American Academy of Pediatrics. Circulation 2006;114(24):2710–38.
96. Tselios K, Sheane BJ, Gladman DD, et al. Optimal monitoring for coronary heart disease risk in patients with systemic lupus erythematosus: a systematic review. J Rheumatol 2016;43(1):54–65.
97. Canas JA, Sweeten S, Balagopal P. Biomarkers for cardiovascular risk in children. Curr Opin Cardiol 2013;28(2):103–14.
98. Salomão RG, de Carvalho LM, Izumi C, et al. Homocysteine, folate, hs-C-reactive protein, tumor necrosis factor alpha and inflammatory proteins: are these biomarkers related to nutritional status and cardiovascular risk in childhood-onset systemic lupus erythematosus? Pediatr Rheumatol 2018; 16(1):4.
99. Pachman LM, Liotta-Davis MR, Hong DK, et al. TNFα-308A allele in juvenile dermatomyositis: association with increased production of tumor necrosis factor α, disease duration, and pathologic calcifications. Arthritis Rheum 2000;43(10): 2368–77.
100. Schwartz T, Sanner H, Gjesdal O, et al. In juvenile dermatomyositis, cardiac systolic dysfunction is present after long-term follow-up and is predicted by sustained early skin activity. Ann Rheum Dis 2014;73(10):1805–10.
101. Schwartz T, Sjaastad I, Flato B, et al. In active juvenile dermatomyositis, elevated eotaxin and MCP-1 and cholesterol levels in the upper normal range are associated with cardiac dysfunction. Rheumatology 2014;53(12):2214–22.
102. Başaran Ö, Çetin İİ, Aydın F, et al. Heart rate variability in juvenile systemic lupus erythematosus patients. Turk J Pediatr 2019;61(5):733–40.
103. Berntsen KS, Tollisen A, Schwartz T, et al. Submaximal exercise capacity in juvenile dermatomyositis after longterm disease: the contribution of muscle, lung, and heart involvement. J Rheumatol 2017;44(6):827–34.
104. Lianza AC, Aikawa NE, Moraes JCB, et al. Long-term evaluation of cardiac function in juvenile idiopathic arthritis under anti-TNF therapy. Clin Exp Rheumatol 2014;32(5):754–9.
105. Al M, Ng L, Tyrrell P, et al. Adipokines as novel biomarkers in paediatric systemic lupus erythematosus. Rheumatology 2008;48(5):497–501.
106. Osaka M, Ito S, Honda M, et al. Critical role of the C5a-activated neutrophils in high-fat diet-induced vascular inflammation. Sci Rep 2016;6(1):21391.
107. Denny MF, Yalavarthi S, Zhao W, et al. A distinct subset of proinflammatory neutrophils isolated from patients with systemic lupus erythematosus induces vascular damage and synthesizes type I IFNs. J Immunol 2010;184(6):3284–97.

108. Duvvuri B, Pachman LM, Morgan G, et al. Neutrophil extracellular traps in tissue and periphery in juvenile dermatomyositis. Arthritis Rheumatol 2020;72(2): 348–58.
109. Garcia-Romo GS, Caielli S, Vega B, et al. Netting neutrophils are major inducers of type I IFN production in pediatric systemic lupus erythematosus. Sci Translational Med 2011;3(73). 73ra20.
110. Tyden H, Lood C, Gullstrand B, et al. Increased serum levels of S100A8/A9 and S100A12 are associated with cardiovascular disease in patients with inactive systemic lupus erythematosus. Rheumatology 2013;52(11):2048–55.
111. Lood C, Tydén H, Gullstrand B, et al. Platelet-derived S100A8/A9 and cardiovascular disease in systemic lupus erythematosus: platelet S100A8/A9 and CVD in SLE. Arthritis Rheumatol 2016;68(8):1970–80.
112. Posadas-Romero C, Torres-Tamayo M, Zamora-González J, et al. High insulin levels and increased low-density lipoprotein oxidizability in pediatric patients with systemic lupus erythematosus: high insulin levels and high LDL oxidizability in SLE. Arthritis Rheum 2004;50(1):160–5.
113. Robinson AB, Tangpricha V, Yow E, et al. Vitamin D status is a determinant of atorvastatin effect on carotid intima medial thickening progression rate in children with lupus: an Atherosclerosis Prevention in Pediatric Lupus Erythematosus (APPLE) substudy. Lupus Sci Med 2014;1(1):e000037.
114. Robinson AB, Tangpricha V, Yow E, et al. Vitamin D deficiency is common and associated with increased C-reactive protein in children and young adults with lupus: an Atherosclerosis Prevention in Pediatric Lupus Erythematosus substudy. Lupus Sci Med 2014;1(1):e000011.
115. Ardoin SP, Schanberg LE, Sandborg CI, et al. Secondary analysis of APPLE study suggests atorvastatin may reduce atherosclerosis progression in pubertal lupus patients with higher C reactive protein. Ann Rheum Dis 2014;73(3): 557–66.
116. Soep JB, Mietus-Snyder M, Malloy MJ, et al. Assessment of atherosclerotic risk factors and endothelial function in children and young adults with pediatric-onset systemic lupus erythematosus: risks for atherosclerosis in pediatric SLE. Arthritis Care Res 2004;51(3):451–7.
117. Raouf J, Idborg H, Englund P, et al. Targeted lipidomics analysis identified altered serum lipid profiles in patients with polymyositis and dermatomyositis. Arthritis Res Ther 2018;20(1):83.
118. Bohr A-H, Pedersen FK, Nielsen CH, et al. Lipoprotein cholesterol fractions are related to markers of inflammation in children and adolescents with juvenile idiopathic arthritis: a cross sectional study. Pediatr Rheumatol 2016;14(1):61.
119. Rochette E, Bourdier P, Pereira B, et al. TNF blockade contributes to restore lipid oxidation during exercise in children with juvenile idiopathic arthritis. Pediatr Rheumatol 2019;17(1):47.
120. Yeh K-W, Lee C-M, Chang C-J, et al. Lipid profiles alter from pro-atherogenic into less atherogenic and proinflammatory in juvenile idiopathic arthritis patients responding to anti TNF-α treatment. PLoS One 2014;9(6):e90757.
121. Sinicato NA, Postal M, Peres FA, et al. Obesity and cytokines in childhood-onset systemic lupus erythematosus. J Immunol Res 2014;2014:162047.
122. Amine B, Ibn Yacoub Y, Rostom S, et al. Prevalence of overweight among Moroccan children and adolescents with juvenile idiopathic arthritis. Joint Bone Spine 2011;78(6):584–6.

123. Zegeye MM, Andersson JSO, Wennberg P, et al. IL-6 as a mediator of the association between traditional risk factors and future myocardial infarction: a nested case-control study. Arterioscler Thromb Vasc Biol 2021;41(4):1570–9.
124. Orione MAM, Silva CA, Sallum AME, et al. Risk factors for juvenile dermatomyositis: exposure to tobacco and air pollutants during pregnancy: juvenile DM risk factors. Arthritis Care Res 2014;66(10):1571–5.
125. França CMP, Sallum AME, Braga ALF, et al. Risk factors associated with juvenile idiopathic arthritis: exposure to cigarette smoke and air pollution from pregnancy to disease diagnosis. J Rheumatol 2018;45(2):248–56.
126. Cozier YC, Barbhaiya M, Castro-Webb N, et al. Relationship of cigarette smoking and alcohol consumption to incidence of systemic lupus erythematosus in a prospective cohort study of Black women. Arthritis Care Res 2019;71(5):671–7.
127. Cui J, Raychaudhuri S, Karlson EW, et al. Interactions between genome-wide genetic factors and smoking influencing risk of systemic lupus erythematosus. Arthritis Rheumatol 2020;72(11):1863–71.
128. Kiyohara C, Washio M, Horiuchi T, et al. Cigarette smoking, alcohol consumption, and risk of systemic lupus erythematosus: a case-control study in a Japanese population. J Rheumatol 2012;39(7):1363–70.
129. Piette E, Foering K, Chang A, et al. Impact of smoking in cutaneous lupus erythematosus. Arch Dermatol 2012;148(3):317–22.
130. Pocovi-Gerardino G, Correa-Rodríguez M, Callejas-Rubio J-L, et al. Beneficial effect of Mediterranean diet on disease activity and cardiovascular risk in systemic lupus erythematosus patients: a cross-sectional study. Rheumatology 2021;60(1):160–9.
131. Correa-Rodríguez M, Pocovi-Gerardino G, Callejas-Rubio J-L, et al. Dietary intake of free sugars is associated with disease activity and dyslipidemia in systemic lupus erythematosus patients. Nutrients 2020;12(4):1094.
132. Dent EL, Broome HJ, Sasser JM, et al. Blood pressure and albuminuria in a female mouse model of systemic lupus erythematosus: impact of long-term high salt consumption. Am J Physiol Regul Integr Comp Physiol 2020;319(4): R448–54.
133. Ray D, Strickland FM, Richardson BC. Oxidative stress and dietary micronutrient deficiencies contribute to overexpression of epigenetically regulated genes by lupus T cells. Clin Immunol 2018;196:97–102.
134. Gorczyca D, Postępski J, Czajkowska A, et al. The profile of polyunsaturated fatty acids in juvenile idiopathic arthritis and association with disease activity. Clin Rheumatol 2017;36(6):1269–79.
135. Marczynski P, Meineck M, Xia N, et al. Vascular inflammation and dysfunction in lupus-prone mice-IL-6 as mediator of disease initiation. Int J Mol Sci 2021;22(5): 2291.
136. Wienke J, Mertens JS, Garcia S, et al. Biomarker profiles of endothelial activation and dysfunction in rare systemic autoimmune diseases: implications for cardiovascular risk. Rheumatology 2021;60(2):785–801.
137. Chang JC, Xiao R, Meyers KE, et al. Nocturnal blood pressure dipping as a marker of endothelial function and subclinical atherosclerosis in pediatric-onset systemic lupus erythematosus. Arthritis Res Ther 2020;22(1):129.
138. Sabio JM, Martinez-Bordonado J, Sánchez-Berná I, et al. Nighttime blood pressure patterns and subclinical atherosclerosis in women with systemic lupus erythematosus. J Rheumatol 2015;42(12):2310–7.

139. Chang JC, Wang Y, Xiao R, et al. Echocardiographic strain analysis reflects impaired ventricular function in youth with pediatric-onset systemic lupus erythematosus. Echocardiography 2020;37(12):2082–90.
140. Su-angka N, Khositseth A, Vilaiyuk S, et al. Carotid intima-media thickness and arterial stiffness in pediatric systemic lupus erythematosus. Lupus 2017;26(9): 989–95.
141. Chow P-C, Ho MH-K, Lee T-L, et al. Relation of arterial stiffness to left ventricular structure and function in adolescents and young adults with pediatric-onset systemic lupus erythematosus. J Rheumatol 2007;34(6):1345–52.
142. Lee W-F, Wu C-Y, Yang H-Y, et al. Biomarkers associating endothelial dysregulation in pediatric-onset systemic lupus erythematous. Pediatr Rheumatol 2019; 17(1):69.
143. Mohan S, Barsalou J, Bradley TJ, et al. Endothelial progenitor cell phenotype and function are impaired in childhood-onset systemic lupus erythematosus. Arthritis Rheumatol 2015;67(8):2257–62.
144. Chung H-T, Huang Y-L, Yeh K-W, et al. Subclinical deterioration of left ventricular function in patients with juvenile-onset systemic lupus erythematosus. Lupus 2015;24(3):263–72.
145. Chang JC, White BR, Elias MD, et al. Echocardiographic assessment of diastolic function in children with incident systemic lupus erythematosus. Pediatr Cardiol 2019;40(5):1017–25.
146. Papadopoulou C, McCann LJ. The vasculopathy of juvenile dermatomyositis. Front Pediatr 2018;6:284.
147. Papadopoulou C, Hong Y, Krol P, et al. The vasculopathy of juvenile dermatomyositis: endothelial injury, hypercoagulability, and increased arterial stiffness. Arthritis Rheumatol 2021;73(7):1253–66.
148. Xu D, Kacha-Ochana A, Morgan GA, et al. Endothelial progenitor cell number is not decreased in 34 children with juvenile dermatomyositis: a pilot study. Pediatr Rheumatol 2017;15(1):42.
149. Wahezi DM, Liebling EJ, Choi J, et al. Assessment of traditional and non-traditional risk factors for premature atherosclerosis in children with juvenile dermatomyositis and pediatric controls. Pediatr Rheumatol 2020;18(1):25.
150. Barth Z, Schwartz T, Flatø B, et al. Association between nailfold capillary density and pulmonary and cardiac involvement in medium to longstanding juvenile dermatomyositis. Arthritis Care Res 2019;71(4):492–7.
151. Picarelli MM, Danzmann LC, Grun LK, et al. Arterial stiffness by oscillometric device and telomere lenght in juvenile idiopathic artrhitis with no cardiovascular risk factors: a cross-sectional study. Pediatr Rheumatol 2017;15(1):34.
152. Obeid J, Nguyen T, Cellucci T, et al. Effects of acute exercise on circulating endothelial and progenitor cells in children and adolescents with juvenile idiopathic arthritis and healthy controls: a pilot study. Pediatr Rheumatol 2015; 13(1):41.
153. Shiff NJ, Brant R, Guzman J, et al. Glucocorticoid-related changes in body mass index among children and adolescents with rheumatic diseases. Arthritis Care Res 2013;65(1):113–21.
154. Schanberg LE, Sandborg C, Barnhart HX, et al. Premature atherosclerosis in pediatric systemic lupus erythematosus: risk factors for increased carotid intima-media thickness in the atherosclerosis prevention in pediatric lupus erythematosus cohort. Arthritis Rheum 2009;60(5):1496–507.
155. Sule S, Fivush B, Neu A, et al. Increased risk of death in pediatric and adult patients with ESRD secondary to lupus. Pediatr Nephrol 2011;26(1):93–8.

156. Atkinson MA, Joo S, Sule S. Hepcidin and arterial.stiffness in children with systemic lupus erythematosus and lupus nephritis: a cross-sectional study. PLoS One 2019;14(3):e0214248.
157. Falaschi F, Ravelli A, Martignoni A, et al. Nephrotic-range proteinuria, the major risk factor for early atherosclerosis in juvenile-onset systemic lupus erythematosus. Arthritis Rheum 2009;43(6):1405–9.
158. Chang JC, Xiao R, Knight AM, et al. A population-based study of risk factors for heart failure in pediatric and adult-onset systemic lupus erythematosus. Semin Arthritis Rheum 2020;50(4):527–33.
159. Leal GN, Silva KF, França CMP, et al. Subclinical right ventricle systolic dysfunction in childhood-onset systemic lupus erythematosus: insights from two-dimensional speckle-tracking echocardiography. Lupus 2015;24(6):613–20.
160. do Prado R, D'Almeida V, Guerra-Shinohara E, et al. Increased concentration of plasma homocysteine in children with systemic lupus erythematosus. Clin Exp Rheumatol 2006;24(5):594–8.
161. Refai TMK, Al-Salem IH, Nkansa-Dwamena D, et al. Hyperhomocysteinaemia and risk of thrombosis in systemic lupus erythematosus patients. Clin Rheumatol 2002;21(6):457–61.
162. Tam L-S, Fan B, Li EK, et al. Patients with systemic lupus erythematosus show increased platelet activation and endothelial dysfunction induced by acute hyperhomocysteinemia. J Rheumatol 2003;30(7):1479–84.
163. Bingham A, Mamyrova G, Rother KI, et al. Predictors of acquired lipodystrophy in juvenile-onset dermatomyositis and a gradient of severity. Medicine 2008; 87(2):70–86.
164. Reiss AB, Carsons SE, Anwar K, et al. Atheroprotective effects of methotrexate on reverse cholesterol transport proteins and foam cell transformation in human THP-1 monocyte/macrophages. Arthritis Rheum 2008;58(12):3675–83.
165. Tao C-Y, Shang J, Chen T, et al. Impact of antimalarial (AM) on serum lipids in systemic lupus erythematosus (SLE) patients: a systematic review and meta-analysis. Medicine 2019;98(14):e15030.
166. Gupta A, Shields KJ, Manzi S, et al. Association of hydroxychloroquine use with reduced risk of incident atrial fibrillation in lupus. Arthritis Care Res 2021;73(6): 828–32.
167. Yang D-H, Leong P-Y, Sia S-K, et al. Long-term hydroxychloroquine therapy and risk of coronary artery disease in patients with systemic lupus erythematosus. J Clin Med 2019;8(6):796.
168. Iudici M, Fasano S, Gabriele Falcone L, et al. Low-dose aspirin as primary prophylaxis for cardiovascular events in systemic lupus erythematosus: a long-term retrospective cohort study. Rheumatology 2016;55(9):1623–30.
169. Fasano S, Pierro L, Pantano I, et al. Longterm hydroxychloroquine therapy and low-dose aspirin may have an additive effectiveness in the primary prevention of cardiovascular events in patients with systemic lupus erythematosus. J Rheumatol 2017;44(7):1032–8.
170. Abel D, Ardoin SP, Gorelik M. The potential role of colchicine in preventing coronary vascular disease in childhood-onset lupus: a new view on an old drug. Pediatr Rheumatol 2021;19(1):15.
171. Yu H-H, Chen P-C, Yang Y-H, et al. Statin reduces mortality and morbidity in systemic lupus erythematosus patients with hyperlipidemia: a nationwide population-based cohort study. Atherosclerosis 2015;243(1):11–8.

172. Ferreira GA, Navarro TP, Telles RW, et al. Atorvastatin therapy improves endothelial-dependent vasodilation in patients with systemic lupus erythematosus: an 8 weeks controlled trial. Rheumatology 2007;46(10):1560–5.
173. Masson W, Rossi E, Mora-Crespo LM, et al. Cardiovascular risk stratification and appropriate use of statins in patients with systemic lupus erythematosus according to different strategies. Clin Rheumatol 2020;39(2):455–62.
174. Wu PW, Rhew EY, Dyer AR, et al. 25-hydroxyvitamin D and cardiovascular risk factors in women with systemic lupus erythematosus. Arthritis Rheum 2009; 61(10):1387–95.
175. Reynolds JA, Haque S, Berry JL, et al. 25-Hydroxyvitamin D deficiency is associated with increased aortic stiffness in patients with systemic lupus erythematosus. Rheumatology 2012;51(3):544–51.
176. Reynolds JA, Haque S, Williamson K, et al. Vitamin D improves endothelial dysfunction and restores myeloid angiogenic cell function via reduced CXCL-10 expression in systemic lupus erythematosus. Sci Rep 2016;6(1):22341.
177. Robinson AB, Thierry-Palmer M, Gibson KL, et al. Disease activity, proteinuria, and vitamin D status in children with systemic lupus erythematosus and juvenile dermatomyositis. J Pediatr 2012;160(2):297–302.
178. Agbalalah T, Hughes SF, Freeborn EJ, et al. Impact of vitamin D supplementation on endothelial and inflammatory markers in adults: a systematic review. J Steroid Biochem Mol Biol 2017;173:292–300.
179. Chew C, Reynolds JA, Lertratanakul A, et al. Lower vitamin D is associated with metabolic syndrome and insulin resistance in systemic lupus: data from an international inception cohort. Rheumatology (Oxford) 2021. https://doi.org/10.1093/rheumatology/keab090. keab090.
180. Tselios K, Gladman DD, Su J, et al. Impact of the new American College of Cardiology/American Heart Association definition of hypertension on atherosclerotic vascular events in systemic lupus erythematosus. Ann Rheum Dis 2020; 79(5):612–7.
181. Juárez-Rojas J, Medina-Urrutia A, Jorge-Galarza E, et al. Pioglitazone improves the cardiovascular profile in patients with uncomplicated systemic lupus erythematosus: a double-blind randomized clinical trial. Lupus 2012;21(1):27–35.
182. Titov AA, Baker HV, Brusko TM, et al. Metformin inhibits the type 1 IFN response in human CD4 + T cells. J Immunol 2019;203(2):338–48.
183. García-Dorta A, Quevedo-Abeledo JC, Rua-Figueroa Í, et al. Beta-cell function is disrupted in patients with systemic lupus erythematosus. Rheumatology (Oxford) 2021;60(8):3826–33.
184. Petri M, Spence D, Bone L, et al. Coronary artery disease risk factors in the Johns Hopkins Lupus Cohort: prevalence, recognition by patients, and preventive practices. Medicine 1992;71(5):291–302.
185. Hollander MC, Sage JM, Greenler AJ, et al. International consensus for provisions of quality-driven care in childhood-Onset systemic lupus erythematosus. Arthritis Care Res 2013;65(9):1416–23.
186. Rochette E, Duché P, Merlin E. Juvenile idiopathic arthritis and physical activity: possible inflammatory and immune modulation and tracks for interventions in young populations. Autoimmun Rev 2015;14(8):726–34.
187. Nader GA, Dastmalchi M, Alexanderson H, et al. A longitudinal, integrated, clinical, histological and mRNA profiling study of resistance exercise in myositis. Mol Med 2010;16(11–12):455–64.

188. Aqel SI, Hampton JM, Bruss M, et al. Daily moderate exercise is beneficial and social stress is detrimental to disease pathology in murine lupus nephritis. Front Physiol 2017;8:236.
189. Perandini LA, Sales-de-Oliveira D, Mello SBV, et al. Exercise training can attenuate the inflammatory milieu in women with systemic lupus erythematosus. J Appl Physiol 2014;117(6):639–47.
190. Barnes J, Nualnim N, Dhindsa M, et al. Macro- and microvascular function in habitually exercising systemic lupus erythematosus patients. Scand J Rheumatol 2014;43(3):209–16.
191. Reis-Neto ET, Silva AE, Monteiro CM, et al. Supervised physical exercise improves endothelial function in patients with systemic lupus erythematosus. Rheumatology 2013;52(12):2187–95.
192. Lelieveld OTHM, Armbrust W, Geertzen JHB, et al. Promoting physical activity in children with juvenile idiopathic arthritis through an internet-based program: results of a pilot randomized controlled trial. Arthritis Care Res 2010;62(5):697–703.
193. Armbrust W, Bos GJFJ, Wulffraat NM, et al. Internet program for physical activity and exercise capacity in children with juvenile idiopathic arthritis: a multicenter randomized controlled trial. Arthritis Care Res 2017;69(7):1040–9.
194. Sule S, Fontaine K. Slow speed resistance exercise training in children with polyarticular juvenile idiopathic arthritis. Open Access Rheumatol 2019;11:121–6.
195. Heale LD, Dover S, Goh YI, et al. A wearable activity tracker intervention for promoting physical activity in adolescents with juvenile idiopathic arthritis: a pilot study. Pediatr Rheumatol 2018;16(1):66.
196. Riisager M, Mathiesen PR, Vissing J, et al. Aerobic training in persons who have recovered from juvenile dermatomyositis. Neuromuscul Disord 2013;23(12):962–8.
197. Omori CH, Silva CAA, Sallum AME, et al. Exercise training in juvenile dermatomyositis. Arthritis Care Res 2012;64(8):1186–94.
198. Carvalho MRP de, Sato EI, Tebexreni AS, et al. Effects of supervised cardiovascular training program on exercise tolerance, aerobic capacity, and quality of life in patients with systemic lupus erythematosus. Arthritis Rheum 2005;53(6):838–44.
199. Yuen HK, Breland HL, Vogtle LK, et al. The process associated with motivation of a home-based Wii Fit exercise program among sedentary African American women with systemic lupus erythematosus. Disabil Health J 2013;6(1):63–8.
200. Abad TO, Sarni RO, da Silva SG, et al. Nutritional intervention in patients with juvenile systemic lupus erythematosus: protective effect against the increase in fat mass. Rheumatol Int 2018;38(6):985–92.
201. da Silva SGL, Terreri MT, Abad TTO, et al. The effect of nutritional intervention on the lipid profile and dietary intake of adolescents with juvenile systemic lupus erythematosus: a randomized, controlled trial. Lupus 2018;27(5):820–7.
202. Moreira MLP, Sztajnbok F, Giannini DT. Relationship between fiber intake and cardiovascular risk factors in adolescents with systemic lupus erythematosus. Rev Paul Pediatr 2021;39:e2019316.
203. Wattiaux A, Bettendorf B, Block L, et al. Patient perspectives on smoking cessation and interventions in rheumatology clinics. Arthritis Care Res 2020;72(3):369–77.
204. Goldstein BI, Carnethon MR, Matthews KA, et al. Major depressive disorder and bipolar disorder predispose youth to accelerated atherosclerosis and early

cardiovascular disease: a scientific statement from the American Heart Association. Circulation 2015;132(10):965–86.
205. Levine GN, Cohen BE, Commodore-Mensah Y, et al. Psychological health, well-being, and the mind-heart-body connection: a scientific statement from the American Heart Association. Circulation 2021;143(10):e763–83.
206. Knight AM, Trupin L, Katz P, et al. Depression risk in young adults with juvenile- and adult-onset lupus: twelve years of followup. Arthritis Care Res 2018;70(3): 475–80.
207. Knight A, Vickery M, Faust L, et al. Gaps in mental health care for youth with rheumatologic conditions: a mixed methods study of perspectives from behavioral health providers. Arthritis Care Res 2019;71(5):591–601.
208. Ardalan K, Adeyemi O, Wahezi DM, et al. Parent perspectives on addressing emotional health for children and young adults with juvenile myositis. Arthritis Care Res 2021;73(1):18–29.
209. Postal M, Lapa AT, Sinicato NA, et al. Depressive symptoms are associated with tumor necrosis factor alpha in systemic lupus erythematosus. J Neuroinflammation 2016;13:5.
210. Jorge A, Lertratanakul A, Lee J, et al. Depression and progression of subclinical cardiovascular disease in systemic lupus erythematosus. Arthritis Care Res 2017;69(1):5–11.
211. Greco CM, Kao AH, Sattar A, et al. Association between depression and coronary artery calcification in women with systemic lupus erythematosus. Rheumatology 2008;48(5):576–81.
212. Greco CM, Li T, Sattar A, et al. Association between depression and vascular disease in systemic lupus erythematosus. J Rheumatol 2012;39(2):262–8.
213. Brown RT, Shaftman SR, Tilley BC, et al. The Health Education for Lupus Study: a randomized controlled cognitive-behavioral intervention targeting psychosocial adjustment and quality of life in adolescent females with systemic lupus erythematosus. Am J Med Sci 2012;344(4):274–82.
214. Connelly M, Schanberg LE, Ardoin S, et al. Multisite randomized clinical trial evaluating an online self-management program for adolescents with juvenile idiopathic arthritis. J Pediatr Psychol 2019;44(3):363–74.
215. Williams EM, Hyer JM, Viswanathan R, et al. Cytokine balance and behavioral intervention; findings from the Peer Approaches to Lupus Self-Management (PALS) project. Hum Immunol 2017;78(9):574–81.
216. Slopen N, Chen Y, Guida JL, et al. Positive childhood experiences and ideal cardiovascular health in midlife: associations and mediators. Prev Med 2017; 97:72–9.
217. Suglia SF, Koenen KC, Boynton-Jarrett R, et al. Childhood and adolescent adversity and cardiometabolic outcomes: a scientific statement from the American Heart Association. Circulation 2018;137(5):e15–28.
218. Baumeister D, Akhtar R, Ciufolini S, et al. Childhood trauma and adulthood inflammation: a meta-analysis of peripheral C-reactive protein, interleukin-6 and tumour necrosis factor-α. Mol Psychiatry 2016;21(5):642–9.
219. Suglia SF, Campo RA, Brown AGM, et al. Social determinants of cardiovascular health: early life adversity as a contributor to disparities in cardiovascular diseases. J Pediatr 2020;219:267–73.
220. Su S, Wang X, Pollock JS, et al. Adverse childhood experiences and blood pressure trajectories from childhood to young adulthood: the Georgia Stress and Heart Study. Circulation 2015;131(19):1674–81.

221. Hornor G, Davis C, Sherfield J, et al. Trauma-informed care: essential elements for pediatric health care. J Pediatr Health Care 2019;33(2):214–21.
222. Cozier YC, Barbhaiya M, Castro-Webb N, et al. Association of child abuse with systemic lupus erythematosus in black women during adulthood. Arthritis Care Res 2021;73(6):833–40.
223. DeQuattro K, Trupin L, Li J, et al. Relationships between adverse childhood experiences and health status in systemic lupus erythematosus. Arthritis Care Res 2020;72(4):525–33.
224. Rubinstein TB, Bullock DR, Ardalan K, et al. Adverse childhood experiences are associated with childhood-onset arthritis in a national sample of US youth: an analysis of the 2016 National Survey of Children's Health. J Pediatr 2020. https://doi.org/10.1016/j.jpeds.2020.06.046.
225. Rubinstein TB, Knight AM. Disparities in childhood-onset lupus. Rheum Dis Clin North America 2020;46(4):661–72.
226. Phillippi K, Hoeltzel M, Robinson AB, et al, for the Childhood Arthritis and Rheumatology Research Alliance (CARRA) Legacy Registry Investigators. Race, income, and disease outcomes in juvenile dermatomyositis. J Pediatr 2017;184:38–44.e1.
227. Chang JC, Xiao R, Burnham JM, et al. Longitudinal assessment of racial disparities in juvenile idiopathic arthritis disease activity in a treat-to-target intervention. Pediatr Rheumatol 2020;18(1):88.
228. Verstappen SMM, Cobb J, Foster HE, et al. The association between low socioeconomic status with high physical limitations and low illness self-perception in patients with juvenile idiopathic arthritis: results From the childhood arthritis prospective study. Arthritis Care Res 2015;67(3):382–9.
229. Brunner HI, Taylor J, Britto MT, et al. Differences in disease outcomes between medicaid and privately insured children: possible health disparities in juvenile rheumatoid arthritis. Arthritis Rheum 2006;55(3):378–84.
230. Barnado A, Carroll RJ, Casey C, et al. Phenome-wide association study identifies marked increased in burden of comorbidities in African Americans with systemic lupus erythematosus. Arthritis Res Ther 2018;20(1):69.
231. Lim SS, Helmick CG, Bao G, et al. Racial disparities in mortality associated with systemic lupus erythematosus — Fulton and DeKalb Counties, Georgia, 2002–2016. MMWR Morb Mortal Wkly Rep 2019;68(18):419–22.
232. Gómez-Puerta JA, Feldman CH, Alarcón GS, et al. Racial and ethnic differences in mortality and cardiovascular events among patients with end-stage renal disease due to lupus nephritis. Arthritis Care Res 2015;67(10):1453–62.
233. Barbhaiya M, Feldman CH, Guan H, et al. Race/ethnicity and cardiovascular events among patients with systemic lupus erythematosus. Arthritis Rheumatol 2017;69(9):1823–31.
234. Maynard JW, Fang H, Petri M. Low socioeconomic status is associated with cardiovascular risk factors and outcomes in systemic lupus erythematosus. J Rheumatol 2012;39(4):777–83.

Disparities in Pediatric Rheumatic Diseases

Alisha M. Akinsete, MD[a], Jennifer M.P. Woo, PhD, MPH[b], Tamar B. Rubinstein, MD, MS[a,*]

KEYWORDS

- Pediatric • Disparities • Health disparities • Social determinants of health • Healthcare • Race • Ethnicity • Gender • Socioeconomic

KEY POINTS

- Health disparities are prevalent across racial/ethnic groups, socioeconomic groups, and geographic areas in pediatric rheumatic diseases.
- Although health disparities in youth with systemic lupus erythematosus (SLE) and JIA have been identified, significant knowledge gaps exist about disparities in other childhood rheumatic diseases.
- Standardizing care is a strategy to decrease disparities, but improved understanding of health care disparities is necessary to develop appropriate interventions and decrease health care inequity in pediatric rheumatology.

INTRODUCTION

Major health disparities exist among youth with rheumatic diseases. Recent studies in pediatric rheumatology found that youth from disadvantaged socioeconomic backgrounds report worse quality of life and experience worse disease outcomes, delays in care, and suboptimal treatment. This aligns with the greater body of health disparity literature that documents the significant impact of social determinants of health (SDoH) on a wide spectrum of health outcomes among children and adolescents.[1] In this review, we discuss the current literature on health and health care disparities affecting youth with rheumatic diseases, intervention studies designed to mitigate the impact of disparities and strategies to achieve health care equity that urgently requires investigation within pediatric rheumatology.

Healthy People 2020 defines a health disparity as "a health difference that is, closely linked with social, economic, and/or environmental disadvantage."[2] Health care

[a] Division of Pediatric Rheumatology, Department of Pediatrics, Children's Hospital at Montefiore/Albert Einstein College of Medicine, 3415 Bainbridge Avenue, Bronx, NY 10467, USA; [b] Epidemiology Branch, National Institute of Environmental Health Sciences, National Institutes of Health, 111 TW Alexander Drive, Research Triangle Park, NC 27709, USA
* Corresponding author.
E-mail address: trubinst@montefiore.org
Twitter: @akinsetemd (A.M.A.); @jmpwoo (J.M.P.W.); @tamarpedsrheum (T.B.R.)

Rheum Dis Clin N Am 48 (2022) 183–198
https://doi.org/10.1016/j.rdc.2021.09.014 rheumatic.theclinics.com

disparities can be largely attributed to the disparate distribution of financial resources available for health spending, as well as structural and institutional barriers that prevent equitable delivery of health services.[2] Although health differences exist across the spectrum of health outcomes, health disparities are those that are systematic, avoidable, unfair, and unjust.[3] Social-ecological models, adapted from Bronfenbrenner's ecological model of human development,[4] can help define nested factors related to familial, individual care, health systems, and broader societal environments that contribute to health and health care disparities in pediatric rheumatology (**Fig. 1**).[5]

Health disparities unjustly affect socially disadvantaged populations who experience barriers to optimal health created by historically-embedded practices of systemic racism and individual and institutional discrimination based on racial/ethnic group, religion, socioeconomic position (SEP), gender, mental health, disability, sexual orientation, and geographic region.[2] SDoH are personal, social, economic, and environmental factors that shape an individual's health[2] and serve as the primary drivers of health and health care disparities among socially disadvantaged groups.[6] Despite their critical role in other diseases (eg, asthma, diabetes, and obesity), research in SDoH in pediatric rheumatology treatment delivery and disease outcomes remains sparse. Robust health and health care disparity research is crucial to appropriately change practice and health policy to address health equity in pediatric rheumatology.

DISPARITIES IN CHILDHOOD-ONSET SYSTEMIC LUPUS ERYTHEMATOSUS

Health disparities in childhood-onset systemic lupus erythematosus (cSLE) have received more research attention than disparities in other pediatric rheumatic diseases. The attention is warranted, as cSLE can be fatal, particularly with suboptimal treatment. Childhood-onset SLE mortality rates are higher among young adults than other age ranges[7] with higher mortality than adult-onset SLE.[8] Morbidity associated with cSLE is particularly high among US young adults of minoritized race/ethnicities. "Minoritized groups" refers to populations systematically devalued or treated

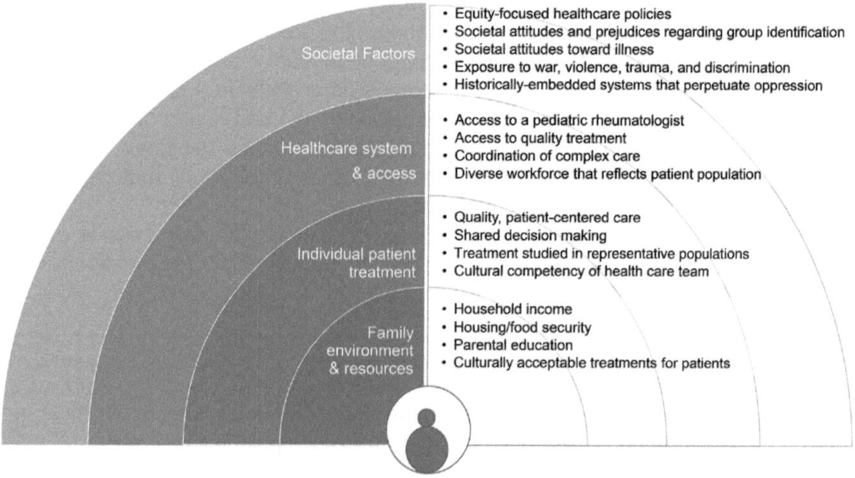

Fig. 1. Modified social-ecological model of contributors to health disparities in pediatric rheumatology potential societal, institutional, individual care, and familial determinants of health disparities among youth with pediatric rheumatic diseases. This conceptual framework is based on Reifsnider and colleagues modified Bronfenbrenner social-ecological model.[5]

subordinately due to sustained systems of oppression and marginalization. In the US, SLE ranks as the fifth cause of death among Black and Hispanic females ages 10 to 25 years old.[9] Despite attention to racial/ethnic disparities, major knowledge gaps exist for other SDoH in cSLE. Few studies have examined income, education, and other factors commonly associated with systemic barriers to health equity.

Health Disparities in Childhood-Onset Systemic Lupus Erythematosus

There are striking differences in disease prevalence and health outcomes across race/ethnicities in both pediatric and adult SLE populations. In cSLE, which is arguably the most studied disease in pediatric rheumatology with regards to health disparities, disparities in mortality—the most critical and most basic indicator of health—have not only persisted in the US but have worsened over time. However, because the most affected populations are often not represented in research studies, important gaps in knowledge exist around the impact of disparities in cSLE among other marginalized populations.

Although Black, Hispanic/Latino, and Asian youth have higher prevalence of cSLE than white youth,[10] the prevalence of cSLE is especially high in indigenous peoples around the globe. This includes American Indian, First Nation Canadian, Maori people of New Zealand, and the Aboriginal people of Australia.[10–14] The highest prevalence of cSLE, like SLE, is documented in Indigenous peoples of North America at 13 per 100,000 or at least 3 times that of the general population.[10,11] Despite the high prevalence of cSLE in indigenous populations, few studies intentionally include indigenous populations who are underrepresented in large cSLE registries and studies.[15]

The largest effort to identify disparities across race/ethnicity in SLE was through the LUMINA study (Lupus in Minorities: Nature vs Nurture) in the US.[16] Although LUMINA primarily examined adults, a proportion of participants were pediatric aged. Data from the LUMINA study established that both Hispanic and Black Americans had higher disease activity scores, worse patient-reported outcomes, and more organ involvement (specifically cardiac and renal). In line with this, Hispanic and Black Americans were treated with higher doses of steroids and with cyclophosphamide, likely indicating worse disease.[17–23]

Indeed, differences in cSLE disease severity between Black and white youth are evident from several other studies, which consistently demonstrate that Black youth are more likely to have the most severe forms of organ involvement associated with SLE, including renal, neurologic, and cardiac disease.[24–26] Furthermore, Black youth with cSLE are more likely to have SLE organ-related disease (renal, neurologic, hematologic, and ocular) than Black adults with adult-onset SLE.[8,27]

Worldwide, nonwhite youth with cSLE have worse disease outcomes than white youth. Black youth from low-resource areas demonstrate the highest rates of end-organ disease and morbidity. In the PULSE cohort from South Africa, Black South African children had more end-organ damage (63% vs 23%) than Black American youth from the Childhood Arthritis and Rheumatology Research Alliance (CARRA) registry, and more Black youth from the PULSE cohort required renal transplantation (8% vs <1%).[28]

Black and Hispanic youth are overrepresented among patients with cSLE who require hospitalization,[7] a marker of increased morbidity and mortality risk; whereas urban youth and youth identifying as non-white/non-Black/"other" are more likely to have longer hospital stays, after accounting for clinical factors such as lupus nephritis.[7] In the US, urban areas are often characterized by greater racial/ethnic heterogeneity, as well as regions of concentrated poverty and economic disadvantage due to historical practices of racial segregation.[29,30] Pockets of increased socioeconomic disadvantage facilitate physical and socioeconomic barriers to access quality health care. Mortality data from the National Center for Health Statistics showed that the mortality rate in the US for patients with SLE ages 0 to 24 was 5.7 times higher in Black youth than white youth in 1995 to 1997 and increased to 6.7 times higher in 2015 to 2017[31]. A recent national study of youth enrolled in Medicaid (an indicator of low income) showed that Black race and hospital located in the southern US were among the strongest risk factors for hospitalization mortality, even after accounting for lupus nephritis and young adult age (age 18–20).[7] The mortality of Black youth with end-stage renal disease (ESRD) from lupus nephritis is twice that of their white counterparts.[10]

Health Care Disparities in Childhood-Onset Systemic Lupus Erythematosus

Health care disparities, specifically disparities in access and treatment, may cause many health disparities observed in cSLE. However, few studies have examined disparities in quality of care, access to care, and cSLE treatment. Studies to date that have attempted to examine health care access and treatment reveals significant disparities in health care along race/ethnicity and income. A study of the CARRA registry found that delays in cSLE diagnosis of greater than 1 year were more common in youth from low-income families. Youth living in a state with a high density of pediatric rheumatologists were more likely to be seen expeditiously.[32] Youth with ESRD from lupus nephritis in the US Renal Data System were less likely to receive renal transplants if they were Black, Hispanic, older, or on Medicaid,[10] suggesting potential structural barriers or bias in the referral of some patients with cSLE for transplant.

Mental health disorders are among the comorbidities most associated with worse quality of life. Approximately a third of youth with cSLE have clinically significant symptoms of depression and/or anxiety.[33] Although, in single-center cohort studies, Black youth appear more affected by mental health disorders,[34] a large study of a national Medicaid sample, showed that Black youth were less likely to be diagnosed with depression or anxiety and less likely to receive pharmacotherapy.[35] Beyond affecting the quality of life, disparities in detecting and treating mental health disorders may have important implications on SLE disease outcomes. For example, depression symptoms are associated with worse medication adherence in youth,[36] whereas in cSLE youth with mental health disorders, mental health treatment, including the use of pharmacotherapy, improves adherence.[37]

DISPARITIES IN JUVENILE IDIOPATHIC ARTHRITIS

Juvenile idiopathic arthritis is the most common pediatric rheumatic disease and is associated with increased risk for morbidity and disability.[38] Youth with JIA from socially disadvantaged backgrounds disproportionally experience this burden, often presenting with more severe disease, reporting poorer disease-related quality of life, and encountering greater delays to treatment by a pediatric rheumatologist.

Health Disparities in Juvenile Idiopathic Arthritis

Overall, the global prevalence rate for JIA is estimated to be 100 to 132 per 100,000.[39,40] Annual incidence rates for JIA range from 1.7 to 196 per 100,000 depending on the country and underlying population and vary even more when stratified by JIA subtypes.[41–47] The highest frequencies of systemic arthritis, a severe JIA subtype associated with greater morbidity than oligoarthritis, are reported among less-developed regions including Southeast Asia, Latin America, Africa, and the Middle East, comprising approximately 20% to 30% of regional reported patients with JIA than white populations in Europe and North America (<10%).[48] Furthermore, in a large US Registry of youth with JIA, a higher proportion of Black (16%) and Hispanic (21%) youth presented with systemic JIA manifestations than white (7%) and non-Hispanic (8%) youth.[49] Similarly, the greatest proportions of rheumatoid factor (RF)-positive polyarthritis JIA, another debilitating JIA subtype, have been reported in Latin America and Southeast Asia,[48] as well as among Indigenous youth of North America.[11,46,50,51] In the US, although rates of polyarthritis JIA were comparable by race/ethnicity, higher proportions of both Black (26%) and Hispanic (23%) youth with JIA were RF-positive than 9% of white and non-Hispanic comparator groups.[49] These patterns suggest that disadvantaged populations may be disproportionally burdened with more severe types of JIA, requiring more aggressive and complex treatment plans when optimal resources and options may be limited.

Although much of the disparities research in JIA evaluate racial/ethnic differences in disease etiology and manifestation, race/ethnicity, a social construct, is often hard to disentangle from measures of SEP due to the persistent racialization of structural and institutional barriers established to maintain and promote social hierarchies.[52] For example, although Black youth had 1.9 times greater odds of joint damage,[49] persistently greater physician- and patient/caregiver-assessed disease activity, and JIA-related pain,[53] they were also more likely to report indicators of low SEP, including annual household income less than $50,000 and reliance on public health insurance. Similarly, children with Medicaid were more likely to present with polyarticular and/or systemic JIA features, as well as present with more active disease and pain than children with private health insurance.[54]

Increased disease activity and morbidity can result in greater disability and reduced quality of life. Low SEP, than high SEP, has been associated with increased disability and decreased quality of life as measured by higher childhood health assessment questionnaire (CHAQ) scores and worse perceived illness.[54,55] Living on a reservation, rather than native North American ancestry, correlated with increased JIA-related disability, supporting the role of SES and place-based factors in race/ethnicity-based health disparities.[56] Racial/ethnic health disparities reveal greater disease severity and morbidity among Black, Hispanic, and Indigenous peoples of the Americas, as well as in Latin American and Southeast Asian countries, which may be largely attributable to socioeconomic factors experienced by disadvantaged groups rather than race/ethnicity alone.

Health Care Disparities in Juvenile Idiopathic Arthritis

Early aggressive treatment of JIA[57–59] may improve treatment response and outcomes, so timely access to quality care is necessary. However, disparities in access to care and treatment among youth with JIA is largely understudied with inferences often made from adults with rheumatoid arthritis, health care practices in other countries, and other pediatric subspecialties.[60]

Socioeconomic factors contribute to social and structural health care access barriers among youth with JIA. In general, children with public insurance are more likely to be denied a subspecialty appointment or experience severe appointment delays than children with private insurance.[61] Furthermore, high parental educational attainment,[62] private insurance,[63] shorter travel distance,[63,64] and residing in low community poverty areas[65] were all associated with earlier access to a rheumatologist for JIA treatment.

Biologic disease-modifying antirheumatic drugs (DMARDs) are instrumental in the treatment of JIA, and early treatment may better reduce disease activity than conventional treatments, particularly among severe JIA cases.[59,66] Whereas disparities in biologic DMARD use is reported among Black adults with rheumatoid arthritis than white counterparts,[67] such disparities have not been described among youth with JIA. Although not designed to examine differences across socio-demographics, studies have reported both higher[49] and lower[53] biologic DMARD use among Black children. Additional research is needed to assess potential disparities in access to and use of DMARDs in racially/ethnically and SEP-diverse populations.

DISPARITIES IN OTHER DISEASES IN PEDIATRIC RHEUMATOLOGY

There is sparse literature identifying health and health care disparities in other pediatric rheumatic diseases. The few studies of juvenile dermatomyositis show a continued pattern of Black and Hispanic youth and youth from low-income families faring worse with delays in diagnosis, increased length of stay during the hospitalization and higher rates of calcinosis.[68–70] Of concern is the growing literature demonstrating important health disparities in adult patients with these diseases, including rheumatic diseases with high morbidity and mortality such as systemic sclerosis[71–75] and sarcoidosis.[76–79]

DISPARITIES IN TRANSITIONAL CARE

The transition period from pediatric rheumatologic care to adult rheumatologic care is particularly fraught with barriers to health care access. In certain diseases, such as cSLE, the transition occurs at a medically and psychologically vulnerable age, resulting in increased mortality and poor outcomes.[8,31,80] Among youth with general chronic disease, Black or Hispanic young adults of lower SEP and non-English speaking are less likely to be prepared to transition to adult rheumatology care.[81]

There are limited rheumatology studies that investigate racial and ethnic differences related to the transition in rheumatology care. A recent large cohort study of privately insured young adults with cSLE found no difference across racial and ethnic groups in experiencing a successful transfer, defined as a visit with an adult rheumatology/nephrology within 12 months after the last pediatric subspecialist visit.[82] A smaller study of youth with cSLE found that lower education and white race was associated with gaps in care during transition.[83]

PEDIATRIC RHEUMATOLOGY WORKFORCE DISPARITIES

Little has been reported on the demographic make-up of pediatric rheumatologists, but a study from 2000 indicated that 95% of the workforce identify as white.[84] The adult workforce, which often services pediatric rheumatology patients, is also highly nondiverse. Underrepresented in medicine (URM) trainees, which include Black or African American, American Indian or Alaska Native, Native Hawaiian or other Pacific Islander, Hispanic or Latino, have increased in most internal medicine subspecialties, but not rheumatology, which remains under 12%.[85]

Discordance in race between clinicians and patients is a risk factor for negative patient-physician interactions and disparate care. One study found that patients with Black SLE report communication that is more hurried and perception of providers using more difficult words than white patients.[86] Further investigations of rheumatologists' implicit biases and the effect on patient treatment and outcomes are needed.

Because of a dearth in pediatric rheumatologists, many youths seek care with adult rheumatologists who are less familiar with the clinical nuances of treating children with rheumatic diseases.[84,87] The American College of Rheumatology Workforce Study projected that the US Pediatric Rheumatology workforce will decrease by 15% to 20% between 2015 and 2025. Furthermore, by 2030, there will be only half the needed pediatric rheumatologists in the US with the Southeast, South Central, and Southwest regions of the US most affected, areas which demographically tend to encompass youth from minority and disadvantaged backgrounds at risk for more severe pediatric rheumatic disease.[88]

With efforts to grow the workforce, an important consideration is increasing the number of pediatric rheumatologists from underrepresented demographics. Key strategies put forth by the US Department of Health and Human Services' Office of Minority Health to address disparities include supporting initiatives to increase a diverse work force and increasing cultural competency of health care workers.[85] This includes educating providers about health care disparities, which is currently not a routine part of rheumatology training; as a result, proposed curriculum to address gaps in knowledge of health disparities s currently being developed.[89]

INTERVENTIONS TO ELIMINATE HEALTH AND HEALTHCARE DISPARITIES

The development and implementation of effective interventions to mitigate health and health care disparities requires an iterative process of identifying, monitoring, and addressing disparities (**Fig. 2**)[90]. Interventions to decrease the gaps in health disparities created by inequities in health care are multifactorial and target individual, community, and macro-environmental factors related to federal policies and systems.[91]

An example of federal programming that successfully targeted disparities[2] is the State Children's Health Insurance Program (sCHIP), federally funded medical insurance for low-income children. The initiation of sCHIP was associated with improved access to primary care for Black and Hispanic children by 9% and 17%, respectively. Moreover, sCHIP implementation was associated with the elimination of previously observed racial/ethnic disparities in unmet needs (delayed or foregone preventive, acute, specialty, emergency care, and required prescriptions). At minimum, pediatric rheumatologists can work with other health care workers, such as nurses and social workers, to secure insurance for patients to help alleviate financial barriers to seeking pediatric rheumatology care.[92]

At an institution and practice level, interventions aim to standardize care, improve provider education, and implement practices that affect vulnerable populations. Addressing SDoH is an important approach to mitigating health care disparities. A study of the implementation of an integrated care management program in a multihospital system in Boston demonstrated both how standardized screening detects challenges in SDoH and how intentionally addressing the needs of vulnerable populations influences quality of care. A team of social workers, nurses, and community health workers were integrated into a rheumatology clinic to address the social needs of patients (eg, transportation challenges, mental health care access, financial insecurity, etc.). Importantly, the study documented the high prevalence of social need in vulnerable adult patients with SLE (97%).[93] Furthermore, the use of a social needs assessment tool has been proposed as an initial step promoting health equity and supporting the equitable distribution of resources to facilitate access to care and thus improve health outcomes. Acceptance of a social needs assessment as part of routine medical care would facilitate a paradigm shift in health care policy acknowledging and starting to address SDoH as crucial drivers of disease progression and prognosis.[94]

In pediatric rheumatology, as in medicine widely, clinicians do not always deliver recommended care despite guidelines.[95–98] Tools that help standardize practice can help reduce disparities in care associated with practitioner implicit bias or variation in institutional practices that contribute to disparate care. In a recent study by Burman and colleagues, investigators created a pediatric lupus care index (p-LuCI) to

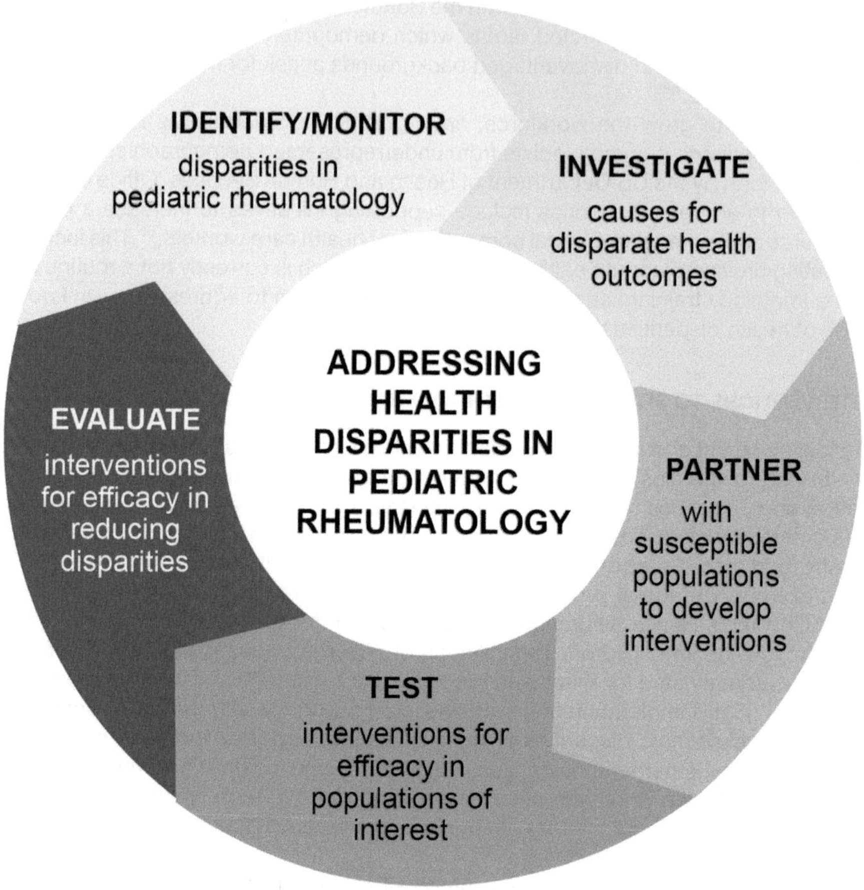

Fig. 2. Addressing health disparities in pediatric rheumatic diseases proposed iterative framework to address health disparities through evidence-based methods. This is modified from a conceptual framework developed by Rashid and colleagues.[90]

help standardize and improve care. The index included standard of care assessments and interventions that should be done at specified times.[99] Completion of the p-LuCI varied based on patient and clinician characteristics, which suggests that greater cultural competency or additional measures may be necessary to ensure the equitable distribution of care. In a JIA implementation study of a clinical decision support tool promoting a treat-to-target approach, Chang and colleagues demonstrated improvement in clinical juvenile arthritis disease activity scores (cJADAS), specifically, among Black children.[53] Importantly, though, it did not close the disparity gap in cJADAS scores between Black and white children. Although tools to standardize care may diminish the impact of provider implicit or explicit biases on care, they are likely not sufficient to fully address health disparities.

AREAS FOR FUTURE STUDIES

Historically, one of the challenges in identifying disparities in pediatric rheumatic diseases stems from a limited body of literature largely based on small single-centered studies without a wide enough lens or enough power to detect differences across sociodemographic groups. Over the past decade, investigators have used administrative datasets and the CARRA registry, leading to a deeper understanding of disparities affecting this patient population. However, there are not enough studies in pediatric rheumatology that have examined even the most basic SDoH, such as income-level and poverty.[15] The continued use of large datasets and registries, such as the CARRA registry, will help advance the field in further identifying disparities in the rarer diseases, as well as further understanding the root causes of disparities in more common pediatric rheumatic diseases. This research will help guide the development of targeted provider- and institution-level interventions and system-level advocacy. Thus, it is critical to ensure that registries truly reflect the diverse pediatric rheumatology patient population and do not systematically exclude hard-to-reach populations.

Indeed, there is a distinct gap in the literature regarding many underrepresented populations. Indigenous youth of the Americas are almost entirely absent despite their greater risk for many rheumatic diseases, including cSLE and polyarticular JIA.[11] Furthermore, the prevalence of pediatric rheumatic disease remains largely unknown due to a lack of rheumatology care among many international populations, particularly in the continent of Africa.[100,101]

A recent systematic review of the participation of underrepresented patients in SLE and rheumatoid arthritis research found that mistrust in providers, inclusion/exclusion criteria that make Black and Hispanic patients ineligible, and lack of community engagement have been barriers to inclusive research in rheumatology.[102] These issues need careful attention in pediatric rheumatology research and are critical to further identify and address disparities. If intervention studies do not include diverse populations or intentionally exclude groups based on language, resources, acceptability, or other barriers, they have the potential to exacerbate health disparities.

Health care disparities among LGBTQ+ (lesbian, gay, bisexual, transgender, questioning, and queer) youth in rheumatology need further investigation. Adolescents reporting minoritized sexual orientation increased from 7.9% in 2009 to 14.3 in 2017.[103] These youth are at increased risk for substance abuse, mental health disorders, and are 3 times more likely to attempt suicide.[103,104] Hence, LGBTQ + issues should be included in research into disparities in pediatric rheumatology and sexual orientation and gender identity should be addressed in clinical encounters with adolescents in the pediatric rheumatology clinic.

SUMMARY

Critical health and health care disparities related to race/ethnicity, SES, and geography have been identified in the most prevalent pediatric rheumatic diseases. However, significant gaps in knowledge exist regarding health disparities associated with rarer pediatric rheumatic diseases and within highly underrepresented demographics. Of note, is the lack of literature investigating health disparities (or even health outcomes) in Indigenous youth with rheumatic diseases, including American Indian youth in the US and First Nation Canadians. Alarmingly, the Indigenous populations of North America have a particularly high prevalence of pediatric rheumatic disease with high morbidity and disability, including SLE and polyarticular JIA.[10,11]

The existence of important health disparities has been identified and is widely recognized in Black Americans over the past several decades as resulting from centuries of systemic and systematic racism and strong racialization of structural and institutional practices. Socioeconomic factors likely serve as influential drivers of observed racial/ethnic disparities in pediatric rheumatic diseases especially in Black youth. Black youth and youth from low SEP households with SLE, JIA, and other rheumatic diseases are more likely to experience greater disease activity and increased morbidity into adulthood.

There exists an urgent need to address and mitigate health and health care disparities within pediatric rheumatology at the individual, institutional, and societal levels. Identification of health disparities is not enough. Little research in pediatric rheumatology has proposed interventions to promote health equity and close gaps in health disparities. The few studies that have investigated strategies to implement standardized treatment have shown limited success in mitigating gaps in health care disparities, let alone gaps in health outcomes. Interventions that specifically target and uplift the care of vulnerable populations may be needed to attain health equity, rather than focusing on the provision of equal care. Strategies that address health and health care disparities on different levels—including practice level changes, improving provider diversity, implementing trainee education to address implicit bias, equitable representation in pediatric rheumatology research, and passing equity-focused health care policy—are crucial to ensuring optimal health and well-being among youth with rheumatic diseases.

CLINICS CARE POINTS

- Evidence of health care and healthcare disparities exist in pediatric rheumatic disease; however, further investigation is necessary to direct interventions to mitigate disparities.
- Black, Hispanic/Latino and Indigenous youth are at increased risk for higher morbidity and more severe disease in several pediatric rheumatic diseases.
- Improving representative inclusion in research and in the pediatric rheumatology workforce is vital to properly address health equity gaps.

ACKNOWLEDGMENTS

This research was supported in part by the Intramural Research Program of the NIH, National Institute of Environmental Health Sciences.

DISCLOSURE

The authors have nothing to disclose.

REFERENCES

1. Oberg C, Colianni S, King-Schultz L. Child Health Disparities in the 21st Century. Curr Probl Pediatr Adolesc Health Care 2016;46(9):291–312.
2. Office of Disease Prevention and Health Promotion. (2010). Phase I report. Healthy People 2020. U.S. Department of Health and Human Services. Available at: https://www.healthypeople.gov/sites/default/files/PhaseI_0.pdf. Accessed March 1, 2021.
3. Braveman PA, Kumanyika S, Fielding J, et al. Health disparities and health equity: the issue is justice. Am J Public Health 2011;101(Suppl 1):S149–55.
4. Brofenbrenner U. Ecological models of human development. International encyclopedia of education. Husten T, Postlethwaite TN (Eds). New York: Elsevier Science. 1994;3(2):1643–7.

5. Reifsnider E, Gallagher M, Forgione B. Using ecological models in research on health disparities. J Prof Nurs 2005;21(4):216–22.
6. Braveman P, Gottlieb L. The social determinants of health: it's time to consider the causes of the causes. Public Health Rep 2014;129(1_suppl2):19–31.
7. Knight AM, Weiss PF, Morales KH, et al. National trends in pediatric systemic lupus erythematosus hospitalization in the United States: 2000-2009. J Rheumatol 2014;41(3):539–46.
8. Tucker LB, Uribe AG, Fernández M, et al. Adolescent onset of lupus results in more aggressive disease and worse outcomes: results of a nested matched case-control study within LUMINA, a multiethnic US cohort (LUMINA LVII). Lupus 2008;17(4):314–22.
9. Yen EY, Singh RR. Brief Report: Lupus—An Unrecognized Leading Cause of Death in Young Females: A Population-Based Study Using Nationwide Death Certificates, 2000–2015. Arthritis Rheumatol 2018;70(8):1251–5.
10. Hiraki LT, Feldman CH, Liu J, et al. Prevalence, incidence, and demographics of systemic lupus erythematosus and lupus nephritis from 2000 to 2004 among children in the US Medicaid beneficiary population. Arthritis Rheum 2012; 64(8):2669–76.
11. Mauldin J, Cameron HD, Jeanotte D, et al. Chronic arthritis in children and adolescents in two Indian health service user populations. BMC Musculoskelet Disord 2004;5:30.
12. Houghton KM, Page J, Cabral DA, et al. Systemic lupus erythematosus in the pediatric North American Native population of British Columbia. J Rheumatol 2006;33(1):161–3.
13. Concannon A, Rudge S, Yan J, et al. The incidence, diagnostic clinical manifestations and severity of juvenile systemic lupus erythematosus in New Zealand Maori and Pacific Island children: the Starship experience (2000-2010). Lupus 2013;22(11):1156–61.
14. Mackie F, Kainer G, Rosenberg A, et al. High rates of SLE (systemic lupus erythematosus) in indigenous children in Australia - an interim report of the Australian Paediatric Surveillance Unit Study (APSU) 2009-2010. J Paediatr Child Health 2011;47:9.
15. Rubinstein TB, Knight AM. Disparities in Childhood-Onset Lupus. Rheum Dis Clin North Am 2020;46(4):661–72.
16. Reveille JD, Moulds JM, Ahn C, et al. Systemic lupus erythematosus in three ethnic groups: I. The effects of HLA class II, C4, and CR1 alleles, socioeconomic factors, and ethnicity at disease onset. LUMINA Study Group. Lupus in minority populations, nature versus nurture. Arthritis Rheum 1998;41(7): 1161–72.
17. Alarcón GS, Rodríguez JL, Benavides G, et al. Systemic lupus erythematosus in three ethnic groups: V. Acculturation, health-related attitudes and behaviors, and disease activity in Hispanic patients from the LUMINA Cohort. Arthritis Rheum 1999;12(4):267–76.
18. Burgos PI, McGwin G, Pons-Estel GJ, et al. US patients of Hispanic and African ancestry develop lupus nephritis early in the disease course: data from LUMINA, a multiethnic US cohort (LUMINA LXXIV). Ann Rheum Dis 2011; 70(2):393–4.
19. Uribe AG, Alarcón GS, Sanchez ML, et al. Systemic lupus erythematosus in three ethnic groups. XVIII. Factors predictive of poor compliance with study visits. Arthritis Care Res 2004;51(2):258–63.

20. Alarcón GS, McGwin JG, Bastian HM, et al. Systemic lupus erythematosus in three ethnic groups. VIII. Predictors of early mortality in the LUMINA cohort. Arthritis Rheum 2001;45(2):191–202.
21. Bastian HM, Alarcon GS, Roseman JM, et al. Systemic lupus erythematosus in a multiethnic US cohort (LUMINA) XL II: factors predictive of new or worsening proteinuria. Rheumatology 2006;46(4):683–9.
22. Alarcón GS, Calvo-Alén J, McGwin G Jr, et al. Systemic lupus erythematosus in a multiethnic cohort: LUMINA XXXV. Predictive factors of high disease activity over time. Ann Rheum Dis 2006;65(9):1168–74.
23. Fernández M, Alarcón GS, Calvo-Alén J, et al. A multiethnic, multicenter cohort of patients with systemic lupus erythematosus (SLE) as a model for the study of ethnic disparities in SLE. Arthritis Rheum 2007;57(4):576–84.
24. Hiraki LT, Benseler SM, Tyrrell PN, et al. Ethnic differences in pediatric systemic lupus erythematosus. J Rheumatol 2009;36(11):2539–46.
25. Chang JC, Xiao R, Mercer-Rosa L, et al. Child-onset systemic lupus erythematosus is associated with a higher incidence of myopericardial manifestations compared to adult-onset disease. Lupus 2018;27(13):2146–54.
26. Harrison MJ, Zühlke LJ, Lewandowski LB, et al. Pediatric systemic lupus erythematosus patients in South Africa have high prevalence and severity of cardiac and vascular manifestations. Pediatr Rheumatol Online J 2019;17(1):76.
27. Bundhun PK, Kumari A, Huang F. Differences in clinical features observed between childhood-onset versus adult-onset systemic lupus erythematosus: a systematic review and meta-analysis. Medicine (Baltimore) 2017;96(37):e8086.
28. Lewandowski LB, Watt MH, Schanberg LE, et al. Missed opportunities for timely diagnosis of pediatric lupus in South Africa: a qualitative study. Pediatr Rheumatol Online J 2017;15(1):14.
29. Massey DS, Tannen J. Suburbanization and Segregation in the United States: 1970-2010. Ethn Racial Stud 2018;41(9):1594–611.
30. Parker K, Horowitz J, Brown A, et al. (2018). What unites and divides urban, suburban and rural communities. Pew Research Center. Available at: https://www.pewresearch.org/social-trends/wp-content/uploads/sites/3/2018/05/Pew-Research-Center-Community-Type-Full-Report-FINAL.pdf. Accessed March 1, 2021.
31. Guo Q, Liang M, Duan J, et al. Age differences in secular trends in black-white disparities in mortality from systemic lupus erythematosus among women in the United States from 1988 to 2017. Lupus 2021;30(5):715–24.
32. Rubinstein TB, Mowrey WB, Ilowite NT, et al. Delays to care in pediatric lupus patients: data from the childhood arthritis and rheumatology research alliance legacy registry. Arthritis Care Res (Hoboken) 2018;70(3):420–7.
33. Rubinstein T, Davis A, Rodriguez M, et al. Addressing mental health in pediatric rheumatology. Curr Treat Options Rheumatol 2018;4(1):55–72.
34. Knight A, Weiss P, Morales K, et al. Depression and anxiety and their association with healthcare utilization in pediatric lupus and mixed connective tissue disease patients: a cross-sectional study. Pediatr Rheumatol Online J 2014;12:42.
35. Knight AM, Xie M, Mandell DS. Disparities in psychiatric diagnosis and treatment for youth with systemic lupus erythematosus: analysis of a National US Medicaid Sample. J Rheumatol 2016;43(7):1427–33.
36. Davis AM, Graham TB, Zhu Y, et al. Depression and medication nonadherence in childhood-onset systemic lupus erythematosus. Lupus 2018;27(9):1532–41.

37. Chang JC, Davis AM, Klein-Gitelman MS, et al. Impact of psychiatric diagnosis and treatment on medication adherence in youth with systemic lupus erythematosus. Arthritis Care Res (Hoboken) 2021;73(1):30–8.
38. Moorthy LN, Peterson MG, Hassett AL, et al. Burden of childhood-onset arthritis. Pediatr Rheumatol Online J 2010;8:20.
39. Oen KG, Cheang M. Epidemiology of chronic arthritis in childhood. Semin Arthritis Rheum 1996;26(3):575–91.
40. Dave M, Rankin J, Pearce M, et al. Global prevalence estimates of three chronic musculoskeletal conditions: club foot, juvenile idiopathic arthritis and juvenile systemic lupus erythematosus. Pediatr Rheumatol Online J 2020;18(1):49.
41. Cardoso I, Frederiksen P, Specht IO, et al. Age and Sex Specific Trends in Incidence of Juvenile Idiopathic Arthritis in Danish Birth Cohorts from 1992 to 2002: A Nationwide Register Linkage Study. Int J Environ Res Public Health 2021; 18(16):8331.
42. Harrold LR, Salman C, Shoor S, et al. Incidence and prevalence of juvenile idiopathic arthritis among children in a managed care population, 1996-2009. J Rheumatol 2013;40(7):1218–25.
43. Modesto C, Anton J, Rodriguez B, et al. Incidence and prevalence of juvenile idiopathic arthritis in Catalonia (Spain). Scand J Rheumatol 2010;39(6):472–9.
44. Thierry S, Fautrel B, Lemelle I, et al. Prevalence and incidence of juvenile idiopathic arthritis: a systematic review. Joint Bone Spine 2014;81(2):112–7.
45. Schinzel V, da Silva SGL, Terreri MT, et al. Prevalence of juvenile idiopathic arthritis in schoolchildren from the city of Sao Paulo, the largest city in Latin America. Adv Rheumatol 2019;59(1):32.
46. Khodra B, Stevens AM, Ferucci ED. Prevalence of Juvenile Idiopathic Arthritis in the Alaska Native Population. Arthritis Care Res (Hoboken) 2020;72(8):1152–8.
47. Shiff NJ, Oen K, Kroeker K, et al. Trends in Population-Based Incidence and Prevalence of Juvenile Idiopathic Arthritis in Manitoba, Canada. Arthritis Care Res (Hoboken) 2019;71(3):413–8.
48. Consolaro A, Giancane G, Alongi A, et al. Phenotypic variability and disparities in treatment and outcomes of childhood arthritis throughout the world: an observational cohort study. Lancet Child Adolesc Health 2019;3(4):255–63.
49. Ringold S, Beukelman T, Nigrovic PA, et al, Investigators CRSP. Race, ethnicity, and disease outcomes in juvenile idiopathic arthritis: a cross-sectional analysis of the Childhood Arthritis and Rheumatology Research Alliance (CARRA) Registry. J Rheumatol 2013;40(6):936–42.
50. Saurenmann RK, Rose JB, Tyrrell P, et al. Epidemiology of juvenile idiopathic arthritis in a multiethnic cohort: ethnicity as a risk factor. Arthritis Rheum 2007; 56(6):1974–84.
51. Rosenberg AM, Petty RE, Oen KG, et al. Rheumatic diseases in Western Canadian Indian children. J Rheumatol 1982;9(4):589–92.
52. Williams DR, Priest N, Anderson NB. Understanding associations among race, socioeconomic status, and health: patterns and prospects. Health Psychol 2016;35(4):407–11.
53. Chang JC, Xiao R, Burnham JM, et al. Longitudinal assessment of racial disparities in juvenile idiopathic arthritis disease activity in a treat-to-target intervention. Pediatr Rheumatol Online J 2020;18(1):88.
54. Brunner HI, Taylor J, Britto MT, et al. Differences in disease outcomes between medicaid and privately insured children: possible health disparities in juvenile rheumatoid arthritis. Arthritis Rheum 2006;55(3):378–84.

55. Verstappen SM, Cobb J, Foster HE, et al. The association between low socio-economic status with high physical limitations and low illness self-perception in patients with juvenile idiopathic arthritis: results from the Childhood Arthritis Prospective Study. Arthritis Care Res (Hoboken) 2015;67(3):382–9.
56. Oen K, Malleson PN, Cabral DA, et al. Early predictors of longterm outcome in patients with juvenile rheumatoid arthritis: subset-specific correlations. J Rheumatol 2003;30(3):585–93.
57. Albers HM, Wessels JAM, Van Der Straaten RJHM, et al. Time to treatment as an important factor for the response to methotrexate in juvenile idiopathic arthritis. Arthritis Care Res 2008;61(1):46–51.
58. Foster HE, Eltringham MS, Kay LJ, et al. Delay in access to appropriate care for children presenting with musculoskeletal symptoms and ultimately diagnosed with juvenile idiopathic arthritis. Arthritis Rheum 2007;57(6):921–7.
59. Huang B, Qiu T, Chen C, et al. Timing matters: real-world effectiveness of early combination of biologic and conventional synthetic disease-modifying antirheumatic drugs for treating newly diagnosed polyarticular course juvenile idiopathic arthritis. RMD Open 2020;6(1):e001091.
60. Tesher MS, Onel KB. The clinical spectrum of juvenile idiopathic arthritis in a large urban population. Curr Rheumatol Rep 2012;14(2):116–20.
61. Bisgaier J, Rhodes KV. Auditing access to specialty care for children with public insurance. N Engl J Med 2011;364(24):2324–33.
62. Shiff NJ, Tucker LB, Guzman J, et al. Factors associated with a longer time to access pediatric rheumatologists in Canadian children with juvenile idiopathic arthritis. J Rheumatol 2010;37(11):2415–21.
63. Agarwal M, Freychet C, Jain S, et al. Factors impacting referral of JIA patients to a tertiary level pediatric rheumatology center in North India: a retrospective cohort study. Pediatr Rheumatol 2020;18(1):21.
64. Tzaribachev N, Benseler SM, Tyrrell PN, et al. Predictors of delayed referral to a pediatric rheumatology center. Arthritis Rheum 2009;61(10):1367–72.
65. Balmuri N, Soulsby WD, Cooley V, et al. Community poverty level influences time to first pediatric rheumatology appointment in Polyarticular Juvenile Idiopathic Arthritis. Pediatr Rheumatol Online J 2021;19(1):122.
66. Tynjala P, Vahasalo P, Tarkiainen M, et al. Aggressive combination drug therapy in very early polyarticular juvenile idiopathic arthritis (ACUTE-JIA): a multicentre randomised open-label clinical trial. Ann Rheum Dis 2011;70(9):1605–12.
67. Suarez-Almazor ME, Berrios-Rivera JP, Cox V, et al. Initiation of disease-modifying antirheumatic drug therapy in minority and disadvantaged patients with rheumatoid arthritis. J Rheumatol 2007;34(12):2400–7.
68. Phillippi K, Hoeltzel M, Byun Robinson A, et al. Race, income, and disease outcomes in juvenile dermatomyositis. J Pediatr 2017;184:38–44.e1.
69. Kwa MC, Silverberg JI, Ardalan K. Inpatient burden of juvenile dermatomyositis among children in the United States. Pediatr Rheumatol 2018;16(1):70.
70. Pachman LM, Hayford JR, Chung A, et al. Juvenile dermatomyositis at diagnosis: clinical characteristics of 79 children. J Rheumatol 1998;25(6):1198–204.
71. Steen V, Domsic RT, Lucas M, et al. A clinical and serologic comparison of African American and Caucasian patients with systemic sclerosis. Arthritis Rheum 2012;64(9):2986–94.
72. Chung MP, Dontsi M, Postlethwaite D, et al. Increased Mortality in Asians With Systemic Sclerosis in Northern California. ACR Open Rheumatol 2020;2(4):197–206.

73. Mayes MD, Lacey JV, Beebe-Dimmer J, et al. Prevalence, incidence, survival, and disease characteristics of systemic sclerosis in a large US population. Arthritis Rheum 2003;48(8):2246–55.
74. Gelber AC, Manno RL, Shah AA, et al. Race and association with disease manifestations and mortality in scleroderma: a 20-year experience at the Johns Hopkins Scleroderma Center and review of the literature. Medicine (Baltimore) 2013; 92(4):191–205.
75. Blanco I, Mathai S, Shafiq M, et al. Severity of systemic sclerosis-associated pulmonary arterial hypertension in African Americans. Medicine (Baltimore) 2014; 93(5):177–85.
76. Baughman RP, Field S, Costabel U, et al. Sarcoidosis in America. Analysis Based on Health Care Use. Ann Am Thorac Soc 2016;13(8):1244–52.
77. Hena KM. Sarcoidosis Epidemiology: Race Matters. Front Immunol 2020;11: 537382.
78. Westney GE, Judson MA. Racial and ethnic disparities in sarcoidosis: from genetics to socioeconomics. Clin Chest Med 2006;27(3):453–62, vi.
79. Ogundipe F, Mehari A, Gillum R. Disparities in sarcoidosis mortality by region, urbanization, and race in the United States: a multiple cause of death analysis. Am J Med 2019;132(9):1062–8.e3.
80. Felsenstein S, Reiff AO, Ramanathan A. Transition of care and health-related outcomes in pediatric-onset systemic lupus erythematosus. Arthritis Care Res (Hoboken) 2015;67(11):1521–8.
81. McManus MA, Pollack LR, Cooley WC, et al. Current status of transition preparation among youth with special needs in the United States. Pediatrics 2013; 131(6):1090–7.
82. Chang JC, Knight AM, Lawson EF. Patterns of healthcare use and medication adherence among youth with systemic lupus erythematosus during transfer from pediatric to adult care. J Rheumatol 2021;48(1):105–13.
83. Son MB, Sergeyenko Y, Guan H, et al. Disease activity and transition outcomes in a childhood-onset systemic lupus erythematosus cohort. Lupus 2016;25(13): 1431–9.
84. Mayer ML, Sandborg CI, Mellins ED. Role of pediatric and internist rheumatologists in treating children with rheumatic diseases. Pediatrics 2004;113(3 Pt 1): e173–81.
85. Jackson CS, Gracia JN. Addressing health and health-care disparities: the role of a diverse workforce and the social determinants of health. Public Health Rep 2014;129(1_suppl2):57–61.
86. Sun K, Eudy AM, Criscione-Schreiber LG, et al. Racial differences in patient-provider communication, patient self-efficacy, and their associations with lupus-related damage: a cross-sectional survey. J Rheumatol 2021;48(7): 1022–8.
87. Correll CK, Spector LG, Zhang L, et al. Barriers and alternatives to pediatric rheumatology referrals: survey of general pediatricians in the United States. Pediatr Rheumatol Online J 2015;13:32.
88. Correll CK, Ditmyer MM, Mehta J, et al. 2015 American College of Rheumatology Workforce Study and Demand Projections of Pediatric Rheumatology Workforce, 2015-2030. Arthritis Care Res 2020.
89. Blanco I, Barjaktarovic N, Gonzalez CM. Addressing Health Disparities in Medical Education and Clinical Practice. Rheum Dis Clin North Am 2020;46(1): 179–91.

90. Rashid JR, Spengler RF, Wagner RM, et al. Eliminating Health Disparities Through Transdisciplinary Research, Cross-Agency Collaboration, and Public Participation. Am J Public Health 2009;99(11):1955–61.
91. Wasserman J, Palmer RC, Gomez MM, et al. Advancing health services research to eliminate health care disparities. Am J Public Health 2019; 109(S1):S64–9.
92. Shone LP. Reduction in Racial and Ethnic Disparities After Enrollment in the State Children's Health Insurance Program. Pediatrics 2005;115(6):e697–705.
93. Taber KA, Williams JN, Huang W, et al. Use of an Integrated Care Management Program to Uncover and Address Social Determinants of Health for Individuals With Lupus. ACR Open Rheumatol 2021;3(5):305–11.
94. Bourgois P, Holmes SM, Sue K, et al. Structural vulnerability: operationalizing the concept to address health disparities in clinical care. Acad Med 2017;92(3): 299–307.
95. Groot N, De Graeff N, Avcin T, et al. European evidence-based recommendations for diagnosis and treatment of childhood-onset systemic lupus erythematosus: the SHARE initiative. Ann Rheum Dis 2017;76(11):1788–96.
96. Ringold S, Weiss PF, Colbert RA, et al. Childhood arthritis and rheumatology research alliance consensus treatment plans for new-onset polyarticular juvenile idiopathic arthritis. Arthritis Care Res (Hoboken) 2014;66(7):1063–72.
97. Mina R, Von Scheven E, Ardoin SP, et al. Consensus treatment plans for induction therapy of newly diagnosed proliferative lupus nephritis in juvenile systemic lupus erythematosus. Arthritis Care Res 2012;64(3):375–83.
98. Otten MH, Anink J, Prince FH, et al. Trends in prescription of biological agents and outcomes of juvenile idiopathic arthritis: results of the Dutch national Arthritis and Biologics in Children Register. Ann Rheum Dis 2015;74(7):1379–86.
99. Burnham JM, Cecere L, Ukaigwe J,et al. Factors associated with variation in pediatric systemic lupus erythematosus care delivery. ACR Open Rheumatol 2021; 3(10):708–714.
100. Henrickson M. Policy challenges for the pediatric rheumatology workforce: Part III. the international situation. Pediatr Rheumatol 2011;9(1):26.
101. Sandhu VK, Hojjati M, Blanco I. Healthcare disparities in rheumatology: the role of education at a global level. Clin Rheumatol 2020;39(3):659–66.
102. Lima K, Phillip CR, Williams J, et al. Factors associated with participation in rheumatic disease-related research among underrepresented populations: a qualitative systematic review. Arthritis Care Res (Hoboken) 2020;72(10):1481–9.
103. Raifman J, Charlton BM, Arrington-Sanders R, et al. sexual orientation and suicide attempt disparities among US adolescents: 2009–2017. Pediatrics 2020; 145(3):e20191658.
104. Fish JN, Baams L. Trends in alcohol-related disparities between heterosexual and sexual minority youth from 2007 to 2015: findings from the youth risk behavior survey. LGBT Health 2018;5(6):359–67.

Pediatric Rheumatic Disease in Lower to Middle-Income Countries

Impact of Global Disparities, Ancestral Diversity, and the Path Forward

Christiaan Scott, MBChB[a], Sujata Sawhney, MD, MRCP, CCT[b], Laura B. Lewandowski, MD, MS[c,*]

KEYWORDS

- Pediatric rheumatology • Lower to middle-income countries • Global health
- Health disparities

KEY POINTS

- Currently, there is a shortage of pediatric rheumatologists in low to middle-income countries, which house most of the world's pediatric population. Without intervention, this disparity will widen.
- Early diagnosis and treatment have improved outcomes for pediatric rheumatologic diseases. However, current access barriers to rheumatology care, medications, diagnostics, research, and training threaten the optimal health of children worldwide.
- There are no treatment guidelines for most pediatric rheumatic diseases in low to middle-income countries and guidelines from high-income countries are inappropriate for resource-limited settings with high rates of endemic infections.
- Collaborative, multitargeted approaches will advance our understanding of pediatric rheumatology worldwide, benefiting the international pediatric rheumatology community in all settings.

INTRODUCTION

Pediatric rheumatologists take care of multisystem autoimmune disease in children. Musculoskeletal diseases such as juvenile idiopathic arthritis (JIA) and childhood

[a] Red Cross War Memorial Children's Hospital, University of Cape Town, Klipfontein Road, Rondebosch, Cape Town, Western Cape, South Africa; [b] Pediatric Rheumatology Division, Institute of Child Health, Sir Ganga Ram Hospital, New Delhi 110022, India; [c] National Institute of Arthritis, Musculoskeletal, and Skin Diseases, NIH, DHHS, 9000 Rockville Pike, Building 10, 12N248, Bethesda, MD 20892-1102, USA
* Corresponding author.
E-mail address: laura.lewandowski@nih.gov

Rheum Dis Clin N Am 48 (2022) 199–215
https://doi.org/10.1016/j.rdc.2021.09.001
0889-857X/22/Published by Elsevier Inc.

systemic lupus erythematosus (cSLE) contribute to the worldwide burden of disability, yet early diagnosis, and treatment limits damage and improves outcomes. Long-term prognosis in pediatric rheumatic diseases (PRDs) is influenced by complex interdependent factors, such as access to care, health care policy, infrastructure, health delivery, and caregiver socioeconomic status.[1] The major global inequality in wealth and health care access means that most of the world's children who live in low and middle-income countries (LMIC) are at risk for poorer outcomes.[2] We will review the current state of rheumatic disease epidemiologic data in LMIC, the impact of health policy, workforce shortages, barriers to building rheumatology capacity, the impact of access to care and research, and discuss models for impactful short-term and long-term change in global health disparities for the future.

MISSING DATA: THE SCOPE OF THE PROBLEM

There is little knowledge of the current burden of PRD worldwide. In places with trained rheumatology providers, there are data on the incidence and prevalence of rheumatic disease. From these statistics, we estimate the number of children expected to have rheumatic disease in places whereby there is no rheumatologist to diagnose and treat these children. The most common prevalence rates for JIA are 1 to 4/1000 children, with a higher prevalence in community surveys than clinic-based studies.[3] Parts of the world with the largest pediatric populations are also countries with the lowest percentage of pediatric rheumatologists (**Fig. 1**).[4] For example, in the Democratic Republic of Congo with nearly 40 million children, there is no in-country or regional access to pediatric rheumatology (PR) and no reports of rheumatic disease. Yet based on the prevalence data, an estimated 160,000 children are living with undiagnosed rheumatic disease. Such approximations are based on the population data and do not account for existing geographic differences in disease.

In the era of the Millennium Development goals (2000–2015), 8 goals set by the United Nations to reduce poverty and increase development, childhood mortality dropped dramatically worldwide, mostly through efforts addressing malnutrition and infectious and tropical diseases.[5] The efforts shifted focus from child survival to improving child health outcomes, which means addressing and managing noncommunicable diseases (NCDs).[6] Indeed, musculoskeletal disease contributes to

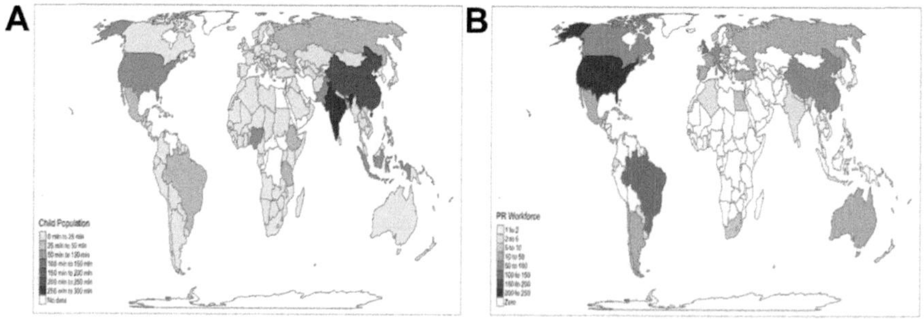

Fig. 1. Mapping the World Pediatric Rheumatology Workforce and the World Pediatric Population. (*A*) The number of children ages 0 to 14 in each country. The map demonstrates that much of the world's pediatric population resides in LMIC,[a] particularly sub-Saharan Africa, South Asia, and Southeast Asia. (*B*) The global distribution of the pediatric rheumatology workforce is concentrated in North America and Europe, largely in HIC.[b] [a] Population data provided by the World Bank.[123] [b] Data aggregated from recent publications and PRINTO resources.[4,27–31,124]

disability-adjusted life years (DALYs), and preventable disability acquired in childhood has lifelong consequences.[2] Suffering from the pain and inflammation of untreated rheumatic disease affects physical and mental health, growth, and development.[7] Therefore, developing systems to identify, diagnose, and treat children with rheumatic disease is imperative. Without trained health care providers to recognize PRDs, the chance for early diagnosis, specialized care, and critical research is lost.

IDEAL CARE MODEL FOR PEDIATRIC RHEUMATOLOGY

Provisions for the care of PRDs should include facilities for both the acutely unwell child and patients with indolent chronic disease.[8] Multidisciplinary PR teams optimally deliver care with access to intensive care and multispecialty facilities on site. Ideal rheumatology care includes early recognition, prompt referral and diagnosis, objective disease activity assessment, use of up-to-date evidence-based treatment pathways, careful follow-up, management of associated comorbidities (eg, infections and osteoporosis), and a smooth transition to adult rheumatology care.[9,10] In high-income countries (HIC), whereby governments spend a high proportion of the gross domestic product on health care infrastructure and delivery, much of this is often possible. However, even in HIC, the unequal distribution of PR providers creates gaps in access to care.[11] With the exception of JIA, there are no disease-specific guidelines for LMIC (vs HIC) despite the vast differences in disease profile, comorbid conditions, and access to therapy that complicate both the diagnosis and treatment of LMIC patients.[12]

ACCESS TO CARE IN LOWER TO MIDDLE-INCOME COUNTRIES

LMIC face extensive challenges delivering optimal care to the child with PRD, particularly resource constraints in all aspects of care. Significant constraints include the lack of trained PR workforce, poor health infrastructure, financial constraints (high cost of care, burden of patients' self-pay, lack of uniform health insurance), high rates of illiteracy and poor health literacy, social barriers such as the stigma of a chronic medical condition, and different government health care priorities. Governments in LMIC focus on the delivery of basic services such as clean drinking water, sanitation, vaccination, and interventions for malnutrition in the setting of virtually absent social services.[13,14]

In most LMIC, adequate facilities for diagnosis and drug treatment for PRD are available only in teaching institutions in large cities. Long distances to travel for specialty care are a major impediment for the early diagnosis of common rheumatic diseases.[14,15] Even the most talented, well-trained rheumatologist is limited by poor access to diagnostics, especially in places with high rates of endemic mimics such as tuberculosis, HIV, and malaria.[15–19] High-medication costs are another barrier to ideal care. The World Health Organization Essential Medicines List (EML) is a critical piece of health policy that shapes medication access for many LMIC.[20,21] Currently, the only medicine approved for juvenile joint disease is aspirin. Aspirin is woefully inadequate to treat the pain and suffering of conditions such as JIA and SLE and does not prevent irreversible inflammatory damage. Recently the Pediatric Task Force for Global Musculoskeletal Health (a virtual global community with a shared vision to "work better together" to improve the lives of children and young people) surveyed PR providers globally to inform an appeal to the WHO to revise the EML for PRD.[22,23] Lack of access to care and effective medications leads to the late recognition and treatment of PRDs. Delays in treatment allow damage (which by definition is irreversible) to skin, joints, muscles, and internal organs increasing the risk of lifelong morbidity and in some cases early mortality. Inadequately managed PRDs that persist into adulthood add to the burden of DALYs, an important outcome measure of musculoskeletal diseases in adults, which has shown a significant worldwide increase in the last decade.[24] With limited health budgets allocated to rheumatologic care, few providers, and inadequate access to medications, it is not surprising that late diagnosis and damage in multiple organs is common for children with PRDs in LMIC.[25,26]

WORKFORCE SHORTAGE

Many LMIC have no trained PR care providers (see **Fig. 1**). The data in **Fig. 1** are based on recently published summaries and databases of PR workforce and may not reflect changes since the time of publication.[4,27–31] In most LMIC, PR shortages reflect severe regional shortages of health care workers and pediatricians in general.[32] In these regions, nonphysician health care providers constitute the bulk of the primary care workforce. Appropriately, they have focused training and effort on the management of common, life-threatening conditions, and noncommunicable chronic conditions are not a priority. In most cases, rheumatology providers are localized in major centers, which create disparities even in countries whereby there are trained rheumatologists. Training opportunities for pediatrics or pediatric subspecialties are also quite limited in many LMIC's, especially in Africa, whereby only one country has PR training available.[32] In places with large pediatric populations and general workforce shortages, subspecialists cover general pediatrics. The COVID-19 pandemic has exacerbated the imbalance of physician workforce shortages in LMIC.[33] The staggering inequalities will not be resolved soon and the goal of a fully functioning PR service in each country is likely not achievable. Alternative models of training in basic rheumatic disease care may offer interim solutions, while allowing for the growth of service lines as part of the general development of health care in LMIC. Individual countries are at different levels of progress and require flexible programs adapted for their particular needs.

ACCESS TO RESEARCH

LMIC often lack critical infrastructure for the successful execution of rheumatology research, despite having interested providers. In HIC, trainees identified funding, access to research infrastructure, time protected from clinical responsibility, and mentorship as the most critical pieces for success in research.[34,35] In addition, early career investigators in Europe and South America have identified additional barriers to embarking on research careers, including statistical support to design and interpret studies, lack of experience writing grants and papers, lack of English proficiency, and lack of mentorship in their area of research interest.[36] The barriers to research training and infrastructure lead to a publication bias, with the vast majority of publications coming from HIC.[37] Despite these barriers, research led by LMIC providers is critical to creating clinical guidelines relevant to their practice setting, given their knowledge of endemic infection types and rates, prevalent PRDs, access to diagnostics and medications.[12] Access to research is an area whereby collaboration between HIC with available tools and trained personnel and LMIC with local expertise could revolutionize the landscape of what we currently understand about the worldwide burden of rheumatic disease.[6,26]

HEALTH DISPARITIES AND ANCESTRAL DIVERSITY IN PEDIATRIC RHEUMATIC DISEASE IN LOWER TO MIDDLE-INCOME COUNTRIES

Epidemiology of pediatric rheumatic diseases in lower to middle-income countries

Most data on PRD in LMIC come from case studies or single-center reports; there are few national registries and no population-based studies.[23] Most of the pediatric rheumatologists work in teaching institutions with appropriate infrastructure for care of complex patients, but the access to care barriers and lack of multicenter data make it hard to understand overall incidence and prevalence of rheumatic disease in LMIC.[38] PRDs occur in patients of all ancestral backgrounds. Some rheumatic diseases are more prevalent in certain ancestral backgrounds: JIA is more common in White patients and SLE in Black and Hispanic patients in HIC.[39–41] Studies from HIC demonstrate differences in disease severity and outcomes for Black patients with rheumatic disease, but the relationships are multifaceted. Race is a social construct without a biological basis. Health disparities in rheumatic disease have complex influences, including socioeconomic factors, effects of systemic racism, genetic susceptibility, and environmental exposures.[42,43] To understand the impact of ancestral genetic diversity on PRD, we need to improve access to care and research in high and low-income settings.[44] The vast majority of genetic studies for rheumatic disease are in HIC, in adult populations of European ancestry. Additionally, strong European ancestry bias in reference genomes and genotyping arrays only compound these issues. A few adult studies have implicated genetic changes which confer risks for specific populations, (ie, APOL1 confers increased risk for poor renal outcomes in SLE patients of African ancestry).[45] We need larger studies encompassing a wider geographic range of PR patients to understand if the genetic associations reported in adult-onset disease are present in diverse childhood-onset cohorts. Further complicating understanding the role of ancestry is the interplay of genetics, epigenetics, and environment. Epigenetic changes that occur because of toxic stress, violence, and trauma disproportionately affect certain racial/ethnic groups in different locations.[46–48] Environmental influences such as pollution and UV light vary widely across geographic locations and are implicated in the pathogenesis of disease.[49–51] Most LMIC report delays in recognition and diagnosis resulting in subsequent damage for most PRDS.[26,52] The interplay of access to care and biological predisposition to severe disease is complex and requires both clinical and translational research investigation. Next, we review the epidemiology of PRDs from LMIC, acknowledging the reporting bias in countries with PR providers.

JUVENILE IDIOPATHIC ARTHRITIS

Juvenile idiopathic arthritis (JIA) is the most prevalent PRD and a leading cause of acquired nontraumatic musculoskeletal disability.[2,53] The diagnosis is based on clinical features and the exclusion of mimicking conditions. There are no serological, histological, genetic, or radiological tests to confirm or exclude the diagnosis. Adding to the difficulty of diagnosis is the fact that several different phenotypes are recognized as JIA subtypes according to the ILAR classification.[54] Although some phenotypes, such as rheumatoid factor positive polyarticular JIA, are early presentations of conditions such as rheumatoid arthritis, others such as oligoarticular JIA or systemic JIA are rare or nonexistent in adults. The frequency of mimicking conditions, the lack of a specific diagnostic test, and confusion with adult diagnostic patterns and criteria complicate the diagnosis of JIA and delay access to care, even in the most well-resourced health care systems.[11,55] It is likely that this combination of factors have led to an underestimation of JIA prevalence in LMIC contributing to the lack of resources dedicated to health care worker training, diagnosis and treatment in LMIC.[12,28,56] Delays in diagnosis and other pressing societal and health care conditions, especially the enormous burden of tuberculosis, human immunodeficiency virus (HIV), and malaria in sub-Saharan Africa and other LMIC regions are likely to contribute to the paucity of data on JIA from LMIC, adding to the perception of rarity.[3,57] Studies estimating prevalence of JIA range globally between 1 and 4/1000 children, with higher prevalence described in community screening studies than in hospital-based studies.[2,57,58] The largest multinational study on outcomes in JIA to date, the EPOCA (Epidemiology, Outcomes and Treatments in JIA) study, enrolled 9081 patients from 130 centers in 49 countries and showed a clear correlation between the wealth and geographic origin of the country and JIA outcomes, with LMIC having poorer outcomes.[59]

In addition, the EPOCA study showed phenotypic differences between countries and regions. Systemic JIA (33%) and enthesitis-related arthritis (29%) make up higher proportions of JIA diagnoses in Southeast Asia, whereas oligoarticular JIA rates are higher in Southern Europe (56%).[59] These findings mirror case series from LMIC such as Brazil, Thailand, India, and South Africa.[60–63] The vast majority of genetic studies in JIA are done in non-Hispanic White patients.[64] Smaller studies in Black and Hispanic populations have confirmed an association with HLA-DRB3 allele in rheumatoid factor positive polyarthritis.[65] An international GWAS on patients with JIA from 9 nations, including 2 LMIC, determined that the genetics of sJIA differs from other JIA patients.[66] Additional studies in globally diverse JIA cohorts will enhance understanding of the genetic spectrum of disease.

Even more, pressing than the lack of research access is the plight of children with JIA living in regions of the world whereby pediatric care is severely constrained or nonexistent and about whom virtually nothing is reported in the literature. Fortunately, the last 2 decades have seen tremendous advances in the care of JIA. Disease-modifying drugs such as methotrexate are widely (though not universally) available, offering opportunities for access to safe and affordable therapy in most parts of the world. However, the revolution in cytokine-targeting biologic drugs and small molecules offers hope for the future, as access is currently severely restricted due to cost, lack of infrastructure, and expertise and risk of comorbidities such as tuberculosis.[22,67] As patent rights for expensive first-generation biologic agents expire, there is steady growth in the availability of biosimilars drugs. Although this reduces direct drug costs, the agents remain relatively expensive and require special handling such as refrigeration, which impedes broad access.

CHILDHOOD-ONSET SYSTEMIC LUPUS ERYTHEMATOSUS

Childhood-onset systemic lupus erythematosus (cSLE) is a chronic, systemic autoimmune disease that is potentially fatal.[68] Approximately 1 of 5 systemic lupus erythematous (SLE) cases has disease onset in the childhood years.[69] cSLE is more severe than adult-onset disease in both HIC and LMIC, and standardized mortality rate is 3 times higher than the general population.[70,71] The incidence and prevalence of cSLE vary widely by geographic location, ancestry, and gender. The definition of cSLE varies by region, with some areas classifying cSLE as onset by 16 years of age and others at 18 or older. This difference contributes to variance in reported incidence and prevalence of disease.[72] Reported rates thus span wide ranges, with an incidence of 0.28 to 2.5/100,000 children and prevalence of 1.89 to 34.1/100,000.[73,74] In less-resourced settings, poor access to care can lead to underdiagnosis, lowering apparent incidence, and prevalence.[75] Global estimates of cSLE suggest that the highest burden is in LMIC with large pediatric populations.[76]

Recent studies demonstrated that cSLE occurs in LMIC and cSLE patients have high disease activity and rates of damage. In a study from South Africa, cSLE patients had higher rates of proliferative lupus nephritis, higher disease activity scores, and higher rates of damage when compared with North American counterparts.[26] A review of patients in India revealed similar patterns with high rates of lupus nephritis and disease damage.[77] High severity of disease translates to high mortality rates. In Tanzania, cSLE was fatal in 50% of identified cases.[75] A comprehensive meta-analysis of worldwide cSLE mortality since 1950 demonstrated that cSLE patients in LMIC have the worst survival rates of SLE patients at any age of onset worldwide.[78] Infections are a leading driver of mortality in SLE in some less-resourced countries, along with lack of access to renal replacement therapy and renal transplant.[77,79]

Few GWAS highlight cSLE. One study conducted in Mexico found an association between the PTPN22 gene (which encodes the cytoplasmic lymphoid-specific phosphatase, a powerful regulator of immune homeostasis) and cSLE, consistent with previous reports of autoimmune disease.[80] Genetic studies assessing the burden of common variants using polygenic risk scores have found differences based on ancestry.[81] Studies of larger, more diverse cSLE populations will enhance understanding of the biologic mechanisms of SLE globally.

JUVENILE DERMATOMYOSITIS

Juvenile dermatomyositis (JDM) is a rare connective tissue disease in children, with a reported incidence of 1.9/million children in the UK and 2.5/million in US.[82,83] The only pooled nation-wide data available from LMIC is a review of 189 JDM patients from a multicenter study in Brazil.[84] A report from India projected 3500 cases of JDM in the country based on a previous prevalence report in HIC.[25] In Northern India, 18 JDM patients seen over a 10-year period had a median delay to diagnosis of over 9 months, reflecting poor access to care.[85] In a multicenter study from Southeast Asia, Malaysia reported the highest percentage (6.9%) of prevalent JDM patients in their registry of patients with rheumatic disease.[23] As most of sub-Saharan Africa does not have PR providers, data on JDM are sparse and come mostly from case reports. A study from Tanzania reported seeing only 4 JDM patients (7.5% of children with PR evaluations) over a 7-year period.[75] Inpatient hospital records from Nigeria reported only one patient with JDM out of 57 PR patients seen over a 5-year period.[86] South Africa has the largest number of PRs in sub-Saharan Africa, and accordingly the highest numbers of reported cases of JDM. A cross-sectional study from 3 hospitals in Cape Town reported 25 JDM patients over a 9-year period, with the achievement of inactive disease in 40%.[87]

Although sparse, the reports of JDM from LMIC demonstrate a pattern of severe disease and high rates of damage. South Africa reported extremely high rates of calcinosis (44%–71% of all patients) and cutaneous vasculitis (43%).[83,87] In a multicenter study in Brazil, calcinosis occurred in 32% of patients.[84] Centers in India have reported up to 27% of patients complicated by calcinosis.[85,88] In studies conducted in India, calcinosis was associated with delay in diagnosis and treatment and with cardiac involvement.[89] Cutaneous damage was reported in greater than 50% of patients in India followed over a 5-year period.[90] Calcinosis raters were lower in a small study from Iran but associated with a polycyclic course.[91] Reports of higher rates of calcinosis and other damage in LMIC reflect poor access to care, as they mirror rates seen in historic cohorts in HIC without treatment. These data on damage and calcinosis support reports from HIC that income disparities lead to adverse outcomes in JDM.[92]

Myositis autoantibodies are not routinely available in LMIC. A few studies report the prevalence of autoantibodies. In India, 30%–50% of JDM children were autoantibody positive.[93] Anti-MJ antibody was present in 22% of JDM patients reported from Argentina and predicted a severe phenotype.[94] Interestingly, environmental pollution is also linked to admissions for PRDs in Brazil.[95] Environmental influences may play a role in many autoimmune diseases, and the link between pollution exposure and autoimmune phenotype warrants further investigation.

Mortality rates for JDM in HIC is 0% to 3%, but higher in all LMIC that reported data. In the multicenter study in Brazil, mortality was 4%.[84] In India, mortality remains high at 11%, due to disease severity, gastrointestinal vasculitis, and infections.[96,97] Infection was the leading cause of death in Indian JDM patients, regardless of age at diagnosis, similar to SLE reports from LMIC.[97,98]

VASCULITIS

Vasculitis in childhood is difficult to diagnose and often requires multidisciplinary care. Vasculitides demonstrate geographic variation in prevalence: Kawasaki's disease (KD) and Takayasu's arteritis are more common in Asian populations and Henoch Schönlein Purpura (HSP) is more common in European populations. ANCA-associated vasculitis is extremely rare in the pediatric population and no data are available from LMIC. There is little epidemiologic data available from LMIC on most vasculitic conditions.

There is an increased awareness about KD in LMIC that may be linked to the reported increase of KD in countries showing rapid industrialization.[99] In a recent report from Southeast Asia on the referral pattern of PRD, systemic vasculitis was a common diagnosis in clinic patients. The most common vasculitis diagnoses were HSP and KD.[23] A study from Chile reported increased hospitalization rates and incidence of KD between 2001 and 2007.[100] A recent report from Latin America discussed the outcome of KD in more than 300 patients over a 10-year period with a recurrence rate of 8% during the first 3 years of follow-up, significantly higher than reported in HIC. This study and others from the region showed a significant delay between the disease onset, diagnosis, and administration of intravenous immunoglobulin (IVIg) with 21.5% of children receiving IVIg after day 10 and only 20% referred with the correct diagnosis. Lack of resources to treat the child with KD in LMIC may result in coronary aneurysm development and a high burden of adult coronary artery disease over the next few decades.[101,102]

In LMIC, there may be a link between Takayasu's arteritis (TA) and tuberculosis.[103,104] One large multicenter series of 71 TA patients from Brazil reported TB in 5 patients. Delay in diagnosis was common, largely due to the misdiagnosis of the patients with either coarctation of aorta or acute rheumatic fever. The presence of aortic regurgitation in patients with both rheumatic fever and TA confounded the diagnosis in many cases.[105] Younger children had an increased diagnostic delay than children over 10 years.[106] The link between tuberculosis and TA may lead to important insights into pathogenesis, especially in TB endemic settings, further highlighting the importance of conducting research in LMIC.

SYSTEMIC SCLEROSIS, LOCALIZED SCLERODERMA, INFLAMMATORY BONE DISEASE

The data addressing rarer PRDs from LMIC are even sparser. Over a 2-year period, out of 900 patients with PRD seen in Singapore, no patient had systemic sclerosis (SSc). In all other Southeast Asian countries, both SSc and localized scleroderma were reported, except in Malaysia whereby 8 of 567 patients seen in the clinic had SSc but there was no patient with localized scleroderma.[23] In one report from Nigeria, 2 (3.5%) hospital admissions were due to SSc.[86] One patient from Malaysia was reported to have inflammatory bone disease in a cohort of more than 4000 PRD patients from Southeast Asia.[23] Rare conditions require trained PRs to make the diagnosis.

FUTURE SOLUTIONS

Currently, there are large global disparities in access to PR care. Even by conservative estimates, there are thousands of children worldwide suffering from PRD without hope of diagnosis or treatment. Without concerted effort to address these issues, the disparities will only widen over time. One such effort is the Pediatric Musculoskeletal Task Force, which is an independent global collaborative network of pediatric rheumatologists, orthopedic surgeons, patients, and caregivers, aimed at addressing unmet needs in pediatric MSK health.[107]

The first issue is the lack of expertise in many LMIC. Without regional or local expertise, there can be no training of a future workforce. PR providers are needed to handle the clinical workload, teaching, and training. However, with fewer practitioners, less trainees get exposure to PR, such exposure early in education is critical to developing future trained providers.[31,108–110] An important step to increase the PR workforce in LMIC is to create short, focused in-person training opportunities for pediatricians interested in rheumatology either bringing experts in to provide training or sending local trainees out of the country. Trainees worldwide feel the burden of extended training time and deferred earning, but in LMIC these barriers block most learners from pursuing this path. Shorter in-person training programs can be supplemented with an online, asynchronous curriculum.[111] The COVID-19 global pandemic accelerated the development of virtual medical education and training; LMIC without access to PR can leverage this new approach.[112–114] There are emerging training models to adapt for local training that can address unmet needs in rheumatology access to care. Recent experience has shown that more can be taught in the virtual space than previously imagined, and training tools and assessments are being developed at an unprecedented pace. The right balance of virtual and in-person training is not defined and may vary with instructors, trainees, prior training, setting, and access to other resources. In any case, virtual learning will not solve large systemic inequities, such as the unequal to access to effective medications and reliable Internet and technology, also known as the digital divide.[115,116] One excellent example of virtual training is Pediatric Musculoskeletal Matters (http://www.pmmonline.org), which encompasses multimedia tools such as modules, images, videos, and training materials and are open access, available in multiple formats including website and app, and used worldwide by providers taking care of children with rheumatic disease.[117] Increasing access to rheumatology educational conferences and continuing medical education efforts in HIC is another key step, especially now that many conferences are virtual or offered as a hybrid participation format.[118,119] Finally, strengthening the education of pediatricians and general practitioners to recognize PRD and refer for further care is an essential step in countries with few providers.[120] Given huge health care challenges facing LMIC, innovative solutions leveraging multiple types of health care providers offers the best medium and long-term solutions to provide affordable and accessible care for children with PRDs. "RightPath," which leverages community physician and triage systems to appropriately identify patients who need subspecialty care, is a model that could be adapted for use in LMIC.[121] A larger robust health system equipped with trained practitioners who recognize PRD may be able to lower barriers for access to specialized care.[107]

The road to funding a larger workforce is a long and difficult path. As we have highlighted, the robust data needed to address the burden of PRD in most LMIC do not exist. Government budgets in LMIC are highly constrained and supported by low GDPs. Health policy is data driven and without epidemiologic data to support funding for PR education, training, clinical care, and research infrastructure, LMIC governments will continue to focus on other priorities.

Telemedicine is an important new avenue to improve access to care. In 2020, telemedicine went from being relatively rare in PR to being a central component of the longitudinal management of chronic autoimmune diseases during a global pandemic. Acknowledging that a careful physical examination is sometimes critical, particularly for initial diagnosis, the adaptation of innovations developed for safety during the pandemic may be useful to increase access to care in LMIC. Many families of children with PRD take on significant costs to attend distant clinics, including missed work and school days, travel expenses, danger of unsafe travel conditions, and arranging care for other children or family members.[14] Telemedicine could reduce the travel burden for longitudinal PR care.[122]

Whatever the approach to reducing the gaps in access to care, acting now is imperative. Lack of access to PR care leads to delays in diagnosis or misdiagnosis for diseases with large morbidity and mortality. As described, the consequences of this gap are high mortality rates for many PRDs in LMIC. In nonfatal cases, children from LMIC suffer high rates of irreversible damage and have poor access to the support needed to address the resulting damage and disability, such as renal replacement therapy, physical therapy, or assistive/adaptive devices.

SUMMARY

Children worldwide do not have adequate access to rheumatology care and medicines. The barriers to PRD diagnosis, treatment, and longitudinal care are much greater in LMIC and pose a complex problem that will require multi-pronged sustained solutions. However, pediatric rheumatologists, drawn to complexity and collaboration, and the worldwide PR community are particularly poised to tackle the problem. The first step is facilitating collaboration between LMIC and HIC to create research and training programs. Such collaboration will require robust support from regional rheumatology organizations (eg, American College of Rheumatology, African League Against Rheumatism) and global research organizations such as Wellcome Trust, Gates Foundation, and others. Successful collaboration will develop innovative methods and transition LMIC partners to independent efforts, whereby providers use their local expertise in government funding, health policy, hospital procedure, endemic infections, and health disparities to drive research and clinical guidelines custom-built for their unique patient population. The path forward requires attention, assessment, creativity, and cooperation to train future generations of PR providers, educators, and researchers in LMIC.

CLINICS CARE POINTS

- The global epidemiology of pediatric rheumatic disease is poorly understood due to paucity of pediatric rheumatologists in LMIC.
- The global shortage of pediatric rheumatology providers contributes to large disparities in accessing pediatric rheumatology care and research.
- Lack of access to care and research in LMIC result in high rates of morbidity and mortality from pediatric rheumatic disease in many places worldwide. Collaborative and innovative solutions must be developed and implemented to reduce severe outcomes in these populations.

DISCLOSURE

Drs L.B. Lewandowski, S. Sawhney, and C. Scott have no financial disclosures or conflicts of interest to declare. The opinions expressed in this article are the author's own and do not reflect the view of the National Institutes of Health, the Department of Health and Human Services, or the United States government.

REFERENCES

1. Consolaro A, Schiappapietra B, Dalprà S, et al. Optimisation of disease assessments in juvenile idiopathic arthritis. Clin Exp Rheumatol 2014;32(5 Suppl 85): S-126–130.
2. Dave M, Rankin J, Pearce M, et al. Global prevalence estimates of three chronic musculoskeletal conditions: club foot, juvenile idiopathic arthritis and juvenile systemic lupus erythematosus. Pediatr Rheumatol 2020;18(1):1–7.
3. Manners PJ, Diepeveen DA. Prevalence of juvenile chronic arthritis in a population of 12-year-old children in urban Australia. Pediatrics 1996;98(1):84–90.
4. Correll CK, Ditmyer MM, Mehta J, et al. 2015 American College of rheumatology workforce study and demand projections of pediatric rheumatology workforce, 2015-2030. Arthritis Care Res 2021. https://doi.org/10.1002/acr.24497.
5. Wang H, Bhutta ZA, Coates MM, et al. Global, regional, national, and selected subnational levels of stillbirths, neonatal, infant, and under-5 mortality, 1980–2015: a systematic analysis for the Global Burden of Disease Study 2015. Lancet 2016;388(10053):1725–74.
6. Migowa A, Colmegna I, Hitchon C, et al. The spectrum of rheumatic in-patient diagnoses at a pediatric hospital in Kenya. Pediatr Rheumatol 2017;15(1):4.
7. Schanberg LE, Anthony KK, Gil KM, et al. Daily pain and symptoms in children with polyarticular arthritis. Arthritis Rheum 2003;48(5):1390–7.
8. Spencer CH. Why should pediatric rheumatology be recognized as a separate subspecialty: an open letter to medical councils and government agencies. Springer; 2007.
9. Tong A, Jones J, Speerin R, et al. Consumer perspectives on pediatric rheumatology care and service delivery: a qualitative study. J Clin Rheumatol 2013; 19(5):234–40.
10. Tunnicliffe DJ, Singh-Grewal D, Craig JC, et al. Healthcare and research priorities of adolescents and young adults with systemic lupus erythematosus: a mixed-methods study. J Rheumatol 2017;44(4):444–51.
11. Foster HE, Eltringham MS, Kay LJ, et al. Delay in access to appropriate care for children presenting with musculoskeletal symptoms and ultimately diagnosed with juvenile idiopathic arthritis. Arthritis Care Res 2007;57(6):921–7.
12. Scott C, Chan M, Slamang W, et al. Juvenile arthritis management in less resourced countries (JAMLess): consensus recommendations from the cradle of humankind. Clin Rheumatol 2019;38(2):563–75.
13. Morton S, Pencheon D, Squires N. Sustainable Development Goals (SDGs), and their implementation: a national global framework for health, development and equity needs a systems approach at every level. Br Med Bull 2017;124(1): 81–90.
14. Lewandowski LB, Watt MH, Schanberg LE, et al. Missed opportunities for timely diagnosis of pediatric lupus in South Africa: a qualitative study 2017;15(1):14.
15. Agarwal M, Freychet C, Jain S, et al. Factors impacting referral of JIA patients to a tertiary level pediatric rheumatology center in North India: a retrospective cohort study. Pediatr Rheumatol 2020;18(1):1–11.

16. Misra DP, Sharma A, Agarwal V. Rheumatology science and practice in India. Rheumatol Int 2018;38(9):1587–600.
17. Olowu WA, Adelusola KA, Adefehinti O, et al. Quartan malaria-associated childhood nephrotic syndrome: Now a rare clinical entity in malaria endemic Nigeria. Nephrol Dial Transplant 2010;25(3):794–801.
18. Foster H, Rapley T. Access to pediatric rheumatology care—a major challenge to improving outcome in juvenile idiopathic arthritis. The J Rheumatol 2010; 37(11):2199–202. https://doi.org/10.3899/jrheum.100910.
19. Bristow S, Jackson D, Shields L, et al. The rural mother's experience of caring for a child with a chronic health condition: An integrative review. J Clin Nurs 2018; 27(13–14):2558–68.
20. Foster HE, Scott C. Update the WHO EML to improve global paediatric rheumatology. Nat Rev Rheumatol 2020;16(3):123.
21. Bazargani YT, Ewen M, de Boer A, et al. Essential medicines are more available than other medicines around the globe. PloS one 2014;9(2):e87576.
22. Scott C, Smith N, James R, et al. Revising the WHO Essential Medicines List for paediatric rheumatology. Pediatr Rheumatol 2021;19(1):1–2.
23. Arkachaisri T, Tang SP, Daengsuwan T, et al. Paediatric rheumatology clinic population in Southeast Asia: are we different? Rheumatology (Oxford) 2017;56(3): 390–8.
24. Sebbag E, Felten R, Sagez F, et al. The world-wide burden of musculoskeletal diseases: a systematic analysis of the World Health Organization Burden of Diseases Database. Ann Rheum Dis 2019;78(6):844–8.
25. Sawhney S, Manners P. The place of pediatric rheumatology in India. Indian J Pediatr 2010;77(9):993–6.
26. Lewandowski LB, Schanberg LE, Thielman N, et al. Severe disease presentation and poor outcomes among pediatric systemic lupus erythematosus patients in South Africa. Lupus 2017;26(2):186–94.
27. Dolezalova P, Anton J, Avcin T, et al. The European network for care of children with paediatric rheumatic diseases: care across borders. Rheumatology (Oxford) 2019;58(7):1188–95.
28. Tangcheewinsirikul S, Tang SP, Smith N, et al. Delivery of paediatric rheumatology care: a survey of current clinical practice in Southeast Asia and Asia-Pacific regions. Pediatr Rheumatol Online J 2021;19(1):11.
29. Reveille JD, Muñoz R, Soriano E, et al. Review of Current Workforce for Rheumatology in the Countries of the Americas 2012-2015. J Clin Rheumatol 2016;22(8): 405–10.
30. Brophy J, Marshall DA, Badley EM, et al. Measuring the Rheumatology Workforce in Canada: A Literature Review. The J Rheumatol 2016;43(6):1121–9.
31. Argraves M, Mehta JJ. Pediatric rheumatology: Not just a little adult workforce issue. Semin Arthritis Rheum 2021;51(5):e13.
32. Harper BD, Nganga W, Armstrong R, et al. Global Gaps in Training Opportunities for Pediatricians and Pediatric Subspecialists. Acad Pediatr 2020;20(6): 823–32.
33. Risko N, Werner K, Offorjebe OA, et al. Cost-effectiveness and return on investment of protecting health workers in low-and middle-income countries during the COVID-19 pandemic. PloS one 2020;15(10):e0240503.
34. Ogdie A, Shah AA, Makris UE, et al. Barriers to and facilitators of a career as a physician-scientist among rheumatologists in the US. Arthritis Care Res 2015; 67(9):1191–201.

35. Jani M, Sepriano A, Mv Onna, et al. SAT0676 SUPPORTING EARLY CAREER RESEARCHERS IN RHEUMATOLOGY AND MUSCULOSKELETAL MEDICINE: RESULTS FROM AN EMERGING EULAR NETWORK (EMEUNET) SURVEY. Ann Rheum Dis 2019;78(Suppl 2):1439–40.
36. Ugarte-Gil MF, Alarcón GS. Medical scientific publications from latin America: a commentary. J Clin Rheumatol 2019;25(4):157–8.
37. Lewandowski LB. Tackling global challenges in pediatric rheumatology. Curr Opin Rheumatol 2020;32(5):414–20.
38. Terreri MT, Campos LM, Okuda EM, et al. Profile of paediatric rheumatology specialists and services in the state of São Paulo. Rev Bras Reumatol 2013; 53(4):346–51.
39. Saurenmann RK, Rose JB, Tyrrell P, et al. Epidemiology of juvenile idiopathic arthritis in a multiethnic cohort: Ethnicity as a risk factor. Arthritis Rheum 2007; 56(6):1974–84.
40. Somers EC, Marder W, Cagnoli P, et al. Population-based incidence and prevalence of systemic lupus erythematosus: the Michigan lupus epidemiology and surveillance program. Arthritis Rheumatol 2014;66(2):369–78.
41. Chakravarty EF, Bush TM, Manzi S, et al. Prevalence of adult systemic lupus erythematosus in California and Pennsylvania in 2000: Estimates obtained using hospitalization data. Arthritis Rheum 2007;56(6):2092–4.
42. Borrell LN, Elhawary JR, Fuentes-Afflick E, et al. Race and genetic ancestry in medicine—a time for reckoning with racism. N Engl J Med 2021;384(5):474–80.
43. Yearby R. Structural racism and health disparities: Reconfiguring the social determinants of health framework to include the root cause. J L Med Ethics 2020; 48(3):518–26.
44. Williams JN, Dall'Era M, Lim SS, et al. Increasing Ancestral Diversity in Systemic Lupus Erythematosus Clinical Studies. Arthritis Care Res 2020. https://doi.org/10.1002/acr.24474.
45. Blazer A, Dey ID, Nwaukoni J, et al. Apolipoprotein L1 risk genotypes in Ghanaian patients with systemic lupus erythematosus: a prospective cohort study. Lupus Sci Med 2021;8(1):e000460.
46. Hoge C, Bowling CB, Lim SS, et al. Association of poverty income ratio with physical functioning in a cohort of patients with systemic lupus erythematosus. The J Rheumatol 2020;47(7):983–90.
47. Gilcrease GW, Padovan D, Heffler E, et al. Is air pollution affecting the disease activity in patients with systemic lupus erythematosus? State of the art and a systematic literature review. Eur J Rheumatol 2020;7(1):31.
48. DeQuattro K, Trupin L, Li J, et al. Relationships between adverse childhood experiences and health status in systemic lupus erythematosus. Arthritis Care Res 2020;72(4):525–33.
49. Alves AGF, de Azevedo Giacomin MF, Braga ALF, et al. Influence of air pollution on airway inflammation and disease activity in childhood-systemic lupus erythematosus. Clin Rheumatol 2018;37(3):683–90.
50. Goulart MFG, Alves AGF, Farhat J, et al. Influence of air pollution on renal activity in patients with childhood-onset systemic lupus erythematosus. Pediatr Nephrol 2020;35(7):1247–55.
51. Barbhaiya M, Costenbader K. Ultraviolet radiation and systemic lupus erythematosus. Lupus 2014;23(6):588–95.
52. Al-Mayouf SM, Hashad S, Khawaja K, et al. Cumulative damage in juvenile idiopathic arthritis: a multi-center study from the Pediatric Rheumatology Arab Group (PRAG). Arthritis Care Res (Hoboken) 2021;73(4):586–92.

53. Palman J, Shoop-Worrall S, Hyrich K, et al. Update on the epidemiology, risk factors and disease outcomes of Juvenile idiopathic arthritis. Best Pract Res Clin Rheumatol 2018;32(2):206–22.
54. Petty RE, Southwood TR, Manners P, et al. International league of associations for rheumatology classification of juvenile idiopathic arthritis: second revision, Edmonton, 2001. The J Rheumatol 2004;31(2):390–2.
55. Aoust L, Rossi-Semerano L, Koné-Paut I, et al. Time to diagnosis in juvenile idiopathic arthritis: a french perspective. Orphanet J rare Dis 2017;12(1):1–5.
56. Tanya M, Teh KL, Das L, et al. Juvenile idiopathic arthritis in Southeast Asia: the Singapore experience over two decades. Clin Rheumatol 2020;39(11):3455–64.
57. Manners PJ, Bower C. Worldwide prevalence of juvenile arthritis why does it vary so much? The J Rheumatol 2002;29(7):1520–30.
58. Abdwani R, Abdalla E, Al Abrawi S, et al. Epidemiology of juvenile idiopathic arthritis in Oman. Pediatr Rheumatol 2015;13(1):1–6.
59. Consolaro A, Giancane G, Alongi A, et al. Phenotypic variability and disparities in treatment and outcomes of childhood arthritis throughout the world: an observational cohort study. Lancet Child Adolesc Health 2019;3(4):255–63.
60. Rocha FAC, Landim J, Aguiar MG, et al. Evaluation of disease activity in a low-income juvenile idiopathic arthritis cohort. Rheumatol Int 2019;39(1):67–71.
61. Vilaiyuk S, Soponkanaporn S, Jaovisidha S, et al. A retrospective study on 158 Thai patients with juvenile idiopathic arthritis followed in a single center over a 15-year period. Int J Rheum Dis 2016;19(12):1342–50.
62. Srivastava R, Phatak S, Yadav A, et al. HLA B27 typing in 511 children with juvenile idiopathic arthritis from India. Rheumatol Int 2016;36(10):1407–11.
63. Weakley K, Esser M, Scott C. Juvenile idiopathic arthritis in two tertiary centres in the Western Cape, South Africa. Pediatr Rheumatol Online J 2012;10(1):35.
64. Hersh AO, Prahalad S. Immunogenetics of juvenile idiopathic arthritis: a comprehensive review. J Autoimmun 2015;64:113–24.
65. Silva-Ramirez B, Cerda-Flores R, Rubio-Pérez N, et al. Association of HLA DRB1 alleles with juvenile idiopathic arthritis in Mexicans. Clin Exp Rheumatol 2010; 28(1):0124–7.
66. Ombrello MJ, Arthur VL, Remmers EF, et al. Genetic architecture distinguishes systemic juvenile idiopathic arthritis from other forms of juvenile idiopathic arthritis: clinical and therapeutic implications. Ann Rheum Dis 2017;76(5): 906–13.
67. Shah R, Dey D, Pietzonka T, et al. Determinants of Use of Biotherapeutics in sub-Saharan Africa. Trends Pharmacol Sci 2021;42(2):75–84.
68. Ardoin SP, Schanberg LE. Paediatric rheumatic disease: lessons from SLE: children are not little adults. Nat Rev Rheumatol 2012;8(8):444–5.
69. Jiménez S, Cervera R, Font J, et al. The epidemiology of systemic lupus erythematosus. Clin Rev Allergy Immunol 2003;25(1):3–11.
70. Mina R, Brunner HI. Pediatric lupus–are there differences in presentation, genetics, response to therapy, and damage accrual compared with adult lupus? Rheum Dis Clin North Am 2010;36(1):53–80, vii-viii.
71. Chen Y-M, Lin C-H, Chen H-H, et al. Onset age affects mortality and renal outcome of female systemic lupus erythematosus patients: a nationwide population-based study in Taiwan. Rheumatology 2014;53(1):180–5.
72. Silva CA, Avcin T, Brunner HI. Taxonomy for systemic lupus erythematosus with onset before adulthood. Arthritis Care Res 2012;64(12):1787–93.
73. Pineles D, Valente A, Warren B, et al. Worldwide incidence and prevalence of pediatric onset systemic lupus erythematosus. Lupus 2011;20(11):1187–92.

74. Hiraki LT, Feldman CH, Liu J, et al. Prevalence, incidence, and demographics of systemic lupus erythematosus and lupus nephritis from 2000 to 2004 among children in the US medicaid beneficiary population. Arthritis Rheum 2012; 64(8):2669–76.
75. Furia FF, Godfrey E, Mwamanenge N, et al. Spectrum of paediatric rheumatic disorders at a tertiary hospital in Tanzania. Pediatr Rheumatol Online J 2020; 18(1):30.
76. Dave M, Rankin J, Pearce M, et al. Global prevalence estimates of three chronic musculoskeletal conditions: club foot, juvenile idiopathic arthritis and juvenile systemic lupus erythematosus. Pediatr Rheumatol 2020;18(1):49.
77. Srivastava P, Abujam B, Misra R, et al. Childhood lupus nephritis in India: Single centre experience over 25 years. Int J Rheum Dis 2015;18:27.
78. Tektonidou MG, Lewandowski LB, Hu J, et al. Survival in adults and children with systemic lupus erythematosus: a systematic review and Bayesian meta-analysis of studies from 1950 to 2016 2017;76(12):2009–16.
79. Rianthavorn P, Prurapark P. Infections in hospitalized children with newly diagnosed systemic lupus erythematosus in underresourced areas. Lupus 2020; 29(11):1475–82.
80. Baca V, Velázquez-Cruz R, Salas-Martínez G, et al. Association analysis of the PTPN22 gene in childhood-onset systemic lupus erythematosus in Mexican population. Genes Immun 2006;7(8):693–5.
81. Webber D, Cao J, Dominguez D, et al. Association of systemic lupus erythematosus (SLE) genetic susceptibility loci with lupus nephritis in childhood-onset and adult-onset SLE. Rheumatology (Oxford) 2020;59(1):90–8.
82. Oddis CV, Conte CG, Steen VD, et al. Incidence of polymyositis-dermatomyositis: a 20-year study of hospital diagnosed cases in Allegheny County, PA 1963-1982. The J Rheumatol 1990;17(10):1329–34.
83. Faller G, Mistry BJ, Tikly M. Juvenile dermatomyositis in South African children is characterised by frequent dystropic calcification: a cross sectional study. Pediatr Rheumatol Online J 2014;12:2.
84. Sato JO, Sallum AM, Ferriani VP, et al. A Brazilian registry of juvenile dermatomyositis: onset features and classification of 189 cases. Clin Exp Rheumatol 2009;27(6):1031–8.
85. Prasad S, Misra R, Agarwal V, et al. Juvenile dermatomyositis at a tertiary care hospital: is there any change in the last decade? Int J Rheum Dis 2013;16(5): 556–60.
86. Olaosebikan BH, Adelowo OO, Animashaun BA, et al. Spectrum of paediatric rheumatic diseases in Nigeria. Pediatr Rheumatol Online J 2017;15(1):7.
87. Okong'o LO, Esser M, Wilmshurst J, et al. Characteristics and outcome of children with juvenile dermatomyositis in Cape Town: a cross-sectional study. Pediatr Rheumatol Online J 2016;14(1):60.
88. Chickermane PR, Mankad D, Khubchandani RP. Disease patterns of juvenile dermatomyositis from Western India. Indian Pediatr 2013;50(10):961–3.
89. Saini I, Kalaivani M, Kabra SK. Calcinosis in juvenile dermatomyositis: frequency, risk factors and outcome. Rheumatol Int 2016;36(7):961–5.
90. Sharma A, Gupta A, Rawat A, et al. Long-term outcome in children with juvenile dermatomyositis: A single-center study from north India. Int J Rheum Dis 2020; 23(3):392–6.
91. Malek A, Raeeskarami SR, Ziaee V, et al. Clinical course and outcomes of Iranian children with juvenile dermatomyositis and polymyositis. Clin Rheumatol 2014;33(8):1113–8.

92. Phillippi K, Hoeltzel M, Byun Robinson A, et al. Race, income, and disease outcomes in juvenile dermatomyositis. J Pediatr 2017;184:38–44.e31.
93. Hussain A, Rawat A, Jindal AK, et al. Autoantibodies in children with juvenile dermatomyositis: a single centre experience from North-West India. Rheumatol Int 2017;37(5):807–12.
94. Espada G, Maldonado Cocco JA, Fertig N, et al. Clinical and serologic characterization of an Argentine pediatric myositis cohort: identification of a novel autoantibody (anti-MJ) to a 142-kDa protein. The J Rheumatol 2009;36(11):2547–51.
95. Vidotto JP, Pereira LA, Braga AL, et al. Atmospheric pollution: influence on hospital admissions in paediatric rheumatic diseases. Lupus 2012;21(5):526–33.
96. Choudhury TA, Singh RG, Usha, et al. Clinicopathologic spectrum of crescentic glomerulonephritis: a hospital-based study. Saudi Journal Kidney Diseases Transplantation : Official Publication Saudi Cent Organ Transplant Saudi Arabia 2014;25(3):689–96.
97. Muhammed H, Gupta L, Lawrence A. Infections are leading cause of in-hospital mortality in Indian patients with inflammatory myopathy. Mechanics 2019;3:7–9.
98. Sartori Vieira C, de Rezende RPV, Mendes Klumb E, et al. Mortality profile related to the spectrum of systemic connective tissue diseases: a retrospective, population-based, case-control study. Lupus 2019;28(12):1498–500.
99. Kushner HI, Macnee RP, Burns JC. Kawasaki disease in India: increasing awareness or increased incidence? Perspect Biol Med 2009;52(1):17–29.
100. Borzutzky A, Hoyos-Bachiloglu R, Cerda J, et al. Rising hospitalization rates of Kawasaki Disease in Chile between 2001 and 2007. Rheumatol Int 2012;32(8):2491–5.
101. Singh S, Sharma A, Jiao F. Kawasaki disease: issues in diagnosis and treatment-a developing country perspective. Indian J Pediatr 2016;83(2):140–5.
102. Newburger JW, Takahashi M, Gerber MA, et al. Diagnosis, treatment, and long-term management of Kawasaki disease: a statement for health professionals from the Committee on Rheumatic Fever, Endocarditis, and Kawasaki Disease, Council on Cardiovascular Disease in the Young, American Heart Association. Pediatrics 2004;114(6):1708–33.
103. Castillo-Martínez D, Amezcua-Castillo LM, Granados J, et al. Is Takayasu arteritis the result of a Mycobacterium tuberculosis infection? The use of TNF inhibitors may be the proof-of-concept to demonstrate that this association is epiphenomenal. Clin Rheumatol 2020;39(6):2003–9.
104. Pedreira ALS, Santiago MB. Association between Takayasu arteritis and latent or active Mycobacterium tuberculosis infection: a systematic review. Clin Rheumatol 2020;39(4):1019–26.
105. Clemente G, Silva CA, Sacchetti SB, et al. Takayasu arteritis in childhood: misdiagnoses at disease onset and associated diseases. Rheumatol Int 2018;38(6):1089–94.
106. Clemente G, Hilario MO, Lederman H, et al. Takayasu arteritis in a Brazilian multicenter study: children with a longer diagnosis delay than adolescents. Clin Exp Rheumatol 2014;32(3 Suppl 82):S128–33.
107. Foster HE, Scott C, Tiderius CJ, et al. Improving musculoskeletal health for children and young people–A 'call to action'. Best Pract Res Clin Rheumatol 2020;34(5):101566.
108. Al Maini M, Al Weshahi Y, Foster HE, et al. A global perspective on the challenges and opportunities in learning about rheumatic and musculoskeletal diseases in undergraduate medical education. Clin Rheumatol 2020;39(3):627–42.

109. Chowichian M, Sonjaipanich S, Charuvanij S. Attitude toward pediatric rheumatology among residency-trained pediatricians. Pediatr Int 2021;63:1162–9. https://doi.org/10.1111/ped.14621.
110. Kolasinski SL, Bass AR, Kane-Wanger GF, et al. Subspecialty choice: Why did you become a rheumatologist? Arthritis Care Res 2007;57(8):1546–51.
111. Lewandowski LB, Schiffenbauer A, Mican JM, et al. Rheumatology capacity building: implementing a rheumatology curriculum for Liberian health-care providers in 2016. Clin Rheumatol 2020;39(3):689–96.
112. Dua AB, Kilian A, Grainger R, et al. Challenges, collaboration, and innovation in rheumatology education during the COVID-19 pandemic: leveraging new ways to teach. Clin Rheumatol 2020;1–7.
113. Bilal S, Shanmugam VK. Enhancing rheumatology education during the COVID-19 pandemic. Rheumatol Int 2021;1–6.
114. El Miedany Y, El Aroussy N, Youssef S, et al. AB1396 Teaching the millennials: using youtube for teaching rheumatology in the standard educational settings. Ann Rheum Dis 2018;77(Suppl 2):1782.
115. Cruz-Jesus F, Oliveira T, Bacao F. The global digital divide: evidence and drivers. J Glob Inf Management (Jgim) 2018;26(2):1–26.
116. Correia A-P. Healing the Digital Divide During the COVID-19 Pandemic. Q Rev Distance Educ 2020;21(1).
117. Smith N, Foster HE, Jandial S. A mixed methods evaluation of the paediatric musculoskeletal matters (PMM) online Portfolio. Pediatr Rheumatol Online J 2021;19(1):85.
118. Sandhu VK, Hojjati M, Blanco I. Healthcare disparities in rheumatology: the role of education at a global level. Clin Rheumatol 2020;39(3):659–66.
119. Faller G, Allen RC. Improving the management of paediatric rheumatic diseases globally. Best Pract Res Clin Rheumatol 2009;23(5):643–53.
120. Khan SEA, Saeed MA, Batool S, et al. A rheumatology curriculum in Pakistan for empowering family physicians and fighting disability. Clin Rheumatol 2020; 39(3):681–7.
121. Smith N, Mercer V, Firth J, et al. RightPath: a model of community-based musculoskeletal care for children. Rheumatol Adv Pract 2020;4(2):rkaa057.
122. Kessler EA, Sherman AK, Becker ML. Decreasing patient cost and travel time through pediatric rheumatology telemedicine visits. Pediatr Rheumatol 2016; 14(1):54.
123. Population ages 0-14, total. World Bank. 2019. Available at: https://data.worldbank.org/indicator/SP.POP.0014.TO. Accessed 1/20/2019.
124. PRINTO. Paediatric Rheumatology International Trials Organization (PRINTO). Available at: www.printo.it. Accessed February 15, 2021.

Ultrasonography in Pediatric Rheumatology

Patricia Vega-Fernandez, MD, MSc, RhMSUS[a], Tracy V. Ting, MD, MSc, RhMSUS[a], Laura Pratt, MD, RhMSUS[b], Christine M. Bacha, MD[c], Edward J. Oberle, MD, RhMSUS[b,*]

KEYWORDS

- Musculoskeletal ultrasonography • Pediatric rheumatology
- Juvenile idiopathic arthritis • Synovitis • Enthesitis

KEY POINTS

- Musculoskeletal ultrasonography (MSUS) can enhance the care of children with juvenile idiopathic arthritis (JIA), and there is early research to identify ways to supplement care in other pediatric rheumatic diseases.
- Pediatric MSUS may improve the detection of arthritis and determine the extent of disease even in clinically "normal" joints, help monitor inflammatory disease activity and response to therapy, and may have a potential role in assessing the risk of disease flare.
- Advances in ultrasonography allow for evaluation of various forms of inflammatory processes in children with JIA, including synovitis, tenosynovitis, and enthesitis.
- Ultrasound-guided intra-articular injections are safe, effective, and well-tolerated in the pediatric population.

INTRODUCTION

Inflammatory arthritis is a frequent finding in pediatric rheumatologic diseases (PRD), including juvenile idiopathic arthritis (JIA). Although JIA remains a clinical diagnosis, imaging can be a useful supplemental tool. Modalities including conventional radiography, ultrasonography, and MRI offer additional objective information both from diagnostic and monitoring standpoints. Owing to growing interest[1,2] and evidence,[3–6] point-of-care musculoskeletal ultrasonography (MSUS) has been increasingly used in pediatric rheumatology clinics. Key features of ultrasonography, including its portability, ease of evaluation (in even very young children), and ability to quickly assess multiple joints, have led to its adoption in clinical practice. Unlike radiography, which is limited to bony changes seen late in arthritis, and MRI, which is costly, may require

[a] Department of Pediatrics, Division of Rheumatology, University of Cincinnati, Cincinnati Children's Hospital Medical Center, 3333 Burnet Avenue MLC 4010, Cincinnati, OH 45229, USA; [b] University of Nebraska Medical Center, 985520 Nebraska Medical Center, Omaha, NE 68198-5520, USA; [c] Division of Rheumatology, Nationwide Children's Hospital, 700 Children's Drive, ED 3013, Columbus, OH 43205, USA
* Corresponding author.
E-mail address: Edward.Oberle@nationwidechildrens.org

Rheum Dis Clin N Am 48 (2022) 217–231
https://doi.org/10.1016/j.rdc.2021.09.009
rheumatic.theclinics.com

sedation, and have variable access, ultrasonography can readily provide clues to subclinical disease activity, monitor treatment response, and guide intra-articular and tendon sheath injections (**Table 1**). Furthermore, MSUS can evaluate synovitis, tenosynovitis, and enthesitis as well as late complications including bony erosions, cartilage thinning, and advanced bony ossification, a feature unique to growing children affected by untreated inflammatory arthritis.[7] An additional key advantage of MSUS is the ability to be performed at the bedside with dynamic motion, thereby offering real-time information to enhance medical decision making at the point of care. However, despite advances in MSUS, there remain key limitations. MSUS is operator dependent and requires appropriate training and machine technology. Certain joints including the spine, sacroiliac joint, and temporomandibular joint (TMJ) are difficult to assess. Furthermore, evidence-based literature regarding standard acquisition and imaging protocols remains limited despite recent advances.[8,9] This review discusses current evidence for the use of MSUS as applied to children with rheumatic disease such as JIA.

HEALTHY JOINTS

Obtaining a thorough understanding of childhood growth and secondary ossification centers is critical to avoid key mistakes in the interpretation of pediatric findings (**Fig. 1**). Established definitions for sonographic features of joints in healthy children are available for guidance (**Table 2**).[10,11] The following MSUS points must be considered when evaluating a healthy joint in children:

- Being aware that increased Doppler signal may reflect normal vascular channels in a growing child.
- Understanding the normal sonoanatomy of the pediatric knee,[12,13] ankle,[13] hip,[14] shoulder,[15] and elbow[16] joints.

Table 1
Comparison of imaging techniques used for evaluation of juvenile idiopathic arthritis

	Conventional Radiograph (X-Ray)	MSUS	MRI
Pros	• Widely available • Painless, fast, and noninvasive • Allows evaluation of erosions (late finding)	• Noninvasive technique suitable for bedside use • No ionizing radiation • Allows for dynamic examination • Time and cost-efficient • Multiregional: possible to examine several joint regions in one session • Assists in procedural guidance	• Most sensitive imaging technique to evaluate for synovial and tendon pathology • Sensitive to cartilage involvement in JIA • Detects bone marrow edema, which has been related to inflammation
Cons	• Radiation risk • Poor visualization of soft tissue and supportive structures (tendons, ligaments)	• Operator and machine dependent • Limited normative data on children • Lack of standardization in pediatric rheumatology • Limited use in TMJ and axial skeleton	• Cost • Time consuming • Sedation might be required • Limit availability • Scoring systems for JIA not available for all joints

Abbreviation: TMJ, temporomandibular joint.

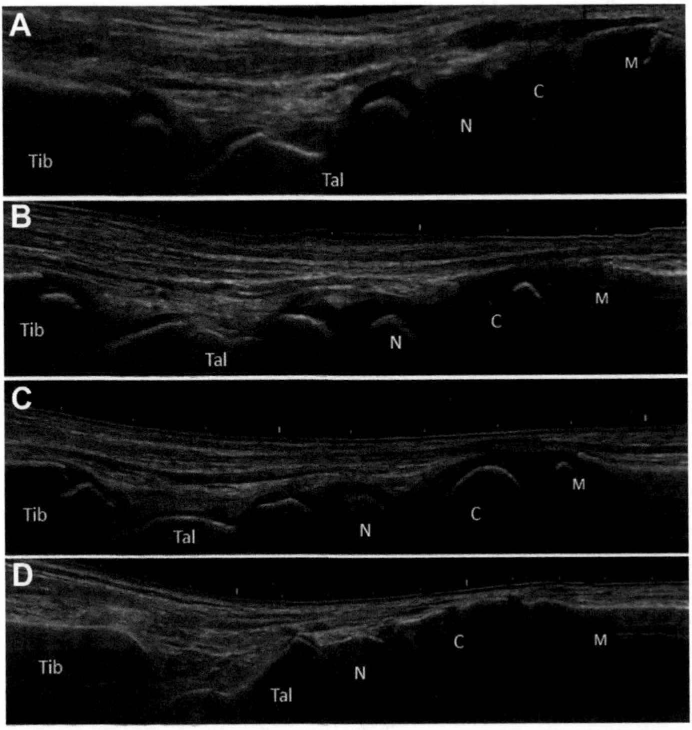

Fig. 1. Sonographic appearance of dorsal longitudinal view of healthy ankle and midfoot during various stages of development. (*A*) 2-year-old; (*B*) 5-year-old; (*C*) 8-year-old; (*D*) 16-year-old. Key: C, cuneiform; M, metatarsal bone; N, navicular; Tal, talus; Tib, tibia.

- Identifying that cartilage[17] and tendon[18] thickness may vary with age and sex.
- Being aware that small physiologic effusions can be seen among healthy children within most joints.[12,17,18]

SYNOVITIS

The clinical joint examination of some children or specific joints can be challenging either due to patient-specific details (body habitus, behavioral concerns, or cooperation) or the complexity of the anatomy being assessed (ie, ankle), respectively. The importance of accurately detecting synovitis is critical to the diagnosis and management of JIA (**Fig. 2**). Pediatric MSUS may improve the detection of arthritis and determine the extent of disease while monitoring response to therapy. Based on these understandings, international experts recommend routine use of MSUS to supplement clinical care.[19]

Despite the use of MSUS to evaluate for synovitis in JIA, earlier publications lacked consistency in defining synovitis and scanning technique to make that determination.[20] The use of descriptors for pathologic conditions found in rheumatoid arthritis (RA), among a fully ossified adult skeleton, had also been extrapolated to use in pediatric diseases without validation (see **Table 2**).[21] These shortcomings led to the need for a standardized definition of ultrasound features in joints of children with synovitis. Owing to the efforts of Pediatric Task Force of the Outcome Measures in Rheumatology (OMERACT) Ultrasound (US) work group, preliminary definitions for synovitis

Table 2
Sonographic definitions used in pediatric musculoskeletal ultrasonography

Definitions for the Normal Child Joint (Validated) (Roth et al,[10] 2015; Collado et al,[11] 2018)	
Hyaline cartilage	The hyaline cartilage will present as a well-defined anechoic structure (with/without bright echoes/dots) that is noncompressible. The cartilage surface can (but does not have to) be detected as a hyperechoic line
Secondary ossification center	With advancing maturity, the epiphyseal secondary ossification center will appear as a hyperechoic structure, with a smooth or irregular surface within the cartilage
Normal joint capsule	A hyperechoic structure that can (but does not have to) be seen over bone, cartilage, and other intra-articular tissue of the joint
Synovial membrane	Under normal circumstances, the thin synovial membrane is undetectable
Growth plate	The ossified portion of articular bone is detected as a hyperechoic line. Interruptions of this hyperechoic line may be detected at the growth plate and at the junction of 2 or more ossification centers. May be intra-articular or extra- articular according to its anatomic location
Physiologic vascularity	Detected by power Doppler within joint structures at any age during growth but is joint and age dependent • Visible within fat pads and unossified structures (physis, cartilage)
Fat pad	Can be detected as an intra-articular structure with heterogeneous echotexture and may show vascularity
Preliminary definitions for synovitis in children (Roth et al,[22] 2017)	
Synovitis	Includes assessment of B-mode and Doppler mode findings Features can be detected on basis of B-mode findings alone: • Synovial effusion • Synovial hypertrophy Cannot be detected based on Doppler findings alone Doppler signals must be detected within synovial hypertrophy to be considered a sign of synovitis
Synovial effusion	An abnormal, intra-articular, anechoic, or hypoechoic material that is displaceable
Synovial hypertrophy	An abnormal, intra-articular, hypoechoic material that is nondisplaceable
Definitions for adult pathology (not validated for children yet frequently used) (Wakefield et al,[21] 2005)	
Bone erosion	An intra-articular discontinuity of the bone surface that is visible in 2 perpendicular planes
Synovial fluid	Abnormal hypoechoic or anechoic (relative to subdermal fat, but sometimes may be isoechoic or hyperechoic) intra-articular material that is displaceable and compressible, but does not exhibit Doppler signal

(*continued on next page*)

Table 2
(*continued*)

Synovial hypertrophy	Abnormal hypoechoic (relative to subdermal fat, but sometimes may be isoechoic or hyperechoic) intra-articular tissue that is nondisplaceable and poorly compressible and that may exhibit Doppler signal
Tenosynovitis	Hypoechoic or anechoic thickened tissue with or without fluid within the tendon sheath, which is seen in 2 perpendicular planes and which may exhibit Doppler signal
Enthesopathy	Abnormally hypoechoic (loss of normal fibrillar architecture) and/or thickened tendon or ligament at its bony attachment (may occasionally contain hyperechoic foci consistent with calcification), seen in 2 perpendicular planes, that may exhibit Doppler signal and/or bony changes including enthesophytes, erosions, or irregularity

Adapted from Oberle, E. Musculoskeletal ultrasound for diagnosis and treatment in juvenile idiopathic arthritis. Curr Treat Options in Rheum. 2017;3:49–62; with permission.

in children now exist (see **Table 2**)[22] with subsequent validation in commonly affected joints.[23] A key component of these definitions is the emphasis on abnormal Doppler signal being limited to the borders of hypertrophied synovium. Normal physiologic flow that is intra-articular but extrasynovial—within surrounding connective tissue—is a frequent misinterpretation for active inflammation.

As the evidence grows for the role of MSUS there remains a need to identify joint-specific pediatric acquisition and scoring protocols as well as the ideal surveillance study. At present the only known published pediatric protocol is for the knee[9]; however, the authors of this review are actively participating in ongoing protocol developments through the Childhood Arthritis and Rheumatology Research Alliance (CARRA) Ultrasound work group on several key joints. Also, although MSUS can be performed on multiple joints at the bedside, to obtain images on all joints is impractical. Identifying a limited number of joints for evaluation is important for both screening and monitoring longitudinally. Collado and colleagues[8] identified a 10-joint protocol noting that ultrasound imaging of the knees, ankles, wrists, elbows and second metacarpophalangeal joint (MCP) joints correctly identified abnormal findings in 42 patients with polyarticular JIA.[8] Further work on the utility of a comprehensive limited MSUS study and its sensitivity to change is ongoing.[24] In regard to scoring, Vojinovic and colleagues[25] described synovitis grading system for children that

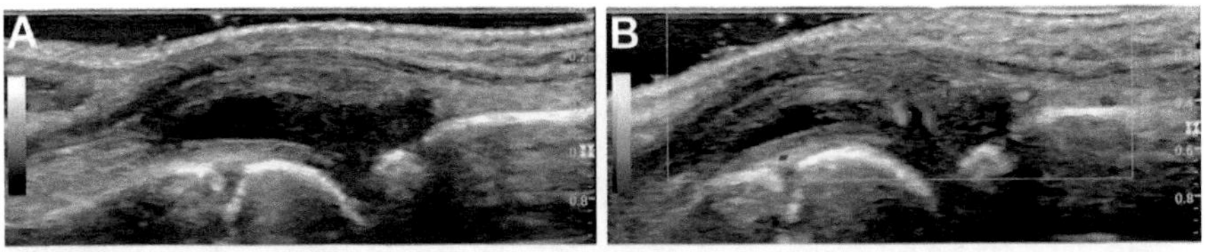

Fig. 2. Dorsal longitudinal scan of the metacarpal joint in a 7-year-old patient with JIA showing effusion and synovial hypertrophy on B-mode (*A*) and hyperemia within expanded synovium (*B*).

includes the absence or presence of Doppler signal, which was found to be reliable, although further studies must evaluate its sensitivity to change.

There is extensive evidence supporting that MSUS is more sensitive than clinical examination in the detection and location of synovitis in children with JIA.[3,6,26–30] This fact is exemplified by the largest of these cross-sectional studies that evaluated 1664 joints in 32 children with JIA.[3] Physical examination led to diagnosis of synovitis in 104 (6.3%) joints when compared with 167 (10%) diagnosed by MSUS. Significantly, 5% (86 of 1560) of clinically normal joints demonstrated ultrasound features of synovitis with the most common areas being the wrist, proximal interphalangeal, subtalar, and metatarsal joints. These joints consistently reveal undetected synovitis across most studies.[6,26,28–30] Abnormal ultrasound findings moderately correlate with swelling on examination, whereas joint tenderness or pain on motion and restricted motion are poor predictors of ultrasound abnormalities. These studies suggest clinical examination alone may incorrectly underestimate the extent of synovitis while inappropriately overdiagnosing unaffected joints.

The long-term implications of the detection of subclinical synovitis are unclear. Abnormal joints on MSUS can progress into clinically active joints.[5] Given that proper detection of joints with active inflammation is essential for both diagnosis of JIA and subtype assignment, as well as therapeutic choices, detection of subclinical synovitis on ultrasonography may impact treatment decisions.[31] However, implementation of imaging into a treat to target strategy in RA has mixed outcomes with larger clinical trials concluding that treating for ultrasound remission does not add to tight clinical care.[32–35] No such trial has been reported in children with JIA to date.

TENOSYNOVITIS

Ultrasonography provides a highly detailed view of tendons giving a clear assessment of the fibrillar structure and surrounding sheath when present. As per the adult OMERACT definition in RA, tenosynovitis may appear as "hypoechoic or anechoic thickened tissue, with or without fluid, within the tendon sheath."[21] Tenosynovitis in children generally has a similar appearance (**Fig. 3**), and the Pediatric US OMERACT work group is currently validating this observation in the pediatric population. High intraobserver concordance for tenosynovitis in wrist and MCP joints has already been demonstrated in B-mode (0.88) and power Doppler (1.0) in pediatric rheumatology.[36]

Tenosynovitis may be underappreciated on clinical examination or misinterpreted as isolated synovitis.[4] MSUS examination of 49 swollen ankles in patients with JIA clinically thought to correspond to isolated tibiotalar synovitis demonstrated sonographic evidence of tenosynovitis in 35 (71%) ankles, with 39% of ankles having tenosynovitis alone. The investigators suggest that ultrasound evaluations should be considered in all swollen ankles of patients with JIA because isolated tenosynovitis may impact

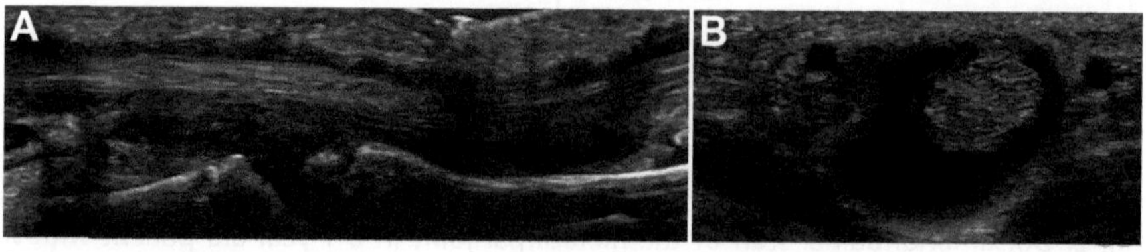

Fig. 3. Longitudinal (*A*) and transverse (*B*) scans of flexor tendon of index finger in a 6-year-old with tenosynovitis.

treatment choices or outcomes, particularly if intra-articular injections were to be performed.[4]

SUBCLINICAL DISEASE AND IMPLICATION FOR DISEASE FLARE

At present, disease remission in JIA is based on the clinical assessment of arthritis as defined by the presence of joint swelling or joint with tenderness and limited range of motion. However, the use of MSUS may allow for a more objective and real-time assessment of disease activity. The presence of subclinical synovitis defined by MSUS in children with JIA has been recognized independently of the joint examined.[3,36–38] Studies looking to investigate the clinical implications of MSUS subclinical synovitis have revealed conflicting results, which may partially be due to variability of definitions used to define abnormal MSUS findings and lack of validated scanning protocols and scoring systems in children (**Table 3**).[39–41]

In 2018, a novel study investigated the ability of MSUS to assess treatment-induced changes in synovial abnormalities in children with new-onset JIA.[42] At 6 months of follow-up, subclinical disease as assessed by MSUS was found in 18.6% of the affected joints at baseline. Standardized response mean values for B-mode of 2.44 and for PD-mode scores of 1.23 from baseline to 6 months indicated a strong sensitivity to change. A limitation of this study was that it excluded the small joints of fingers and toes, which are joints commonly involved in JIA. Also, the inclusion of any synovial abnormality on MSUS as a sign of subclinical disease could have led to an overestimation of disease burden.

Caution should be exercised when interpreting the results of mentioned studies. Given the differences of the natural history of disease among all JIA categories, it seems appropriate to use a homogeneous sample when looking to investigate the prognostic role of MSUS in JIA. Studies have included subjects with all JIA categories but systemic JIA. Furthermore, validated and reliable pediatric-specific MSUS scanning protocols and scoring systems are required for further research in pediatric

Table 3
Summary of study findings on risk of flare in clinically inactive patients

	Study Procedures	Outcome
Magni-Manzoni et al,[39] 2013	• 39 JIA with CID for at >3 months • 52 joints US at enrollment • Follow-up until JIA flare or for at least 2 y of CID	US abnormalities at enrollment did not predict flare of synovitis
De Lucia et al,[40] 2018	• 88 JIA with CID for >3 mo • 44 joints US at enrollment • Follow-up for 4 y	Abnormal US increased risk of flare (OR = 3.8, 95% CI 1.2–11.5)
Nieto-Gonzalez et al,[41] 2019	• 56 JIA with CID undergoing TNFi tapering • 22 joint, 8 tendon US at enrollment and 6 mo • Follow-up for 1 y	Abnormal US did not predict flares when TNFi tapering was applied

Abbreviations: CI, confidence interval; CID, clinical inactive disease; OR, odds ratio; TNFi, tumor necrosis factor inhibitors; US, ultrasonography.

rheumatology MSUS, such as the recently published knee scanning protocol with scoring system proposed by the CARRA Ultrasound work group.[9] In summary, the significance of subclinical synovitis at the time of clinical remission still needs to be defined.

ENTHESITIS

Enthesitis is inflammation at the insertion of a tendon, ligament, joint capsule, or fascia onto the bone and is clinically defined by tenderness at these sites. Accurate diagnosis in patients with new inflammatory arthritis ensures proper classification of the disease, which aids treatment and prognosis. Findings of enthesitis on ultrasonography can include loss of the normal fibrillar echotexture and thickening of the tendon[43] (**Fig. 4**). To date there are no standard, validated definitions of the components of enthesitis or a reliable scoring system for Doppler activity with enthesitis in pediatric rheumatology.

Doppler signals within the insertion site close to the bone are considered specific for enthesitis, yet children's entheses may show physiologic vascularization, which confounds interpretation of sonographic enthesitis.[44] Identification of other sonographic findings of enthesitis such as enthesophytes, erosions, and calcifications may support the presence or absence of entheseal inflammation. The evaluation of these abnormalities in children can be difficult due to age-related variation of the bone-cartilage surface.[45] Normative data are in varying stages of development.[18] Despite the lack of agreed-upon definitions, several studies have reported on the sensitivity of MSUS to detect enthesitis in pediatric patients with JIA (**Table 4**).[46–48] Overall, the literature regarding enthesitis evaluated with MSUS in pediatric patients remains limited, and further investigation is needed to define normal and pathologic changes to the entheses at different stages of development.

PROCEDURAL GUIDANCE

One of the more common reasons for pediatric rheumatologists to perform ultrasonography is procedural guidance for intra-articular injections[49] (**Fig. 5**). MSUS is used to target complex anatomic spaces that may not be amenable to blind injections and to direct injections to the precise areas of pathology. Previous publications have highlighted the value of ultrasound-guided injections, particularly in the wrist and ankle, with follow-up to confirm improvement or resolution of disease activity.[50–52] In 2 reports by Laurell and colleagues,[50,51] more than half of patients with JIA and clinically active arthritis of the wrist or ankle had multiple compartments involved by MSUS assessment. Following ultrasound-guided steroid injections, 80% of wrists

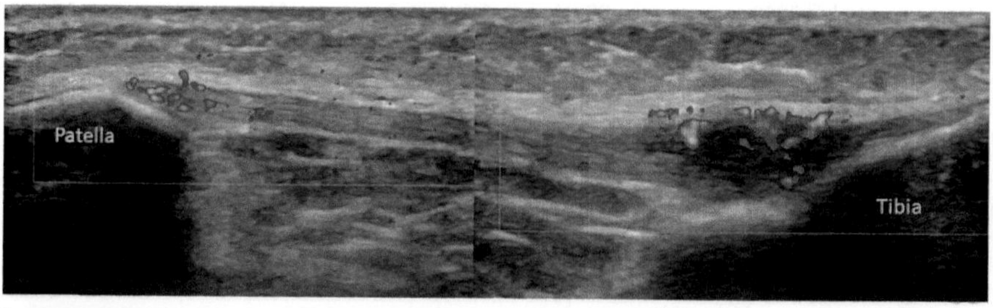

Fig. 4. Longitudinal scan of patellar ligament demonstrating enthesitis of both insertions in an adolescent with psoriatic arthritis.

Table 4
Summary of study findings on musculoskeletal ultrasonography sensitivity for enthesitis detection

Study	Remarkable Findings
Jousse-Joulin et al,[46] 2011	• Found that 50% of sites with sonographic evidence of enthesitis were clinically missed on physical examination
Weiss et al,[47] 2014	• Demonstrated the sensitivity of MSUS to detect subclinical enthesitis in pediatric patients with JIA • Abnormal findings on MSUS were most detected at the insertion of the quadriceps (30%), common extensor (12%), and Achilles (10%) tendons
Shenoy & Aggarwal,[48] 2016	• Compared the accuracy of MSUS and clinical examination in JIA-enthesitis related arthritis • More entheseal sites were found abnormal by MSUS than by clinical examination • Concordance rate between MSUS and clinical examination was 89.4% with discordance at the tibial tuberosity, superior patellar pole, and Achilles entheseal sites

and 72% of ankles had resolution of active arthritis on follow-up. Appropriate safety and tolerability of ultrasound-guided injections is reported with an age-weight-joint-based protocol,[53] including smaller joints like the midfoot and tendon sheaths.[54] Ultrasound-guided injection of the TMJ has also been reported as safe and effective,[55,56] even though MSUS is not currently the preferred imaging modality for diagnosis of TMJ disease.[57,58]

Ultrasonography Beyond Juvenile Idiopathic Arthritis

Although most of the literature on MSUS use by pediatric rheumatologists has focused on JIA, a few studies suggest potential additional uses for other PRD. In inflammatory myositis, changes in muscle echogenicity have been suggested to correlate with active disease by strength assessment.[59] Habers and colleagues[59] assessed muscle echogenicity by MSUS at disease diagnosis or flare and repeated assessments for 12 months. Echogenicity initially increased after starting treatment, suggesting muscle edema, but decreased and normalized within 6 to 12 months. Childhood Myositis Assessment Scale (CMAS) improved in this period, but it improved more quickly than MSUS findings. The investigators suggest that change in echogenicity may be an indicator of occult muscle disease because it improves more slowly than CMAS.

In localized scleroderma, changes in echogenicity and vascularity in the dermis, hypodermis, and deep tissues have all been shown with ultrasonography.[60]

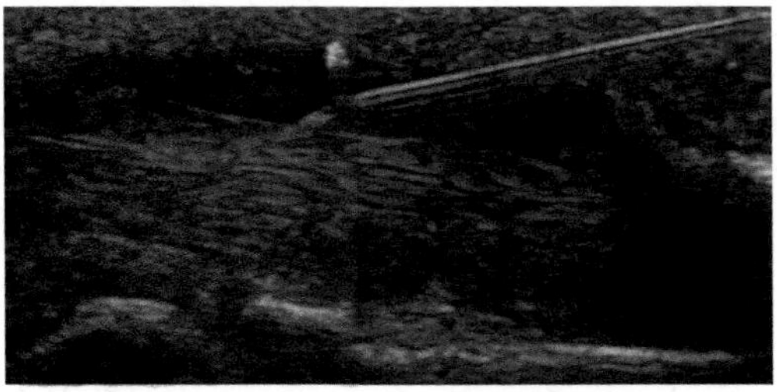

Fig. 5. Direct, in-plane ultrasound-guided injection of tendon sheath.

Echogenicity in active lesions can range from hypoechoic to hyperechoic findings when compared with inactive lesions or the contralateral side. Similarly, active lesions can show increased or decreased vascularity on Doppler assessment. Initial efforts to standardize ultrasound imaging acquisition and interpretation in localized scleroderma are reported by Li and colleagues.[60] Further study is needed to characterize potential MSUS findings in this patient population.

In juvenile Sjögren syndrome, Hammenfors and colleagues[61] report that pathologic changes on major salivary gland ultrasound correlate with clinical symptoms such as hyposalivation and clinical salivary gland enlargement and additional diagnostic findings such as autoantibody status. Reported changes on ultrasound imaging included increased salivary gland heterogeneity compared with a normal homogeneous-appearing gland and increased number of hypoechoic changes in the glands. Additional work is needed in these areas to confirm appropriate use and establish guidelines for MSUS as a diagnostic tool in Sjögren syndrome.

EDUCATION AND RESEARCH

Although pediatric rheumatology fellowship programs have been moving toward adopting routine MSUS education for all trainees, many pediatric centers continue to be without certified ultrasonographers. Given the reliance of MSUS on operator skillsets, it is critical that those performing and evaluating ultrasound studies have a sound level of training. Thus, to fill the void, multiple organizations worldwide have varying programs for teaching general MSUS, with a few geared toward pediatrics. In North America, these include a more rigorous program offered through the Ultrasound School of North American Rheumatologists (USSONAR) and 1- to 3-day courses offered through the American College of Rheumatology (ACR), CARRA, and the Canadian Rheumatology Ultrasound Society (CRUS), as well as through other regional educational centers. Basic pediatric-focused ultrasonographic training is limited and has been offered through USSONAR, CARRA, and ACR; however, despite growing interest, these programs fill quickly and advanced programming in pediatrics is lacking. Internationally, several organizations including the European League Against Rheumatism (EULAR), the PanAmerican League of Associations for Rheumatology (PANLAR), and the Asia Pacific League of Associations for Rheumatology (APLAR) also offer training. Self-directed educational Web sites are also available, including a pediatric-focused site.[62] The ACR offers certification for MSUS training indicating a high level of preparedness and skill; however, pediatric-specific MSUS training certification does not exist. When available, it should require additional knowledge of healthy joint sonoanatomy. Therefore, a growing need for additional pediatric focused MSUS training exists.

MSUS may be crucial to future research in JIA and other pediatric rheumatic diseases. The ability to assess subclinical synovitis would offer important supplemental information for both diagnosis and treatment efficacy. However, research in MSUS that goes beyond generation of definitions and validations of sensitivity to detect pathologic findings is critically needed. Work to develop MSUS scanning and scoring protocols in children is ongoing. Once established, further validation will be needed with current gold standards (ie, MRI). At present there remain a small number of ACR MSUS-certified pediatric rheumatologists who can devote time for this important research.

SUMMARY

The advantages of incorporating musculoskeletal ultrasonography into the care of pediatric patients with rheumatic diseases, particularly JIA, has become more evident over the last few years. Given its ability to identify subclinical disease, localize inflammatory processes to specific structures, and monitor response to therapy, use of MSUS has the potential to positively influence patient outcomes. However, with evaluation of pediatric musculoskeletal features still being a newer application of this technology, further work is needed to understand the long-term implications and potential impact of identifying subclinical disease and treating to a target of ultrasound remission rather than clinical remission. Until then, the importance of wider availability of pediatric-specific MSUS education and the need for adherence to validated sonographic definitions and protocols cannot be overstated.

CLINICS CARE POINTS

- Musculoskeletal ultrasonography is more sensitive than the clinical examination in identifying inflammatory processes within the joints of children and helps localize inflammation to the synovium, tendon, and/or enthesis.
- The presence of subclinical synovitis as determined by ultrasonography has been recognized in JIA. However, the significance of this finding in the treatment and prognosis of children with JIA needs to be further clarified.
- Ultrasound-guided intra-articular injections are safe, effective, and well-tolerated in the pediatric population.
- Additional uses of MSUS in pediatric rheumatology have been suggested in inflammatory myositis, localized scleroderma, and juvenile Sjögren syndrome, but further study is needed to better characterize abnormal findings and standardize imaging protocols and reporting in these diseases.

DISCLOSURE

E.J. Oberle and P. Vega-Fernandez are mentors for USSONAR. The other authors have nothing to disclose.

REFERENCES

1. Magni-Manzoni S. Ultrasound in juvenile idiopathic arthritis. Pediatr Rheumatol Online J 2016;14(1):33.
2. Lanni S, De Lucia O, Possemato N, et al. Musculoskeletal ultrasound in paediatric rheumatology: the Italian perspective. Clin Exp Rheumatol 2016;34(5):957–8.
3. Magni-Manzoni S, Epis O, Ravelli A, et al. Comparison of clinical versus ultrasound-determined synovitis in juvenile idiopathic arthritis. Arthritis Rheum 2009;61(11):1497–504.
4. Rooney ME, McAllister C, Burns JF. Ankle disease in juvenile idiopathic arthritis: ultrasound findings in clinically swollen ankles. J Rheumatol 2009;36(8):1725–9.
5. Janow GL, Panghaal V, Trinh A, et al. Detection of active disease in juvenile idiopathic arthritis: sensitivity and specificity of the physical examination vs ultrasound. J Rheumatol 2011;38(12):2671–4.
6. Pascoli L, Wright S, McAllister C, et al. Prospective evaluation of clinical and ultrasound findings in ankle disease in juvenile idiopathic arthritis: importance of ankle ultrasound. J Rheumatol 2010;37(11):2409–14.
7. Windschall D, Collado P, Vojinovic J, et al. Age-Related Vascularization and Ossification of Joints in Children: An International Pilot Study to Test Multiobserver Ultrasound Reliability. Arthritis Care Res (Hoboken) 2020;72(4):498–506.

8. Collado P, Naredo E, Calvo C, et al. Reduced joint assessment vs comprehensive assessment for ultrasound detection of synovitis in juvenile idiopathic arthritis. Rheumatology (Oxford) 2013;52(8):1477–84.
9. Ting TV, Vega-Fernandez P, Oberle EJ, et al. Novel Ultrasound Image Acquisition Protocol and Scoring System for the Pediatric Knee. Arthritis Care Res (Hoboken) 2019;71(7):977–85.
10. Roth J, Jousse-Joulin S, Magni-Manzoni S, et al. Definitions for the sonographic features of joints in healthy children. Arthritis Care Res (Hoboken) 2015;67(1):136–42.
11. Collado P, Windschall D, Vojinovic J, et al. Amendment of the OMERACT ultrasound definitions of joints' features in healthy children when using the DOPPLER technique. Pediatr Rheumatol Online J 2018;16(1):23.
12. Windschall D, Trauzeddel R, Haller M, et al. Pediatric musculoskeletal ultrasound: age- and sex-related normal B-mode findings of the knee. Rheumatol Int 2016;36(11):1569–77.
13. Keshava SN, Gibikote SV, Mohanta A, et al. Ultrasound and magnetic resonance imaging of healthy paediatric ankles and knees: a baseline for comparison with haemophilic joints. Haemophilia 2015;21(3):e210–22.
14. Trauzeddel RF, Lehmann H, Windschall D, et al. Age-dependent arthrosonographic reference values of the hip joint in healthy children and adolescents - a cross-sectional multicenter ultrasound study. Pediatr Radiol 2017;47(10):1329–36.
15. Trauzeddel R, Windschall D, Trauzeddel RF, et al. Arthrosonographic reference values of the shoulder joint in healthy children and adolescents: a cross-sectional multicentre ultrasound study. Klin Padiatr 2017;229(5):293–301.
16. Trauzeddel R, Lehman H, Trauzeddel RF, et al. Age dependent ultrasound B-mode findings of the elbow joint in healthy children and adolescents. Rheumatol Int 2019;39(6):1007–18.
17. Collado P, Vojinovic J, Nieto JC, et al. Toward Standardized Musculoskeletal Ultrasound in Pediatric Rheumatology: Normal Age-Related Ultrasound Findings. Arthritis Care Res (Hoboken) 2016;68(3):348–56.
18. Chauvin NA, Ho-Fung V, Jaramillo D, et al. Ultrasound of the joints and entheses in healthy children. Pediatr Radiol 2015;45(9):1344–54.
19. Colebatch-Bourn AN, Edwards CJ, Collado P, et al. EULAR-PReS points to consider for the use of imaging in the diagnosis and management of juvenile idiopathic arthritis in clinical practice. Ann Rheum Dis 2015;74(11):1946–57.
20. Collado P, Jousse-Joulin S, Alcalde M, et al. Is ultrasound a validated imaging tool for the diagnosis and management of synovitis in juvenile idiopathic arthritis? A systematic literature review. Arthritis Care Res (Hoboken) 2012;64(7):1011–9.
21. Wakefield RJ, Balint PV, Szkudlarek M, et al. Musculoskeletal ultrasound including definitions for ultrasonographic pathology. J Rheumatol 2005;32(12):2485–7.
22. Roth J, Ravagnani V, Backhaus M, et al. Preliminary Definitions for the Sonographic Features of Synovitis in Children. Arthritis Care Res (Hoboken) 2017;69(8):1217–23.
23. Rossi-Semerano L, Breton S, Semerano L, et al. Application of the OMERACT synovitis ultrasound scoring system in juvenile idiopathic arthritis: a multicenter reliability exercise. Rheumatology (Oxford) 2021;60(8):3579–635.
24. Vega-Fernandez P, Ting TV, Oberle EJ, et al. The MUSICAL pediatric ultrasound examination - a comprehensive, reliable, time efficient assessment of synovitis. Arthritis Care Res (Hoboken) 2021. https://doi.org/10.1002/acr.24759.

25. Vojinovic J, Magni-Manzoni S, Collado P, et al. SAT0636 Ultrasonography definitions for synovitis grading in children: the omeract pediatric ultrasound task force. Ann Rheum Dis 2017;76(Suppl 2):1015.
26. Breton S, Jousse-Joulin S, Cangemi C, et al. Comparison of clinical and ultrasonographic evaluations for peripheral synovitis in juvenile idiopathic arthritis. Semin Arthritis Rheum 2011;41(2):272–8.
27. Hendry GJ, Gardner-Medwin J, Steultjens MP, et al. Frequent discordance between clinical and musculoskeletal ultrasound examinations of foot disease in juvenile idiopathic arthritis. Arthritis Care Res (Hoboken) 2012;64(3):441–7.
28. Haslam KE, McCann LJ, Wyatt S, et al. The detection of subclinical synovitis by ultrasound in oligoarticular juvenile idiopathic arthritis: a pilot study. Rheumatology (Oxford) 2010;49(1):123–7.
29. Karmazyn B, Bowyer SL, Schmidt KM, et al. US findings of metacarpophalangeal joints in children with idiopathic juvenile arthritis. Pediatr Radiol 2007;37(5):475–82.
30. Lanni S, Bovis F, Ravelli A, et al. Delineating the application of ultrasound in detecting synovial abnormalities of the subtalar joint in juvenile idiopathic arthritis. Arthritis Care Res (Hoboken) 2016;68(9):1346–53.
31. Nieto-Gonzalez JC, Monteagudo I, Vargas-Henny L, et al. Impact of musculoskeletal ultrasound on clinical practice in paediatric rheumatology. Clin Exp Rheumatol 2015;33(4):583–7.
32. Dale J, Stirling A, Zhang R, et al. Targeting ultrasound remission in early rheumatoid arthritis: the results of the TaSER study, a randomised clinical trial. Ann Rheum Dis 2016;75(6):1043–50.
33. Haavardsholm EA, Aga AB, Olsen IC, et al. Ultrasound in management of rheumatoid arthritis: ARCTIC randomised controlled strategy trial. BMJ 2016;354:i4205.
34. Paulshus Sundlisaeter N, Aga AB, Olsen IC, et al. Clinical and ultrasound remission after 6 months of treat-to-target therapy in early rheumatoid arthritis: associations to future good radiographic and physical outcomes. Ann Rheum Dis 2018;77(10):1421–5.
35. Sundin U, Aga AB, Skare O, et al. Conventional versus ultrasound treat to target: no difference in magnetic resonance imaging inflammation or joint damage over 2 years in early rheumatoid arthritis. Rheumatology (Oxford) 2020;59(9):2550–5.
36. Ventura-Rios L, Faugier E, Barzola L, et al. Reliability of ultrasonography to detect inflammatory lesions and structural damage in juvenile idiopathic arthritis. Pediatr Rheumatol Online J 2018;16(1):58.
37. Rebollo-Polo M, Koujok K, Weisser C, et al. Ultrasound findings on patients with juvenile idiopathic arthritis in clinical remission. Arthritis Care Res (Hoboken) 2011;63(7):1013–9.
38. Lanni S, Marafon DP, Civino A, et al. Comparison between clinical and ultrasound assessment of the ankle region in juvenile idiopathic arthritis. Arthritis Care Res (Hoboken) 2021;73(8):1180–6.
39. Magni-Manzoni S, Scire CA, Ravelli A, et al. Ultrasound-detected synovial abnormalities are frequent in clinically inactive juvenile idiopathic arthritis, but do not predict a flare of synovitis. Ann Rheum Dis 2013;72(2):223–8.
40. De Lucia O, Ravagnani V, Pregnolato F, et al. Baseline ultrasound examination as possible predictor of relapse in patients affected by juvenile idiopathic arthritis (JIA). Ann Rheum Dis 2018;77(10):1426–31.
41. Nieto-Gonzalez JC, Rodriguez A, Gamir-Gamir ML, et al. Can ultrasound-detected subclinical synovitis be an indicator of flare recurrence in juvenile

idiopathic arthritis remission patients on tapered TNFi? Clin Exp Rheumatol 2019; 37(4):705–12.
42. Lanni S, van Dijkhuizen EHP, Vanoni F, et al. Ultrasound changes in synovial abnormalities induced by treatment in juvenile idiopathic arthritis. Clin Exp Rheumatol 2018;36(2):329–34.
43. Weiss PF, Chauvin NA, Roth J. Imaging in Juvenile Spondyloarthritis. Curr Rheumatol Rep 2016;18(12):75.
44. Roth J, Stinson SE, Chan J, et al. Differential pattern of Doppler signals at lower-extremity entheses of healthy children. Pediatr Radiol 2019;49(10):1335–43.
45. Windschall D, Malattia C. Ultrasound imaging in paediatric rheumatology. Best Pract Res Clin Rheumatol 2020;34(6):101570.
46. Jousse-Joulin S, Breton S, Cangemi C, et al. Ultrasonography for detecting enthesitis in juvenile idiopathic arthritis. Arthritis Care Res (Hoboken) 2011;63(6): 849–55.
47. Weiss PF, Chauvin NA, Klink AJ, et al. Detection of enthesitis in children with enthesitis-related arthritis: dolorimetry compared to ultrasonography. Arthritis Rheumatol 2014;66(1):218–27.
48. Shenoy S, Aggarwal A. Sonologic enthesitis in children with enthesitis-related arthritis. Clin Exp Rheumatol 2016;34(1):143–7.
49. Magni-Manzoni S, Collado P, Jousse-Joulin S, et al. Current state of musculoskeletal ultrasound in paediatric rheumatology: results of an international survey. Rheumatology (Oxford) 2014;53(3):491–6.
50. Laurell L, Court-Payen M, Nielsen S, et al. Ultrasonography and color Doppler in juvenile idiopathic arthritis: diagnosis and follow-up of ultrasound-guided steroid injection in the ankle region. A descriptive interventional study. Pediatr Rheumatol Online J 2011;9(1):4.
51. Laurell L, Court-Payen M, Nielsen S, et al. Ultrasonography and color Doppler in juvenile idiopathic arthritis: diagnosis and follow-up of ultrasound-guided steroid injection in the wrist region. A descriptive interventional study. Pediatr Rheumatol Online J 2012;10:11.
52. Young CM, Horst DM, Murakami JW, et al. Ultrasound-guided corticosteroid injection of the subtalar joint for treatment of juvenile idiopathic arthritis. Pediatr Radiol 2015;45(8):1212–7.
53. Young CM, Shiels WE 2nd, Coley BD, et al. Ultrasound-guided corticosteroid injection therapy for juvenile idiopathic arthritis: 12-year care experience. Pediatr Radiol 2012;42(12):1481–9.
54. Peters SE, Laxer RM, Connolly BL, et al. Ultrasound-guided steroid tendon sheath injections in juvenile idiopathic arthritis: a 10-year single-center retrospective study. Pediatr Rheumatol Online J 2017;15(1):22.
55. Parra DA, Chan M, Krishnamurthy G, et al. Use and accuracy of US guidance for image-guided injections of the temporomandibular joints in children with arthritis. Pediatr Radiol 2010;40(9):1498–504.
56. Habibi S, Ellis J, Strike H, et al. Safety and efficacy of US-guided CS injection into temporomandibular joints in children with active JIA. Rheumatology (Oxford) 2012;51(5):874–7.
57. Weiss PF, Arabshahi B, Johnson A, et al. High prevalence of temporomandibular joint arthritis at disease onset in children with juvenile idiopathic arthritis, as detected by magnetic resonance imaging but not by ultrasound. Arthritis Rheum 2008;58(4):1189–96.

58. Zwir LF, Terreri MT, do Amaral ECA, et al. Is power Doppler ultrasound useful to evaluate temporomandibular joint inflammatory activity in juvenile idiopathic arthritis? Clin Rheumatol 2020;39(4):1237–40.
59. Habers GE, Van Brussel M, Bhansing KJ, et al. Quantitative muscle ultrasonography in the follow-up of juvenile dermatomyositis. Muscle Nerve 2015;52(4): 540–6.
60. Li SC, Liebling MS, Ramji FG, et al. Sonographic evaluation of pediatric localized scleroderma: preliminary disease assessment measures. Pediatr Rheumatol Online J 2010;8:14.
61. Hammenfors DS, Valim V, Bica B, et al. Juvenile Sjögren's Syndrome: Clinical Characteristics With Focus on Salivary Gland Ultrasonography. Arthritis Care Res 2020;72(1):78–87.
62. Roth J, Windschall D, Malattia C, et al. Ped-MUS. In: Ped-MUS Steering Committee. 2020. Available at: https://www.ped-mus.com/. Accessed October 18, 2020.

The Promises and Perils of Social Media for Pediatric Rheumatology

Jonathan S. Hausmann, MD[a,b,*], Elissa R. Weitzman, ScD, MSc[c,d,e]

KEYWORDS

• Social media • Pediatric rheumatology • Self-help groups • Digital technology
• Patient support organizations • Research

KEY POINTS

- Social media has revolutionized and empowered communities of people living with rare diseases, including children with pediatric rheumatic diseases, and given a voice to groups that would have otherwise lacked the opportunity to meet and exchange information and support.
- Online platforms have become important alternative and complementary layers of the health information and psychosocial support ecosystem for patients with chronic illnesses and caregivers.
- Social media have been a research asset: successfully tracking epidemics, enrolling large numbers of patients with rare diseases into research studies, and providing insights into patient perceptions about diseases and their medications.
- Multiple challenges exist: privacy and confidentiality issues, generating knowledge from large amounts of online data, integrating social media into the electronic health records, and harnessing social media to improve patient outcomes.

Conflict of Interest: J.S. Hausmann: salary support from the Childhood Arthritis and Rheumatology Research Alliance (CARRA), consulting for Novartis, Pfizer, Biogen, all unrelated to this work. E.R. Weitzman: none.
Funding: J. S. Hausmann receives funding from the Rheumatology Research Foundation. E. R. Weitzman receives funding from the following grants: NIAMS/NIH R21 U19 AR069522-01, NIAMS/NIH AR070944-01A1, NIAMS/NIH R21AR070944-01A1.
[a] Program in Rheumatology, Division of Immunology, Boston Children's Hospital, 300 Longwood Avenue, Fegan 6, Boston, MA 02115, USA; [b] Division of Rheumatology and Clinical Immunology, Beth Israel Deaconess Medical Center, Boston, MA, USA; [c] Division of Adolescent/Young Adult Medicine, Boston Children's Hospital, Boston, MA, USA; [d] Department of Pediatrics, Harvard Medical School, Boston, MA, USA; [e] Computational Health Informatics Program, Boston Children's Hospital, Boston, MA, USA
* Corresponding author. 300 Longwood Avenue, Fegan 6, Boston, MA 02115.
E-mail address: jonathan.hausmann@childrens.harvard.edu

Rheum Dis Clin N Am 48 (2022) 233–243
https://doi.org/10.1016/j.rdc.2021.09.005 rheumatic.theclinics.com

INTRODUCTION

Social media are online platforms that allow users to interact with each other through text, images, or videos. Over the last 10 years, their use has increased dramatically by people of all ages. This popularization of social media has revolutionized and empowered communities of people living with rare diseases, giving voices to groups that would have otherwise lacked the opportunity to meet and exchange information and support.

Pediatric rheumatic diseases (PRDs) are rare diseases, which by definition affect fewer than 200,000 people in the United States. The development of social media has enabled families of children with similar PRDs to meet and support each other regardless of geographic distance. Clinicians and researchers have also leveraged social media to obtain health information from their patients and to engage with these rare disease communities for research. Although social media has many valuable aspects, using it in health care and health research is complex and requires attention to issues of privacy, confidentiality, and safety.

This article reviews the promises and perils of social media related to health, focusing on their potential use to support research and care of children with PRD. The authors rely heavily on data from the use of social media by children and families with nonpediatric rheumatic health conditions, as this field is only beginning to enter the social media arena.

SOCIAL MEDIA

Since the advent of social media in the early 2000s, the types and numbers of platforms that allow user interaction have increased exponentially. These social media platforms include those that target various audiences from professional (LinkedIn) to personal (Facebook), as well as blogging platforms where people share articles they have written (Medium) and microblogging platforms where those same messages are much shorter (Twitter). In addition to sharing text, social media platforms allow sharing of videos (YouTube), photos (Instagram), and even workouts (Strava). There are also sites where users curate and collect content found across the Internet onto a single location (Pinterest). More recently, platforms have emerged that enable posting and sharing of ephemeral posts (Snapchat) and short-form videos (TikTok). Not surprisingly, social media platforms also target users with chronic medical conditions, including those that support exchange among specific sets of health conditions (TuDiabetes) or a wide array of health concerns (PatientsLikeMe).

The use of social media has grown steadily over time. The Pew Research Center estimates that 72% of US adults use some type of social media, but this varies by age (ie, as high as 90% of those aged 18 to 29, and down to 40% of those aged 65 and older).[1] Social media usage patterns are dynamic, with continual development of new sites, platforms, and applications. Among large established platforms, YouTube is the most popular and used by 73% of all adult social media users, followed closely by Facebook, used by 69%. However, among 18- to 24-year-olds, Instagram and Snapchat are especially common, used by 75% and 73% of young adults, respectively. Young people, in particular, are “poly-platform” users–with multiple profiles and accounts.

Facebook is probably the most common social media platform used by parents of children with rare diseases. In a recent study of the 4246 rare disorders that present in childhood, researchers found 6398 active support groups, representing 826 of the most well-known and prevalent rare diseases [2]. The authors found that the number of disease groups has increased continuously over time, and many were available in multiple languages. Most (69%) of support groups were private, which allows access to the group only after approval by a group administrator. The overwhelming popularity of private over public groups, likely reflects parents' desire for a private environment in which to discuss aspects of their child's health.

PROMISES OF SOCIAL MEDIA

Use by Families of Children with Health Concerns

Before the advent of social media, families obtained information about their child's disease primarily from their health care providers.[3] As information became more accessible on the Internet, families gained direct access to medical organizations, journals, and health news Web sites. This stage is referred to as Web 1.0, where the information flowed unidirectionally from established entities to consumers. The advent of Web 2.0, when social media were born, allowed users to interact with the online material and with each other, and to develop and share their own content and perspectives.

While a clinician can provide expert guidance about a disease during the clinical visit, they may not have the time–or know-how–to provide the support and affirmation that many patients and families require. Families of children with health care problems may turn to each other and to online communities to address unmet needs for the kind of information, support, and guidance that can be derived from a shared first-hand experience. As such, online platforms have become important alternative and complementary layers of the health information and psychosocial support ecosystem. Turning to online communities, Facebook groups, and other social media platforms is especially common among parents of children with rare conditions, who may struggle to identify the nature of their child's health problem and find adequate support and guidance.[4,5] Families with children with unusual symptoms or undiagnosed diseases also use online communities for help in finding a potential diagnosis and emotional support during the stressful diagnostic odyssey.[5,6] Once a diagnosis is made, online patient support groups can provide psychosocial support and help prepare families for the future, especially regarding schooling, health insurance, and medications. Families may find that engaging with others facing similar health conditions can help them navigate the complexity of services and systems that may be useful and necessary to manage their child's health condition.

Social media engagement can provide families with informational and psychosocial support and empower them with insights that they can then carry into and enrich their interactions with their health care providers. Many online groups have professional advisory boards or groups of experts working to curate accurate content.[7] The psychosocial support they provide families of children with chronic health conditions is also invaluable. One study of mothers of children with chronic illnesses noted that online communication was essential in helping to manage the mothers' emotions regarding their child's diagnosis.[4] Online support can decrease feelings of parental isolation, improve disease-related knowledge, and enhance parents' understanding of issues not often discussed in the clinic.[8]

The knowledge and empowerment families receive from social media can enable them to make better medical decisions. Parents often verify and clarify with their health care providers what they learn about from their online networks, and these actions can improve the parent/provider relationship.[8] Studies have shown that patients and families often make treatment decisions and change their behavior based on what they learn from these online groups.[8–10]

In a recent study of parents of children with PRD contacted online through patient support organizations, almost all (98.7%) reported using Facebook to read about other families with children with similar conditions.[11] These online interactions decreased the parent's feelings of isolation and normalized the diagnosis of a PRD in their child. In addition, parents reported that these online interactions translated into changes in their management of their child's symptoms, medication side effects, and the psychosocial impact of these diseases on their children. Notably, almost half the parents surveyed reported that online discussions affected decision making about which medication(s) to use to treat their child's illness, demonstrating that online discussions have real-world impact on clinical care.

Social media enable like-minded patient and family communities to collaborate and become strong advocates to improve the care and awareness of rare diseases, increase research funding, and influence health policy decisions. These online communities have helped to obtain orphan drug designation for the treatment of rare diseases, encouraged health care insurers to provide coverage to pay for drugs, and ensured in many instances that patients can receive the drugs regardless of the families' ability to pay.[7]

Use by Adolescents and Young Adults

Although many children with PRDs may be too young to participate in social media (social media platforms generally require users to be ages 13 and above), adolescents and young adults (AYAs) with PRD have the potential to benefit significantly from online interactions. As of 2018, 95% of adolescents (ages 13–18) had access to a smartphone (and thereby to social media). Almost half (45%) stated they were online "almost constantly," and another 44% accessed the Internet "several times a day."[12]

In a study of otherwise healthy AYAs attending a primary care clinic, 98% reported using at least 1 social media platform within the prior month. Half endorsed posting information about their health on these platforms, most commonly regarding mood, wellness, and acute medical conditions.[13] Reasons for sharing health-related information included the desire to connect with others with similar conditions and seek advice and support. Notably, only a quarter of participants thought social media were a valuable source of health information, and most did not want to connect with their health care teams through social media. They preferred, instead, to communicate with their health care team through text messaging.

AYAs with chronic health conditions, on the other hand, may have more reasons to participate in online health communities than otherwise healthy groups. Through online platforms, patients may help each other obtain self-management skills, ultimately improving outcomes and reducing costs.[14] Studies of AYAs with type 1 diabetes showed improved disease management and glycemic control in those who participated in online communities that fostered peer-to-peer exchange and offered psychosocial support.[15] A meta-analysis of social media interventions showed that most were successful in improving health outcomes.[16]

In pediatric rheumatology, Scalzi and colleagues (2018) tested the benefits of engaging in a disease-centered social media forum versus using a private journal to improve self-management skills among AYAs with systemic lupus erythematosus.[17] The study provided all participants with a Web-based educational program about lupus. Those randomized to the social media forum showed improvement in medication adherence, measures of self-efficacy, a sense of agency, and community and empowerment, compared with those randomized to the private journal. The success of the social media support group cohort suggests that future interventions that create or engage online communities may be particularly valuable in improving the care of AYAs with PRD.

Use by Clinicians and Researchers

Clinicians and researchers can also leverage social media to improve patient and population health. For example, in addition to the physical examination and laboratory data obtained from patients during clinical encounters, clinicians may one day utilize a person's digital phenotype (ie, their interactions with social media) to obtain a more comprehensive view of their experience of illness.[18] Although this concept is in its nascent stages, the hope is that data from social media and fitness trackers may be used to monitor patients' health between visits and potentially detect disease flares at an earlier stage.

As an example, the frequency of use and sentiment expressed in social media may predict disease flares. In 1 study of AYAs with various inflammatory conditions, patients reported that time spent on Facebook during a disease flare or hospitalization more than doubled to 11 hours per day compared with 5 hours per day during periods of low disease activity.[19] Thus, frequent use of social media may be a proxy for disease activity in these AYAs and could be used to initiate earlier interventions.

Social media can also be used to better understand patient beliefs regarding treatments, and to evaluate real-world data regarding drug efficacy and side effects. One group sought to study patient perceptions of disease-modifying antirheumatic drugs (DMARDs) on social media. They analyzed millions of social media posts and found 54,742 that referred to DMARDs.[20] The authors showed that biologic and targeted synthetic DMARDs had an overall positive sentiment from the public, primarily because of their efficacy. In contrast, methotrexate and sulfasalazine had slightly negative sentiments because of side effects. These types of studies are helpful to highlight the concerns of the patient community, allowing health care providers to better inform patients about common drug side effects and provide preemptive education regarding the online perspectives patients may find about the drug.

Researchers have also successfully leveraged social media to enroll participants in research studies. This is especially helpful for research on rare diseases, in which large numbers of participants may be difficult to reach in the clinic setting. Successful recruitment of patients with rare diseases online has included studies in congenital heart disease[21] and hemophilia.[22] A recent study of parents of children with PRD contacted through social media and patient support organizations found that Facebook was the most-used platform for recruiting patients.[11] This enrollment method was particularly beneficial for enrolling children with especially rare PRDs compared to those with more common conditions such as juvenile rheumatoid arthritis (JIA).

More recently, the COVID-19 Global Rheumatology Alliance launched a patient experience survey to parents of children with PRD to understand better the pandemic's impact on the child's health.[23] By leveraging social media platforms and patient support organizations, more than 400 parents of children with PRD from around the world participated in the study and completed an online survey regarding their experiences during the pandemic. This study again highlights the feasibility and cost-effectiveness of leveraging online groups to conduct large-scale research studies.

Social media have also been used to broadcast public health messages. The benefits of utilizing this medium are its low cost and extensive reach. Messages can easily reach even vulnerable populations such as youth and racial and ethnic minorities, who are commonly present online. Public health messages through social media platforms can leverage social support, memes, and influencers (popular users on social media), which can improve a health campaign's reach and public engagement.[24] Research has shown the efficacy of these platforms to enhance knowledge regarding health topics such as skin cancer.[25] Also, positive behavior change has been shown to take place through social media programs.[26]

Social media platforms have also been leveraged for public health surveillance.[27] For instance, Twitter has been used to identify restaurants that may have been responsible for foodborne infections,[28] track Chikungunya outbreaks throughout Europe,[29] and to describe the spread of SARS-CoV-2 around the world.[30] Researchers recently utilized digital data streams from Twitter as early indicators of coronavirus disease 2019 (COVID-19) activity, and they were able to anticipate confirmed cases and deaths by 2 to 3 weeks.[31]

PERILS OF SOCIAL MEDIA

Privacy

Although there are many valuable aspects of health-related social media use by patients, families, clinicians, and researchers, ensuring privacy and safety is challenging for patients, families, and clinicians. Protecting pediatric populations is essential; however, privacy protections safeguarding youth are often missing or lax. Persons of color and members of other marginalized groups may also be at particular risk, as disclosure of identifying information and health problems can be stigmatizing or result in discrimination. Risks from breach of privacy or disclosure of health information may be especially acute in the United States, where eligibility for obtaining insurance, health care, employment, and housing could be jeopardized by such disclosures.

Privacy of personal health information may be of concern to adolescents and young adults, as most do not want to share their online lives with their health care teams.[13,19] Projects attempting to use a patient's digital phenotype to improve health will have to overcome such barriers.

Safety and Accuracy

Social media have also contributed to the diffusion of health-related misinformation (false information shared without the intent of causing harm) and disinformation (false information knowingly created to cause doubt, confusion, or harm). Disinformation is promoted to create fear, anxiety, and mistrust in institutions.[32] Campaigns of misinformation are particularly harmful to people who are scared and doubtful, who are more susceptible to believing them. Not surprisingly, misinformation may often be more popular online than health information that is accurate.

Inaccurate health information may drive the uptake of unproven therapies, as occurred with hydroxychloroquine during the early phase of the COVID-19 pandemic,[33] and may encourage patients to avoid effective treatments. For instance, the online misinformation regarding vaccines may have led to decreased vaccination rates in developed countries.[34] More recently, studies have shown that reading misinformation about the COVID-19 vaccine lowers a person's likelihood to receive a vaccine, which has severe implications for public health, especially in achieving herd immunity and putting a stop to the pandemic.

The accuracy of self-reported health data found on social media also has its limitations. Although patients and their families are best for reporting PROs and quality of life measures, they may struggle to recall more specific aspects regarding procedures or treatments.[21] Researchers may not be able to verify the patients' self-reported medical conditions. Nevertheless, studies have shown that self-reported data obtained from these platforms generally align with a patient's medical records[35] and the data gathered from patients usually match those obtained under clinical settings. .[13]

Also, those with poorer health or more severe illness may be more likely to post on social media sites related to health, more likely to consume health content online,[13] or post more frequently when they are ill, thus biasing health information found on social media sites.[19] Thus, it is possible that negative impressions about health may spread to others online, as emotional states can be transferred on Facebook,[36] and negative health behaviors such as smoking and obesity spread in social networks.[37,38]

Psychological Impacts for Caregivers and Clinicians

Informational needs may differ between caregivers. For example, although some people become empowered with increasing information, others may experience unpleasant feelings, sorrow, or added anxiety, especially when presented with information about disease-related complications or death of other children with similar conditions.[4] Similar effects were found in a study exploring returning research results to study participants from the Childhood Arthritis and Rheumatology Research Alliance (CARRA) Registry.[39] Authors found that this information could be affirming for some participants and allowed them to feel that their experiences in managing their child's disease were validated. However, reading the results presented an informational burden for other participants, raising more questions than answers and requiring more ability than they had to understand it.

Clinicians often view their patient's excursions into social media in a negative light. Reasons vary, and may include feeling that their expertise is being questioned, concern about misinformation patients may find online, or that they do not have enough time to discuss and evaluate this information with their patients in the clinic.[8]

Health Disparities

Social media support groups may potentially exacerbate existing health disparities experienced by racial, ethnic, and other minorities, because those who join patient support groups tend to be middle- and upper-income, educated, married, suburban whites.[40] Whether these disparities exist in online patient support communities is unknown. Compared with whites, older adults from racial and ethnic minorities are less likely to use technology such as social media related to their health,[41] which may inadvertently put them at a disadvantage in receiving informational and emotional support. Fortunately, the use of social media for younger people of racial and ethnic minorities appears to be equivalent to those of whites; they may actually even be more likely to engage in online activism.[42]

OPPORTUNITIES

Teaching critical thinking skills and health literacy to patients and families can provide them with tools to better assess the accuracy of health messages found online. Highlighting the potential negative bias of online health information may allow patients and families to put the information they read into perspective. It is also essential to tailor the amount and type of health information that patients or families may want to see online.

Simple techniques can prevent the inadvertent sharing of misinformation. Studies show that in general, people want to avoid spreading misinformation and can tell truth from fiction. However, when deciding to share content, they may focus on social validation and reinforcement, rather than the story's accuracy.[43] A simple nudge prompting people to consider the accuracy of the content before they share it decreased the rate of disseminating false information. At the same time, social media companies have also begun to more aggressively flag or remove health misinformation and provide links to reliable health content.[44,45]

Box 1
Examples of reliable online resources for children with pediatric rheumatic diseases and their families

General rheumatology web sites and support organizations

- American College of Rheumatology: rheumatology.org
- Arthritis Foundation: arthritis.org
- Childhood Arthritis and Rheumatology Research Alliance (CARRA): carragroup.org
- National Association of Rare Disorders: rarediseases.org
- RareConnect: rareconnect.org

Disease-specific Web sites and support organizations

- Autoinflammatory Alliance: autoinflammatory.org
- CRMO Foundation: crmofoundation.org
- CureJM: curejm.org
- Lupus Foundation of America: lupus.org
- Scleroderma Foundation: scleroderma.org
- Sjogren's foundation: sjogrens.org
- Spondylitis Association of America: spondylitis.org
- Systemic Autoinflammatory Disease (SAID) Support: saidsupport.org
- Systemic JIA Foundation systemicjia.org
- Vasculitis Foundation: vasculitisfoundation.org

Physicians should be educated on the value of online interactions for patients and families and to combat physician mistrust of online health information. Rather than asking patients and families not to look for health information online, clinicians should refer them to reliable sources of information and effective support groups instead (**Box 1**). Guiding patients to find accurate health information online is a new responsibility for physicians in this digital age.[46] Taking it a step further, clinicians may also become involved in curating or creating accurate health content and refuting inaccurate information encountered online.

SUMMARY

Despite all the issues and polarization that social media have created, these platforms are here to stay. Clinicians must become more familiar with social media platforms so they can guide their patients and families to find accurate health content and receive the emotional support they desire. Social media can be a blessing for families of children with rare diseases, as parents and patients are using these platforms to collaborate, advocate, and support each other. Adolescents and young adults with chronic health conditions are also meeting each other online, sharing their lives, and learning from each other, often with objective improvements in their disease management. Instead of supplementing medical care, clinicians should view these outlets as complementary to the care they provide in the clinic. Social media provide emotional support and informational resources that clinicians may not be able to provide during the clinic visit. For researchers, social media have successfully tracked epidemics, enrolled large numbers of patients with rare diseases into research studies, and provided new insights into patient perceptions about diseases and medications. The use of health-related social media research will only continue to expand in the future, but issues of privacy and confidentiality regarding online health information need to be solved. Incorporating social media data into clinical care will also require overcoming multiple challenges: making sense of the data, being able to integrate it with information in the electronic health record, and ultimately using it to improve patient outcomes.

CLINICS CARE POINTS

- Children with pediatric rheumatic diseases and their families are engaging with each other through online networks.
- Rather than discourage these behaviors, clinicians should find ways to guide patients and families to find accurate health content, and to receive the emotional support they desire.
- Clinicians should help develop critical thinking skills and health literacy in their patients and families to help them interpret online information.
- Clinicians should consider taking part in online conversations by creating or curating accurate health content, and by partnering with patient support organizations.

REFERENCES

1. Social Media Fact Sheet. Pew Research Center. Available at: https://www.pewresearch.org/internet/fact-sheet/social-media/?menuItem=d102dcb7-e8a1-42cd-a04e-ee442f81505a. Accessed April 22, 2021.
2. Titgemeyer SC, Schaaf CP. Facebook support groups for rare pediatric diseases: quantitative analysis. Jmir Pediatr Parent 2020;3(2):e21694.
3. Berenbaum F. The social (media) side to rheumatology. Nat Rev Rheumatol 2014;10(5):314–8.
4. Glenn AD. Using online health communication to manage chronic sorrow: mothers of children with rare diseases speak. J Pediatr Nurs 2015;30(1):17–24.
5. Tozzi AE, Mingarelli R, Agricola E, et al. The internet user profile of Italian families of patients with rare diseases: a Web survey. Orphanet J Rare Dis 2013;8(1):76.
6. Hausmann JS, Lomax KG, Shapiro A, et al. The patient journey to diagnosis and treatment of autoinflammatory diseases. Orphanet J Rare Dis 2018;13(1):156.
7. Black AP, Baker M. The impact of parent advocacy groups, the Internet, and social networking on rare diseases: the IDEA League and IDEA League United Kingdom example. Epilepsia 2011;52(s2):102–4.
8. Benetoli A, Chen TF, Aslani P. How patients' use of social media impacts their interactions with healthcare professionals. Patient Educ Couns 2018;101(3):439–44.
9. Frost J, Massagli M. PatientsLikeMe the case for a data-centered patient community and how ALS patients use the community to inform treatment decisions and manage pulmonary health. Chron Resp Dis 2009;6(4):225–9.
10. Huber J, Maatz P, Muck T, et al. The effect of an online support group on patients' treatment decisions for localized prostate cancer: an online survey. Urol Oncol Semin Orig Invest 2017;35(2):37.e19–28.
11. Hausmann J, Del Gaizo V, Magane K, et al. Health–related social media use by parents of children with rheumatic diseases [abstract]. Arthritis Rheumatol 2019;71(suppl 10). Available at: https://acrabstracts.org/abstract/health-related-social-media-use-by-parents-of-children-with-rheumatic-diseases/. Accessed July 12, 2021.
12. Anderson M, Teens JJ. Social Media & Technology 2018. Pew Research Center. Available at: https://www.pewresearch.org/internet/2018/05/31/teens-social-media-technology-2018/2031. Accessed July 1, 2021.
13. Hausmann JS, Touloumtzis C, White MT, et al. Adolescent and young adult use of social media for health and its implications. J Adolesc Health 2017;60(6):714–9.
14. Bodenheimer T, Lorig K, Holman H, et al. Patient self-management of chronic disease in primary care. JAMA 2002;288(19):2469–75.

15. Weitzman E, Wisk L. In: Klonoff D, Kerr D, Mulvaney S, editors. Using social media to support type 1 diabetes management and outcomes for adolescents and young adults: areas of promise and challenge. Diabetes Digital Health; 2020. https://doi.org/10.1016/B978-0-12-817485-2.00008-0.
16. Sawesi S, Rashrash M, Phalakornkule K, et al. The impact of information technology on patient engagement and health behavior change: a systematic review of the literature. Jmir Med Inform 2016;4(1):e1.
17. Scalzi LV, Hollenbeak CS, Mascuilli E, et al. Improvement of medication adherence in adolescents and young adults with SLE using web-based education with and without a social media intervention, a pilot study. Pediatr Rheumatol 2018;16(1):18.
18. Jain SH, Powers BW, Hawkins JB, et al. The digital phenotype. Nat Biotechnol 2015;33(5):462–3.
19. Nardi LD, Trombetta A, Ghirardo S, et al. Adolescents with chronic disease and social media: a cross-sectional study. Arch Dis Child 2020;105(8):744–8.
20. Sharma C, Whittle S, Haghighi PD, et al. Mining social media data to investigate patient perceptions regarding DMARD pharmacotherapy for rheumatoid arthritis. Ann Rheum Dis 2020;79(11):1432–7.
21. Schumacher KR, Stringer KA, Donohue JE, et al. Social media methods for studying rare diseases 2014. 133(5):e1345-e1353. DOI: 10.1542/peds.2013-2966.
22. DiBenedetti DB, Coles TM, Sharma T, et al. Assessing patients' and caregivers' perspectives on stability of factor VIII products for haemophilia A: a web-based study in the United States and Canada. Haemophilia 2014;20(4):e296–303.
23. Hausmann J, Kennedy K, Surangiwala S, et al. Early impacts of the COVID-19 pandemic on children with pediatric rheumatic diseases. European Journal of Rheumatology, 2021 (accepted manuscript).
24. Kostygina G, Tran H, Binns S, et al. Boosting health campaign reach and engagement through use of social media influencers and memes. Soc Media Soc 2020; 6(2). 2056305120912475.
25. Gough A, Hunter RF, Ajao O, et al. Tweet for behavior change: using social media for the dissemination of public health messages. Jmir Public Heal Surveill 2017; 3(1):e14.
26. Laranjo L, Arguel A, Neves AL, et al. The influence of social networking sites on health behavior change: a systematic review and meta-analysis. J Am Med Inform Association 2015;22(1):243–56.
27. Brownstein JS, Freifeld CC, Madoff LC. Digital disease detection — Harnessing the web for public health surveillance. N Engl J Med 2009;360(21):2153–7.
28. Harris JK, Mansour R, Choucair B, et al. Health department use of social media to identify foodborne illness - Chicago, Illinois, 2013-2014. MMWR Morb Mortal Wkly Rep 2014;63(32):681–5.
29. Rocklöv J, Tozan Y, Ramadona A, et al. Using big data to monitor the introduction and spread of Chikungunya, Europe, 2017 - Volume 25, Number 6—June 2019 - Emerging Infectious Diseases journal - CDC. Emerg Infect Dis 2019;25(6): 1041–9.
30. Bisanzio D, Kraemer MUG, Brewer T, et al. Geolocated Twitter social media data to describe the geographic spread of SARS-CoV-2. J Trav Med 2020;27(5): taaa120.
31. Kogan NE, Clemente L, Liautaud P, et al. An early warning approach to monitor COVID-19 activity with multiple digital traces in near real time. Sci Adv 2021; 7(10):eabd6989.

32. Wang Y, McKee M, Torbica A, et al. Systematic literature review on the spread of health-related misinformation on social media. Soc Sci Med 2019;240:112552.
33. Sattui SE, Liew JW, Graef ER, et al. Swinging the pendulum: lessons learned from public discourse concerning hydroxychloroquine and COVID-19. Expert Rev Clin Immu 2020;16(7):1–8.
34. Loomba S, Figueiredo A de, Piatek SJ, et al. Measuring the impact of COVID-19 vaccine misinformation on vaccination intent in the UK and USA. Nat Hum Behav 2021;5(3):337–48.
35. Randell RL, Long MD, Cook SF, et al. Validation of an internet-based cohort of inflammatory bowel disease (CCFA Partners). Inflamm Bowel Dis 2014;20(3):541–4.
36. Kramer ADI, Guillory JE, Hancock JT. Experimental evidence of massive-scale emotional contagion through social networks. Proc Natl Acad Sci U S A 2014;111(24):8788–90.
37. Christakis NA, Fowler JH. The spread of obesity in a large social network over 32 years. N Engl J Med 2007;357(4):370–9.
38. Christakis NA, Fowler JH. The collective dynamics of smoking in a large social network. N Engl J Med 2008;358(21):2249–58.
39. Weitzman ER, Magane KM, Wisk LE. How returning aggregate research results impacts interest in research engagement and planned actions relevant to health care decision making: cohort study. J Med Internet Res 2018;20(12):e10647.
40. Mandell DS, Salzer MS. Who joins support groups among parents of children with autism? Autism 2007;11(2):111–22.
41. Mitchell UA, Chebli PG, Ruggiero L, et al. The digital divide in health-related technology use: the significance of race/ethnicity. Gerontologist 2018;59(1):6–14.
42. Auxier B. Social media continue to be important political outlets for Black Americans. Pew Research Center. Available at: https://www.pewresearch.org/fact-tank/2020/12/11/social-media-continue-to-be-important-political-outlets-for-black-americans/. Accessed April 22, 2021.
43. Pennycook G, McPhetres J, Zhang Y, et al. Fighting COVID-19 misinformation on social media: experimental evidence for a scalable accuracy-nudge intervention. Psychol Sci 2020;31(7):770–80.
44. Updates to our work on COVID-19 vaccine misinformation. Twitter. Available at: https://blog.twitter.com/en_us/topics/company/2021/updates-to-our-work-on-covid-19-vaccine-misinformation.html. Accessed April 22, 2021.
45. Combating COVID-19 misinformation across our apps. Facebook. Available at: https://about.fb.com/news/2020/03/combating-covid-19-misinformation/. Accessed April 22, 2021.
46. Pho K. Guiding patients online is a new physician responsibility for the digital age. KevinMD. Available at: https://www.kevinmd.com/blog/2011/03/guiding-patients-online-physician-responsibility-digital-age.html. Accessed April 22, 2021.

Using the Electronic Health Record to Enhance Care in Pediatric Rheumatology

Alysha J. Taxter, MD, MSCE[a,*], Marc D. Natter, MD[b,c]

KEYWORDS

- Electronic health record • HITECH • Cures act • Interoperability
- Clinical research informatics • Pediatric rheumatology

KEY POINTS

- The HITECH Act and the 21st Century Cures Act have advanced implementation of electronic health records, interoperability, information use, and data exchange
- Recently adopted, open standards for EHR data interchange (FHIR, SMART) offer powerful, new mechanisms for data sharing that are well suited for pediatric rheumatology research
- Community involvement is needed to optimize the efficiency of EHR-based data entry forms for pediatric rheumatic diseases

INTRODUCTION

Pediatric rheumatology practitioners devote considerable effort to distilling relevant data from diverse—and frequently voluminous—sources of information. Although a detailed medical interview and specialized physical examination are important pillars in the process of the diagnosis and management of childhood-onset rheumatic conditions, the ability to rapidly review and efficiently glean key facts and patterns from the medical record remain critically important prerequisites to the delivery of timely, efficient, and effective care. Furthermore, advancements in the evidence-based treatment of these uncommon to rare diseases require access to larger patient populations than are available at any one clinical site and entail the collection and analysis of complex sets of multisite, and often multisource, diagnostic and treatment data. The electronic health record (EHR), sometimes referred to as electronic medical

[a] Nationwide Children's Hospital, 700 Children's Drive, Columbus, OH 43205, USA; [b] Computational Health Informatics Program, Boston Children's Hospital, 300 Longwood Avenue BCH3187, Boston, MA 02115, USA; [c] Mass General Hospital for Children, 55 Fruit Street, Boston, MA 02114, USA
* Corresponding author.
E-mail address: Alysha.Taxter@nationwidechildrens.org

https://doi.org/10.1016/j.rdc.2021.08.004

record or patient health record, offers a powerful tool for fulfilling these requirements. In this review, we explore the capabilities for and challenges of applying EHR technology to improve pediatric rheumatology practice and research, summarized in **Table 1**.

HISTORICAL CONTEXT: ELECTRONIC HEALTH RECORDS

The EHR evolved[1] from efforts in the 1950s to 1970s to accomplish 2 distinct advancements: (1) converting paper-based patient registration and billing systems to more useable and efficiently linked electronic hospital information systems, and (2) advancing adoption and usability of a problem-oriented approach to medical documentation.[2,3] The advent of the microcomputer era in the 1980s and 1990s saw a much broader dissemination of EHR software, with a shift in focus from "home-grown" EHR systems focusing on clinical needs to offerings by commercial vendors, particularly in the United States, with a focus on EHR systems designed to optimize fee-for-services reimbursement. By the early 2000s, these factors were widely recognized as barriers contributing to system-level inefficiencies and safety concerns.[4]

The Health Information Technology for Economic and Clinical Health (HITECH) Act, which was enacted in the United States in 2009 as part of the American Recovery and Reinvestment Act (ARRA), introduced new, functional metrics of clinical and public health usability for the EHR termed "Meaningful Use."[5,6] A summary of the contemporary timeline of milestones pertinent to EHR system advancement is outlined in **Fig. 1**. In 2016, the US 21st Century Cures Act was enacted to support the next iteration of electronic health information use, access, and exchange, with a goal of improving information exchange for providers and patients, while also supporting software developers to create vendor-agnostic health information applications.[7] This law mandates an openly available, standardized, nonproprietary set of application programming interfaces (APIs) to facilitate health data exchange. For example, an application on a patient's smartphone could use this API to request the patient's latest blood pressure measurements obtained by their physician, while an EHR from another hospital system where the patient was seen at a later date could likewise use the same API to obtain the same blood pressure measurement, along with other data about the treatments the patient was prescribed.

The key requirement to such data exchange is the availability of publicly defined sets of APIs which are universally supported throughout the EHR systems. Another standardization mandate is adoption of the Fast Healthcare Interoperability Resources (FHIR) approach—an openly available, electronic health data resources framework established by Health Level Seven International (HL7).[8,9] A companion standard, the Sustainable Medical Apps Reusable Technology (SMART) framework, was also recently adopted as a model approach for building apps that are reuseable ("write an app once, have it run anywhere"), which readily interconnects to the EHR ecosystem via FHIR.[10,11] The Cures Act also led to the definition of an initial Core Data Set for Interoperability (USCDI), which is composed of classes of data elements designed to enable medication and allergy reconciliations, problem list reconciliation, care transitions, and electronic case reporting.[7,12,13] In 2022, expansion of the Core Data Set to classify all health care data elements in standardized formats, both structured and unstructured, is planned. The Cures Act promotes such access by prohibiting the practice of information blocking, whereas proprietary restrictions and excessive costs for obtaining timely access to one's own health data are no longer allowable, improving the ability of patients, providers, and researchers to gain access to health data. See **Box 1** for links to additional health information technology and EHR resources.

Table 1
High priority EHR capabilities for improving clinical practice, quality of care, and clinical research in pediatric rheumatology, with a summary of current applications and challenges

Problem	EHR Capability	Application to Pediatric Rheumatology	Challenges
Rapid Documentation	• Note functionality • Template utilization • Specialized forms	• Epic's PR-COIN SmartForm, homunculus documentation, and disease activity score calculations • Developments in Natural Language Processing	Most notes contain unstructured data, lack of standardization, documentation tools not readily implemented, insufficient end-user training, provider burnout
Patient Engagement	• Patient-portal access	Ability to obtain patient-generated data: • Questionnaires/patient-reported outcomes • Computer adaptive testing • Home monitoring tools (applications, smart devices) • Graphical depictions of data such as timeline views	Not yet universally implemented, utilization often requires technical sophistication of users
Interoperability: EHR data interfacing with medical apps, registries, and other clinical research	• Standardized data elements and data fields • Fast Healthcare Interoperability Resources (FHIR)	• Export and real-time access to clinical data and PROs collected within the EHR	Standard data elements not universally used, FHIR-EHR and FHIR-Registry interfaces in early stages of development or do not yet exist
Access to knowledge: pediatric rheumatology treatment guidelines, Consensus Treatment Plans (CTP), Treat to Target (T2T)	• Clinical Decision Support	• Ability to build clinician advisories leveraging existing EHR data	Not always readily designed, integrated, or implemented using currently deployed technology

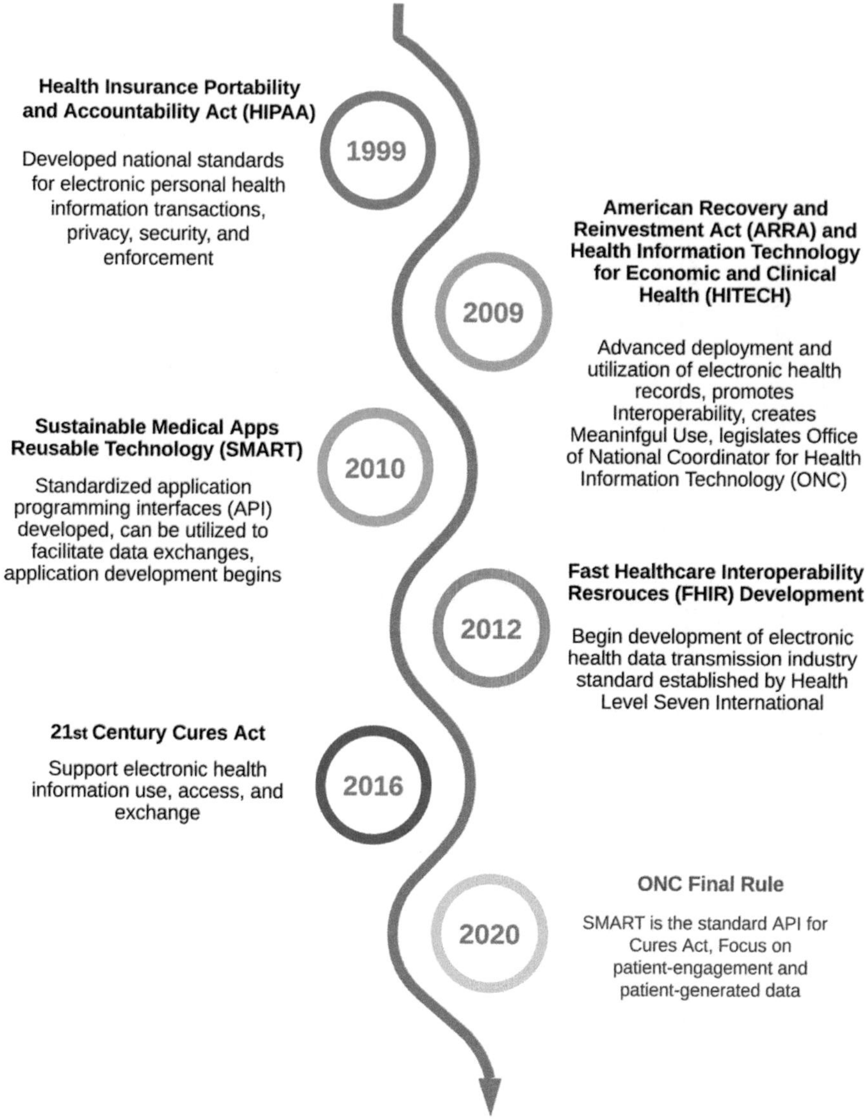

Fig. 1. History of EHRs: contemporary milestones from the 1990s through 2020s.

ELECTRONIC HEALTH RECORD CAPABILITIES FOR IMPROVING CLINICAL PRACTICE, QUALITY OF CARE, AND CLINICAL RESEARCH IN PEDIATRIC RHEUMATOLOGY

Efficient Documentation: Getting Data into the Electronic Health Record So That It Can Be Meaningfully Accessed

There are multiple sources of personal health information, including medical history, medications, results of tests, imaging, pathology reports, patient-reported outcomes, and so forth—most all of which should be housed within a patient's medical record if it is to be truly comprehensive and longitudinal. A large proportion of these data elements are best represented and stored in the EHR within structured data fields,

Box 1
Useful Web sites and available resources

- Health Information Technology: https://www.healthit.gov/
- Health Level 7 (HL7) Fast Healthcare Interoperability Resources (FHIR): http://hl7.org/fhir/index.html
- Health Insurance Portability and Accountability Act: https://www.hhs.gov/hipaa/for-professionals/security/index.html
- Meaningful Use: https://www.cdc.gov/ehrmeaningfuluse/
- SMART on FHIR: https://smarthealthit.org

also called discrete or coded fields, which are ideal for representing classes of data suited to standardization. Examples include body temperature, blood pressure, pain scores, and laboratory results. Structured data fields also readily support features such as alerts, for example, if data entered falls outside of prespecified ranges, such as a heart rate of 1 or 1000. Although a great many coding systems have been designed for health data standardization,[14,15] only a handful are in widespread usage, for example, Logical Observation Identifiers Names and Codes (LOINC) for laboratory and clinical observations, Systematized Nomenclature of Medicine Clinical Terms (SNOMED) for clinical findings, Current Procedural Terminology (CPT) for specifying medical services and procedures provided, RxNorm for generic and branded medications, and International Classification of Disease (ICD) for diagnostic billing codes. Although the use of structured data is advantageous for reporting and research, manually recording such data is often a burdensome task for the EHR user faced with completing a myriad of separate multiselect fields, drop-down lists, and checkboxes, particularly when injudiciously designed forms result in markedly increased documentation time, a leading cause of provider burnout.[16] The usual alternative—unstructured data such as typed or dictated clinical notes, or free-text medication instructions—is more convenient and remains ubiquitious[17] but problematic when the goal is data reuse for clinical reporting or research purposes. Although unstructured text can be transformed into structured data by using, for instance, natural language processing (NLP) tools, the accurate extraction of complex concepts—particularly important temporal relationships between concepts—remains challenging.

Pediatric rheumatologists spend an average of 26 minutes per outpatient encounter completing chart review and documentation tasks.[18] How can currently available (and future) EHR capabilities be used for improving documentation efficiency in pediatric rheumatology practice and research? In the adult rheumatology realm, one of the earlier specialty-specific EHR customizations has been the joint homunculus. This data entry concept has been adapted to multiple different EHR platforms and typically offers a combination of point-and-click plus discrete data entry; currently, a pediatric-specific version has been developed by at least one major EHR vendor in collaboration with pediatric rheumatologists. Another useful approach is the development of pediatric rheumatology disease-specific EHR forms, an approach first adopted and put into practice in pediatric rheumatology by the Pediatric Rheumatology Care & Outcomes Improvement Network (PR-COIN),[19] a quality improvement network. In this approach, Epic Systems Corporation (Verona, WI) SmartForms were developed for multiple aspects of juvenile arthritis care and enable streamlined entry of subspecialty and disease-specific data.

Patient Engagement: Enabling Direct Entry of Data About Patients, by Patients and Their Caregivers

Several modalities have been developed to enable direct entry of self (or proxy) reported data into the EHR, including use of in-clinic mobile devices, free-standing kiosks, and more recently Web-based or mobile platforms that interconnect with patient "portals" to the EHR. Capturing patient data at the time of patient care can inform clinical decision-making and engages patients and families in their care.[20] Similarly, dashboards can be created and used at point-of-care, displayed to patients and families, catalyzing more data-driven conversations about a patient's symptoms, progress, and outcomes using a combination of patient- and provider-captured and laboratory clinical data.[21,22] An example of currently available Patient Timeline Dashboard functionality from Epic Systems Corporation software is seen in **Fig. 2**.

Particular challenges arise regarding PROs for use in pediatric rheumatology, however, as some of the most potentially useful measures of physical function and pain interference have only been recently validated and are not yet in widespread

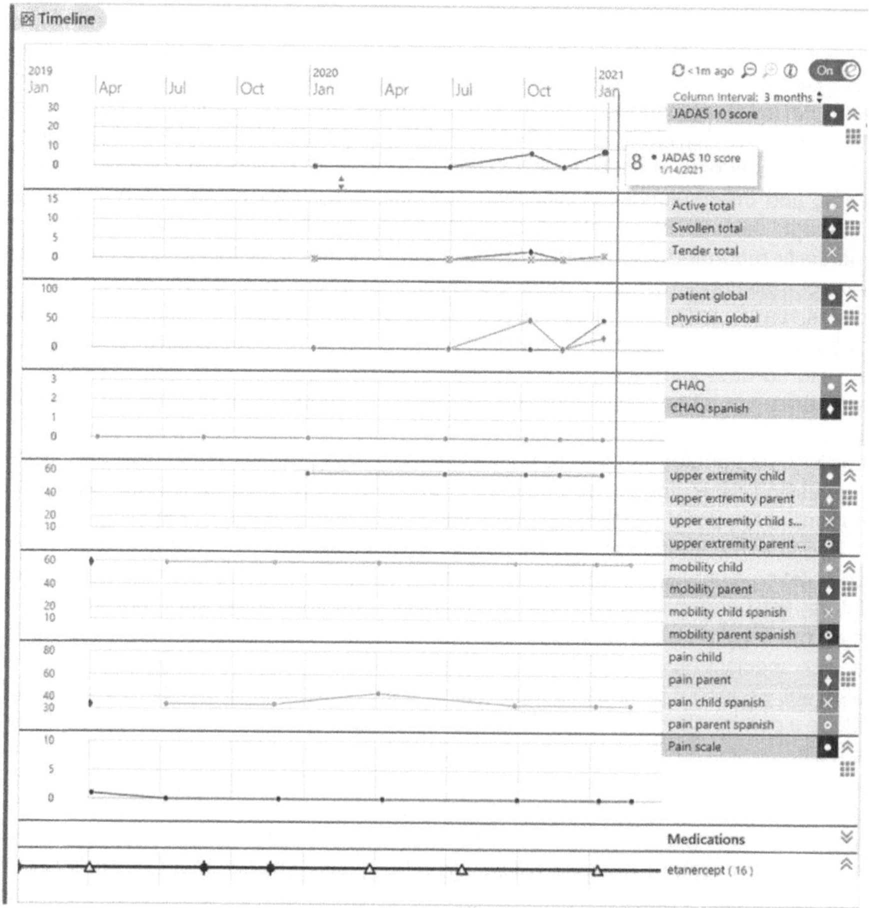

Fig. 2. Patient-Engagement Dashboard displaying patient-reported, provider-reported, and clinical data over time. © 2021 Epic Systems Corporation. Used with permission.

use.[23–25] In addition, the burden on patients when answering more lengthy surveys can be considerable and results in decreased usage and missing data in full-length PRO instruments. A time-saving solution to this problem is computer-adaptive testing (CAT), which provides automated survey abbreviation by selecting a subset of survey items based on answers to preceding item responses. Although CAT PROs have recently been programmed into many EHR systems, particularly the NIH-funded Patient-Reported Outcomes Measurement Information Systems (PROMIS) CAT instruments,[26] clinical interpretation of such PROs in pediatric rheumatology has remained largely untested. Fortunately, a focus of the recent NIH funded Advancing the Science of Pediatric Patient Reported Outcomes for Children with Chronic Disease (PEPR) study[27] is validation and calibration of pediatric-specific, disease agnostic PROMIS measures, including CAT surveys, in pediatric rheumatology cohorts.

Interoperability: Reusing Clinical Data for Research and Quality Improvement

With the advent of large, multicenter, longitudinal investigator-sponsored research and quality improvement network studies in pediatric rheumatology, for example, the Childhood Arthritis and Rheumatology Research Network (CARRA) Registry, PR-COIN, Pediatric Rheumatology InterNational Trials Organization (PRINTO),[19,28–30] and others, a particularly sought-after capability is the elimination of double data entry of identical, or highly similar, data into both EHR and external study data collection platforms. Although EHR to disease registry data transfer is a specific provision of the Cures Act, multiple barriers remain to the time and cost-effective integration of EHR data for direct research registry usage. Prior, well-funded efforts in other subspecialties including pediatric Inflammatory Bowel Disease[31] and pediatric Pulmonary Hypertension Network[32] highlight that in addition to EHR data accessibility, maintaining data integrity (data provenance and accurate data element mapping) introduces considerable challenges. For regulated clinical trials in particular, formal assurance of data provenance, auditing, and security, for example, as per US 21 CFR 11, must also be satisfied.

Data integrity is necessary when designing EHRs to interface with research and quality improvement networks. One aspect of data integrity—data provenance, or the origin and lineage of data—is particularly critical to ensuring the truth and validity of data collected. For example, if a patient designates a pain score of 5.5 on a visual analog scale in a PRO platform used by the EHR, but the number is rounded to a whole number on transfer of the PRO results to an EHR, this value is no longer correct. Understanding the flow of the data from the source to the EHR, and then to a secondary research database, often depends on the capability to inspect audit records from intermediate systems and may be required to adjudicate otherwise unexplained differences in study observations.[33] Accurate data element mapping represents a related domain of challenges—for instance, when determining medication history, available data elements in an EHR can include medication order entry data, medication administration records, pharmacy data, and medication reconciliation data. These elements all inform different aspects of medication history, leading to the expectation that a direct mapping of actual medication start and stop dates is feasible. However, in the outpatient setting, data most often obtained during routine medication reconciliation inaccurately conflate medication order dates with start dates and dates of recording of discontinued medications with stop dates. Finally, data may be simply missing. It has been estimated that medication records, for instance, are commonly inaccurate and incomplete nearly 50% of the time.[34,35] Clearly, although the potential of clinical data reuse for research and reporting is very promising, there are many potential pitfalls when repurposing clinical data for research.[33]

Nonetheless, successful examples of clinical data reuse for research exist. The Rheumatology Clinical Registry (RCR), developed by the American College of Rheumatology as a quality improvement tool, and which became the Rheumatology Informatics System for Effectiveness (RISE),[36] is a successful model of a "data-in-once" platform used by adult rheumatology practices to track and compare quality measures, including those mandated by Medicare and Medicaid Services (CMS). As part of the RISE Learning Collaborative,[37] the PR-COIN quality improvement network also leverages EHR-based data integration, using the Epic Systems Corporation EHR software for direct entry into their database, along with options to electronically transfer data from other EHR vendors into the database. At the same time, the CARRA Registry, an investigator-sponsored, FDA Phase 4 postmarketing surveillance network that includes multiple substudies and clinical trials, has moved forward to a data warehousing strategy based on the FHIR data interchange standard and is now piloting a project in which EHR data available in PCORnet Common Data Model format[38] is exported from pre-existing PCORnet data warehouses, converted into FHIR format, and then linked to subject-level CARRA Registry data from participating sites.[39]

Access to Knowledge: Using Electronic Health Record Data at Point of Care for Clinical Decision Support

Clinical decision support (CDS) uses a combination of individual patient information and decision algorithms (typically using rule-based approaches but sometimes machine-generated models) to recommend particular actions that are anticipated to improve care. Examples of CDS aids include pop-up alerts to providers that a vaccine may be due, suggested order sets based on a presenting symptom or risk factor, and alerts based on data a clinician may be otherwise unaware of, such as a prolonged QTc interval and potential medication interaction. Although CDS aids can be a powerful tool when judiciously applied within provider workflows, they can otherwise become "nag" screens to be ignored or inculcate a false sense of reassurance when a warning is erroneously absent. Key tenets of optimal application of CDS is proposed by Bates' "Ten Commandments"[40] (**Box 2**) and the CDS "Five Rights" (getting the right information, to the right person, in the right intervention format, through the right channel, at the right time).[41] At present, few pediatric rheumatology-specific examples of CDS appear to be in progress, but we introduce the concept here given its likely future promise in advancing implementation science in pediatric rheumatology, as discussed in more detail below.

CONCLUSIONS AND FUTURE DIRECTIONS

Current advances in EHR capabilities, although promising, have yet to translate to widely disseminated improvements in clinical practice, quality of care, and clinical research in pediatric rheumatology. This lack of progress is, of course, not unique to pediatric rheumatology, but in our opinion exacts a disproportionately negative impact on a subspecialty whose focus on the diagnosis and treatment of uncommon to rare diseases necessitates close collaboration, standardization, and sharing of data to conduct adequately powered studies. Although we and others believe that the roots of these shortcomings reflect the current EHR-health care ecosystem rather than actual technological barriers,[42] we posit that a new window of opportunity for rapid EHR ecosystem change is emerging—one catalyzed by phase-in of the US HITECH Act requirements for health care data sharing and accessibility, recent streamlining of outpatient evaluation and management documentation requirements by the US Centers for Medicare and Medicaid Services, and a rapid adoption of patient portals

Box 2
Ten commandments for effective clinical decision support

1. Speed Is Everything
2. Anticipate Needs and Deliver in Real Time
3. Fit into the User's Workflow
4. Little Things Can Make a Big Difference
5. Recognize that Physicians Will Strongly Resist Stopping
6. Changing Direction Is Easier than Stopping
7. Simple Interventions Work Best
8. Ask for Additional Information Only When You Really Need It
9. Monitor Impact, Get Feedback, and Respond
10. Manage and Maintain Your Knowledge-based Systems

Data from Bates DW, Kuperman GJ, Wang S, et al. Ten commandments for effective clinical decision support: making the practice of evidence-based medicine a reality. *J Am Med Inform Assoc.* 2003;10(6):523-530; with permission.

and telemedicine in context of the COVID-19 pandemic. We are optimistic that these recent developments, if accompanied by a renewed commitment of time and resources by stakeholders in the pediatric rheumatology community, ongoing collaboration with EHR vendors, and steady commitment of the regulatory community to incentivize continuing beneficial EHR ecosystem change,[43,44] will provide many new opportunities to use health information technology, EHRs, and new interoperability standards and technologies to inform, streamline, and ultimately improve care, research, and outcomes in pediatric rheumatology. Specifically, we believe that focusing efforts of the pediatric rheumatology community toward progress of the EHR ecosystem in the following areas is likely to have the most impact on the practice of pediatric rheumatology in the next decade:

1. "Data in"—*a comprehensive effort to standardize a core set of data elements and data collection forms within and across EHR platforms for pediatric rheumatic diseases should be prioritized*. At present, one of the authors (AT) is working with an EHR vendor to incorporate the CARRA Registry data elements into the data model of their EHR platform. This effort should be expanded to include other EHR platforms and pediatric rheumatic diseases not currently encompassed in the CARRA Registry, along with inclusion of terminology standardization across the international community (eg, SNOMED-CT and LOINC data element mapping enhancements for pediatric rheumatology). In parallel, current efforts to adapt EHR data entry forms from their adult rheumatology counterparts should be expanded wherever feasible across major EHR vendors, with consideration to using vendor-specific form builders that can be shared among EHR installations (eg, centrally available Epic SmartForms) as well as making use of vendor-agnostic, standardized app-building approaches (eg, SMART and other FHIR-based app frameworks), for "data-in-once" capture of both clinical practice and clinical research data.
2. "Data out"—*leveraging "Data In" standardizations to create real-time data conduits from the EHR into clinical research registries and trials, quality improvement*

databases, and patient-facing health dashboards in pediatric rheumatology. Although established by the Cures Act, the real-world use of standardized FHIR APIs for EHR data access faces many hurdles. We believe that a unified approach of the pediatric rheumatology community to prioritize and partner with other subspecialty groups, EHR vendors, and regulatory and standards-making bodies can accelerate the use and availability of EHR data interfaces for this purpose. As examples, the REDCap Consortium is actively developing multifaceted EHR integration modules based on FHIR,[45] and the authors have been directly involved in efforts to develop, demonstrate, and disseminate implementations of the FHIR standard for ensuring US 21 CFR 11-compliant usage for clinical trials.[46] Building new clinical trials and quality improvement projects in pediatric rheumatology on these and similar data interchange frameworks is likely to accelerate the achievement of "data-in-once" repurposing from the EHR.

3. *"Grass-roots" EHR workflow process improvement*. We believe there is a clear opportunity to leverage the EHR to improve EHR user workflows, providing downstream benefits for improving clinical care and clinical research. EHRs are highly complex suites of software that tend to be so granularly configurable and comprehensive that their usage frequently results in cognitive overload to users. Compounding this issue, the relative underrepresentation of pediatric rheumatology providers, compared with other general and subspecialty providers, means that many institutions lack a depth of expertise when configuring pediatric rheumatology-specific views and related subspecialty functionality in their EHR systems. However, from ad-hoc reports and the experience of an interinstitutional pilot project by the author (AT), we find that short-term, expert user-guided EHR workflow analysis and improvement projects can result in the rapid adoption of incremental, but substantive, time-saving approaches to interacting with EHR systems. To more widely disseminate these benefits, we believe that a pediatric rheumatology 'EHR Corps' of EHR vendor-specific "super-user" experts could be assembled to collaboratively enhance workflows across the subspecialty. Such a group could provide cross-institutional expertise and advisement when building, customizing, deploying, and maintaining EHR functionality at an individual institutional level.
4. *CDS for pediatric rheumatology* is easily the most underdeveloped EHR capability at present, largely due to the current paucity of evidence supporting specific, individualized treatment algorithms for childhood-onset rheumatic diseases. The inadequacy of the evidence base is well recognized, and 2 broad initiatives—Consensus Treatment Plans (CTPs)[47] developed by CARRA, and Treat to Target (T2T)[48]—focus respectively on determining which standardized approaches (CTPs) best improves care, or quantifying how single empirically designed, target-driven approaches (T2T) improves care. Although CARRA has developed multiple, disease-specific CTPs for polyarticular and systemic-onset juvenile idiopathic arthritis, systemic lupus erythematosus with nephritis and juvenile dermatomyositis among other diseases, knowledge of and adherence to these CTPs appears to vary widely, as individual CTPs are not delivered in real-time nor are captured in EHR-based workflows. Likewise, T2T assessments and decision point logic have had very limited implementation in the EHR at present. Nonetheless, the data elements needed to provide decision support assistance are, or could be, captured within the EHR, enabling subsequent development of a spectrum of pediatric rheumatology-specific CDS tools ranging from basic, rule-based decision aids to advanced, machine learning predictive algorithms.

SUMMARY

The EHR ecosystem is undergoing rapid evolution, most recently in response to new rules and regulations promulgated by the US HITECH legislation of 2009 and 21st Century Cures Act of 2016, which together promote enhanced information use, access, and exchange for providers and patients, and support vendor-agnostic application development in health information technology. Pediatric rheumatology stands to benefit by pursuing focused approaches to improving EHR-based user workflows and strategies for data repurposing supported by new technology standards, particularly implementations of Fast Healthcare Interoperability Resources (FHIR) and Sustainable Medical Apps Reusable Technology (SMART) based strategies that facilitate data transfer from EHR to collaborative registries and quality improvement efforts. With proper software design and workflow reinvention, there are ready opportunities to standardize data capture to be used for combined patient care and clinical research, integrate patient-reported outcomes into clinical care, and incorporate consensus treatment plans and treat-to-target decision support tools into the EHR for pediatric rheumatology.

CLINICS CARE POINTS

- TheHITECH and the 21st Century Cures Act advanced implementation of electronic health records, interoperability, information use, and exchange.
- New technology for data interchange exists, including FHIR and SMART standards, but are not routinely used or implemented for pediatric rheumatology research.
- There is an opportunity to standardize electronic data input and output, to leverage the EHR for both patient care and research, and to develop and integrate clinical decision support into pediatric rheumatology specific applications.

FUNDING

Dr. A.J. Taxter receives salary support from CARRA as her role as the CARRA Informatics Associate.

DISCLOSURE

Dr A.J. Taxter is a volunteer member of the Epic Rheumatology Steering Board. Dr M.D. Natter has nothing to disclose.

REFERENCES

1. McDonald CJ, Hripcsak G. Electronic health record systems. 4th edition. London: Springer; 2014.
2. Weed LL. Medical records that guide and teach. N Engl J Med 1968;278(11): 593–600.
3. Weed LL. Medical records that guide and teach. N Engl J Med 1968;278(12): 652–7, concl.
4. Institute of Medicine (US). Committee on data standards for patient safety. Key capabilities of an electronic health record system: letter report. Washington (DC): National Academies Press (US); 2003. Available at: https://www.ncbi.nlm.nih.gov/books/NBK221802/. Accessed March 1, 2021.

5. Centers for Disease Control and Prevention. Public Health and Promoting Interoperability Programs. 2019. Available at: https://www.cdc.gov/ehrmeaningfuluse/. Accessed February 10, 2021.
6. Blumenthal D, Tavenner M. The "meaningful use" regulation for electronic health records. N Engl J Med 2010;363(6):501–4.
7. Office of the national coordinator for health information technology. Health IT; 2021. Available at: https://www.healthit.gov/. Accessed February 10, 2021.
8. Mandl KD, Kohane IS. No small change for the health information economy. N Engl J Med 2009;360(13):1278–81.
9. Hussain MA, Langer SG, Kohli M. Learning HL7 FHIR Using the HAPI FHIR Server and Its Use in Medical Imaging with the SIIM Dataset. J Digit Imaging 2018;31(3):334–40.
10. SMART. SMART Health IT. 2021. Available at: https://smarthealthit.org/. Accessed March 1, 2021.
11. Mandel JC, Kreda DA, Mandl KD, et al. SMART on FHIR: a standards-based, interoperable apps platform for electronic health records. J Am Med Inform Assoc 2016;23(5):899–908.
12. Pageler NM, Webber EC, Lund DP. Implications of the 21st Century Cures Act in Pediatrics. Pediatrics. 2021 Mar;147(3):e2020034199. doi: 10.1542/peds.2020-034199.
13. Federal Register. 21st Century Cures Act: interoperability, information blocking, and the ONC health IT certification Program 2020. Available at: https://www.federalregister.gov/documents/2020/05/01/2020-07419/21st-century-cures-act-interoperability-information-blocking-and-the-onc-health-it-certification. Accessed February 10, 2021.
14. Whetzel PL, Noy NF, Shah NH, et al. BioPortal: enhanced functionality via new Web services from the National Center for Biomedical Ontology to access and use ontologies in software applications. Nucleic Acids Res 2011;39(Web Server issue):W541–5.
15. National Institutes of Health National Library of Medicine. Unified medical language system. 2016. Available at: https://www.nlm.nih.gov/research/umls/knowledge_sources/metathesaurus/index.html. Accessed March 3, 2021.
16. Dymek C, Kim B, Melton GB, et al. Building the evidence-base to reduce electronic health record-related clinician burden. J Am Med Inform Assoc 2021 Apr 23;28(5):1057–61. https://doi.org/10.1093/jamia/ocaa238.
17. Johnson KE, Kamineni A, Fuller S, et al. How the provenance of electronic health record data matters for research: a case example using system mapping. EGEMS (Wash DC) 2014;2(1):1058.
18. Overhage JM, Johnson KB. Pediatrician Electronic health record time use for outpatient encounters. Pediatrics 2020;146(6):e20194017.
19. Harris JG, Bingham CA, Morgan EM. Improving care delivery and outcomes in pediatric rheumatic diseases. Curr Opin Rheumatol 2016;28(2):110–6.
20. Gerhardt WE, Mara CA, Kudel I, et al. Systemwide implementation of patient-reported outcomes in routine clinical care at a children's hospital. Jt Comm J Qual Patient Saf 2018;44(8):441–53.
21. Opipari-Arrigan L, Dykes DMH, Saeed SA, et al. Technology-enabled health care collaboration in pediatric chronic illness: pre-post interventional study for feasibility, acceptability, and clinical impact of an electronic health record-linked platform for patient-clinician partnership. JMIR Mhealth Uhealth 2020;8(11):e11968.
22. Batalden M, Batalden P, Margolis P, et al. Coproduction of healthcare service. BMJ Qual Saf 2016;25(7):509–17.

23. Cunningham NR, Kashikar-Zuck S, Mara C, et al. Development and validation of the self-reported PROMIS pediatric pain behavior item bank and short form scale. Pain 2017;158(7):1323–31.
24. Jones JT, Carle AC, Wootton J, et al. Validation of patient-reported outcomes measurement information system short forms for use in childhood-onset systemic lupus erythematosus. Arthritis Care Res (Hoboken) 2017;69(1):133–42.
25. Mara CA, Kashikar-Zuck S, Cunningham N, et al. Development and psychometric evaluation of the PROMIS pediatric pain intensity measure in children and adolescents with chronic pain. J Pain 2021;22(1):48–56.
26. Health Measures. Health measures. 2021. Available at: https://www.healthmeasures.net. Accessed March 2, 2021.
27. Childhood Arthritis and Rheumatology Research Alliance. Advancing the science of pediatric patient reported outcomes for children with chronic disease (PEPR). 2021. Available at: https://carragroup.org/research-registry/projects/pepr. Accessed March 1, 2021.
28. Beukelman T, Kimura Y, Ilowite NT, et al. The new Childhood Arthritis and Rheumatology Research Alliance (CARRA) registry: design, rationale, and characteristics of patients enrolled in the first 12 months. Pediatr Rheumatol Online J 2017; 15(1):30.
29. Brunner HI, Rider LG, Kingsbury DJ, et al. Pediatric Rheumatology Collaborative Study Group - over four decades of pivotal clinical drug research in pediatric rheumatology. Pediatr Rheumatol Online J 2018;16(1):45.
30. Ruperto N, Martini A. Network in pediatric rheumatology: the example of the Pediatric Rheumatology International Trials Organization. World J Pediatr 2008;4(3): 186–91.
31. Crandall W, Kappelman MD, Colletti RB, et al. ImproveCareNow: the development of a pediatric inflammatory bowel disease improvement network. Inflamm Bowel Dis 2011;17(1):450–7.
32. National Institutes of Health. Research Portfolio Online Reporting Tools (RePORT). 2021. Available at: https://projectreporter.nih.gov/project_info_description.cfm?aid=9769939&icde=53811326. Accessed March 2, 2021.
33. Hersh WR, Weiner MG, Embi PJ, et al. Caveats for the use of operational electronic health record data in comparative effectiveness research. Med Care 2013;51(8 Suppl 3):S30–7.
34. Abdulghani KH, Aseeri MA, Mahmoud A, et al. The impact of pharmacist-led medication reconciliation during admission at tertiary care hospital. Int J Clin Pharm 2018;40(1):196–201.
35. Motulsky A, Weir DL, Couture I, et al. Usage and accuracy of medication data from nationwide health information exchange in Quebec, Canada. J Am Med Inform Assoc 2018;25(6):722–9.
36. Francisco M, Johansson T, Kazi S. Overview of the American College of Rheumatology's electronic health record-enabled registry: the rheumatology informatics system for effectiveness. Clin Exp Rheumatol 2016;34(5 Suppl 101):S102–4.
37. University of California San Francisco. RISE learning collaborative. 2020. Available at: https://risepro.ucsf.edu/learn-more/. Accessed March 1, 2021.
38. The National Patient-Centered Clinical Research Network. Data. 2021. Available at: https://pcornet.org/data/. Accessed March 1, 2021.
39. Childhood arthritis and rheumatology research Alliance. Limit JIA; 2021. Available at: https://carragroup.org/research-registry/projects/limit-jia. Accessed March 1, 2021.

40. Bates DW, Kuperman GJ, Wang S, et al. Ten commandments for effective clinical decision support: making the practice of evidence-based medicine a reality. J Am Med Inform Assoc 2003;10(6):523–30.
41. Sirajuddin AM, Osheroff JA, Sittig DF, et al. Implementation pearls from a new guidebook on improving medication use and outcomes with clinical decision support. Effective CDS is essential for addressing healthcare performance improvement imperatives. J Healthc Inf Manag 2009;23(4):38–45.
42. Institute of Medicine (US) Roundtable on Evidence-Based Medicine. The Learning Healthcare System: Workshop Summary. Olsen L, Aisner D, McGinnis JM, editors. Washington (DC): National Academies Press (US); 2007. PMID: 21452449.
43. Gordon WJ, Mandl KD. The 21st century cures act: a competitive apps market and the risk of innovation blocking. J Med Internet Res 2020;22(12):e24824.
44. Mandl KD, Kohane IS. Data Citizenship under the 21st Century Cures Act. N Engl J Med 2020;382(19):1781–3.
45. NIH Collaboratory Living Textbook of Pragmatic Clinical Trials. Playing with FHIR–innovative use cases for the new REDCap EHR integration module (Paul Harris, PhD) 2019. Available at: https://rethinkingclinicaltrials.org/news/october-18-2019-playing-with-fhir-innovative-use-cases-for-the-new-redcap-ehr-integration-module-paul-harris-phd/. Accessed March 2, 2021.
46. HL7 FHIR. Patient reported outcomes FHIR implementation guide. 2018. Available at: http://www.hl7.org/fhir/us/patient-reported-outcomes/2018Sep/. Accessed March 2, 2021.
47. Ringold S, Nigrovic PA, Feldman BM, et al. The childhood arthritis and rheumatology research alliance consensus treatment plans: toward comparative effectiveness in the pediatric rheumatic diseases. Arthritis Rheumatol 2018;70(5): 669–78.
48. Ravelli A, Consolaro A, Horneff G, et al. Treating juvenile idiopathic arthritis to target: recommendations of an international task force. Ann Rheum Dis 2018; 77(6):819–28.

The Emerging Telehealth Landscape in Pediatric Rheumatology

Rajdeep Pooni, MD, MS*, Tzielan Lee, MD

KEYWORDS

- Pediatric rheumatology • Telehealth • Telemedicine • Digital health
- Health services delivery

KEY POINTS

- Telemedicine programs are of particular importance given the need for an increase in access to pediatric rheumatology providers.
- The recent COVID-19 pandemic dramatically changed telehealth policies and use of telemedicine in the ambulatory setting and has provided an opportunity to evaluate the more general use of telemedicine in pediatric rheumatology practice.
- Further research on telemedicine programs in pediatric rheumatology is needed to evaluate the impact on clinical outcomes, research, patient acceptability, and health disparities.

INTRODUCTION

The COVID-19 pandemic caused a major shift in health care delivery models, particularly in the ambulatory care space.[1,2] Pediatric rheumatology providers largely operate in the outpatient setting and follow patients closely and regularly because of the chronic nature of pediatric rheumatic diseases. During the pandemic, most providers were forced to incorporate virtual visits—synchronous remote encounters between patients and healthcare providers[3]—to provide direct care to their patients that they would have normally seen in an in-person setting. As such, pediatric rheumatologists had to learn how to quickly adapt their in-person clinical practices, including examination and assessment of disease activity, to this digital space. Moving forward, telemedicine may have ongoing potential in pediatric rheumatology care because of a growing workforce shortage. Recent workforce trends indicate that fewer trainees are selecting pediatric subspecialties such as rheumatology as

Division of Allergy, Immunology and Rheumatology, Department of Pediatric Rheumatology, Stanford Children's Health, Stanford University School of Medicine, 700 Welch Road, Suite 301, Palo Alto, CA 94304, USA
* Corresponding author.
E-mail address: rpooni@stanford.edu

Rheum Dis Clin N Am 48 (2022) 259–270
https://doi.org/10.1016/j.rdc.2021.08.005
rheumatic.theclinics.com

a career, and that this will result in a decline in the number of pediatric rheumatologists.[4] Understanding barriers to telemedicine use in pediatric rheumatology specifically, and how to implement successful telemedicine programs for chronic disease management across large geographic areas is of the utmost importance, particularly in light of this continuing gap. In addition, understanding how telemedicine fits into the context of pediatric rheumatology practice and research to meet the goals of patients, providers, and researchers will be of critical importance.[5] This review highlights the potential impact of telemedicine in pediatric rheumatology care and considerations for its future use.

BACKGROUND

There is a clear workforce shortage in the field of pediatric rheumatology[6]: many children and young people with pediatric rheumatic diseases live a considerable distance from a pediatric rheumatologist.[7] This in turn, may result in gaps in disease management, and/or suboptimal care received from nonpediatric rheumatology providers to fill this need. Concerns regarding this issue have been previously highlighted in both pediatric and adult rheumatology communities, especially in remote or rural communities where there is a real concern for delays in diagnosis and adequate treatment.[8]

Telemedicine, the use of telecommunications and information technology to provide access to health assessment, diagnosis, intervention, and consultation across a distance,[9] has long been touted as one potential avenue to bridge these care gaps. Telehealth includes a broader scope of remote clinical and nonclinical services[10] that may be similarly applicable (**Table 1**). Telemedicine has been demonstrated to be successful in other pediatric use cases, including but not limited to pediatric psychiatry,[11] pediatric cardiology,[12] and pediatric endocrinology.[13] Despite this, there have been barriers to further implementation of telemedicine in both general pediatric and subspecialty care. Licensing requirements, provider interest, and training resources are among the greatest barriers identified in starting new pediatric telehealth programs,

Table 1
Common telehealth terms and definitions[52,53]

Terms	Definitions
Telehealth	Methods for enhancing health care, public health, or health education delivery and support using telecommunications technologies
Telemedicine	Delivery of health care services, by health care professionals using information and communication technologies to exchange of health information for diagnosis, treatment, and prevention of disease (synchronous)
Store and forward	Exchange of recorded patient health information between providers or between a patient and a provider (asynchronous)
Chat-based interactions	Online or mobile app communications that transmit a patient's personal health data, vital signs, diagnostic images, or other health data for a health care provider to review
Remote patient monitoring	Use of electronic devices to record a patient's health data for a provider to receive and evaluate at a later time
mHealth	Health-related applications and programs used on mobile phones and other smart devices

along with poor or nonexistent insurance reimbursement.[14] Additional barriers included policy issues (such as privacy and data security), personnel training, information quality, and service quality.[15] Determining how these potential barriers impact the implementation of telehealth programs in pediatric rheumatology would be of value to inform its future use, but to date, there have been relatively few studies of telemedicine use in pediatric rheumatology.

IMPACT OF HEALTH POLICY ON TELEMEDICINE USE

Health policy, both at a national level and state level (within the United States), has directly impacted the utilization of telemedicine services. In 1996, the Health Insurance Portability and Accountability Act (HIPAA) was enacted to protect personal health information (PHI) but the HIPAA Privacy Rule, enacted in 2000, established national standards to how personal medical records, health care clearinghouses, and providers conduct health care transactions electronically.[16] In 2009, the Health Information Technology for Economic and Clinical Health (HITECH) Act accelerated the use of health information technologies and encouraged adoption of the electronic health record (EHR) to improve interoperability, reduce health care costs, and improve patient care and outcomes (see Chapter X: "Using the Electronic Health Record in Pediatric Rheumatology" in this issue).[17] In addition, 2020 was a year notable for many changes in health care delivery and health care policy. Owing to the COVID-19 Public Health Emergency Declaration, HIPAA flexibilities allowed for providers to use popular video chat applications to deliver care and waivers set provisions for practicing across state lines, allowing patients to receive care in their home location, and providing reimbursement for new and established patient visits alike.[18] With the passage of these policies, we have seen an unparalleled growth of telehealth services and rapid expansion of telemedicine to support direct patient to provider care in multiple settings including inpatient, urgent care, general pediatric, and pediatric subspecialty care.[19]

From a policy standpoint, there remains some uncertainty about whether national regulatory policies will remain or change following the COVID-19 pandemic. There have been varying recommendations for policymakers and insurers regarding reimbursement criteria, billing codes, and payment models, and incentivizing patient-centered telehealth technologies.[20] In addition, there is a need for ongoing evaluation of telemedicine[21] focusing on quality and safety measures.[22] The American College of Rheumatology (ACR) recently put forth a telemedicine policy statement that supports the ongoing use of telemedicine as a part of clinical care, but also notes the importance of studying the clinical outcomes of remote care.[23] Pediatric rheumatologists must pay close attention to these policies, and advocate for legislative changes that may affect their ability to provide virtual care to their patients with pediatric rheumatic disease.

"VIRTUALIZABILITY" OF PEDIATRIC RHEUMATOLOGY CARE

In addition to institutional and legislative barriers, pediatric rheumatologists have long been concerned about the ability to conduct telemedicine visits with their patients that are of high quality, which also appropriately and safely assess the clinical status of patients. A recent Childhood Arthritis and Rheumatology Research Alliance (CARRA) survey on the use of telemedicine during the COVID-19 pandemic found that 65.7% of pediatric rheumatologists felt they were not able to elicit all the information needed to make a clinical assessment on a telemedicine visit.[24] Another study found that pediatric rheumatologists' main concerns regarding adopting telemedicine in practice included being able to perform an accurate physical examination (including a musculoskeletal examination), obtaining vital signs, communication issues between the provider and patient, difficulties obtaining laboratories or imaging quickly when there is an urgent clinical need, and being able to provide ancillary needs such as nursing or social work support at the time of the visit.[25] Other pediatric-specific considerations include adolescent confidentiality,[26] ability to conduct pubertal and/or developmental examinations,[27] and being able to collaborate with families/caregivers in the health care process.[28]

Despite these concerns, pediatric rheumatologists recognize the great potential of telemedicine to address the pressing access issues. Patient/family burdens—including the expense and time needed to travel, work time, and school time lost (of particular importance in pediatric chronic care)—have been shown to decrease with the utilization of telemedicine for pediatric rheumatology follow-up visits.[29] It has also been found that although patients and caregivers may initially prefer in-person pediatric rheumatology clinic visits, as familiarity with telemedicine increased, so did patient and caregiver acceptability of this care modality.[30] However, although there may be clear advantages in terms of patient access and time and cost-savings associated with telemedicine care, there is currently very limited data on the quality of these visits and reliability of the physical examination (especially the musculoskeletal examination) in pediatric rheumatology care.

HOW TO ADAPT TELEMEDICINE TO PEDIATRIC RHEUMATOLOGY CARE

As discussed earlier, the COVID-19 pandemic resulted in the sudden deployment of telemedicine visits across the United States and abroad. Pediatric rheumatologists and patients were forced to rapidly adapt to this modality of care. In doing so, the need for additional research and guidance regarding best practices for telemedicine in pediatric rheumatology has become glaringly apparent. This includes providing telemedicine-specific training for providers, clinical staff, and patient/families, identifying visit types and patient factors that can result in successful telemedicine visits, generating models/algorithms that may automate these processes, and adapting the musculoskeletal examination (a critical component of many pediatric rheumatology visits) and other physical examination components for virtual care.

The patient-provider relationship is of particular importance as it may affect health outcomes. It is known that among vulnerable patients, such as those who are uninsured, having a good relationship with their provider allows patients to help make clinical decisions in line with their preferences.[31] In addition, relational factors between providers and caregivers/patients may influence shared-decision making in the clinical setting.[32] It is not known specifically how telemedicine influences the relationship between provider and patient or provider and caregiver, but best practices that foster physician connection with their patients should be created and implemented in all pediatric rheumatology telemedicine visits. Recently, a set of clinician practices that promote humanism and meaningful connection during virtual encounters, the "Tele-Presence 5," has been proposed to do just this (**Fig. 1**). Adopting this or a similar best practice in pediatric chronic care telemedicine visits should be considered.

Presently, there are no specific guidelines as to which pediatric rheumatology patients should be seen in-person or through telemedicine visits. It is often at the discretion of the provider or patient/family, and is partially influenced by institutional or regional practices. In a recent CARRA-wide survey of pediatric rheumatologists,[24] most providers felt that urgent visits were generally best suited for in-person visits, but there was no overall consensus regarding other visit types (eg, new patient consultations/visits, injection teaching). As pediatric rheumatology continues to move

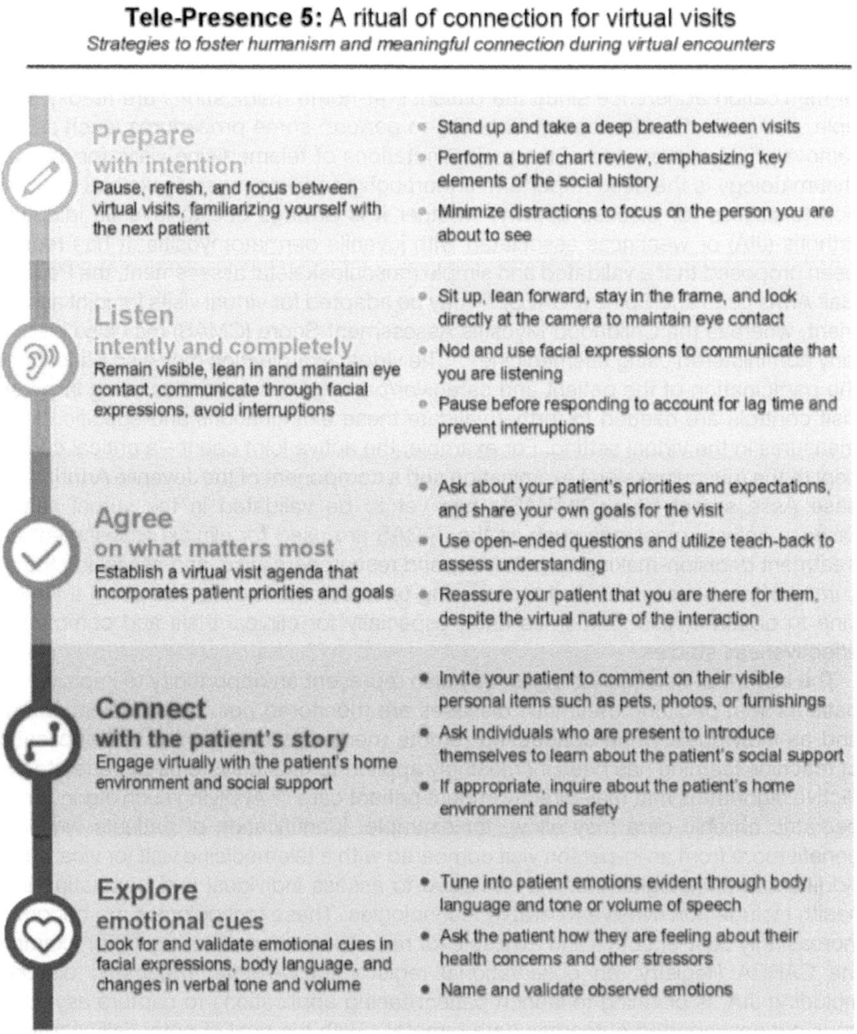
Tele-Presence 5: A ritual of connection for virtual visits
Strategies to foster humanism and meaningful connection during virtual encounters
Prepare
with intention
Pause, refresh, and focus between virtual visits, familiarizing yourself with the next patient
Stand up and take a deep breath between visits
Perform a brief chart review, emphasizing key elements of the social history
Minimize distractions to focus on the person you are about to see
Listen
intently and completely
Remain visible, lean in and maintain eye contact, communicate through facial expressions, avoid interruptions
Sit up, lean forward, stay in the frame, and look directly at the camera to maintain eye contact
Nod and use facial expressions to communicate that you are listening
Pause before responding to account for lag time and prevent interruptions
Agree
on what matters most
Establish a virtual visit agenda that incorporates patient priorities and goals
Ask about your patient's priorities and expectations, and share your own goals for the visit
Use open-ended questions and utilize teach-back to assess understanding
Reassure your patient that you are there for them, despite the virtual nature of the interaction
Connect
with the patient's story
Engage virtually with the patient's home environment and social support
Invite your patient to comment on their visible personal items such as pets, photos, or furnishings
Ask individuals who are present to introduce themselves to learn about the patient's social support
If appropriate, inquire about the patient's home environment and safety
Explore
emotional cues
Look for and validate emotional cues in facial expressions, body language, and changes in verbal tone and volume
Tune into patient emotions evident through body language and tone or volume of speech
Ask the patient how they are feeling about their health concerns and other stressors
Name and validate observed emotions

Fig. 1. From Tele-Presence 5 https://med.stanford.edu/presence/initiatives/stanford-presence-5/tele-presence-5.html. These recommendations for virtual visits were adapted from Zulman DM & Verghese A, et al. Practices to foster physician presence and connection with patients in the clinical encounter. JAMA 2020; 323(1):70-81.

forward with virtual care, we will need to define the following: (1) determining when it is advantageous to supplement virtual care with traditional in-person clinical visits; (2) automating scheduling processes to promote efficiency; (3) ensuring safety and avoid harm for our patients participating in virtual care; (4) ensuring social equity in telemedicine; and (5) determining which outcome measures should be used when assessing the quality of telemedicine visits. It has been previously proposed that the application of machine learning to real-life digital health interventions may hold some promise in improving health care delivery processes[33,34] such as telemedicine, but pediatric rheumatologists will still need to define specific quality and safety measures in order for such technologies to be usefully applied to our patient population.

For many specialties, the telemedicine platform may actually provide additional information to the provider that may not be available during in-person visits; a recent study demonstrated that these novel adaptations can include improved assessment of medication adherence since the patient's at-home medications are readily available, and patient and/or caregiver ability to perform some procedures (such as cast removal).[35] However, one of the major limitations of telemedicine visits for pediatric rheumatology is the need to perform a thorough hands-on musculoskeletal examination to assess for disease activity, whether it is arthritis due to juvenile idiopathic arthritis (JIA) or weakness associated with juvenile dermatomyositis. It has recently been proposed that a validated and simple musculoskeletal assessment, the Pediatric Gait Arms Legs and Spine (pGALS),[36] may be adapted for virtual visits for joint assessment, whereas the Childhood Myositis Assessment Score (CMAS) may also be similarly administered using telemedicine.[37] The virtual examination may also benefit from the participation of the patient and caregiver/parent. Further studies using in-person visit controls are needed to further validate these examinations and specific clinical measures in the virtual setting. For example, the active joint count—a critical component of the musculoskeletal examination and a component of the Juvenile Arthritis Disease Assessment Score (JADAS)—has yet to be validated in the virtual setting. Disease activity measures such as the JADAS are used for clinical assessment and treatment decision-making by providers and researchers alike, and assessing the accuracy of such measures performed using telemedicine is critical to using telemedicine to obtain clinical outcomes data, especially for clinical trials and comparative effectiveness studies.

The advent of new technologies may also represent an opportunity to improve how patients with pediatric rheumatic diseases are monitored both on a population level and as individuals when conducting remote medical assessments. The application of machine learning has been increasingly applied to health systems to generate predictive algorithms that may directly impact patient care.[38] Applying such algorithms in pediatric chronic care may allow, for example, identification of patients who may benefit more from an in-person visit compared with a telemedicine visit (or vice versa). Additional technologies that may be used to assess individual and population-level health include noninvasive wearable technologies. These technologies are becoming increasingly cost-effective and available for remote-health monitoring.[39] For example, the CARRA Registry, an observational registry for pediatric rheumatic diseases including JIA, is planning to launch patient-facing applications to capture asynchronous patient-reported outcomes data remotely, with the goal of potentially capturing additional clinical data between in-person and telemedicine clinical visits. There are also increasing use cases for the support of a remote examination with a joint range of motion.[40,41] Pediatric rheumatologists may be able to use such technologies to improve the accuracy of a remote musculoskeletal examination in the future.

TELEMEDICINE OUTCOMES

A critical issue for pediatric rheumatology and health systems, in general, is that there are no universally applied quality measures for telemedicine visits. Institutional frameworks have suggested evaluating domains such as clinical quality and safety when evaluating institutional digital health programs. The American Academy of Pediatrics Section on Telehealth Care's SPROUT (Supporting Pediatric Research in Outcomes and Utilization of Telehealth) has conceptualized a telehealth evaluation profile that focuses on 4 measurement domains: (1) health outcomes, (2) health delivery (quality and cost), (3) experience, and (4) program implementation and key performance indicators.[42] Pediatric rheumatologists must begin to define specialty-specific quality measures that may be applied in our patient population. This could include using disease activity measures such as the Systemic Lupus Erythematous Disease Activity Index (SLEDAI) or Juvenile Arthritis Disease Activity Score (JADAS) to evaluate the impact of telemedicine on disease activity. Definitions of telemedicine failures could include criteria for "near misses" (patients who were seen via telemedicine but then subsequently needed to be seen urgently or in the emergency room before their next regularly scheduled appointment) or "telemedicine failures" (patients who were admitted following a telemedicine visit due to suboptimal evaluation during a telehealth session). These are not currently used outcome measures, but could be considered in evaluating the impact of telemedicine on the quality of clinical visits in pediatric chronic care.

PATIENT ADAPTATIONS TO TELEMEDICINE

Caregiver involvement, as well as patient perception and participation in virtual visits, are important aspects of pediatric rheumatology and chronic pediatric care in general. Previous evaluations of the caregiver perception of telemedicine visits in pediatric rheumatology were unfavorable, but at the time of that study, only 8% of those surveyed had familiarity with telemedicine.[30] A more recent study evaluating the patient and caregiver experience of telemedicine in pediatric subspecialty care (including pediatric rheumatology) illustrated that although many patients and caregivers found both monetary and nonmonetary value in telemedicine, virtual visits did introduce a new role for the caregiver with a new set of expectations.[43] This new role includes the ability, and responsibility, of the parent/caregiver to be able to report vital signs, details of the physical examination and other pertinent clinical information to their provider. As we continue to move forward with telemedicine as a part of pediatric rheumatology practice, we will need to find ways to provide patients and their caregivers with clear guidance and expectations for the virtual examination and visit. This may include best practices, examination guides for the musculoskeletal examination, previsit questionnaires that include documentation of critical data elements including vitals or other measurements, and other at-home tools that can be used to improve the clinical assessment when conducting virtual visits. Using the patient/parent partnerships in pediatric rheumatology research and quality improvement networks such as CARRA and PR-COIN (Pediatric Rheumatology Care & Outcomes Improvement Network) to help develop these tools is more critical now than ever.

IMPACT OF TELEMEDICINE ON PEDIATRIC RHEUMATOLOGY RESEARCH

The COVID-19 pandemic also had unintended consequences on clinical research. Many of these changes had to do with how resources were allocated (eg, suspension of research during the pandemic because of overwhelming clinical needs and institution of antiviral protocols), while others were functional due to shifting away from in-person study team and patient visits.[44] Other unintended consequences on the research included difficulty collecting patient-reported outcomes and complete data (including a musculoskeletal assessment) necessary for disease activity assessments (such as the Juvenile Arthritis Disease Activity Score or the Systemic Lupus Disease Activity Index) during telehealth visits. The reluctance of patients and families to go to the hospital for clinical visits also impacted clinical trial and registry visits, biospecimen collection and laboratory testing for safety monitoring and disease assessment. Although one study suggested that the COVID-19 pandemic may have accelerated and improved remote monitoring in clinical studies through the use of telehealth and other e-technologies,[45] a recent survey among PR-COIN sites found that very few sites were able to collect patient-reported outcomes, specifically survey measures such as the Childhood Health Assessment Questionnaire (CHAQ) or Patient-Reported Outcomes Measurement Information System (PROMIS) measures for visits conducted via telemedicine.[46] Although this may initially appear to be a discouraging statistic, this turn toward remote medicine represents an opportunity to develop strategies that will eventually improve research methods and enable researchers to reach and enroll more patients remotely for clinical studies, and to improve remote data collection. This will be critical for all pediatric rheumatology research. Indeed, there are initiatives underway to be able to use applications to remotely collect patient-reported outcomes data as well as developing clinical informatics tools to be able to integrate electronic health record (EHR) into clinical research (see EHR chapter).

IMPACT OF TELEMEDICINE ON HEALTH DISPARITIES AND PEDIATRIC RHEUMATOLOGY CARE

Although telemedicine has the ability to increase access by decreasing travel time and time lost from school and work for many patients and families, its inherent reliance on technology may introduce new vulnerabilities and exacerbate disparities in care for many pediatric patients and their families.[47] Difficulties accessing the needed technology—ranging from availability of high-speed Internet[48] to access to necessary hardware[49,50] to digital health literacy[51]—may impact segments of the patient population and introduce new gaps in care. Given the promise that telemedicine holds for promoting access to pediatric rheumatologists for many patients, we need to be able to use telemedicine without introducing new disparities in health care.

SUMMARY

There is great potential in the implementation of telemedicine programs for pediatric rheumatology. Further research is needed to fully assess its impact on clinical outcomes, research, and health disparities. Continued assessment of patient and parental acceptability of this digital health care delivery model is of the utmost importance. We must also consider the overall goals and impact of telemedicine use in pediatric rheumatology and ensure that such programs are designed to increase health care access and promote social equity. We are in a unique situation because of the pandemic to be able to learn from our early experiences of telemedicine programs and must leverage this opportunity to expand the reach of pediatric rheumatology care and research to our patients.

CLINICS CARE POINTS

- Telemedicine may be a valuable health care delivery tool for clinicians to reach patients remotely and increase access, but more studies are needed to evaluate its impact on clinical outcomes and health disparities.
- There is a need to develop quality and safety measures for the use of telemedicine programs in pediatric rheumatology.
- Patient and parent acceptability must be considered in telemedicine programs in pediatric rheumatology care.

DISCLOSURE

The authors have nothing to disclose.

REFERENCES

1. MehrotraAteev, RayKristin MB,LB, Anne B. Rapidly converting to "virtual practices": outpatient care in the era of covid-19. NEJM catalyst innovations in care delivery. 2020. Available at: https://catalyst.nejm.org/doi/full/10.1056/CAT.20.0091. Accessed February 28 2021.
2. CDC. Healthcare Workers. Centers for disease control and prevention. 2020. Available at: https://www.cdc.gov/coronavirus/2019-ncov/hcp/guidance-hcf.html. Accessed February 28 2021.
3. Telehealth Basics [Internet]. ATA. Available at: https://www.americantelemed.org/resource/why-telemedicine/. Accessed February 27 2021.
4. Future challenges in pediatric rheumatology: the role of Graduate Medical Education (GME) [Internet]. ACR Meeting Abstracts. Available at: https://acrabstracts.org/abstract/future-challenges-in-pediatric-rheumatology-the-role-of-graduate-medical-education-gme/. Accessed February 27 2021.
5. Totten AM, McDonagh MS, Wagner JH. The evidence base for telehealth: reassurance in the face of rapid expansion during the COVID-19 pandemic [Internet]. Rockville (MD): Agency for Healthcare Research and Quality (US); 2020 (AHRQ Methods for Effective Health Care). Available at: http://www.ncbi.nlm.nih.gov/books/NBK557174/. Accessed February 28 2021.
6. Henrickson M. Policy challenges for the pediatric rheumatology workforce: Part II. Health care system delivery and workforce supply. Pediatr Rheumatol 2011;9(1):24. Available at: https://doi.org/10.1186/1546-0096-9-23. Accessed July 23, 2020.
7. Mayer ML, Mellins ED, Sandborg CI. Access to pediatric rheumatology care in the United States. Arthritis Care & Research 2003;49(6):759–65. Available at: https://onlinelibrary.wiley.com/doi/abs/10.1002/art.11462. Accessed February 28 2019.
8. Lennep DS, Crout T, Majithia V. Rural health issues in rheumatology: a review. Curr Opin Rheumatol 2020;32(2):119–25. Available from: https://journals.lww.com/10.1097/BOR.0000000000000694. Accessed February 13, 2021.
9. Majerowicz A, Tracy S. Telemedicine: Bridging Gaps in Healthcare Delivery. J AHIMA 2010;81(5):52–53,56. Available at: http://library.ahima.org/doc?oid=100028. Accessed February 13, 2021.
10. What is telehealth? How is telehealth different from telemedicine? | HealthIT.gov [Internet]. Available at: https://www.healthit.gov/faq/what-telehealth-how-telehealth-different-telemedicine. Accessed February 13, 2021.
11. Thomas JF, Novins DK, Hosokawa PW, et al. The use of telepsychiatry to provide cost-efficient care during pediatric mental health emergencies. Psychiatr Serv 2018;69(2):161–8.
12. Maia MR, Castela E, Pires A, et al. How to develop a sustainable telemedicine service? A Pediatric Telecardiology Service 20 years on - an exploratory study. BMC Health Serv Res 2019;19. Available at: https://www.ncbi.nlm.nih.gov/pmc/articles/PMC6757431/. Accessed November 3 2020.
13. Prahalad P, Tanenbaum M, Hood K, et al. Diabetes technology: improving care, improving patient-reported outcomes and preventing complications in young people with Type 1 diabetes. Diabet Med 2018;35(4):419–29. Available at:

https://onlinelibrary.wiley.com/doi/abs/10.1111/dme.13588. Accessed February 13 2021.

14. Olson CA, McSwain SD, Curfman AL, et al. The current pediatric telehealth Landscape. Pediatrics 2018;141(3). Available at: https://pediatrics.aappublications.org/content/141/3/e20172334. Accessed October 28 2020.
15. Burke BL, Hall RW. Care the SOT. Telemedicine: pediatric applications. Pediatrics 2015;136(1):e293–308. Available at: https://pediatrics.aappublications.org/content/136/1/e293. Accessed October 23 2020.
16. Security and HIPAA | AAAAI [Internet]. The American Academy of Allergy, Asthma & Immunology. Available at: https://www.aaaai.org/practice-resources/running-your-practice/practice-management-resources/Telemedicine/HIPAA. Accessed February 13 2021.
17. Doarn CR, Pruitt S, Jacobs J, et al. Federal Efforts to define and advance telehealth—a work in progress. Telemed J E Health 2014;20(5):409–18. Available from: https://www.ncbi.nlm.nih.gov/pmc/articles/PMC4011485/. Accessed February 13 2021.
18. Policy changes during <span class="text-no-wrap">COVID-19</span> | Telehealth.HHS.gov [Internet]. Available at: https://telehealth.hhs.gov/providers/policy-changes-during-the-covid-19-public-health-emergency/. Accessed February 13 2021.
19. Mann DM, Chen J, Chunara R, et al. COVID-19 transforms health care through telemedicine: evidence from the field. J Am Med Inform Assoc 2020. Available from: https://www.ncbi.nlm.nih.gov/pmc/articles/PMC7188161/. Accessed May 18 2020.
20. Five ways—beyond current policy—to truly integrate telehealth into primary care practices | health affairs blog [Internet]. Available at: https://www.healthaffairs.org/do/10.1377/hblog20200903.597561/full/. Accessed February 13, 2021.
21. Chang H. Evaluation framework for telemedicine using the logical framework approach and a fishbone diagram. Healthc Inform Res 2015;21(4):230–8.
22. Telehealth should be expanded—if it can address today's health care challenges | health affairs [Internet]. Available at: https://www.healthaffairs.org/do/10.1377/hblog20200916.264569/full/?utm_medium=email&utm_source=hat&utm_campaign=blog&utm_content=agrawal&. Accessed September 27, 2020.
23. The ACR releases new telemedicine position statement [Internet]. The rheumatologist. Available at: https://www.the-rheumatologist.org/article/the-acr-releases-new-telemedicine-position-statement/. Accessed February 13, 2021.
24. Pooni R, Ronis T, Lee T. Telemedicine Use by pediatric rheumatologists during the COVID-19 pandemic. Pediatr Rheumatol Online J 2021;19(1):93.
25. Pooni R, Sandborg C, Lee T. Building a viable telemedicine presence in pediatric rheumatology. Pediatr Clin North Am 2020;67(4):641–5.
26. Carlson JL, Goldstein R. Using the electronic health record to conduct adolescent telehealth visits in the time of COVID-19. J Adolesc Health 2020;67(2):157–8. Available at: https://www.ncbi.nlm.nih.gov/pmc/articles/PMC7275171/. Accessed November 10, 2020.
27. Regelmann MO, Conroy R, Gourgari E, et al. Pediatric endocrinology in the time of COVID-19: considerations for the rapid implementation of telemedicine and management of pediatric endocrine Conditions. Horm Res Paediatr 2020;93(6):343–50. Available at: https://www.karger.com/Article/FullText/513060. Accessed February 13 2021.
28. Sauers-Ford HS, Hamline MY, Gosdin MM, et al. Acceptability, usability, and effectiveness: a qualitative study evaluating a pediatric telemedicine program.

Acad Emerg Med 2019;26(9):1022–33. Available at: https://www.onlinelibrary.wiley.com/doi/abs/10.1111/acem.13763. Accessed February 13 2021.
29. Kessler EA, Sherman AK, Becker ML. Decreasing patient cost and travel time through pediatric rheumatology telemedicine visits. Pediatr Rheumatol Online J 2016;14. Available at: https://www.ncbi.nlm.nih.gov/pmc/articles/PMC5029100/. Accessed August 6 2019.
30. Bullock DR, Vehe RK, Zhang L, et al. Telemedicine and other care models in pediatric rheumatology: an exploratory study of parents' perceptions of barriers to care and care preferences. Pediatr Rheumatol Online J 2017;15. Available from: https://www.ncbi.nlm.nih.gov/pmc/articles/PMC5504634/. Accessed August 6 2019.
31. Kamimura A, Higham R, Rathi N, et al. Patient-provider relationships among vulnerable patients: the association with health literacy, continuity of care, and self-rated health. J Patient Exp 2020;7(6):1450–7.
32. Boland L, Graham ID, Légaré F, et al. Barriers and facilitators of pediatric shared decision-making: a systematic review. Implement Sci 2019;14(1):7. Available at: https://doi.org/10.1186/s13012-018-0851-5. Accessed September 29, 2020.
33. Triantafyllidis AK, Tsanas A. Applications of machine learning in real-life digital health interventions: review of the literature. J Med Internet Res 2019;21(4):e12286.
34. Smith M, Sattler A, Hong G, et al. From code to bedside: implementing artificial intelligence using quality improvement methods. J Gen Intern Med 2021. Available at: https://doi.org/10.1007/s11606-020-06394-w. Accessed February 14, 2021.
35. Pooni R, Pageler NM, Sandborg C, et al. Pediatric subspecialty telemedicine use from the patient and provider perspective. Pediatr Res. 2021 Mar 22:1–6. doi: 10.1038/s41390-021-01443-4.
36. Foster HE, Jandial S. pGALS - paediatric gait arms legs and spine: a simple examination of the musculoskeletal system. Pediatr Rheumatol Online J 2013;11(1):44.
37. Shenoi S, Hayward K, Curran ML, et al. Telemedicine in pediatric rheumatology: this is the time for the community to embrace a new way of clinical practice. Pediatr Rheumatol Online J 2020;18(1):85.
38. Mortazavi BJ, Downing NS, Bucholz EM, et al. Analysis of machine learning techniques for heart failure readmissions. Circ Cardiovasc Qual Outcomes 2016;9(6):629–40.
39. Majumder S, Mondal T, Deen MJ. Wearable Sensors for remote health monitoring. Sensors (Basel) 2017;17(1). Available from: https://www.ncbi.nlm.nih.gov/pmc/articles/PMC5298703/. Accessed February 27, 2021.
40. Ramkumar PN, Haeberle HS, Navarro SM, et al. Mobile technology and telemedicine for shoulder range of motion: validation of a motion-based machine-learning software development kit. J Shoulder Elbow Surg 2018;27(7):1198–204.
41. Bell KM, Onyeukwu C, McClincy MP, et al. Verification of a portable motion tracking system for remote management of physical rehabilitation of the knee. Sensors (Basel) 2019;19(5):1021.
42. Chuo J, Macy ML, Lorch SA. Strategies for evaluating telehealth. Pediatrics 2020;146(5). Available at: https://pediatrics.aappublications.org/content/146/5/e20201781. Accessed February 15, 2021.
43. Pooni R, Pageler NM, Khalsa U, et al. Pediatric Subspecialty use of Telemedicine during COVID-19: The Patient and Caregiver Perspective (unpublished data).

44. Tuttle KR. Impact of the COVID-19 pandemic on clinical research. Nat Rev Nephrol 2020;16(10):562–4. Available at: https://www.nature.com/articles/s41581-020-00336-9. Accessed Feb 15 2021.
45. COVID-19 and its impact on the future of clinical trial Execution [Internet]. Applied Clinical Trials Online. Available from: https://www.appliedclinicaltrialsonline.com/view/covid-19-and-its-impact-on-the-future-of-clinical-trial-execution. Accessed February 15, 2021.
46. Goh I, Bullock D, Taylor J, et al. Exploring pediatric Tele-rheumatology practices during COVID-19: A Survey of the PRCOIN Network. Front Pediatr 2021;9:642460.
47. Katzow MW, Steinway C, Jan S. Telemedicine and health disparities during COVID-19. Pediatrics 2020;146(2). Available at: https://pediatrics.aappublications.org/content/146/2/e20201586. Accessed February 15, 2021.
48. Wilcock AD, Rose S, Busch AB, et al. Association between broadband internet availability and telemedicine use. JAMA Intern Med 2019;179(11):1580–2. Available at: https://www.ncbi.nlm.nih.gov/pmc/articles/PMC6664376/. Accessed February 15, 2021.
49. Smith WR, Atala AJ, Terlecki RP, et al. Implementation guide for rapid integration of an outpatient telemedicine program during the COVID-19 Pandemic. J Am Coll Surg 2020;231(2):216–22.e2. Available at: https://www.ncbi.nlm.nih.gov/pmc/articles/PMC7192116/. Accessed April 13, 2021.
50. Eberly LA, Kallan MJ, Julien HM, et al. Patient characteristics associated with telemedicine access for primary and specialty ambulatory care during the COVID-19 Pandemic. JAMA Netw Open 2020;3(12). Available at. https://www.ncbi.nlm.nih.gov/pmc/articles/PMC7772717/. Accessed April 13, 2021.
51. Smith B, Magnani JW. New technologies, new disparities: the intersection of electronic health and digital health literacy. Int J Cardiol 2019;292:280–2. Available from: https://www.ncbi.nlm.nih.gov/pmc/articles/PMC6660987/. Accessed February 15, 2021.
52. Telehealth Basics [Internet]. ATA. Available at: https://www.americantelemed.org/resource/why-telemedicine/. Accessed February 27, 2021.
53. CDC. Telehealth Interventions to improve chronic disease | cdc.gov [Internet]. Centers for Disease Control and Prevention. 2020. Available at: https://www.cdc.gov/dhdsp/pubs/telehealth.htm. Accessed February 27, 2021.

Biomarkers in Childhood-Onset Systemic Lupus Erythematosus

Ellen M. Cody, MD[a,*], Hermine I. Brunner, MD, MSc, MBA[b]

KEYWORDS

• Biomarkers • Pediatric • Lupus • SLE • Childhood-onset SLE

KEY POINTS

- Current markers of disease activity for lupus, particularly lupus nephritis, are inadequate, prompting research into new biomarkers.
- Of the many single urinary protein biomarkers of lupus nephritis studied, all lack the sensitivity or specificity to replace a kidney biopsy. Current studies are moving toward combinatorial urinary biomarker panels.
- Newer biomarkers are based on the pathogenesis of lupus, such as neutrophil extracellular traps , microRNA, and changes in gene methylation.

BACKGROUND

SLE (lupus) is a chronic autoimmune disease with substantial personal and public health impact. Lupus nephritis (LN) remains the most severe complication of SLE, accounting for sizable morbidity, mortality, and end-stage renal disease (ESRD).[1] SLE with onset in adolescence or younger is termed cSLE.[2] The incidence and prevalence of SLE varies widely between populations, with higher disease prevalence observed among African American and Asian populations.[3,4] An estimated 20% of SLE cases commence during childhood, and renal involvement occurs in 50% to 70% of patients with cSLE, hence more common than in adult-onset SLE.[3,5] Notably, about 10% of children with proliferative LN progress to ESRD within 5 years of diagnosis.[3] Patients with cSLE tend to have more severe disease courses compared with adult-onset SLE, and this results in higher accumulation of disease- and therapy-related damage, especially chronic corticosteroid use.[3] The new 2019 American College of Rheumatology/European League against Rheumatism Classification Criteria for SLE can be applied

[a] Division of Pediatric Nephrology, Cincinnati Children's Hospital Medical Center, 3333 Burnet Avenue, MC 7022, Cincinnati, OH 45229-3930, USA; [b] Division of Rheumatology, Department of Pediatrics, Cincinnati Children's Hospital Medical Center, University of Cincinnati College of Medicine, 3333 Burnet Avenue, MC 4010, Cincinnati, OH 45229-3930, USA
* Corresponding author.
E-mail address: emcody13@gmail.com

Rheum Dis Clin N Am 48 (2022) 271–285
https://doi.org/10.1016/j.rdc.2021.09.003
rheumatic.theclinics.com

to cSLE and may assist with diagnosis.[6] Measures to track cSLE activity (or degree of inflammation) include clinical indices such as the SLE Disease Activity Index (SLEDAI) and the British Isles Lupus Activity Group index. For diagnosing LN specifically, kidney biopsies continue to be necessary. Currently available laboratory tests to estimate cSLE and LN activity include erythrocyte sedimentation rate; complement components C3 and C4, anti–double-stranded DNA antibodies, estimated glomerular filtration rate, urine sediment, and degree of proteinuria are all poor biomarkers.[1,3,7–9] It is important to note that early treatment improves the prognosis of LN, and there is a strong association between delayed diagnosis and higher incidence of ESRD.[10] Thus, there remains a critical need for new biomarkers to better diagnose, monitor response to therapy and relapse, and accurately assess clinical end points during trials. The current review provides a brief discussion on the frequently studied biomarkers and new biomarkers in cSLE.

DEFINING A BIOMARKER

The US Food and Drug Administration and National Institutes of Health (NIH) Biomarker Working Group defines a biomarker as "an indicator of normal biological processes, pathogenic processes, or biological responses to an exposure or intervention, including therapeutic interventions." There are numerous types of biomarkers depending on their intended application. Examples include diagnostic biomarkers, that is, those that support the diagnosis of a disease or disease process, and prognostic biomarkers, that is, biomarkers that are able to anticipate the future course of a disease.[11] The quality of a biomarker depends on whether it can be measured reliably, precisely, and repeatedly, with limited overlap between diseased and nondiseased status.[11,12] It is important for a biomarker to establish its clinical relevance and to study whether it can and serve as a surrogate for a clinical endpoint.[13] Advantages to using biomarkers, particularly in clinical trials, are that biomarkers can be measured repeatedly and more frequently than the primary endpoint, hence provide interim evidence about safety and efficacy of the intervention.[13]

Statistics for diagnostic tests such as receiver operator characteristic (ROC) curves can assess the quality of a biomarker. ROC curves plot the sensitivity for all possible values of specificity for the test results. The area under the ROC curve (AUC) summarizes the overall diagnostic accuracy of the test. An AUC of 1 represents a perfectly accurate test, and an AUC of 0.5 represents a test that does not discriminate patients with or without disease, whereas values of 0.7 to 0.8 are considered acceptable, 0.8 to 0.9 excellent, and greater than 0.9 outstanding, respectively.[14] Positive predictive value (PPV) and negative predictive value (NPV) of biomarker measurements provide additional estimates about the value of a biomarker, whereas correlation coefficients are sometimes used in support of biomarker adequacy.

LUPUS NEPHRITIS BIOMARKERS

Biomarker discovery focuses on renal disease, particularly in pediatrics, given the limited number of comorbid conditions, such as diabetes or primary hypertension that might affect the relationship between LN and biomarker measurements. Kidney biopsies are the gold standard for diagnosing and monitoring LN.[15] However, kidney biopsies are a costly, invasive, and painful procedure requiring sedation, with potential procedure-related complications such as hematoma, blood loss, and rarely, more severe sequelae.[16] Besides traditional measurement of albumin, various proteins excreted in the urine were evaluated for their potential to reflect the renal inflammatory milieu. **Table 1** summarizes the most studied proteins. Notably, no single biomarker

Table 1
Most studied proteins

Biomarker	Biological Function	Disease Association	Author	Combinatorial Panel
MCP-1/CCL2	• Recruitment of monocytes and lymphocytes to inflammation • Expressed by mesangial cells, podocytes, monocytes; Goilav et al,[42] 2015	• Active vs inactive nephritis • Poor renal outcomes • Distinguish ISN/RPS Classifications • Biopsy correlations: endocapillary hypercellularity, tubular cell flattening, necrosis, high LN-AI, high TIAI	Marks et al,[43] 2008 Watson et al,[44] 2012 Marks et al,[45] 2010 Brunner et al,[17] 2016 Smith et al,[18] 2017 Smith et al,[19] 2018	RAIL—Brunner et al,[17] 2016
NGAL	• Expressed in renal tubular cells follow ischemic or nephrotoxic injury • Seems to be a part of protective antiapoptotic mechanism to limit tubule damage and enhance proliferation; Brunner et al,[46] 2012	• LN vs no LN • Correlation between urinary levels of NGAL and severity of LN • Increase in urinary NGAL up to 3 mo before worsening of LN • Rapidly induced by active inflammation in LN, promptly declines with therapy • Predicts renal flare with higher sensitivity and specificity than dsDNA titers	Rubinstein et al,[47] 2010 Hammad et al,[48] 2013 Brunner et al,[49] 2006 Hinze et al,[50] 2009 Smith et al,[18] 2017 Smith et al,[19] 2018	RAIL—Brunner et al,[17] 2016
Ceruloplasmin	• Copper-containing ferroxidase that can transform ferrous iron, highly damaging to kidney tubules, high levels associated with renal tissue remodeling	• Differentiates active vs inactive LN • Correlates with SLEDAI-R score, mesangial proliferation, capillary proliferation, fibrinoid necrosis, biopsy activity index score • Differs between responders and nonresponders	Suzuki et al,[52] 2009 Brunner et al,[46] 2012 Brunner et al,[51] 2017 Smith et al,[18] 2017 Smith et al,[19] 2018	RAIL—Brunner et al,[17] 2016 EMD Smith et al,[18] 2017; Smith et al,[19] 2018; Smith et al,[20] 2019

(*continued on next page*)

Table 1
(*continued*)

Biomarker	Biological Function	Disease Association	Author	Combinatorial Panel
Transferrin	• Main iron-transporting protein in the blood, enters the glomerular filtrate • Retrieved by specific receptor-mediated uptake in kidney tubular system, so tubular injury will lead to increased urinary TF concentration; Brunner et al,[46] 2012	• Increased as early as 3 mo before a flare • Differentiates LN vs non-LN • Increased in those with high NIH-AI • Associated with mesangial proliferation, capillary proliferation, cellular crescents, and biopsy index score • Differs between responders and nonresponders	Suzuki et al,[52] 2009 Brunner et al,[46] 2012 Brunner et al,[51] 2017 Smith et al,[18] 2017 Smith et al,[19] 2018	EMD Smith et al,[18] 2017; Smith et al,[19] 2018; Smith et al,[20] 2019
AGP[a]	• Produced by epithelial cells • Thought to play role in regulating dynamic properties of glomerular capillary wall by reducing permeability toward macromolecules such as albumin; Brunner et al,[46] 2012	• Differentiates LN vs no LN • Increased as early as 3 mo before a flare • Increased in those with high TIAI • Correlates with SLEDAI-R score, mesangial proliferation, cellular crescents, biopsy activity index score • Differs between responders and nonresponders	Suzuki et al,[52] 2009 Brunner et al,[46] 2012 Smith et al,[18] 2017 Smith et al,[19] 2018	EMD Smith et al,[18] 2017; Smith et al,[19] 2018; Smith et al,[20] 2019
LPGDS[b]	• Involved in nitric oxide regulation and induction of apoptosis in the kidney	• Significantly different between active and inactive LN urine • Increased at least 3 mo before worsening clinical LN • Markedly elevated in urine of patients whose biopsy showed endocapillary hypercellularity • Correlates with SLEDAI-R score	Suzuki et al,[52] 2009 Brunner et al,[51] 2017 Smith et al,[18] 2017 Smith et al,[19] 2018	EMD Smith et al,[18] 2017; Smith et al,[19] 2018; Smith et al,[20] 2019

		• Marked difference in response status for pure class V LN; Brunner et al,[51] 2017		
Adiponectin	• Present on endothelium of intrarenal vasculature • Has antiinflammatory properties • Urinary concentrations increase with kidney injury	• Differs with active LN vs active non-LN lupus • Good accuracy for predicting LN damage status • Increased in the urine with both high NIH-AI and TIAI	Brunner et al,[53] 2019	RAIL—Brunner et al,[17] 2016
VCAM-1	• Cell surface protein, mediates adherence of inflammatory cells to target cells • Found to be elevated in murine models of LN, particularly in endothelial cells, cortical tubules, and glomerular cells	• Limited individual studies in children • Significantly higher in LN vs no LN • Adult studies have shown higher levels of VCAM-1 in active vs inactive LN, as well as activity status, and correlation to renal pathology activity index	Smith et al,[18] 2017 Smith et al,[19] 2018 Gasparin et al,[54] 2020 Singh et al,[55] 2012	

Abbreviations: dsDNA, double stranded DNA; MCP-1, monocyte chemoattractant protein 1; NGAL, neutrophil gelatinase–associated lipocalin; NIH-AI, National Institutes of Health activity index; RAIL, renal activity index of lupus; TF, transferrin; TIAI, tubulointerstitial activity index; VCAM, vascular cell adhesion molecule 1.

[a] A-1 acid glycoprotein.

[b] Lipocalin-type prostaglandin D synthase.

has emerged consistently to be of high quality to better diagnose and monitor cSLE, particularly LN.[10]

COMBINATORIAL BIOMARKER PANELS FOR LUPUS NEPHRITIS

Combinations of biomarkers improve the accuracy with which a disease process can be estimated. Examples include complete blood count, where low hemoglobin in combination with a high RDW and a low MCV is suggestive of iron deficiency anemia. However, low hemoglobin alone does not differentiate acute hemorrhage or thalassemia from iron deficiency.

The renal activity index of lupus (RAIL) is an algorithm calculated from the urine concentrations of 6 combinatorial biomarkers. They are monocyte chemoattractant protein 1 (MCP-1), neutrophil gelatinase–associated lipocalin (NGAL), kidney inflammation molecule 1 (KIM-1), adiponectin, ceruloplasmin, and hemopexin. These urinary proteins best predicted tubulointerstitial activity index status and NIH activity index (NIH-AI) status, with an RAIL score greater than or equal to 0.39 correctly identifying 90% of all cases with high LN-activity as defined by an NIH-AI score of 10 or higher, with a false-positive rate of 14%.[17]

Another proposed urinary biomarker panel consists of alpha-1-acid glycoprotein (AGP), ceruloplasmin (CP), lipocalin-like prostaglandin D synthase (LPGDS), and transferrin (TF). Assessed in combination, these biomarkers when used in patients with biopsy-proven LN had an AUC of 0.920 in the discovery cohort (UK JSLE Cohort), 0.991 in the validation cohort (Einstein Lupus Cohort), with no additional improvement of accuracy from the addition of MCP-1 or vascular cell adhesion molecule 1 (VCAM-1). Urinary TF and NGAL did not differentiate patients with active LN from those with inactive LN.[18] On repeat validation in another (South African Pediatric Lupus Cohort), the biomarker panel performed perfectly (AUC of 1) in that higher levels of each individual urinary biomarker were present in active LN (AGP, ceruloplasmin, LPGDS, transferrin and VCAM-1). There was no difference between the MCP-1 levels in patients with active LN and those with inactive LN.[19] The group further evaluated the biomarkers longitudinally and demonstrated that AGP was best suited to predict upcoming LN flares, and CP was the single best biomarker to anticipate renal remission.[20]

Koutsonikoli and colleagues[7] investigated 4 potential serum biomarkers in children with LN for their association to renal and extra renal disease activity, namely antibodies against nucleosomes (NCS), C1q, glomerular basement membrane (GBM), and serum high-mobility group box 1 protein (HMGB1). All 4 biomarkers were significantly more abundant in patients with LN than healthy controls or patients without LN. HMGB1 levels correlated with LN activity, with a PPV of 64.3% and an NPV of 100%. The combination of anti-NCS, anti-GBM, and HMGB1 had a PPV of 92.9% in predicting the presence of LN in cSLE.

CLINICAL USE OF URINARY BIOMARKERS

Currently, the only urinary biomarkers approved for clinical use in lupus are urinalysis and urine protein to creatinine ratio. However, several novel urine biomarkers, including cystatin-C, NGAL, and KIM-1, that are investigated in LN have been approved for surveillance of other kidney diseases. Achieving biomarker qualification of some or several of the proposed LN biomarker panels requires large validation studies, best done in the context of clinical trials. Progress to move RAIL biomarkers into clinical use has been achieved with the development of novel LUMINEX multiplex assay that allows for the measurement of most of the RAIL biomarkers within 24 hours.[21]

PATHOPHYSIOLOGY-BASED BIOMARKERS

Research into the pathogenesis of cSLE has highlighted the role of environmental exposures in the setting of genetic predisposition to trigger autoimmunity that ultimately results in the clinical presentation of cSLE as demonstrated in **Fig. 1**.[22] Particularly, studies of the dysregulation of T-cell subsets that support a proinflammatory milieu in SLE have yielded several candidate biomarkers that might prove useful to identify specific phenotypes of cSLE.[3,5]

Interferon Signature

One finding thought to be involved in the pathogenesis of SLE is the increased expression of interferon (IFN) regulated genes in blood and tissues, coined a "high IFN signature". In fact, there are monogenic forms of lupus that are linked to activation of type 1 IFN pathway.[23] A high IFN signature is more prominent in early onset disease, with up to 90% of children with cSLE displaying a high IFN signature.[24,25] In a study that investigated the usefulness IFN-alpha to serve as a biomarker, serum levels of IFN-alpha of 26 patients with cSLE were significantly higher than in healthy children, with the highest levels observed with active cSLE as opposed to inactive cSLE or inactive LN. However, there was no difference in patients with versus without LN.[26]

Banchereau and colleagues[27] performed gene expression profiling of 158 patients with cSLE and proposed a "lupus fingerprint," consisting of IFN responsive genes and genes related to histones and neutrophils, among others. This combinatorial biomarker was highly reproducible, and the expression of IFN responsive gene

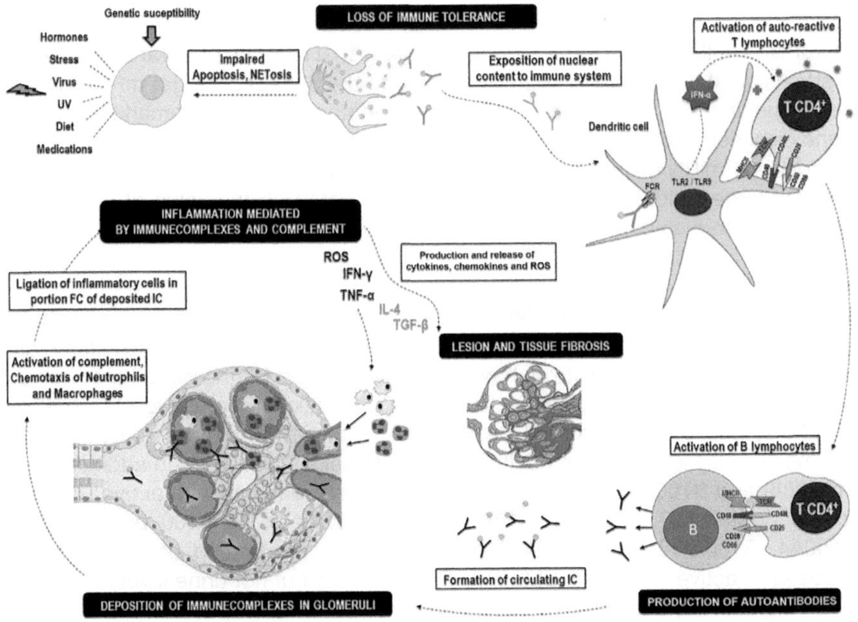

Fig. 1. Pathogenesis of lupus nephritis. (*From* Pinheiro SVB, Dias RF, Fabiano RCG, Araujo SA, Silva A. Pediatric lupus nephritis. J Bras Nefrol. 2019;41(2):252-65.)

lessened with mycophenolate and cyclophosphamide treatment. Another proposed blood-based biomarker is SIGLEC1 (sialic acid–binding immunoglobulin-like lectin 1).[28] This cell surface protein is part of the IFN signature in both adults and children with SLE. Serum levels of SIGLEC1 were more abundant in cSLE than disease controls, which included juvenile idiopathic arthritis, arthralgias, familial mediterranean fever. The serum levels also correlated with changes of the SLEDAI scores ($r = 0.33$, $P = .001$). Conversely, changes in the levels of C3, C4, and anti-double stranded DNA (dsDNA) antibody all failed to be significantly associated with cSLE activity (P values > 0.05). However, SIGLEC1 did not differentiate between patients with cSLE with different organ involvement such as LN or neuropsychiatric disease.

Methylation

Variation of DNA methylation, particularly hypomethylation, has been linked to lupus pathogenesis. Likely studied due to the association of hydralazine and procainamide (DNA methylation inhibitors) with drug-induced lupus, the methylation status of adults with SLE is altered in dendritic cells, T cells, and B cells compared with healthy controls.[29] Recent research suggests a cSLE-specific methylation signature consisting of 21 CpG sites affecting 15 genes with differential loss of DNA methylation across 4 specific cell lineages (CD4 + T cells, CD8 + T cells, B cells, and neutrophils.[30] This methylation signature captures hypomethylation of genes involved in the IFN signaling pathway. The degree of hypomethylation correlates with disease activity and distinguished patients with cSLE from healthy controls. Besides hypomethylation, there is hypermethylation of the promoter region of the FOXP3 gene in cSLE. Hypermethylation of FOXP3 promoter region, among others,[30] has the potential to affect the activity and maturation of regulatory T cells and the maintenance of self-tolerance.[31] Pending further validation, DNA methylation may prove to be a diagnostic biomarker for cSLE and its inflammatory burden.

MicroRNAs

MicroRNAs (miRNAs) are small, noncoding RNAs that regulate posttranscriptional and posttranslational gene expression by binding to the 3′-UTR of target mRNA. Urinary, tissue-specific and blood-based miRNAs are another potential biomarker of autoimmune diseases, including cSLE and SLE.[29,32] **Table 2** summarizes the large number of proposed miRNAs that might prove to be biomarkers for cSLE and SLE. Clearly stringent large validation studies are needed to establish the value of any of these mRNAs to serve as biomarkers for diagnosis or disease course.

S100 Proteins

S100 proteins are a family of proteins that are produced by neutrophils, macrophages, and renal endothelial cells. Once released, S100 proteins propagate the inflammatory response. Various S100 proteins have been investigated for the potential to serve as biomarkers of various pediatric inflammatory conditions. Serum levels of S100A, S100A8/9, and S100A12 are all positively correlated with extrarenal cSLE activity and their levels higher than in healthy controls (P values all <0.01). In addition, serum S100A8/9 and S100A12 protein levels were higher in patients with active LN than in healthy controls (P values <0.012). The urine levels of all S100 proteins tested (S100A4, S100A8/9 and S100A12) were higher in the setting of active renal as opposed to active extrarenal SLE ($P < .0001$). Serum but not urine levels of S100A8/A9 are significantly increased in patients with cSLE when compared with healthy controls, with the highest levels of serum S100A8/9 levels occurring in patients with cSLE with active LN.[33] Both serum and urinary S100A12 concentrations are significantly

Table 2
Proposed microRNAs that might prove to be biomarkers for childhood-onset systemic lupus erythematosus and systemic lupus erythematosus

Author	Study Type	Comparison Groups	MiRNA	Results
Zheng et al,[32] 2019	Meta-analysis (17 studies)17 studies Plasma Adults	SLE vs healthy controls	Pooled analysis, 42 unique miRNA miRNA-21	*Pooled* sensitivity 71%, specificity 81% (AUC 0.88), *miRNA-21* sensitivity 68%, specificity 77% (AUC 0.83)
Su et al,[56] 2018	Next-generation sequencing Plasma and whole blood Adults	LN vs non-N	miR-125a-5p miR-146a-5p miR-221-3p	*P* < .05 for all 3 miRNA
Garcia-Vives et al,[57] 2020	Comparative analyses Urinary exosomal miRNA Adults	Responders vs nonresponders at flare and 1 y posttreatment	miR-31-5p miR-107 miR-135b-5p	Responder group: 2.68x change *miR-31-5p* 2.74x change for *miR-107* Upregulation of all 3 miRNA in responder group *miR-135b-5p* correlated inversely with degree of proteinuria, strongest in nonresponders (r = −0.61, *P* = .008) *miR-135b-5p* distinguishes responder from nonresponder at flare: sensitivity 77.8%, specificity 71.4% (AUC 0.783)
Sole et al,[58] 2019	Comparative analyses Urinary pellet and exosomes Adults	Active LN vs healthy controls	miR-29c miR-200a miR-21 miR-410 miR-150	*miR-21*, *miR-150* overexpressed in LN (6.6x and 2.3x, respectively) *miR-21-5p*, *miR-150*, *miR-29c* strongly correlated with renal chronicity (r = 0.565, r = 0.840, r = −0.559, respectively)

(*continued on next page*)

Table 2
(continued)

Author	Study Type	Comparison Groups	MiRNA	Results
				miR-21, *miR-150* increased according to degree of CI (13.3, 4.8 fold change, respectively) *miR-150*: sensitivity 96%, specificity 83% (AUC 0.970) to distinguish CI *miR-29c*/*miR-150*/*miR-21*: sensitivity 94.4%, specificity 99.8% (AUC 0.996) to distinguish CI, multimarker positive LN patients had lower renal survival rates (*P* = .027)
Cai et al,[59] 2019	Comparative analyses Tissue Pediatric	LN vs healthy controls	miR-145	miR-145 in renal vessels decreased with more severe vascular lesions (*P* < .05)
Zhu et al,[60] 2014	Comparative analyses Blood Pediatric	SLE vs healthy controls	miR-629 miR-525-5p miR-516a-3p	All 3 correlated with SLEDAI score (r = 0.809, r = 0.776, r = 0.792, respectively) All 3 upregulated during active disease, returned to normal after treatment

elevated in patients with cSLE as compared with healthy pediatric controls, again particularly in the setting of active LN.[33] In another study, S100A8/9, S100A4, S100A12, and S100A6 were studied and all were elevated in the urine of patients with active LN compared with those with active extra-renal SLE. All urinary S100 levels decreased with improving LN activity (P = .03), and median levels of S100A4 protein were higher in patients with ISN/RPS classes III/IV compared with class V LN (P = .03).[34] Overall, S100 proteins are promising candidate biomarkers of inflammation caused by SLE and LN and may be useful for following patients longitudinally.

Neutrophil Extracellular Traps

Formed through the efficient, non-inflammatory clearance of neutrophils, termed "NETosis"[35,36], neutrophil extracellular traps (NETs) are fibrous networks that extend from the membranes of activated neutrophils and are composed of decondensed chromatin DNA. NETs are triggers for the production of type I IFNs and increased NETosis occurs in the setting of multiple autoimmune diseases.[37] Aberrant clearance of neutrophils and NET formation may play a role in the pathogenesis of SLE and may be a diagnostic biomarker for LN.[36] In a study of NETs-associated markers in adults, patients with SLE showed decreased NETolytic activity and corresponding increased levels of NET-associated markers.[38] Notably, deficient NETolytic activity and NET-associated elastase activity can be corrected in vitro, and a single report suggests that such "NET assay" allows for the differentiation of patients with cSLE from healthy controls with 100% accuracy.[35] As with several other candidate biomarkers, variation in NET formation does not align with specific organ involvement with cSLE, such as the presence of LN or neuropsychiatric involvement.[35] Taken together, although aberrant NETosis is a recognized feature of SLE, the value of measuring NET burden and NETolytic activity to differentiate SLE from other rheumatic diseases is unknown, as is their value to prognosticate cSLE disease course.

COMPLEMENT SPLIT PRODUCTS

Although regularly measured to assess SLE disease activity, complement components C3 and C4 are inferior to functional assays of complement cascade activation or the measurement of complement split products. Using cytometry to measure C4d levels on erythrocytes and B cells (cell-bound complement activation products, CB-CAP) has been proposed as a sensitive assay to assist in the diagnosis of SLE.[39] Likewise, CB-CAP, especially if assessed together with antinuclear antibodies, anti-dsDNA and anti-Sm levels, can predict the progression of probable to classifiable SLE as per the ACR/EULAR classification criteria.[40] iC3b is the breakdown product of C3b, which corresponds to complement activation via the classic, lectin and alternative pathways. Its evaluation, expressed as ratio of blood iC3b to serum C3 levels, may serve as a tool to estimate complement activation. However, the iC3b:C3 ratio seems comparable with anti-dsDNA antibody levels in differentiating patients with a SLEDAI score of greater than 4 from those with low scores (both AUC = 0.66) and somewhat better than levels of C3 or C4 (both AUC $\leq$ 0.65). A high iC3b/C3 ratio has been associated with the diagnosis of LN, hence could be a biomarker to support the diagnosis of LN.[41]

SUMMARY

The field of lupus biomarkers, particularly cSLE biomarkers, continues to be an active area of research spurred by better understanding of disease pathophysiology. Promising biomarkers are gene based including the IFN signature and methylation status as well as blood-based biomarkers, such as NETs, S100 proteins, and complement split products. However, the newer biomarkers still require extensive study in additional patient cohorts prior to use in clinical care. Biomarkers of LN activity are the furthest along in that several identified urine biomarkers and biomarker panels seem to accurately capture active renal inflammation and anticipate the course of LN. Introduction into clinical care depends on commercial platforms to test biomarkers quickly to provide point-of care support for medical decision-making.

CLINICS CARE POINTS

- Early diagnosis of cSLE is critical for improving outcomes and reducing morbidity and mortality.
- Current biomarkers are insufficient, prompting extensive study into new urine and blood based biomarkers.
- Current biomarkers under investigation include NETS, S100, complement split products, urinary biomarker panels require further study prior to introduction into clinical care.

DISCLOSURE

E.M. Cody: no disclosures. H.I. Brunner: speaking fees for Novartis and Roche (both >$10,000) and GlaxoSmithKline (<$10,000); Consultancies/honoraria (<$10,000): AbbVie, Astra Zeneca-Medimmune, Biogen, Boehringer, Bristol-Myers Squibb, Celgene, Eli Lilly, EMD Serono, Genzyme, GlaxoSmithKline, F. Hoffmann-La Roche, Merck, Novartis, R-Pharm, Sanofi. The Cincinnati Children's Hospital, where HBR works as a full-time public employee, has received contributions (>$10,000 each) from the following industries in the past 3 years: Bristol-Myers Squibb, Eli Lilly, GlaxoSmithKline, F. Hoffmann-La Roche, Janssen, Novartis, and Pfizer. This funding has been reinvested for the research activities of the hospital in a fully independent manner, without any commitment to third parties. Dr Brunner's time is supported by the National Institute of Arthritis and Musculoskeletal and Skin Diseases, NIH (grant P30-AR-076316).

REFERENCES

1. Gergianaki I, Bortoluzzi A, Bertsias G. Update on the epidemiology, risk factors, and disease outcomes of systemic lupus erythematosus. Best Pract Res Clin Rheumatol 2018;32(2):188–205.
2. Silva CA, Avcin T, Brunner HI. Taxonomy for systemic lupus erythematosus with onset before adulthood. Arthritis Care Res (Hoboken) 2012;64(12):1787–93.
3. Aggarwal A, Srivastava P. Childhood onset systemic lupus erythematosus: how is it different from adult SLE? Int J Rheum Dis 2015;18(2):182–91.
4. Oni L, Wright RD, Marks S, et al. Kidney outcomes for children with lupus nephritis. Pediatr Nephrol 2020;1377–85.
5. Borgia RE, Silverman ED. Childhood-onset systemic lupus erythematosus: an update. Curr Opin Rheumatol 2015;27(5):483–92.
6. Aljaberi N, Nguyen K, Strahle C, et al. The performance of the new 2019-eular/acr classification criteria for systemic lupus erythematosus in children and young adults. Arthritis Care Res (Hoboken) 2020;580–5.
7. Koutsonikoli A, Trachana M, Farmaki E, et al. Novel biomarkers for the assessment of paediatric systemic lupus erythematosus nephritis. Clin Exp Immunol 2017;188(1):79–85.

8. Malvar A, Pirruccio P, Alberton V, et al. Histologic versus clinical remission in proliferative lupus nephritis. Nephrol Dial Transplant 2017;32(8):1338–44.
9. Mina R, Abulaban K, Klein-Gitelman MS, et al. Validation of the lupus nephritis clinical indices in childhood-onset systemic lupus erythematosus. Arthritis Care Res (Hoboken) 2016;68(2):195–202.
10. Tektonidou MG, Dasgupta A, Ward MM. Risk of end-stage renal disease in patients with lupus nephritis, 1971-2015: a systematic review and Bayesian meta-analysis. Arthritis Rheumatol 2016;68(6):1432–41.
11. BEST (Biomarkers, EndpointS, and other Tools) Resource. FDA-NIH Biomarker Working Group: Silver Spring (MD)2016. Available at: https://www.ncbi.nlm.nih.gov/books/NBK326791/.
12. Califf RM. Biomarker definitions and their applications. Exp Biol Med (Maywood) 2018;243(3):213–21.
13. Strimbu K, Tavel JA. What are biomarkers? Curr Opin HIV AIDS 2010;5(6):463–6.
14. Mandrekar JN. Receiver operating characteristic curve in diagnostic test assessment. J Thorac Oncol 2010;5(9):1315–6.
15. Anders HJ, Rovin B. A pathophysiology-based approach to the diagnosis and treatment of lupus nephritis. Kidney Int 2016;90(3):493–501.
16. Sun YS, Sun IT, Wang HK, et al. Risk of complications of ultrasound-guided renal biopsy for adult and pediatric patients with systemic lupus erythematosus. Lupus 2018;27(5):828–36.
17. Brunner HI, Bennett MR, Abulaban K, et al. Development of a novel renal activity index of lupus nephritis in children and young adults. Arthritis Care Res (Hoboken) 2016;68(7):1003–11.
18. Smith EM, Jorgensen AL, Midgley A, et al. International validation of a urinary biomarker panel for identification of active lupus nephritis in children. Pediatr Nephrol 2017;32(2):283–95.
19. Smith EMD, Lewandowski LB, Jorgensen AL, et al. Growing international evidence for urinary biomarker panels identifying lupus nephritis in children - verification within the South African Paediatric Lupus Cohort. Lupus 2018;27(14):2190–9.
20. Smith EMD, Eleuteri A, Goilav B, et al. A Markov Multi-State model of lupus nephritis urine biomarker panel dynamics in children: Predicting changes in disease activity. Clin Immunol 2019;198:71–8.
21. Cody EM, Bennett MR, Gulati G, et al. Successful urine multiplex bead assay to measure lupus nephritis activity. Kidney Int Rep 2021;1949–60.
22. Pinheiro SVB, Dias RF, Fabiano RCG, et al. Pediatric lupus nephritis. J Bras Nefrol 2019;41(2):252–65.
23. Lo MS. Insights Gained From the Study of Pediatric Systemic Lupus Erythematosus. Front Immunol 2018;9:1278.
24. Smith EMD, Lythgoe H, Midgley A, et al. Juvenile-onset systemic lupus erythematosus: update on clinical presentation, pathophysiology and treatment options. Clin Immunol 2019;209:108274.
25. Ronnblom L, Leonard D. Interferon pathway in SLE: one key to unlocking the mystery of the disease. Lupus Sci Med 2019;6(1):e000270.
26. Kanakoudi-Tsakalidou F, Farmaki E, Tzimouli V, et al. Simultaneous changes in serum HMGB1 and IFN-alpha levels and in LAIR-1 expression on plasmatoid dendritic cells of patients with juvenile SLE. New therapeutic options? Lupus 2014;23(3):305–12.
27. Banchereau R, Hong S, Cantarel B, et al. Personalized Immunomonitoring Uncovers Molecular Networks that Stratify Lupus Patients. Cell 2016;165(3):551–65.

28. Stuckrad SLV, Klotsche J, Biesen R, et al. SIGLEC1 (CD169) is a sensitive biomarker for the deterioration of the clinical course in childhood systemic lupus erythematosus. Lupus 2020;29(14):1914–25.
29. Wu H, Chang C, Lu Q. The Epigenetics of Lupus Erythematosus. Adv Exp Med Biol 2020;1253:185–207.
30. Yeung KS, Lee TL, Mok MY, et al. Cell lineage-specific genome-wide DNA methylation analysis of patients with paediatric-onset systemic lupus erythematosus. Epigenetics 2019;14(4):341–51.
31. Hanaei S, Sanati G, Zoghi S, et al. The status of FOXP3 gene methylation in pediatric systemic lupus erythematosus. Allergol Immunopathol (Madr) 2020;48(4):332–8.
32. Zheng X, Zhang Y, Yue P, et al. Diagnostic significance of circulating miRNAs in systemic lupus erythematosus. PLoS one 2019;14(6):e0217523.
33. Donohue SJ, Midgley A, Davies JC, et al. Differential analysis of serum and urine S100 proteins in juvenile-onset systemic lupus erythematosus (jSLE). Clin Immunol 2020;214:108375.
34. Turnier JL, Fall N, Thornton S, et al. Urine S100 proteins as potential biomarkers of lupus nephritis activity. Arthritis Res Ther 2017;19(1):242.
35. El-Ghoneimy DH, Hesham M, Hasan R, et al. The behavior of neutrophil extracellular traps and NADPH oxidative activity in pediatric systemic lupus erythematosus: relation to disease activity and lupus nephritis. Clin Rheumatol 2019;38(9):2585–93.
36. Lee KH, Kronbichler A, Park DD, et al. Neutrophil extracellular traps (NETs) in autoimmune diseases: a comprehensive review. Autoimmun Rev 2017;16(11):1160–73.
37. Barnado A, Crofford LJ, Oates JC. At the Bedside: Neutrophil extracellular traps (NETs) as targets for biomarkers and therapies in autoimmune diseases. J Leukoc Biol 2016;99(2):265–78.
38. Jeremic I, Djuric O, Nikolic M, et al. Neutrophil extracellular traps-associated markers are elevated in patients with systemic lupus erythematosus. Rheumatol Int 2019;39(11):1849–57.
39. Kalunian KC, Chatham WW, Massarotti EM, et al. Measurement of cell-bound complement activation products enhances diagnostic performance in systemic lupus erythematosus. Arthritis Rheum 2012;64(12):4040–7.
40. Ramsey-Goldman R, Alexander RV, Massarotti EM, et al. Complement activation in patients with probable systemic lupus erythematosus and ability to predict progression to American College of Rheumatology–classified systemic lupus erythematosus. Arthritis Rheumatol 2020;72(1):78–88.
41. Kim AHJ, Strand V, Sen DP, et al. Association of Blood Concentrations of Complement Split Product iC3b and Serum C3 With Systemic Lupus Erythematosus Disease Activity. Arthritis Rheumatol 2019;71(3):420–30.
42. Goilav B, Putterman C, Rubinstein TB. Biomarkers for kidney involvement in pediatric lupus. Biomark Med 2015;9(6):529–43.
43. Marks SD, Williams SJ, Tullus K, et al. Glomerular expression of monocyte chemoattractant protein-1 is predictive of poor renal prognosis in pediatric lupus nephritis. Nephrol Dial Transplant 2008;23(11):3521–6.
44. Watson L, Midgley A, Pilkington C, et al. Urinary monocyte chemoattractant protein 1 and alpha 1 acid glycoprotein as biomarkers of renal disease activity in juvenile-onset systemic lupus erythematosus. Lupus 2012;21(5):496–501.

45. Marks SD, Shah V, Pilkington C, et al. Urinary monocyte chemoattractant protein-1 correlates with disease activity in lupus nephritis. Pediatr Nephrol 2010;25(11): 2283–8.
46. Brunner HI, Bennett MR, Mina R, et al. Association of noninvasively measured renal protein biomarkers with histologic features of lupus nephritis. Arthritis Rheum 2012;64(8):2687–97.
47. Rubinstein T, Pitashny M, Levine B, et al. Urinary neutrophil gelatinase-associated lipocalin as a novel biomarker for disease activity in lupus nephritis. Rheumatology (Oxford) 2010;49(5):960–71.
48. Hammad A, Mosaad Y, Elhanbly S, et al. Urinary neutrophil gelatinase-associated lipocalin as a marker of severe lupus nephritis in children. Lupus 2013;22(5): 486–91.
49. Brunner HI, Mueller M, Rutherford C, et al. Urinary neutrophil gelatinase-associated lipocalin as a biomarker of nephritis in childhood-onset systemic lupus erythematosus. Arthritis Rheum 2006;54(8):2577–84.
50. Hinze CH, Suzuki M, Klein-Gitelman M, et al. Neutrophil gelatinase-associated lipocalin is a predictor of the course of global and renal childhood-onset systemic lupus erythematosus disease activity. Arthritis Rheum 2009;60(9):2772–81.
51. Brunner HI, Bennett MR, Gulati G, et al. Urine biomarkers to predict response to lupus nephritis therapy in children and young adults. J Rheumatol 2017;44(8): 1239–48.
52. Suzuki M, Wiers K, Brooks EB, et al. Initial validation of a novel protein biomarker panel for active pediatric lupus nephritis. Pediatr Res 2009;65(5):530–6.
53. Brunner HI, Gulati G, Klein-Gitelman MS, et al. Urine biomarkers of chronic kidney damage and renal functional decline in childhood-onset systemic lupus erythematosus. Pediatr Nephrol 2019;34(1):117–28.
54. Gasparin AA, de Andrade NPB, Hax V, et al. Urinary soluble VCAM-1 is a useful biomarker of disease activity and treatment response in lupus nephritis. BMC Rheumatol 2020;4(1):67.
55. Singh S, Wu T, Xie C, et al. Urine VCAM-1 as a marker of renal pathology activity index in lupus nephritis. Arthritis Res Ther 2012;14(4):R164.
56. Su YJ, Lin IC, Wang L, et al. Next generation sequencing identifies miRNA-based biomarker panel for lupus nephritis. Oncotarget 2018;9(46):27911–9.
57. Garcia-Vives E, Sole C, Moline T, et al. The urinary exosomal miRNA expression profile is predictive of clinical response in lupus nephritis. Int J Mol Sci 2020; 21(4):1372–90.
58. Sole C, Moline T, Vidal M, et al. An exosomal urinary miRNA signature for early diagnosis of renal fibrosis in lupus nephritis. Cells 2019;8(8):773–90.
59. Cai Z, Xiang W, Peng X, et al. MicroRNA-145 Involves in the pathogenesis of renal vascular lesions and may become a potential therapeutic target in patients with juvenile lupus nephritis. Kidney Blood Press Res 2019;44(4):643–55.
60. Zhu J, Huang X, Su G, et al. High expression levels of microRNA-629, microRNA-525-5p and microRNA-516a-3p in paediatric systemic lupus erythematosus. Clin Rheumatol 2014;33(6):807–15.

Role of Environment in Pediatric Rheumatic Diseases

Colleen K. Correll, MD, MPH

KEYWORDS

- Environmental risk factors • Juvenile idiopathic arthritis
- Systemic lupus erythematosus • Juvenile dermatomyositis
- Pediatric rheumatic diseases

KEY POINTS

- Evidence linking environmental risk factors for pediatric rheumatic diseases is lacking, but these risk factors are important to the understanding of disease pathogenesis and prevention.
- Commonly studied risk factors include infections, perinatal factors, household exposures, air pollution, and dietary factors.
- Juvenile idiopathic arthritis (JIA) is the pediatric rheumatic disease for which most environmental risk research has been conducted, but many study findings conflict and no consistently strong risk factors have been identified, likely due to limitations of the study design and small sample sizes.
- Low levels of vitamin D were common in most diseases, but causality has been difficult to determine.
- We are likely to see an increase in the study of the microbiome and metabolomics in pediatric rheumatic diseases research.

INTRODUCTION

Like most autoimmune diseases, pediatric rheumatic diseases (PRD) are thought to be caused by a complex combination of interactions between genetic and environmental factors. Yet, environmental epidemiologic studies are lacking compared with genetic studies.[1–3] This scarcity is likely due to the challenges of studying environmental exposures in human diseases. These studies often rely on older methods including questionnaires, geographic data, and assessment of one or a few risk factors at a time; this results in study limitations and/or confounding, including recall bias and difficulties identifying temporality, causality, and dose-response relationships between exposures and disease onset. In addition, the rarity and heterogeneity of PRD makes

Pediatric Rheumatology, Allergy, & Immunology, Academic Office Building, 2450 Riverside Ave S AO-10, Minneapolis, MN 55454, USA
E-mail address: corr0250@umn.edu

Rheum Dis Clin N Am 48 (2022) 287–304
https://doi.org/10.1016/j.rdc.2021.09.007
rheumatic.theclinics.com

environmental epidemiologic research even more challenging. Commonly studied environmental risk factors for PRDs include infections, perinatal exposures, air pollutants, household exposures, ultraviolet radiation (UVR), diet, and nutrition. More recently, adverse childhood events (ACEs) have been recognized as risk factors for PRD. Here we review what is known about environmental risk factors for PRD, focusing on juvenile idiopathic arthritis (JIA), childhood-onset systemic lupus erythematosus (cSLE), and juvenile dermatomyositis (JDM).

JUVENILE IDIOPATHIC ARTHRITIS

JIA is an umbrella term of a group of diseases that are all characterized by chronic arthritis starting in childhood. JIA is the most common chronic PRD, yet pathogenesis remains unclear.[4] JIA encompasses 7 subtypes on clinical phenotype.[5] Because many of these 7 subtypes are unique diseases, studies often focus on one or a few subtypes, resulting in smaller samples sizes and making research more challenging. However, based on newer and more sophisticated genomic studies of JIA and adult rheumatoid arthritis (RA), these 7 subtypes may actually fall into 4 major clusters of arthritis.[6] For future research studies, using these 4 clusters may provide adequate homogeneity within groups and better sample sizes. Studies of adult RA have demonstrated smoking and silica to be strong environmental risk factors[7]; however, finding strong environmental risk factors across repeated studies in JIA has posed more challenge.

In terms of PRD environmental epidemiology research, JIA is the most studied, and a few reviews on this topic have been published previously.[8–10] Results from many of these studies have found weak or no associations, and study results often conflict, leading to unclear answers as to what role the environment plays. Infection has long been thought to be a potential risk factor for JIA, although confirming this has been challenging. Studies have demonstrated that infections early in life[11] and antibiotic usage may be associated with increased risk of JIA onset.[12,13] Another study demonstrated that streptococcal infection may increase the risk of flare in JIA,[14] and the common childhood viruses, parvovirus and Epstein-Barr virus (EBV), were found to be associated with JIA in some studies but not others.[15–22] Maternal and perinatal risk factors, including cesarean delivery, prematurity, maternal tobacco exposure, and lack of breastfeeding, have been associated with JIA risk in some studies,[11,23–36] but many of these findings have not been reproducible. In addition, studies of sibship and birth order[37–39] and seasonality and air pollution have also demonstrated unclear or conflicting results.[40–46] One study found secondhand smoke exposure to be a risk factor.[30] Another study found that increased sun exposure was associated with a decreased risk of JIA.[47] A study investigating animal exposure as a risk factor for oligoarticular JIA found no association.[48] In terms of diet and nutrition, two separate studies found cow's milk allergy and heavy metals in fish as possible risk factors for JIA.[49,50] Moreover, although low levels of vitamin D have been seen in children with JIA, it is challenging to determine causation.[51–53] Two studies have shown life stressors as being associated with JIA, and we are likely to see more studies of this topic as ACEs and their effect on health is prioritized in research and health care.[54,55] **Table 1** summarizes several key findings from environmental studies of JIA based on risk factors.

Microbiome and metabolomic research is beyond the scope of this review, but it should be mentioned that "omics" research is an important and rapidly growing area of research in many autoimmune diseases including JIA.[56–61] Several studies have demonstrated that patients with JIA have a unique gut flora compared with

Table 1
Highlighted studies of environmental risk factors associated with juvenile idiopathic arthritis

Authors	Country and/or Data Source Year	Study Design and Population	Exposure/Method of Determination	Key Findings and Outcomes; OR (95% CI)
Mason et al[36]	US 1995	CC Oligoarticular and polyarticular JIA Cases = 54 HC = 79	Breastfeeding	All JIA: 0.4 (0.2–0.8) Oligoarticular: 0.3 (0.1–0.9) Polyarticular: 0.6 (0.2–1.7)
Jaakkola and Gissler[31]	Finland, Medical Birth Registry 2005	Retrospective cohort All JIA Cases = 31	Heavy prenatal smoke exposure	Girls with JIA: 6.8 (2.0–22.9)
Carlens et al[11]	Sweden 2009	CC All JIA Cases = 3334 HC = 13,336	Perinatal and early life infections	Infections in first year of life: 1.9 (1.7–2.1)
Horton et al[13]	United Kingdom 2015	Nested CC All JIA Cases = 152 HC = 1520	Previous antibiotic exposure	Any antibiotic: 2.1 (1.2–3.5) >5 antibiotic courses: 3.0 (1.6–5.6)
Shenoi et al[25]	United States 2016	CC All JIA Cases = 225 HC = 138	Early life exposures	Prematurity: 1.8 (1.2–2.7)
Thorsen et al[52]	Denmark 2017	CC Oligoarticular and polyarticular JIA Cases = 300 HC = 300	Low vitamin D level at birth from blood spot	1.2 (0.9–1.6)
França et al[30]	Brazil 2018	CC Maternal questionnaire and tropospheric pollutant data All JIA Cases = 66 HC = 124	Smoke exposure by maternal self-report and air pollution	Intrauterine smoke exposure: 3.4 (1.5–8.1) Maternal employment: 0.06 (0.02–0.2) Ideal maternal weight gain: 0.34 (0.2–0.8) Secondhand smoke exposure: after birth: 3.6 (1.8–7.3) Ozone exposure during the second year of life: 2.8 (1.2–6.4)
Rubinstein et al[54]	US National Survey of Children's Health 2020	Cross-sectional	ACEs	≥4 ACEs: 9.4 (4.0–22.1)

Abbreviations: CC, case-control study; CI, confidence intervals; HC, healthy control; OR, odds ratio.

healthy controls. These studies support the idea that gut flora may be altered by the environment, which then leads dysregulation of the immune system and ultimately autoimmune disease. We are likely to learn more about the effects of gut health on JIA in the coming years.

CHILDHOOD SYSTEMIC LUPUS ERYTHEMATOSUS

SLE is a chronic, multisystem inflammatory disease with an incidence of 5 to 20 per million people in the United States, and approximately 10% to 20% of cases start in childhood.[62] Much of what we know about the environmental impacts on SLE comes from adult studies.[63] Risk factors identified in these adult studies that may be relevant to cSLE include EBV,[64] occupational exposures including solvents and silica,[65,66] UVR (as a risk for disease flare),[67] cigarette smoking,[68] and exogenous hormone therapy.[69] In addition, some adult SLE studies have identified early life exposures as potential triggers for adult-onset SLE. One study of adult women with SLE found that early life exposures to frequent pesticide use and extended residence on a farm from early childhood were risk factors for SLE.[70] Another recent study found that child abuse was associated with adult-onset SLE in black women.[71] Many studies have demonstrated that adult and pediatric patients with SLE have lower levels of vitamin D, but the role vitamin D plays in disease onset or activity is less clear.[67,72–75] **Table 2** highlights studies specific to cSLE.

JUVENILE DERMATOMYOSITIS

Juvenile dermatomyositis (JDM) is a rare PRD with an incidence of 3 per million and is characterized by inflammatory muscle and skin disease.[81] Studies support the idea that a preceding illness may trigger JDM onset, but identification of specific pathogens has posed more challenge.[82–88] Several studies have demonstrated that UVR has been associated with disease onset or activity.[89–91] Maternal smoking and maternal exposure to air pollutants may also be risk factors.[92] Similar to JIA and SLE, there is some suggestion that low vitamin D levels may be associated with increased risk of idiopathic inflammatory myositis in adult and pediatric patients, but causality is unclear.[80,93] **Table 3** highlights findings from environmental studies of JDM.

OTHER PEDIATRIC RHEUMATIC DISEASES

Juvenile scleroderma: A large multinational study of juvenile localized scleroderma (n = 750) surveyed pediatric rheumatologists and dermatologists about specific events before disease onset and found that 13% reported a specific trigger (such as mechanical trauma or infection) before disease onset.[96] Although this was an impressively large study, it was limited by lack of a control group and possible recall bias. Adult systemic sclerosis studies have found silica, asbestos, and some organic solvents as risk factors for disease onset, although it is not clear what role these play in pediatric disease.[97,98]

Chronic recurrent multifocal osteomyelitis (CRMO): Although there is a fair amount of published literature regarding the genetic contribution to CRMO, little is known about the role the environment plays in disease pathogenesis.[99]

Pediatric vasculitis: There is a scarcity of published data on environmental risk factors for childhood-onset antineutrophil cytoplasm antibody-associated vasculitis in adults or children, but a systematic review found silica and other pollutants, infection, and UVR as the potential risk factors.[100] However, there is a relatively large amount of published data describing seasonality and environmental risk factors for Kawasaki

Table 2
Environmental factors associated with risk of childhood-onset systemic lupus erythematosus

Authors	Country and/ or Data Source, Year	Study Design and Population	Exposure/Method of Determination	Key Findings and Outcomes [Listed as OR (95% CI) Unless Otherwise Noted]
Infectious				
Tsai et al[21]	China 1995	CC Cases = 20 HC = 20	EBV and CMV genome in leukocytes	EBV positivity: Cases: 3/20 (15%) HC: 0/20 (0%) CMV positivity: Cases: 5/20 (25%) HC: 2/20 (10%) ORs not calculated
James et al[76]	United States 1997	CC Cases (included children and young adults) = 117 HC = 153	EBV seroconversion	49.9 (9.3, 1025)
Perinatal				
Conde et al[77]	Brazil 2018	CC Cases = 30 controls = 86	Maternal self-reported air pollutants during pregnancy and after birth	Maternal occupational exposure: 13.5 (2.5–72.4) Maternal smoking during pregnancy: 8.6 (1.6–47) Prematurity: 15.8, (1.9–135.3) Secondhand smoke exposure: 9.1 (1.8–42.1)

(continued on next page)

Table 2
(continued)

Authors	Country and/or Data Source, Year	Study Design and Population	Exposure/Method of Determination	Key Findings and Outcomes [Listed as OR (95% CI) Unless Otherwise Noted]
Household/atmosphere				
Alves et al[78]	Brazil 2017	Prospective cohort Assessed air pollution as trigger for airway inflammation and cSLE disease activity Cases = 9, 108 consecutive measurements	Air pollution measured by passive samplers for nitrogen dioxide, fine particulate matter, and a data logger for temperature and humidity. Measured for 4-wk cycles every 2.5 mo for 1 year	Increase in fine particulate matter associated with risk of SLEDAI-2K $\geq$ 8: 1.5 (1.1, 1.8)
Goulart et al[79]	Brazil 2020	Prospective cohort Assessed air pollution as trigger for cSLE renal activity Cases = 9 108 consecutive appointments	Air pollution measured by passive samplers for nitrogen dioxide, fine particulate matter, and a data logger for temperature and humidity	Increased levels of fine particulate matter associated with increased dsDNA and urine protein and decreased C3 levels
Vitamin D				
Wright et al[75]	US 2009	CC Cases = 38 HC = 207	Serum vitamin D	36.8% cSLE vs 9.2% HC, had 25(OH)D <10 ng/mL $P < .001$) Greater SLE disease activity index scores in those with 25(OH)D < 20 ng/mL ($P = .01$)

Robinson et al[80]	United States 2012	Cohort JDM = 21 SLE = 37	Serum 25(OH)D levels	Excluding patients with proteinuria, no associations were seen
Stagi et al[72]	Italy 2014	CC Cases = 45 HC = 109	Serum vitamin D level	cSLE had lower vitamin D vs HC. Active SLE had lower levels than inactive
Peracchi et al[73]	Brazil 2014	CC Cases = 30 HC = 30	Serum vitamin D	97% cases vs 77% HC had 25(OH)D levels <32 ng/mL ($P < .001$) Low vitamin D level not associated with disease activity
Lin et al[74]	Taiwan 2016	Retrospective cohort Cases = 35	Serum vitamin D levels were compared between patients with active vs inactive cSLE	Lower [25(OH)D] levels were seen in those with active vs inactive disease: (12.0 ± 7.2 ng/mL vs 15.4 ± 7.4 ng/mL, $P = .005$)

Abbreviations: 25(OH)D, 25-hydroxyvitamin D; CC, case control study; CI, confidence interval; CMV, cytomegalovirus; dsDNA, double-stranded DNA; HC, healthy controls; OR, odds ratio; SLEDAI-2K, Systemic Lupus Erythematosus Disease Activity Index 2000.

Table 3
Environmental factors associated with risk of juvenile dermatomyositis

Authors	Country and/or Data Source, Year	Study Design and Population	Exposure/Method of Determination	Key Findings and Outcomes [Listed as OR (95% CI) Unless Otherwise noted]
Infectious				
Koch et al[82]	United States 1976	CC Questionnaire data Childhood polymyositis Cases = 42 HC = 42	Variety of environmental exposures assessed through self-report, including household size, birth order, perinatal exposures, prior infections, immunizations, animal exposure, population density	No significant associations found Possible increase in preceding streptococcal exposure, but statistical analysis not done 20 cases vs 13 HC exposed to streptococcal infections
Christensen et al[84]	United States 1986	CC JDM cases = 12 JIA cases = 24 Controls = 2192 (controls were hospitalized children with presumed viral infection)	Coxsackie B virus (measured as complement fixing antibody titers to coxsackie B viral antigens)	83% of JDM had positive titers vs 25% with JIA and 25% controls
Pachman et al[83]	United States 1995	CC JDM cases = 20 Age-matched controls with neuromuscular disease = 20	Compared differences in antibodies in serum to several viral and bacterial infections, and compared differences in coxsackie virus and enterovirus in muscle tissue by muscle biopsy	No difference in infectious studies in serum or muscle tissue between cases and controls

Pachman et al[88]	United States 1997	CC Structured interview, collecting exposure data, and measured antibody titers in serum to some infectious agents JDM = 80 JIA = 40 HC = 23	Variety of environmental exposures Antibody titers in serum to *Toxoplasma gondii*, HSV coxsackievirus B	63% JDM vs 42% HC reported illness 3 mo before onset ($P = .013$) No associations in: household smoking, population density, animal exposure, insect bites, stressors, economic status, school or daycare attendance, toxic substances, titers to *T gondii*, HSV, or coxsackievirus B
Pachman et al[85]	United States 2005	Cohort, JDM cases = 286 Parent interviews and medical record review	Infection 3 months before JDM symptom onset	57% had respiratory complaints, 30% gastrointestinal symptoms, and 63% had received antibiotics 3 mo before JDM symptom onset No comparison group
Mamyrova et al[86]	Childhood Myositis Heterogeneity Study 2005	CC JDM = 62 HC = 62 Measured viral serology and DNA	Parvovirus B19	No differences found between cases and controls
Zheng et al[87]	China 2019	CC 27 = JDM 30 = HC EBV infection tested on newly diagnosed patients with JDM	Anti-EBV IgG antibodies	Higher positive rate of EBNA-IgG ($P < .0001$) and EBV capsid antigen-IgG ($P < .05$) compared with HC

(*continued on next page*)

Table 3
(*continued*)

Authors	Country and/or Data Source, Year	Study Design and Population	Exposure/Method of Determination	Key Findings and Outcomes [Listed as OR (95% CI) Unless Otherwise noted]
Perinatal				
Koch et al[82]	United States 1976	CC Childhood polymyositis cases = 42 HC = 42	Many perinatal environmental exposures assessed through self-report	No associations found
Orione et al[92]	Brazil 2014	CC Maternal questionnaire and tropospheric pollutant data JDM = 20 HC = 56	Maternal environmental inhalation Exposure and concentrations of inhaled particulate matter during pregnancy	Maternal smoking: 13.3 (1.2–144.3) Occupational exposure: (35.4 (2.0–632.8) CO exposure in the third trimester: 12.2 (1.3–116.0)
Household/Atmosphere				
Vegosen et al[94]	United States 2007	CC 307 juvenile-onset IIM 3942 HC; 668 adult-onset IIM 6991 HC	Seasonality of birth dates	No difference in overall birth distribution Seasonality seen in some subgroups: Hispanic patients with juvenile-onset IIM, JDM, and p155 antibody, and juvenile-onset IIM and allele DRB1*0301
Shah et al[89] (Childhood Myositis Heterogeneity Collaborative Study Group)	United States 2013	298 juvenile-onset IIM Compared UV radiation exposure in month before symptom onset in JDM vs polymyositis	UV radiation	JDM vs polymyositis increased per unit of highest UV index in the month before symptom onset: 1.18 (1.0–1.4)

Mamyrova et al[95]	United States/ Canada 2017	Online survey JDM cases = 164 Adult dermatomyositis cases = 46	Self-reported environmental exposures associated with disease flare	Sun exposure: OR = 2.2 (1.2–4.3) NSAID use: OR = 1.9 (1.2–3.4) No other associations found.
Neely et al[91]	**CARRA Legacy Registry** United States 2019	Cross-sectional Mean UV index in month before symptom onset in subject's zip code JDM cases 522	Mean UV index association with calcinosis and other indicators of severe disease	Overall, no association between UV index and calcinosis In African Americans, inverse association between UV index and calcinosis
Vitamin D				
Robinson et al[80]	United States 2012	Cohort JDM = 21 SLE = 37	Serum 25(OH)D levels on disease activity	Excluding subjects with proteinuria, serum 25(OH)D levels were inversely associated with disease activity in JDM

Abbreviations: 25(OH)D, 25-hydroxyvitamin D; CARRA, Childhood Arthritis and Rheumatology Research Alliance; CC, case-control study; CI, confidence interval; EBNA, Epstein-Barr nuclear antigen; HC, healthy controls; HSV, herpes simplex virus; IIM, idiopathic inflammatory myopathy; NSAID, nonsteroidal anti-inflammatory drug; OR, odds ratio.

disease.[101] The role of environment in Kawasaki disease is beyond the scope of this article; however, insights from Kawasaki disease research may lead to new understandings of chronic systemic vasculitis in children.

DISCUSSION AND SUMMARY

Identifying environmental risk factors for PRD is important because reducing or eliminating these exposures may prevent disease onset and/or flare and may lead to better understanding of pathogenesis and treatment targets. Infections, antibiotics, prematurity, and smoke exposure may be associated with increased risk of JIA, but additional studies are needed to confirm these findings. Infections, maternal smoke exposure, and other air pollutants and UVR may increase the risk of cSLE and JDM onset or flare. Vitamin D deficiency was commonly seen in PRD, but causality is unclear. Environmental epidemiology studies are important but have been relatively scarce in PRD research, and this is likely due to the known challenges of environmental exposure studies coupled with the rarity of PRDs. As we continue to build multicenter collaborative research platforms and use high-technology research methods, we will be better able to address the role the environment plays in PRD.

The use of high-technology methods in genomics and related research has led to an increasing understanding of the immunopathogenesis of PRD. However, similar high-technology studies of environmental factors or gene-environment relationships have been lagging behind. It is important to note, however, that the study of the microbiome in relationship to adult rheumatic disease and PRD is gaining momentum, as we continue to learn more about the role of gut health in these diseases.[59,102,103] More attention has been focused on metabolomics, epigenetics, and adverse childhood events in relationship to chronic disease, and we are likely to see more of these studies in PRD on the horizon.[104–106]

CLINICS CARE POINTS

- Although not necessarily causal, vitamin D deficiency is common in patients with PRD. Therefore testing for vitamin D deficiency and supplementation when necessary should be considered in patients with PRD.
- UVR has been associated with disease onset, activity, and/or flare in both SLE and JDM, and thus discussion about sun protection with these patients is important.
- Antibiotic usage in early childhood has been associated with increased risk of developing JIA, therefore antibiotics should be used judiciously in the general pediatric population.

DISCLOSURE

The author has nothing to disclose.

REFERENCES

1. Hersh AO, Prahalad S. Immunogenetics of juvenile idiopathic arthritis: A comprehensive review. J Autoimmun 2015;64:113–24.
2. Catalina MD, Owen KA, Labonte AC, et al. The pathogenesis of systemic lupus erythematosus: Harnessing big data to understand the molecular basis of lupus. J Autoimmun 2020;110. https://doi.org/10.1016/j.jaut.2019.102359.

3. Rothwell S, Chinoy H, Lamb JA. Genetics of idiopathic inflammatory myopathies: Insights into disease pathogenesis. Curr Opin Rheumatol 2019;31(6): 611–6.
4. Sacks JJ, Helmick CG, Luo Y-H, et al. Prevalence of and annual ambulatory health care visits for pediatric arthritis and other rheumatologic conditions in the United States in 2001-2004. Arthritis Rheum 2007;57(8):1439–45.
5. Petty RE, Southwood TR, Manners P, et al. International league of associations for rheumatology classification of juvenile idiopathic arthritis: second revision, edmonton, 2001. J Rheumatol 2004;31(2):390–2.
6. Nigrovic PA, Raychaudhuri S, Thompson SD. Review: genetics and the classification of arthritis in adults and children. Arthritis Rheumatol 2018;70(1):7–17.
7. Salliot C, Nguyen Y, Boutron-Ruault M-C, et al. Environment and lifestyle: their influence on the risk of RA. J Clin Med 2020;9(10):3109.
8. Ellis JA, Munro JE, Ponsonby A-L. Possible environmental determinants of juvenile idiopathic arthritis. Rheumatology (Oxford) 2010;49(3):411–25. Available at: http://ovidsp.ovid.com/ovidweb.cgi?T=JS&PAGE=reference&D=med5&NEWS=N&AN=19965974.
9. Berkun Y, Padeh S. Environmental factors and the geoepidemiology of juvenile idiopathic arthritis. Autoimmun Rev 2010;9(5):A319–24. Available at: http://ovidsp.ovid.com/ovidweb.cgi?T=JS&PAGE=reference&D=med5&NEWS=N&AN=19932890.
10. Horton DB, Shenoi S. Review of environmental factors and juvenile idiopathic arthritis. Open Access Rheumatol Res Rev 2019;11:253–67.
11. Carlens C, Jacobsson L, Brandt L, et al. Perinatal characteristics, early life infections and later risk of rheumatoid arthritis and juvenile idiopathic arthritis. Ann Rheum Dis 2009;68(7):1159–64.
12. Arvonen M, Virta LJ, Pokka T, et al. Repeated exposure to antibiotics in infancy: a predisposing factor for juvenile idiopathic arthritis or a sign of this group's greater susceptibility to infections? J Rheumatol 2015;42(3):521–6. Available at: http://ovidsp.ovid.com/ovidweb.cgi?T=JS&PAGE=reference&D=medl&NEWS=N&AN=25320218.
13. Horton DB, Scott FI, Haynes K, et al. Antibiotic exposure and juvenile idiopathic arthritis: a case-control study. Pediatrics 2015;136(2):e333–43.
14. Barash J, Goldzweig O. Possible role of streptococcal infection in flares of juvenile idiopathic arthritis. Arthritis Rheum 2007;57(5):877–80.
15. Söderlund M, von Essen R, Haapasaari J, et al. Persistence of parvovirus B19 DNA in synovial membranes of young patients with and without chronic arthropathy. Lancet 1997;349(9058):1063–5.
16. Oğuz F, Akdeniz C, Ünüvar E, et al. Parvovirus B19 in the acute arthropathies and juvenile rheumatoid arthritis. J Paediatr Child Health 2002;38(4):358–62.
17. Gonzalez B, Larrañaga C, León O, et al. Parvovirus B19 may have a role in the pathogenesis of juvenile idiopathic arthritis. J Rheumatol 2007;34(6).
18. Weissbrich B, Süß-Fröhlich Y, Girschick HJ. Seroprevalence of parvovirus B19 IgG in children affected by juvenile idiopathic arthritis. Arthritis Res Ther 2007;9(4):R82.
19. Aghighi Y, Gilani Sh M, Razavi M, et al. Juvenile rheumatoid arthritis in children with Ebstein Barr virus infection. Pakistan J Biol Sci PJBS 2007;10(20):3638–43. Available at: http://www.ncbi.nlm.nih.gov/pubmed/19093474. Accessed January 10, 2017.
20. Fong S, Miller JJ, Moore TL, et al. Frequencies of Epstein-Barr virus-inducible IgM anti-IgG B lymphocytes in normal children and children with juvenile

rheumatoid arthritis. Arthritis Rheum 1982;25(8):959–65. Available at: http://www.ncbi.nlm.nih.gov/pubmed/6288055. Accessed January 10, 2017.
21. Tsai YT, Kao YF, Chiang BL, et al. Detection of epstein-barr virus and cytomegalovirus genome in white blood cells from patients with juvenile rheumatoid arthritis and childhood systemic lupus erythematosus. Int Arch Allergy Immunol 1995;106(3):235–40.
22. Massa M, Mazzoli F, Pignatti P, et al. Proinflammatory responses to self HLA epitopes are triggered by molecular mimicry to Epstein-Barr virus proteins in oligoarticular juvenile idiopathic arthritis. Arthritis Rheum 2002;46(10):2721–9.
23. Kristensen K, Henriksen L. Cesarean section and disease associated with immune function. J Allergy Clin Immunol 2016;137(2):587–90.
24. Sevelsted A, Stokholm J, Bønnelykke K, et al. Cesarean section chronic immune disorders. Pediatrics 2015;135(1):e92–8.
25. Shenoi S, Shaffer ML, Wallace CA. Environmental risk factors and early-life exposures in juvenile idiopathic arthritis: a case–control study. Arthritis Care Res 2016;68(8):1186–94.
26. Ellis JA, Ponsonby A-L, Pezic A, et al. CLARITY – ChiLdhood Arthritis Risk factor Identification sTudY. Pediatr Rheumatol 2012;10(1):37.
27. Bell SW, Shenoi S, Nelson JL, et al. Juvenile idiopathic arthritis in relation to perinatal and maternal characteristics: a case control study. Pediatr Rheumatol 2017;15(1):36.
28. Räisänen L, Viljakainen H, Sarkkola C, et al. Perinatal risk factors for pediatric onset type 1 diabetes, autoimmune thyroiditis, juvenile idiopathic arthritis, and inflammatory bowel diseases. Eur J Pediatr 2021. https://doi.org/10.1007/s00431-021-03987-3.
29. Shenoi S, Bell S, Wallace CA, et al. Juvenile idiopathic arthritis in relation to maternal prenatal smoking. Arthritis Care Res (Hoboken) 2015;67(5):725–30.
30. França CMP, Sallum AME, Braga ALF, et al. Risk factors associated with juvenile idiopathic arthritis: Exposure to cigarette smoke and air pollution from pregnancy to disease diagnosis. J Rheumatol 2018;45(2):248–56.
31. Jaakkola JJK, Gissler M. Maternal smoking in pregnancy as a determinant of rheumatoid arthritis and other inflammatory polyarthropathies during the first 7 years of life. Int J Epidemiol 2005;34(3):664–71.
32. Rocha FAC, Landim JIVD, Nour ML, et al. Long-term breastfeeding influences disease activity in a low-income juvenile idiopathic arthritis cohort. Clin Rheumatol 2019;38(8):2227–31.
33. Kindgren E, Fredrikson M, Ludvigsson J. Early feeding and risk of Juvenile idiopathic arthritis: A case control study in a prospective birth cohort. Pediatr Rheumatol 2017;15(1). https://doi.org/10.1186/s12969-017-0175-z.
34. Hyrich KL, Baildam E, Pickford H, et al. Influence of past breast feeding on pattern and severity of presentation of juvenile idiopathic arthritis. Arch Dis Child 2016;101(4):348–51.
35. Rosenberg AM. Evaluation of associations between breast feeding and subsequent development of juvenile rheumatoid arthritis. J Rheumatol 1996;23(6):1080–2.
36. Mason T, Rabinovich CE, Fredrickson DD, et al. Breast feeding and the development of juvenile rheumatoid arthritis. J Rheumatol 1995;22(6):1166–70. Available at: http://www.ncbi.nlm.nih.gov/pubmed/7674248. Accessed January 8, 2017.
37. Miller J, Ponsonby A-L, Pezic A, et al. Sibling Exposure and Risk of Juvenile Idiopathic Arthritis. Arthritis Rheumatol (Hoboken, Nj) 2015;67(7):1951–8.

38. Prahalad S, Fraser AM, O'Brien E, et al. Lack of association between birth order and juvenile idiopathic arthritis. Arthritis Rheum 2003;48(10):2989–90.
39. Epidemiology of juvenile chronic arthritis: risk dependent on sibship, parental income, and housing - PubMed. Available at: https://pubmed.ncbi.nlm.nih.gov/10405951/. Accessed February 27, 2021.
40. Berkun Y, Lewy H, Padeh S, et al. Seasonality of birth of patients with juvenile idiopathic arthritis. Clin Exp Rheumatol 2015;33(1):122–6.
41. Seasonal variation in systemic onset juvenile rheumatoid arthritis in Israel - PubMed. Available at: https://pubmed.ncbi.nlm.nih.gov/10332988/. Accessed February 27, 2021.
42. Feldman BM, Birdi N, Boone JE, et al. Seasonal onset of systemic-onset juvenile rheumatoid arthritis. J Pediatr 1996;129(4):513–8.
43. Lindsley CB. Seasonal variation in systemic onset juvenile rheumatoid arthritis. Arthritis Rheum 1987;30(7):838–9.
44. Zeft AS, Prahalad S, Schneider R, et al. Systemic onset juvenile idiopathic arthritis and exposure to fine particulate air pollution. Clin Exp Rheumatol 2016;34(5):946–52.
45. Zeft AS, Prahalad S, Lefevre S, et al. Juvenile idiopathic arthritis and exposure to fine particulate air pollution. Clin Exp Rheumatol 2009;27(5):877–84.
46. Vidotto JP, Pereira LAA, Braga ALF, et al. Atmospheric pollution: Influence on hospital admissions in paediatric rheumatic diseases. Lupus 2012;21(5): 526–33.
47. Chiaroni-Clarke RC, Munro JE, Pezic A, et al. Association of increased sun exposure over the life-course with a reduced risk of juvenile idiopathic arthritis. Photochem Photobiol 2019;95(3):867–73.
48. Radon K, Windstetter D, Poluda D, et al. Exposure to animals and risk of oligoarticular juvenile idiopathic arthritis: A multicenter case-control study. BMC Musculoskelet Disord 2010;11. https://doi.org/10.1186/1471-2474-11-73.
49. Arvonen M, Virta LJ, Pokka T, et al. Cow's Milk Allergy in Infancy and Later Development of Juvenile Idiopathic Arthritis: A Register-Based Case-Control Study. Am J Epidemiol 2017;186(2):237–44.
50. Kindgren E, Guerrero-Bosagna C, Ludvigsson J. Heavy metals in fish and its association with autoimmunity in the development of juvenile idiopathic arthritis: A prospective birth cohort study. Pediatr Rheumatol 2019;17(1). https://doi.org/10.1186/s12969-019-0344-3.
51. Finch SL, Rosenberg AM, Vatanparast H. Vitamin D and juvenile idiopathic arthritis. Pediatr Rheumatol 2018;16(1). https://doi.org/10.1186/s12969-018-0250-0.
52. Thorsen SU, Pipper CB, Alberdi-Saugstrup M, et al. No association between vitamin D levels around time of birth and later risk of developing oligo- and polyarticular juvenile idiopathic arthritis: a Danish case–cohort study. Scand J Rheumatol 2017;46(2):104–11.
53. Marini F, Falcini F, Stagi S, et al. Study of vitamin D status and vitamin D receptor polymorphisms in a cohort of Italian patients with juvenile idiopathic arthritis. Sci Rep 2020;10(1). https://doi.org/10.1038/s41598-020-74861-9.
54. Rubinstein TB, Bullock DR, Ardalan K, et al. Adverse childhood experiences are associated with childhood-onset arthritis in a national sample of US youth: an analysis of the 2016 national survey of children's health. J Pediatr 2020;226: 243–50.e2.
55. Neufeld KM, Karunanayake CP, Maenz LY, et al. Stressful life events antedating chronic childhood arthritis. J Rheumatol 2013;40(10):1756–65.

56. Verwoerd A, Ter Haar NM, de Roock S, et al. The human microbiome and juvenile idiopathic arthritis. Pediatr Rheumatol Online J 2016;14(1):55. https://doi.org/10.1186/s12969-016-0114-4.
57. Arvonen M, Berntson L, Pokka T, et al. Gut microbiota-host interactions and juvenile idiopathic arthritis. doi:10.1186/s12969-016-0104-6
58. Majumder S, Aggarwal A. Juvenile idiopathic arthritis and the gut microbiome: Where are we now? Best Pract Res Clin Rheumatol 2019;33(6):101496.
59. Manasson J, Blank RB, Scher JU. The microbiome in rheumatology: Where are we and where should we go? Ann Rheum Dis 2020;79(6):S727–33.
60. Holers VM. Insights from populations at risk for the future development of classified rheumatoid arthritis. Rheum Dis Clin North Am 2014;40(4):605–20.
61. Cassotta M, Forbes-Hernandez TY, Cianciosi D, et al. Nutrition and rheumatoid arthritis in the 'omics' era. Nutrients 2021;13(3):1–25.
62. Lim SS, Bayakly AR, Helmick CG, et al. The incidence and prevalence of systemic lupus erythematosus, 2002-2004: The Georgia Lupus Registry. Arthritis Rheumatol (Hoboken, Nj) 2014;66(2):357–68.
63. Parks CG, de Souza Espindola Santos A, Barbhaiya M, et al. Understanding the role of environmental factors in the development of systemic lupus erythematosus. Best Pract Res Clin Rheumatol 2017;31(3):306–20.
64. Hanlon P, Avenell A, Aucott L, et al. Systematic review and meta-analysis of the sero-epidemiological association between Epstein-Barr virus and systemic lupus erythematosus. Arthritis Res Ther 2014;16(1). https://doi.org/10.1186/ar4429.
65. Cooper GS, Wither J, Bernatsky S, et al. Occupational and environmental exposures and risk of systemic lupus erythematosus: Silica, sunlight, solvents. Rheumatology 2010;49(11):2172–80.
66. Parks CG, Cooper GS. Occupational exposures and risk of systemic lupus erythematosus: A review of the evidence and exposure assessment methods in population-and clinic-based studies. Lupus 2006;15(11):728–36.
67. Barbhaiya M, Costenbader KH. Ultraviolet radiation and systemic lupus erythematosus. Lupus 2014;23(6):588–95.
68. Costenbader KH, Kim DJ, Peerzada J, et al. Cigarette smoking and the risk of systemic lupus erythematosus: a meta-analysis. Arthritis Rheum 2004;50(3): 849–57.
69. Costenbader KH, Feskanich D, Stampfer MJ, et al. Reproductive and menopausal factors and risk of systemic lupus erythematosus in women. Arthritis Rheum 2007;56(4):1251–62.
70. Parks CG, D'Aloisio AA, Sandler DP. Early life factors associated with adult-onset systemic lupus erythematosus in women. Front Immunol 2016;7(MAR). https://doi.org/10.3389/fimmu.2016.00103.
71. Cozier YC, Barbhaiya M, Castro-Webb N, et al. Association of child abuse with systemic lupus erythematosus in black women during adulthood. *Arthritis Care Res (Hoboken)* March 2020. https://doi.org/10.1002/acr.24188.
72. Stagi S, Cavalli L, Bertini F, et al. Vitamin D levels in children, adolescents, and young adults with juvenile-onset systemic lupus erythematosus: A cross-sectional study. Lupus 2014;23(10):1059–65.
73. Peracchi OAB, Terreri MTRA, Munekata RV, et al. Low serum concentrations of 25-hydroxyvitamin D in children and adolescents with systemic lupus erythematosus. Braz J Med Biol Res 2014;47(8):721–6.

74. Lin TC, Wu JY, Kuo ML, et al. Correlation between disease activity of pediatric-onset systemic lupus erythematosus and level of vitamin D in Taiwan: A case–cohort study. J Microbiol Immunol Infect 2018;51(1):110–4.
75. Wright TB, Shults J, Leonard MB, et al. Hypovitaminosis D is associated with greater body mass index and disease activity in pediatric systemic lupus erythematosus. J Pediatr 2009;155(2):260–5.
76. James JA, Kaufman KM, Farris AD, et al. An increased prevalence of Epstein-Barr virus infection in young patients suggests a possible etiology for systemic lupus erythematosus. J Clin Invest 1997;100(12):3019–26.
77. Conde PG, Farhat LC, Braga ALF, et al. Are prematurity and environmental factors determinants for developing childhood-onset systemic lupus erythematosus? Mod Rheumatol 2018;28(1):156–60.
78. Alves AGF, de Azevedo Giacomin MF, Braga ALF, et al. Influence of air pollution on airway inflammation and disease activity in childhood-systemic lupus erythematosus. Clin Rheumatol 2018;37(3):683–90.
79. Goulart MFG, Alves AGF, Farhat J, et al. Influence of air pollution on renal activity in patients with childhood-onset systemic lupus erythematosus. Pediatr Nephrol 2020;35(7):1247–55.
80. Robinson AB, Thierry-Palmer M, Gibson KL, et al. Disease activity, proteinuria, and vitamin D status in children with systemic lupus erythematosus and juvenile dermatomyositis. J Pediatr 2012;160(2):297–302.
81. Mendez EP, Lipton R, Ramsey-Goldman R, et al. US incidence of juvenile dermatomyositis, 1995-1998: results from the National Institute of Arthritis and Musculoskeletal and Skin Diseases Registry. Arthritis Rheum 2003;49(3):300–5.
82. Koch MJ, Brody JA, Gillespie MM. Childhood polymyositis: A case-control study. Am J Epidemiol 1976;104(6):627–31.
83. Pachman LM, Litt DL, Rowley AH, et al. Lack of detection of enteroviral rna or bacterial dna in magnetic resonance imaging–directed muscle biopsies from twenty children with active untreated juvenile dermatomyositis. Arthritis Rheum 1995;38(10):1513–8.
84. Christensen ML, Pachman LM, Schneiderman R, et al. Prevalence of coxsackie b virus antibodies in patients with juvenile dermatomyosiTIS. Arthritis Rheum 1986;29(11):1365–70.
85. Packman LM, Lipton R, Ramsey-Goldman R, et al. History of infection before the onset of juvenile dermatomyositis: Results from the National Institute of Arthritis and Musculoskeletal and Skin diseases research registry. Arthritis Care Res 2005;53(2):166–72.
86. Mamyrova G, Rider LG, Haagenson L, et al. Parvovirus B19 and onset of juvenile dermatomyositis [6]. J Am Med Assoc 2005;294(17):2170–1.
87. Zheng Q, Zhu K, Gao CN, et al. Prevalence of Epstein–Barr virus infection and characteristics of lymphocyte subsets in newly onset juvenile dermatomyositis. World J Pediatr 2019. https://doi.org/10.1007/s12519-019-00314-7.
88. Pachman LM, Hayford JR, Hochberg MC, et al. New-onset juvenile dermatomyositis: comparisons with a healthy cohort and children with juvenile rheumatoid arthritis. Arthritis Rheum 1997;40(8):1526–33.
89. Shah M, Targoff IN, Rice MM, et al. Ultraviolet radiation exposure is associated with clinical and autoantibody phenotypes in Juvenile myositis. Arthritis Rheum 2013;65(7):1934–41.
90. Mamyrova G, Rider LG, Ehrlich A, et al. Environmental factors associated with disease flare in juvenile and adult dermatomyositis. Rheumatology (Oxford) 2017 Aug 1;56(8):1342–7. https://doi.org/10.1093/rheumatology/kex162.

91. Neely J, Long CS, Sturrock H, et al. Association of short-term ultraviolet radiation exposure and disease severity in juvenile dermatomyositis: results from the childhood arthritis and rheumatology research alliance legacy registry. Arthritis Care Res 2019;71(12):1600–5.
92. Orione MAM, Silva CA, Sallum AME, et al. Risk Factors for Juvenile Dermatomyositis: Exposure to Tobacco and Air Pollutants During Pregnancy. Arthritis Care Res (Hoboken) 2014;66(10):1571–5.
93. Azali P, Helmers SB, Kockum I, et al. Low serum levels of vitamin D in idiopathic inflammatory myopathies. Ann Rheum Dis 2013;72(4):512–6.
94. Vegosen LJ, Weinberg CR, O'Hanlon TP, et al. Seasonal birth patterns in myositis subgroups suggest an etiologic role of early environmental exposures. Arthritis Rheum 2007;56(8):2719–28.
95. Rider LG, Wu L, Mamyrova G, et al. Environmental factors preceding illness onset differ in phenotypes of the juvenile idiopathic inflammatory myopathies. Rheumatology 2010;49(12):2381–90.
96. Zulian F, Athreya BH, Laxer R, et al. Juvenile localized scleroderma: clinical and epidemiological features in 750 children. An international study. Rheumatology 2006;45(5):614–20.
97. Marie I, Gehanno JF. Environmental risk factors of systemic sclerosis. Semin Immunopathol 2015;37(5):463–73.
98. Ouchene L, Muntyanu A, Lavoué J, et al. Toward understanding of environmental risk factors in systemic sclerosis. J Cutan Med Surg 2020. https://doi.org/10.1177/1203475420957950.
99. Zhao Y, Ferguson PJ. Chronic nonbacterial osteomyelitis and chronic recurrent multifocal osteomyelitis in children. Pediatr Clin North Am 2018;65(4):783–800.
100. Scott J, Hartnett J, Mockler D, et al. Environmental risk factors associated with ANCA associated vasculitis: a systematic mapping review. Autoimmun Rev 2020;19(11). https://doi.org/10.1016/j.autrev.2020.102660.
101. Burns JC, Herzog L, Fabri O, et al. Seasonality of kawasaki disease: a global perspective. PLoS One 2013;8(9). https://doi.org/10.1371/journal.pone.0074529.
102. Arvonen M, Vänni P, Sarangi AN, et al. Microbial orchestra in juvenile idiopathic arthritis: Sounds of disarray? Immunol Rev 2020;294(1):9–26.
103. Rosenbaum JT, Silverman GJ. The microbiome and systemic lupus erythematosus. N Engl J Med 2018;378(23):2236–7.
104. Priori R, Scrivo R, Brandt J, et al. Metabolomics in rheumatic diseases: The potential of an emerging methodology for improved patient diagnosis, prognosis, and treatment efficacy. Autoimmun Rev 2013;12(10):1022–30.
105. Surace AEA, Hedrich CM. The role of epigenetics in autoimmune/inflammatory disease. Front Immunol 2019;10(JULY). https://doi.org/10.3389/fimmu.2019.01525.
106. Akbaba TH, Sag E, Balci-Peynircioglu B, et al. Epigenetics for clinicians from the perspective of pediatric rheumatic diseases. Curr Rheumatol Rep 2020;22(8). https://doi.org/10.1007/s11926-020-00912-9.

Precision Medicine

Towards Individualized Dosing in Pediatric Rheumatology

Stephen J. Balevic, MD, MHS[a,b,*],
Anna Carmela P. Sagcal-Gironella, MD, MS[c,d,e]

KEYWORDS

• Precision medicine • Pharmacokinetics • Therapeutics • Clinical pharmacology
• DMARDs

KEY POINTS

- Current dosing paradigms in children with rheumatic disease fail to account for the wide between-patient variability in drug absorption, distribution, metabolism, and elimination.
- Several strategies exist to optimize dosing for biologic and non-biologic DMARDs, including therapeutic drug monitoring, pharmacogenomics, and the use of pharmacokinetic/pharmacodynamic models.
- When encountering treatment failure, it is important to consider whether drug exposure is adequate (dosing, medication adherence) before considering other reasons for treatment failure.

INTRODUCTION

Over the past several decades, biologics and targeted small molecule disease-modifying antirheumatic drugs (DMARDs) have revolutionized the treatment of pediatric rheumatic diseases. Currently, there are 10 biologic or small molecule therapeutics with US Food and Drug Administration (FDA) indications for the treatment of a pediatric rheumatic disease, including the first FDA-approved medication for pediatric systemic lupus erythematosus (SLE).[1] Despite increases in the number of available therapeutics, many children continue to experience active inflammatory disease and treatment failure. For example, approximately 1 in 4 children with juvenile idiopathic

[a] Department of Pediatrics, Duke University, Durham, NC, USA; [b] Duke Clinical Research Institute, Durham, NC, USA; [c] Department of Pediatrics, Hackensack Meridian School of Medicine, Nutley, NJ, USA; [d] Division of Pediatric Rheumatology, Joseph M. Sanzari Children's Hospital, 30 Prospect Avenue, WFAN 3rd Floor, Hackensack, NJ 07601, USA; [e] K. Hovnanian-Children's Hospital, Neptune, NJ, USA
* Corresponding author. Duke University Medical Center, 2301 Erwin Road, CHC, T-Level, Durham, NC 27710, USA.
E-mail address: Stephen.balevic@duke.edu

Rheum Dis Clin N Am 48 (2022) 305–330
https://doi.org/10.1016/j.rdc.2021.09.010
rheumatic.theclinics.com

arthritis (JIA) fails to respond to treatment with a first biologic DMARD and requires transition to a second biologic.[2] In addition, approximately half of children with SLE in the PLUTO trial did not reach the primary efficacy endpoint despite treatment with intravenous belimumab in addition to standard of care.[3]

One reason for treatment failure is the lack of dosing paradigms to account for wide between-patient variability in drug pharmacokinetics (PK) because of developmental changes or genetic polymorphisms that effect drug absorption, distribution, metabolism, and elimination. Relevant developmental changes are reviewed and summarized in other publications.[4] As an example, young infants have higher gastric pH compared with older children and adults, potentially reducing absorption of weakly acidic drugs like methotrexate (MTX).[4] In addition, children have a progressive decrease in total body water relative to fat as they age, which results in an increased volume of distribution for lipid-soluble drugs like hydroxychloroquine (HCQ). Furthermore, significant changes in glomerular filtration, the activity of hepatic drug–metabolizing enzymes, and expression or activity of drug transporters can alter drug clearance and change the dosage of medication required to maintain steady state concentrations needed for drug effectiveness.[4] As a result, the half-lives of drugs in children vary widely from those in adults, depending on age (**Fig. 1**).[5]

In addition to physiologic changes, there is genetic variability in the function of many drug-metabolizing enzymes and transporters. Thiopurine methyltransferase (TPMT) is perhaps the best-recognized example of a polymorphic drug-metabolizing enzyme in rheumatology, although common genetic mutations increasingly are recognized in enzymes that influence response or toxicity to cyclophosphamide, MTX, HCQ, allopurinol, and others. As a result of growing recognition that enzyme polymorphisms significantly influence effective dosing, the FDA has included pharmacogenomic information in greater than 200 drug labels.[6]

Collectively, the failure of current dosing strategies to account for developmental and genetic variability affecting PK reduces drug effectiveness, highlighting the

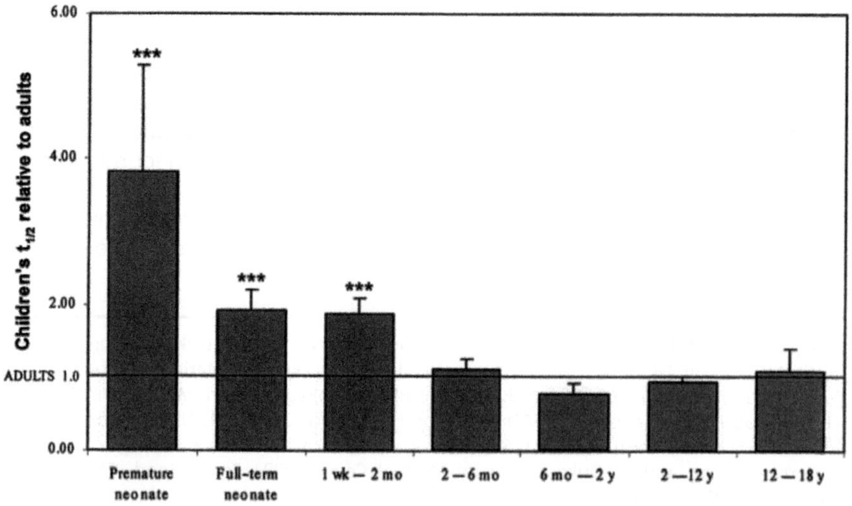

Fig. 1. Differences in drug half-lives ($t_{½}$) between adults and children receiving common therapeutics. (*From* Ginsberg G, Hattis D, Sonawane B, et al. Evaluation of child/adult pharmacokinetic differences from a database derived from the therapeutic drug literature. Toxicol Sci 2002;66:185 to 200 (see Fig. 1 in original).)

significant need to individualize dosing for children with rheumatic diseases through precision medicine. In order to raise awareness of precision dosing strategies for pediatric rheumatic diseases, this review addresses the following 3 topics: (1) review of precision medicine from a clinical pharmacology perspective and key concepts governing drug exposure and response in children; (2) examples of precision dosing biologic drugs; and (3) examples of precision dosing synthetic DMARDs.

PRECISION MEDICINE, A CLINICAL PHARMACOLOGY PERSPECTIVE

The most common dosing schemes for DMARDs in children are normalizing by weight (eg, milligrams/kilograms or milligrams/square meter) or binning, where a flat dosage is administered based on body weight range (ie, 15–30 kg). Unfortunately, neither approach produces consistent drug exposure throughout childhood. For example, scaling by weight (eg, milligrams/kilograms) falsely assumes a linear relationship between dosage and body size, whereas, in reality, growth and maturation in children are heterogeneous and nonlinear throughout childhood.[7] There are rapid changes in the capacity of most drug-metabolizing enzymes during the first year(s) of life, with relatively less change during late childhood and adolescence.[8] As a result, normalizing by body weight often underestimates dosage for young children due to their naturally lower body weight, potentially resulting in therapeutic failure.[9] A pertinent example in pediatric rheumatology was the failed infliximab trial, where children were administered the same weight-based dosage of infliximab used in adults, resulting in lower serum drug levels, underestimation of the treatment effect, and worse infusion reactions.[10–12]

For clinicians, common dosing pitfalls include the belief that administering a medication has a dichotomous effect (ie, "either it works or it doesn't"), or alternatively, the belief that there is 1 effective dose for each rheumatic disease. In reality, drug dosage is a surrogate for the concentration of drug at the site of action. Depending on the concentration of drug at the site of action, pharmacologic and clinical responses may vary. Accordingly, there are several strategies to optimizing pharmacologic response, including (1) PK/pharmacodynamic (PD) model–guided dosing, (2) therapeutic drug monitoring (TDM), and (3) pharmacogenomics.

Population Pharmacokinetic/Pharmacodynamic Model–guided Dosing

Modeling and simulation are powerful tools to optimizing dosing and are used extensively by industry and the FDA to support drug labeling.[13] Most pediatric rheumatologists, however, are unfamiliar with PK/PD modeling. PK quantifies the effect of the body on a drug (eg, metabolizing or excreting a drug) whereas PD quantifies the effect the drug has on the body (eg, clinical or pharmacologic effect).[14] Using mathematical modeling, PK and PD can be combined and advanced statistics used to identify the dose required to achieve the desired drug response.[15] A population PK/PD approach takes the model 1 step further by quantifying between-patient variability and identifying the reasons, or covariates, that explain the variability (eg, body mass index, creatinine, and concomitant medications).[14] By leveraging a population PK/PD model, a clinician or pharmacist uses an individual patient's covariates to identify a truly personalized dosage. Furthermore, clinicians can add individual patient drug levels (eg, TDM) to the model for better accuracy. As an example of this approach, investigators developed a population PK model for infliximab in children with inflammatory bowel disease (IBD).[16] They found that by including an individual patient's weight, albumin, antidrug antibody level (ATI), and erythrocyte sedimentation rate (ESR) in the model, they could predict infliximab concentrations precisely (**Fig. 2**).[16] Moreover,

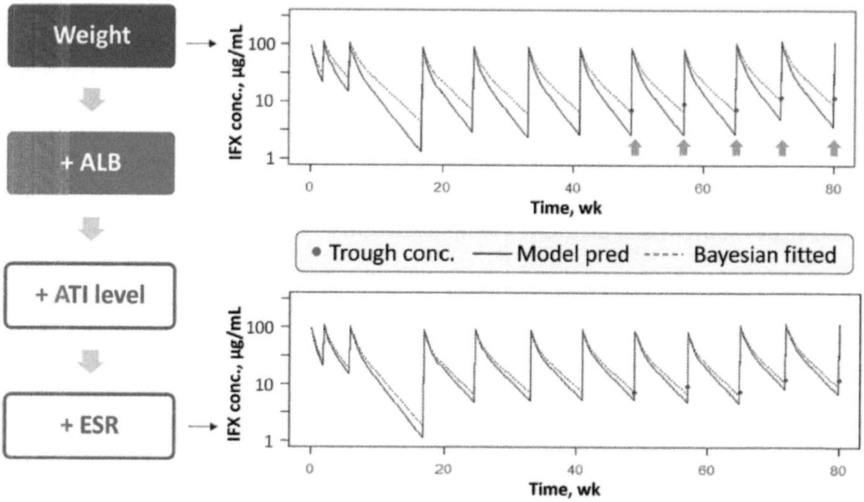

Fig. 2. Example of population PK model-directed dosing for infliximab. Stepwise covariate analysis for a representative patient case. The example shows how well the model-predicted PK profile overlaid with the actual observations. The addition of serum albumin concentration, ATI category, and ESR improved the prediction of the observed IFX trough concentrations (B) in comparison with the base model, which included body weight as a covariate (A). The orange arrows highlight how the base model was not as accurate in predicting IFX trough concentrations, especially at greater than 40 weeks. Alb, albumin; conc, concentration; pred, prediction. (*From* Bauman LE, Xiong Y, Mizuno T, et al. Improved Population Pharmacokinetic Model for Predicting Optimized Infliximab Exposure in Pediatric Inflammatory Bowel Disease. Inflamm Bowel Dis 2020;26:429-39.;(Figure 1 in original).)

by including a patient's actual infliximab trough level in the model, they demonstrated improved accuracy of model predictions. The final PK model could individualize dosing for infliximab and obtain target trough concentrations in pediatric IBD.[16]

Major challenges to implementing population PK/PD modeling in the clinical setting include the sheer complexity of the modeling, lack of in-depth pharmacology training during medical school, and lack of time for clinicians or pharmacists to conduct the simulations. Recently, researchers have focused on developing software that allows a simple, point-of-care solution to individualize a patient's dose based on existing PK/PD models.[15] For example, InsightRx (https://www.insight-rx.com) is an online platform that currently supports individualized dosing for adalimumab, MTX, infliximab, tacrolimus, and intravenous immunoglobulin.[17] Clinicians are able to enter specific patient information and the relevant covariates (eg, age and weight) and identify a model-directed starting dose. Current InsightRX models, however, were not developed specifically for children with rheumatic disease.

Although available software platforms are a significant innovation in dosing, the models are only as strong as the studies used to derive them. To implement PK/PD model–guided dosing on a wide scale, the rheumatology research community must invest in further PK/PD studies for both existing and new therapeutics and educate the community on PK, PD, and the pharmacologic principles guiding model interpretation. Although a review of drug metabolism is outside the scope of this article, there are excellent public resources (eg, PharmGKB) that provide evidence-based summaries of pharmacogenomics, including detailed metabolic pathways, clinical annotations, and dosing guidance for individual drugs.[18]

Therapeutic Drug Monitoring

TDM is the practice of measuring drug concentrations, usually in blood, to determine whether a concentration is sufficient to achieve response or limit toxicity.[19] Based on the measured drug level, the dosage then is either increased or decreased to achieve the target concentration. TDM is a promising strategy to individualize dose, because most drugs show a stronger correlation between whole-blood or serum/plasma levels and pharmacologic response compared with dose alone. For example, measuring trough concentrations of tacrolimus is considered standard of care, because adjusting dosage based on trough concentrations improves outcome (lower rates of acute organ transplant rejection) while also reducing toxicity.[20] Less commonly, TDM can involve measuring a biomarker of response (ie, a PD marker)—for example, the total white blood cell count to guide cyclophosphamide dosing or the international normalized ratio for warfarin. Historically, TDM was reserved for drugs with narrow therapeutic indices, unacceptable toxicity, or wide interindividual variability in dosage requirements.[19] It increasingly is recognized, however, that TDM may have a role in optimizing dosing for a wide range of therapeutics where PK is variable. In addition to optimizing dosage, TDM is a helpful tool to identify medication nonadherence. For example, multiple studies have suggested that monitoring HCQ concentration in whole blood or serum can identify medication nonadherence accurately.[21,22] Moreover, by counseling lupus patients who had low HCQ blood levels, investigators found that adherence to HCQ improved by 24%.[23]

To apply TDM in clinical practice, it is important to recall that drug concentration changes throughout the dosing interval. Accordingly, it is important to identify when in the dosing interval (eg, peak, trough, or random) a sample is drawn. In addition, drug concentration can be measured in several matrices, including whole blood, plasma, and serum. Some drugs preferentially partition in 1 matrix, meaning that drug levels in whole blood may or may not be comparable to plasma and/or serum. Lastly, there are several ways to measure drug exposure, including a single, static measurement (eg, peak or trough); average concentration; and total exposure (by calculating the area under the time vs concentration curve [AUC] [**Fig. 3**).

There are several potential challenges implementing TDM for DMARDs on a wide scale. First, there are no commercially available assays to measure the blood

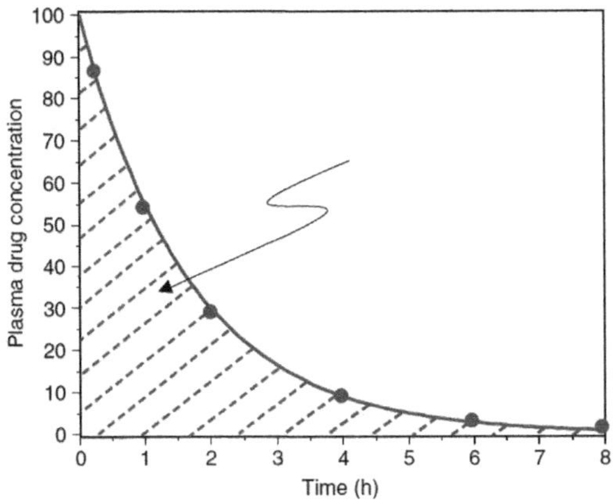

Fig. 3. AUC. (*From* Tirona R, Kim R. Introduction to Clinical Pharmacology. In: Clinical and Translational Science: Principles of Human Research. Robertson D, Williams GH, editors. San Diego: Elsevier Science & Technology; 2008. Figure 22.5 in original).

concentration of commonly used DMARDs. Second, target drug concentration often is unknown. In addition, achieving a target drug or biomarker concentration does not guarantee response. Lastly, a clinician may not know how to adjust a dose to achieve a given target concentration. Despite these potential limitations, PK/PD modeling easily identifies the association between dose, drug concentration, and response. Such modeling is a standard part of a new drug application to FDA but is not always publicly available.[24] Accordingly, there is a clear need for further research into target drug levels for DMARDs and whether the target level from adults can be extrapolated to children.

Pharmacogenomics

Broadly, pharmacogenomics is the study of how common genetic variants (ie, polymorphisms) are associated with drug exposure and response.[18] Genes that code for drug-metabolizing enzymes, drug transporters, and drug receptors often contain relevant polymorphisms. Based on genotype and the specific drug of interest, an individual patient's phenotype (eg, rapid metabolizer or slow metabolizer) and subsequent dosage needs can be determined. There are multiple commercially available platforms that investigators and clinicians can use to identify critical polymorphisms.[25]

Although pharmacologists have long known that enzymes are responsible for metabolizing synthetic or small molecule DMARDs, only recently has there been awareness of their substantial genetic variability. For example, cytochrome P450 (CYP) 2D6—which metabolizes more than 25% of all drugs on the market—has more than 160 variants.[26] Each variant may be associated with increased or decreased metabolism and subsequent high or low drug concentrations in the body. The clinical implications of the variants are far from trivial; CYP2D6 ultrarapid metabolizers (1%–10% of the white population)[27] have died from respiratory depression after receiving codeine.[28] Also, polymorphisms in drug metabolizing enzymes usually follow ancestral inheritance and could be responsible for observed racial disparities in treatment response for rheumatic diseases.

EXAMPLES OF PRECISION DOSING FOR BIOLOGIC DRUGS

To individualize dosing for biologics, it is necessary to understand (1) the causes of PK variability between individual patients; (2) the exposure-response relationship between biologic drug levels and outcomes; and (3) the target concentrations needed to obtain the desired outcome. The term, *biologics*, can refer to a multitude of different therapeutics (eg, blood products and vaccines); the term, *biologic*, in this review refers to protein-based therapeutics, in particular monoclonal antibodies.

Brief Primer on Biologic Pharmacokinetics

As large molecules, biologics used to treat rheumatic diseases must be administered parentally, either subcutaneously or intravenously. When given subcutaneously, biologics are absorbed slowly and move via convection through lymphatic vessels and into systemic circulation.[29] There is wide variability between patients in the degree of absorption and drug bioavailability after subcutaneous injection, meaning varying amounts of the administered dose reach the systemic circulation.[29,30] Elimination of monoclonal antibodies is unique compared with small molecules; monoclonal antibodies are cleared predominantly through intracellular catabolism via the reticuloendothelial system and by forming complexes with either target antigens (eg, tumor necrosis factor [TNF]-α and interleukin [IL]-6) or antidrug antibodies (ADAs).[29,30] As a result, many biologics display both linear PK and nonlinear PK, where drug exposure may increase disproportionately with higher dosages. Studies consistently demonstrate that the development of ADAs results in lower drug levels and worse clinical outcomes for multiple biologics.[31–34] For example, patients with antibodies to adalimumab had significantly lower European League Against Rheumatism (EULAR) response rates and significantly lower change in the Disease Activity Score in 28 Joints (DAS28) after treatment.[32]

The unique clearance pathways for biologics result in significant clinical implications. Patients with high antigen levels (eg, TNF-α) may have higher drug clearance, resulting in shorter drug half-lives and lower trough concentrations.[29,30] For example, adults with RA and high C-reactive protein (CRP) at baseline (a surrogate for inflammatory disease and antigenic burden) have a 47% reduction in infliximab half-life (14 days to 8 days).[35] Additionally, adults with RA and high baseline TNF-α concentrations are significantly more likely to have undetectable infliximab trough concentrations compared with patients with low TNF-α at baseline.[36] Monoclonal antibodies can be protected from intracellular catabolism by binding to the neonatal Fc receptor (FcRn), although other endogenous immunoglobulins (including rheumatoid factor) also are competing for the receptor.[37] Accordingly, children who are rheumatoid factor positive or have higher endogenous immunoglobulin concentrations may have higher clearance of monoclonal antibodies.

In addition to differences in baseline antigen levels and endogenous proteins that influence biologic drug clearance, several other patient characteristics may have an impact on the PK of biologic drugs, including body weight and size, sex, age, concomitant medications (eg, MTX), polymorphisms in the FcRn, and renal function (anakinra only).[29,30] **Tables 1** and **2** highlight the effect of various clinical characteristics on drug PK and overall strategies to optimize dosing.

Assay differences for assessing biologic levels may result in different target concentrations across studies. Accordingly, before adopting TDM for biologics in clinical practice, clinicians first should identify the commercial assay they intend to use and ensure the target concentrations from the literature (discussed later) use the same or similar assays. Readers are referred to other sources that review assays in the context of TDM for biologic drugs.[61]

Optimal Dosing Strategies for Biologics

Although a majority of data characterizing the exposure-response relationship for biologics come from the adult literature, there are consistent observations across

Table 1
Clinical characteristics effecting pharmacokinetics[35,36,38–48]

Drug	Clearance	Volume of Distribution
Adalimumab	Age, ADA, MTX, rheumatoid factor, CRP, sex, weight	Weight
Etanercept	**Body surface area, sex**	**Weight**
Infliximab	CRP, MTX, ADA, TNF-α	Weight
Tocilizumab	Body surface area, sex, high-density lipoprotein	Total protein, albumin
Canakinumab	**Weight, albumin**	**Weight**
Anakinra	Weight, creatinine clearance	Weight
Abatacept	Weight	Weight

Bold represents data in pediatric rheumatic diseases.

Table 2
Selected data supporting optimal dosing strategies

Drug	Therapeutic Drug Modeling and Pharmacokinetic/ Pharmacodynamic Modeling	Pharmacogenomics
Adalimumab	• Adalimumab levels correlated with change in DAS28 and EULAR response. Optimal cutoff trough concentration 1.274 μg/mL at 6 mo[33] • Median serum adalimumab trough levels (6.9 μg/mL) were higher in RA patients in remission.[49] • Adalimumab trough level of 5 μg/mL for EULAR good response in RA (91% sensitivity; 43% specificity)[50] • In adults with RA, EULAR good responders had higher serum adalimumab levels compared with moderate or nonresponders.[32]	• FcRn genotype was associated with lower levels of adalimumab and infliximab in patients with IBD.[51] • In RA, polymorphisms in the TNF-α and IL-6 genes associated with response to etanercept[52] • In spondyloarthritis, polymorphisms in the TNF-α gene associated with response to etanercept[53]
Etanercept	• Etanercept levels correlated with change in DAS28 and EULAR response. Optimal cutoff trough concentration 1.274 μg/mL at 6 mo[33] • Etanercept levels correlated with change in DAS28 at 3 mo (r = −0.50; P = .03). Etanercept concentration of 3.1 μg/mL at 3 mo predicted DAS28 response at 6 mo (87% sensitivity; 67% specificity).[54] • Etanercept levels significantly higher in EULAR good responders compared with both moderate responders and nonresponders (median 3.7 mg/L, 3.1 mg/L, and 2.8 mg/L, respectively)[55] • Target troughs for remission were 1.34 μg/mL for adalimumab (sensitivity 81.9%; specificity 81%) and 1.56 μg/mL for etanercept (sensitivity 71.1%; specificity 71.4%).[49]	
Infliximab	• Progressively higher serum trough concentrations of infliximab in RA patients were associated with larger ACR responses, reduction in CRP, and less radiographic joint damage.[56] • In patients with RA, 48% with infliximab trough concentrations >10 μg/mL achieved an ACR 50 or greater.[56]	

(*continued on next page*)

Table 2
(*continued*)

Drug	Therapeutic Drug Modeling and Pharmacokinetic/ Pharmacodynamic Modeling	Pharmacogenomics
	• EULAR responders had significantly higher median serum trough infliximab concentrations than nonresponders (3.6 mg/L vs 0.5 mg/L).[35]	
Tocilizumab	• Pooled data from 4 RCTs (n = 2243) showed adults with RA and AUC <100 μg/mL*h had lower ACR 20/50/70 and higher DAS28 scores.[57] • The effective tocilizumab concentration at which a 50% maximum DAS28 response was observed was 3.7 μg/mL.[57] • RA patients with tocilizumab concentrations >10 μg/mL had significantly lower DAS28, ESR, and CRP.[50] • Clinical remission or low disease activity was higher in RA patients with detectable trough levels of tocilizumab. Recommended minimum serum tocilizumab concentration of 3.48 μg/mL to obtain clinical remission[58]	• In RA, polymorphisms in the IL-6 receptor were associated with poor swollen joint counts and EULAR response.[59] • In RA, polymorphisms in IL-6 receptor were associated with low disease activity at 12 mo.[60]

multiple drug classes that higher biologic dosages (resulting in higher drug levels) are associated with improved outcomes (see **Table 2**). For example, a clinical trial in RA patients who were not responding to infliximab, at 3 mg/kg, were randomized to receive infliximab, at 1.5-mg/kg dosage increments; the study found that greater than 80% of patients who received higher infliximab dosages experienced at least a 20% improvement in disease activity without a higher incidence of adverse events.[62] Similarly, a clinical trial in pediatric Crohn disease found that children initially nonresponsive to adalimumab achieved remission 31% of the time dosed every 2 weeks and response 57% of the time when dosing was escalated to weekly.[63] For children with autoinflammatory diseases, the FDA drug label for canakinumab suggests increasing the dosage if clinical response is not adequate.[39] It also is well recognized that children with systemic JIA and/or macrophage activation syndrome may respond progressively better with higher doses of anakinra.[64] Furthermore, a PK/PD model for tocilizumab suggested an additional 14% of adults with RA would achieve DAS28 remission if tocilizumab dosage were increased from 4 mg/kg to 8 mg/kg.[57]

Despite accumulating evidence of an exposure-response relationship for biologics in rheumatic diseases, target concentrations for many biologics in children are unknown, and current TDM and PK/PD modeling strategies assume that achieving the comparable adult target levels will be similarly efficacious in children. Despite this potential limitation, the FDA recently published data confirming similar exposure-response between adults and children with RA and JIA.[65] Nevertheless, it is clear from the ATTRACT trial that "target concentrations" depend partly on the desired response and may vary from individual to individual. In addition, differences in target concentrations between studies likely are due to differences in drug measurement assays, concomitant medications, and underlying population characteristics.

Most of the few examples of concentration-guided clinical trials for infliximab have conflicting results. A clinical trial of infliximab in IBD randomized participants to either traditional infliximab maintenance dosing or concentration-guided dosing (3–7 μg/mL).[66] The investigators found no difference in clinical remission at 1 year (likely due to flaws with the study design where both treatment groups received initial dosage optimization based on trough levels) but nevertheless observed that patients receiving concentration-guided dosing had significantly fewer flares. An abstract presented at the 2020 American College of Rheumatology (ACR) annual meeting showed that adults with a variety of conditions (rheumatoid arthritis, psoriasis, spondyloarthritis, and IBD) did not have higher remission rates using TDM (target 3–8 μg/mL) compared with usual care.[67] Heterogeneity in design and relatively low target concentrations, however, limit the studies' generalizability.

PRECISION DOSING FOR NONBIOLOGIC DISEASE-MODIFYING ANTIRHEUMATIC DRUGS

Unlike most biologic DMARDs, nonbiologic DMARDs, such as HCQ, MTX, mycophenolate mofetil (MMF), and azathioprine (AZA), often are subject to hepatic drug metabolism and/or renal elimination. Both biologic and nonbiologic DMARDs, however, share high interindividual variability in the degree of drug exposure and response at any dosage. The high interindividual variability for nonbiologic DMARDs is due, in part, to genetic polymorphisms that have an impact on drug-metabolizing enzymes, target receptors, and drug transporters. Accordingly, the precision medicine principles used for biologic DMARDs can be applied to nonbiologic DMARDs, including TDM and pharmacogenomics. **Table 3** highlights specific data supporting precision medicine approaches for several nonbiologic DMARDs.

Genetic variation can affect individual drug metabolism and response in 2 key areas: activation and elimination.[97] Broadly, nonbiologic DMARDs can be classified as (1) a prodrug, requiring metabolism to an active metabolite to exert its pharmacologic effect, or (2) an active drug; in which case metabolism of the drug usually (but not always) is associated with conversion to an inactive metabolite and loss of therapeutic effect. For example, if a gene variant in a drug-metabolizing enzyme is associated with a loss of function, then conversion of a prodrug like MMF to its active metabolite mycophenolic acid (MPA) is reduced, potentially decreasing both efficacy and toxicity. If the gene variant were associated with increased function, however, then conversion of MMF to MPA would be increased, potentially leading to increased efficacy or toxicity.[98] In addition, when there is loss of function of a gene variant encoding an enzyme that mediates drug elimination, the variant may lead to increased drug levels, which is of particular concern in drugs with a narrow therapeutic window.[97,98]

Optimal Dosing Strategies for Nonbiologic Disease-modifying Antirheumatic Drugs

Therapeutic drug monitoring and pharmacogenomics for mycophenolate mofetil

Recent data in both children and adults with SLE show that MMF dosing based on weight or body surface does not reliably correlate with the conversion and

Table 3
Therapeutic drug monitoring and pharmacogenomic studies of selected nonbiologic disease-modifying antirheumatic drugs[50]

Reference	Study Type	Sample Size	Patient Characteristics	Main Findings
Mycophenolate Mofetil				
Neumann et al,[68,69] 2008	Prospective, consecutive, unblinded	38	26 ANCA vasculitis 12 SLE	MPA trough concentrations ≥3.5 mg/L associated with sustained remission
Zahr et al,[70] 2010	Prospective, consecutive, single blinded, single center	71	26 active SLE (mean SLEDAI ± SD): 11.6 ± 4.4 45 inactive SLE: 1.9 ± 1.6	12-h MPA AUC ≥35 mg*h/L correlated with decreased clinical activity
Lertdumrongluk et al,[69,71] 2010	Prospective, unblinded	18	Active lupus nephritis (class III/IV)	12-h MPA AUC >45 mg*h/L associated with improved outcomes 12-h MPA AUC correlated well with trough (C0) and MPA level 1 h postdose (C1) Enteric-coated mycophenolate sodium has different PK.
Sagcal-Gironella et al,[72] 2011	Prospective, unblinded, PK/PD evaluation	19	Pediatric SLE Time-adjusted mean BILAG pre-MMF 9.8 ± 5.4 BILAG post-MMF 5.8 ± 3.7	12-h MPA AUC ≥ mg*h/L correlated with improved disease control based on BILAG Inverse relationship between MPA AUC and IMPDH activity, supporting the use of IMPDH as a PD target
Fukuda et al,[73] 2012	Prospective, unblinded, PK/PG evaluation	32	Pediatric renal transplant recipients	UGT1A9-440C>T, UGT2B7-900A>G, and MRP2-24T>C polymorphisms correlated with increased MPA AUC
Kittanamongkolchai et al,[69,74] 2013	Prospective, unblinded	19	Active lupus nephritis (class III/IV)	MPA level 1 h postdose (C1) >13 mg/L associated with better disease outcomes
Woillard et al,[75] 2014	Retrospective	36	Pediatric SLE 16 active disease (SLEDAI >6)	MPA AUC >45 mg*h/L L correlated with disease control

(*continued on next page*)

Table 3
(continued)

Reference	Study Type	Sample Size	Patient Characteristics	Main Findings
Sagcal-Gironella et al,[76] 2014	Prospective, unblinded, PK/PG evaluation	18	Pediatric SLE	UGT1A9-440T (−331C) or UGT2B7-900G polymorphism was associated with reduced clearance and higher MPA AUC. UGT1A9-275A polymorphism showed relatively increased clearance.
Yap et al,[77] 2020	Prospective, unblinded PK/PG evaluation	88	Adult SLE (stable disease)	ABCC2 rs2273697 A/G polymorphism correlated with lowed MPA AUC
Chen et al,[78] 2020	Retrospective, cross-sectional	67	Pediatric SLE 25 Active disease (SLEDAI $\geq$ 6)	12-h MPA AUC $\geq$39 mg*h/L, MPA trough concentration >1.01 mg/L associated with lowest risk for active disease
Godron-Dubrasquet et al,[79] 2020	Retrospective	27	Pediatric lupus nephritis	MPA AUC >45 mg*h/L associated with better response rate
Hydroxychloroquine				
Zahr et al,[80] 2021	Retrospective	55	Pediatric SLE	HCQ blood concentration lower in children with active vs inactive lupus (536 ng/mL $\pm$ 294 ng/mL vs 758 ng/mL $\pm$ 490 ng/mL)
Munster et al,[81] 2002	6-wk, double-blind trial, 3 dosing arms (400 mg/d, 800 mg/d, or 1200 mg/d), followed by 18-wk open-label treatment at 400 mg/d	123	Rheumatoid arthritis	No target HCQ concentration identified There was correlation between disease improvement and HCQ concentration. There was correlation between GI adverse effects and elevated HCQ concentration.
Costedoat-Chalumeau et al,[69,82] 2006	Longitudinal, blinded, PK/PD evaluation	143	SLE 23 with SLEDAI 12.4 $\pm$ 7.5	HCQ >1000 ng/mL associated with decreased exacerbation

Costedoat-Chalumeau et al,[70,84] 2007	Prospective, blinded	203	SLE	HCQ <130 ng/mL associated with nonadherence. HCQ >205 ng/mL unable to distinguish intermittent vs complete adherence
Costedoat-Chalumeau et al,[69,83] 2013	Prospective, randomized, double-blind, placebo-controlled, multicenter	171	SLE with stable disease and SELENA-SLEDAI ≤12	HCQ >1000 ng/mL associated with fewer disease flares but dose escalation based on concentration did not correlate with disease activity.
Ting et al,[84] 2012	Prospective	70	Pediatric SLE	HCQ <100 ng/mL associated with nonadherence
Jallouli et al,[85] 2015	Retrospective	509	SLE On HCQ 400 mg/d	HCQ <200 ng/mL associated with poor adherence and excluded from analysis No association between ethnicity or smoking with HCQ concentration No PK drug-drug interaction with CYP inhibitors/inducers nor antacids Higher HCQ concentrations in patients with chronic renal insufficiency
Mok et al,[86] 2016	Longitudinal, consecutive	276	SLE	HCQ >500 ng/mL considered as minimal therapeutic level and correlated with lower disease activity and fewer disease flares in patients in clinical and serologic remission.
Balbi et al,[87] 2020	Prospective	60	Pediatric lupus nephritis	HCQ ≤573 ng/mL predicted flare within 6 mo.
Methotrexate				
Dervieux et al,[88] 2004	Cross-sectional, single center	108	RA	Suggested optimal RBC MTX PG levels >60 nmol/L and may be used in TDM

(*continued on next page*)

Table 3
(*continued*)

Reference	Study Type	Sample Size	Patient Characteristics	Main Findings
Dervieux et al,[89] 2005	Cross-sectional, observational study, multicenter	226	RA	Lower RBC MTX PG levels (median 40 nmol/L) and a lower pharmacogenetic index (median 2) were associated with a higher number of joint counts, higher disease activity, and higher modified Health Assessment Questionnaire.
Becker et al,[90] 2010	Cross-sectional analysis, single center	99	JIA	There was a 40-fold interindividual variability of MTX PG total concentration. Seven individual subtypes of MTX PG metabolites were identified. The route of administration contributed to the variability in concentration of most MTX PGs.
Becker et al,[91] 2011	Cross-sectional analysis, single center	104	JIA	There was an association between MTX PGs and adverse effects (LFT elevation and GI side effects). No association between MTX PGs and active arthritis
Bulatovic et al,[92] 2012	Longitudinal study design with derivation and validation cohorts	183	JIA	A prediction model consisting of clinical (ESR) and genetic variables (SNPs in genes coding for enzymes involved in MTX metabolism) of clinical nonresponse to MTX in JIA was proposed and validated.

Pastore et al,[93] 2015	Prospective	69	JIA	The most common functional variants of ATIC, ITPA, and SLC19A1 genes were associated with clinical response to MTX defined as remission stable for a 6-mo period, as ACRPed score and as change in JADAS.
Calasan et al,[94] 2015	Prospective	113	JIA	Long chain erythrocyte MTX PGs were associated with lower JADAS-27 at 3 mo and during 1 y of MTX treatment.
de Rotte et al,[95] 2015	Longitudinal study design with derivation and validation cohorts	102	RA	An increase in erythrocyte-MTX PG concentration was associated with a decreased DAS28 over 9 mo in 2 cohorts.
Azathioprine				
Askanase et al[96]	Prospective	50	SLE	Mean concentration of 6-TGN of 159 pmol/8 $\times 10^8$ RBCs was associated with efficacy. Maximum of 3.5 mg/kg/d required to achieve the proposed target 6-TGN concentrations in IBD of 235–450 pmol/8 $\times 10^8$ RBCs

Abbreviations: ABCC2, adenosine triphosphate-binding cassette subfamily C member 2; ATIC, 5-aminoimidazole-4-carboxamide ribonucleotide transformylase; ITPA, inosine-triphosphate-pyrophosphatase; MRP2, multidrug resistance-associated protein 2; SLC19A1, solute-liquid-carrier-19A1; ANCA, anti-neutrophil cytoplasmic antibody; SLEDAI, Systemic Lupus Erythematosus Disease Activity Index; LFT, liver function test; ACR Ped score, American College of Rheumatology Pediatric Score; JADAS, Juvenile Arthritis Disease Activity Score; JADAS-27, Juvenile Arthritis Disease Activity Score 27-reduced joint count.

subsequent clinical response to MPA.[99–101] Because of the poor correlation between MMF weight-based dosing and MPA concentrations, TDM using MPA trough concentrations or AUC of the time concentration profile is a promising approach to optimizing dosing and achieving maximal clinical efficacy with minimal toxicity.[100,102,103] Potential challenges to the regular use of MPA concentrations to guide MMF dosing, however, include the determination of the appropriate MPA exposure target (ie, AUC using samples collected over 12 hours vs 24 hours or at other specific time points, or the use of trough concentrations) and the difficulty translating an MPA exposure target into an MMF dosage change. To overcome these barriers, 2 studies in childhood-onset SLE propose using PK models or bayesian estimators (BEs) to determine MPA AUC using 1 blood sample collected at 3 time points (20 minutes, 60 minutes, and 180 minutes).[75,99] Overall, preliminary evidence suggests targeting an MPA AUC of greater than 30 mg*h/L to 45 mg*h/L (see **Table 3**) for optimal response. To help guide MMF dosing to achieve these target exposure levels, there are Web/cloud-based services, which provide similar BE of MPA AUC based on population PK models, such as InsightRX, MW Pharm (https://www.mwpharm.nl/mwpharm.htm), and Limoges University Hospital (https://pharmaco.chu-limoges.fr).[104] The programs are available for clinical use and typically require input of patient-specific data, such as clinical characteristics (eg, weight), drug concentrations, and administration time and dose.

Pharmacogenomics also may help optimize MMF dosing. UDP-glucuronosyltransferases (UGTs) inactivate MPA in multiple organs; studies done in pediatric renal transplant and pediatric SLE patients[73,76] show that specific variants in UGTs are associated with MPA AUC and clearance. Future studies that evaluate the UGT variants for inclusion in PK/PD models and BEs may allow for precise estimation of optimal MMF dosing.

Therapeutic drug monitoring and pharmacogenomics for methotrexate

There is wide variability in the MTX dose required by individual patients to achieve disease control and remission.[105,106] In JIA, significant intraindividual and interindividual variability in MTX concentrations have been noted after oral and subcutaneous administration.[107] The observation that children require higher MTX doses to maintain disease control in comparison to adult RA patients has led to studies showing the age dependence of oral MTX PK.[108] MTX has a short plasma half-life of elimination (approximately 6 hours) and is taken up rapidly by different cells.[106] As a result, MTX plasma concentrations do not correlate well with disease activity.[109] Instead, polyglutamated forms of MTX (MTX polyglutamates [PGs]), found in red blood cells, are a better marker for MTX drug exposure given their long half-life and anti-inflammatory effects.[106] Several studies in RA and JIA show a direct relationship between the concentration of MTX PGs and disease control.[90–92,94,95] Accordingly, TDM using MTX PGs is a promising strategy to optimizing dosage. Early studies in RA[88,89] identified optimal MTX PG concentrations of greater than 60 nmol/L for TDM, although studies are ongoing to confirm this target exposure level in JIA.

Although TDM using MTX PG concentrations are a promising strategy to optimize dosing, there are several limitations to implementing TDM for MTX in clinical practice. First, MTX PG concentrations take a long time to attain steady state, which limit the ability to use TDM to guide initial MTX dosing and assessing early treatment adherence.[106] Target concentrations also may differ between different diseases (eg, JIA vs childhood-onset SLE). Accordingly, additional research in children is needed to clarify optimal MTX PG concentrations in various disease settings and the required dosage to obtain the target concentrations.

As summarized in **Table 3**, genetic variation in the folate pathway influencing purine synthesis,[110,111] cellular transport of MTX and folate,[92,112–114] and MTX excretion[115] correlate with clinical response or toxicity in JIA. In an effort to apply PG to clinical practice, a prediction model was developed and validated in 104 JIA patients consisting of clinical (ESR) and genetic variables (single-nucleotide polymorphisms [SNPs] in genes coding for enzymes involved in MTX metabolism). Using the model, a total risk score was generated ranging from 0 to 11; a cutoff of 3 or more provided a positive predictive value of 83% and negative predictive value of 41% for treatment failure.[92] If replicated, the model may be an important tool to implement in clinical practice, particularly as rheumatologists become more comfortable ordering and interpreting pharmacogenetic tests. In addition, SNPs in amino-imidazole carboxamide ribonucleotide transformylase and ADORA2a, an adenosine receptor correspond with higher concentrations of long-chain MTX PGs.[91] Long-chain MTX PGs also correlate with MTX-induced gastrointestinal (GI)-related adverse effects and elevated transaminases in children with JIA.[91] It, therefore, is possible that testing for genotypes associated with MTX disposition may identify children at risk for poor MTX tolerance, suggesting implementation of alternative treatment strategies.

Therapeutic drug monitoring and pharmacogenomics for azathioprine

AZA has complex drug disposition with multiple relevant metabolites that can be measured in clinical practice, including 6-thioguanine nucleotide (6-TGN) and 6-methylmercaptopurine (6-MMP); 6-TGN concentrations correlate with increased response (>235 pmol/8 $\times$ 10^8 red blood cells [RBCs])[116] in IBD and increased risk for myelotoxicity (>450 pmol/8 $\times$ 10^8 RBCs). In addition, concentrations of 6-MMP greater than 5700 pmol/8 $\times$ 10^8 RBCs are associated with hepatotoxicity.[106] A study in 50 adults with SLE showed a mean 6-TGN concentration of 159 pmol/8 $\times$ 10^8 RBCs predicted efficacy and a maximum dose of 3.5 mg/kg/d was required to achieve 6-TGN concentrations between 235 pmol/8 $\times$ 10^8 to 450 pmol/8 $\times$ 10^8 RBCs. Although the limited available studies are encouraging, further prospective trials are needed to better characterize the safe and effective AZA metabolite concentrations in children with rheumatic disease before specific dosing guidance is recommended.

Screening for genetic variations in TPMT can identify patients at risk for myelotoxicity.[117,118] In addition, up to 31% of patients preferentially produce 6-MMP instead of 6-TGN.[119] This metabolic shunting indicates thiopurine resistance and increased hepatotoxicity.[120] A single measurement of TPMT genotype prior to treatment, however, may not fully characterize toxicity risk, because enzyme activity fluctuates over time and can be inhibited or induced by other concomitant medications.[69] Accordingly, assays that measure TPMT function instead of genotype may be more accurate in guiding initial dosing, after which dosing can be further refined through TDM by measuring 6-TGN and 6-MMP concentrations.

Therapeutic drug monitoring for hydroxychloroquine

Several observational studies suggest an association between HCQ blood concentrations and disease activity in systemic or cutaneous lupus.[82,106,121] In addition, a multicenter controlled trial (Plaquenil LUpus Systemic Study (PLUS))[83] in adults with SLE investigated the strategy of increasing HCQ dosing to achieve a blood concentration of at least 1000 ng/mL. Unfortunately, dose escalation did not reduce flare rate except in a subset of patients without early disease flares who consistently achieved target concentrations. Investigators also determined that whole-blood HCQ concentrations less than 130 ng/mL to 200 ng/mL were associated with nonadherence to HCQ.[29,122,123] Low serum HCQ concentrations ($\leq$100 ng/mL) were associated with increased disease activity and preterm birth in a cohort of pregnant women with SLE.[21] There are few data addressing HCQ TDM in children, but large (100-fold) variability in drug concentrations is observed and preliminary data found that SLE flare rates over 1 year were numerically (but not statistically) higher in children with serum concentrations less than or equal to 100 ng/mL.[124] In addition, a retrospective study of 55 children with SLE found that 87.6% of children with whole-blood HCQ levels greater than 750 ng/mL had inactive lupus.[80] Only 3 of the 55 children experienced retinal toxicity, and there did not appear to be a clear association with whole-blood levels. Ongoing clinical trials may help clarify the therapeutic window and optimal dosing of HCQ in children (NCT04358302). Ultimately, PK/PD models for HCQ in both children and adults are needed to definitively characterize HCQ dosages needed for maximal effectiveness while minimizing the risk of retinal toxicity.

PRECISION MEDICINE FOR OPTIMIZING THERAPY IN PEDIATRIC RHEUMATOLOGY

Achieving disease control in children with rheumatic disease as early as possible is critical to improving outcomes; for example, 96% of children with systemic JIA who achieve inactive disease by 1 month continue to maintain remission at 1 year, compared with only 47% who do not achieve inactive disease by 1 month.[125] Because children are at risk for long-term toxicity from chronic immunomodulation, there is an urgent need to optimize the dosage of medications needed for clinical efficacy, while minimizing toxicity. Recent advances in clinical pharmacology have elucidated mechanisms of intraindividual and interindividual variability in drug exposure and response for biologic and nonbiologic DMARDs, opening a potentially fruitful avenue to individualize dosing in children with rheumatic disease. High-quality, prospective PK/PD and pharmacogenomics studies are essential, however, to close existing knowledge gaps and provide clinicians with the practical guidance needed to optimize dosing for individual children.

CLINICS CARE POINTS

- Current dosing paradigms in children with rheumatic disease fail to account for the wide between-patient variability in drug absorption, distribution, metabolism, and elimination.
- Several strategies exist to optimize dosing for biologic and nonbiologic DMARDs, including TDM, pharmacogenomics, and the use of PK/PD models.
- When encountering treatment failure, it is important to consider whether drug exposure is adequate (dosing and medication adherence) before considering other reasons for treatment failure, such as differences in disease phenotype/biology, incorrect underlying diagnosis, and other causes.

DISCLOSURE

S.J. Balevic receives support from the National Institutes of Health (5R01-HD076676–04, 1R01HD083003–01, HHSN275201000003I, HHSN275201800003I, 1 K23 AR075874-01A1, and HHSN272201500006I 5U24-TR001608–03), FDA (5U18FD006298–03), PCORI, the Rheumatology Research Foundation's Scientist Development Award, the Thrasher Research Fund, the Childhood Arthritis and Rheumatology Research Alliance, and consulting for UCB.

REFERENCES

1. Guzman M, Hui-Yuen JS. Management of pediatric systemic lupus erythematosus: focus on belimumab. Drug Des Devel Ther 2020;14:2503–13.
2. Kearsley-Fleet L, Heaf E, Davies R, et al. Frequency of biologic switching and the outcomes of switching in children and young people with juvenile idiopathic arthritis: a national cohort study. Lancet Rheumatol 2020;2:e217–26.
3. Ruperto N, Abud-Mendoza C, Viola DO, et al. The pluto study: intravenous belimumab in children with systemic lupus erythematosus. Ann Rheum Dis 2019;78:764–5.
4. Kearns GL, Abdel-Rahman SM, Alander SW, et al. Developmental pharmacology–drug disposition, action, and therapy in infants and children. N Engl J Med 2003;349:1157–67.
5. Ginsberg G, Hattis D, Sonawane B, et al. Evaluation of child/adult pharmacokinetic differences from a database derived from the therapeutic drug literature. Toxicol Sci 2002;66:185–200.
6. US Food and Drug Administration. Table of pharmacogenomic biomarkers in drug labeling. Avilable at: https://www.fda.gov/drugs/science-and-research-drugs/table-pharmacogenomic-biomarkers-drug-labeling. Accessed June 7, 2021.
7. Balevic SJ, Cohen-Wolkowiez M. Innovative study designs optimizing clinical pharmacology research in infants and children. J Clin Pharmacol 2018;58(Suppl 10):S58–72.
8. Cella M, Knibbe C, Danhof M, et al. What is the right dose for children? Br J Clin Pharmaco 2010;70:597–603.
9. Johnson TN. The problems in scaling adult drug doses to children. Arch Dis Child 2008;93:207–11.
10. Balevic SJ, Becker ML, Cohen-Wolkowiez M, et al. Clinical trial design in juvenile idiopathic arthritis. Paediatr Drugs 2017;19:379–89.
11. Lovell DJ, Ruperto N, Giannini EH, et al. Advances from clinical trials in juvenile idiopathic arthritis. Nat Rev Rheumatol 2013;9:557–63.
12. Ruperto N, Lovell DJ, Cuttica R, et al. A randomized, placebo-controlled trial of infliximab plus methotrexate for the treatment of polyarticular-course juvenile rheumatoid arthritis. Arthritis Rheum 2007;56:3096–106.
13. US Food and Drug Administration. Guidance for industry: population pharmacokinetics 1999. Available at: https://www.fda.gov/downloads/Drugs/GuidanceComplianceRegulatoryInformation/Guidances/UCM072137.pdf. Accessed March 8, 2018.
14. Yang X, Sherwin CM, Yu T, et al. Pharmacokinetic modeling of therapies for systemic lupus erythematosus. Expert Rev Clin Pharmacol 2015;8:587–603.
15. Vinks AA, Emoto C, Fukuda T. Modeling and simulation in pediatric drug therapy: application of pharmacometrics to define the right dose for children. Clin Pharmacol Ther 2015;98:298–308.
16. Bauman LE, Xiong Y, Mizuno T, et al. Improved population pharmacokinetic model for predicting optimized infliximab exposure in pediatric inflammatory bowel disease. Inflamm Bowel Dis 2020;26:429–39.
17. InsightRX. Drug modules. Available at: https://www.insight-rx.com/product/drug-modules. Accessed March 30, 2021.
18. Whirl-Carrillo M, McDonagh EM, Hebert JM, et al. Pharmacogenomics knowledge for personalized medicine. Clin Pharmacol Ther 2012;92:414–7.

19. Kang JS, Lee MH. Overview of therapeutic drug monitoring. Korean J Intern Med 2009;24:1–10.
20. Brunet M, van Gelder T, Asberg A, et al. Therapeutic drug monitoring of tacrolimus-personalized therapy: second consensus report. Ther Drug Monit 2019;41:261–307.
21. Balevic SJ, Green TP, Clowse MEB, et al. Pharmacokinetics of hydroxychloroquine in pregnancies with rheumatic diseases. Clin Pharmacokinet 2019;58: 525–33.
22. Costedoat-Chalumeau N, Houssiau F, Izmirly P, et al. A prospective international study on adherence to treatment in 305 patients with flaring SLE: assessment by drug levels and self-administered questionnaires. Clin Pharmacol Ther 2019; 106:374–82.
23. Durcan L, Clarke WA, Magder LS, et al. Hydroxychloroquine blood levels in systemic lupus erythematosus: clarifying dosing controversies and improving adherence. J Rheumatol 2015;42:2092–7.
24. US Food and Drug Administration. General clinical pharmacology considerations. Guidance for industry 2014. Available at: https://www.fda.gov/downloads/Drugs/GuidanceComplianceRegulatoryInformation/Guidances/UCM425885.pdf. Accessed August 14, 2018.
25. Deeken J. The Affymetrix DMET platform and pharmacogenetics in drug development. Curr Opin Mol Ther 2009;11:260–8.
26. National Institute of General Medical Sciences. Pharmacogenomics. Available at: https://www.nigms.nih.gov/education/fact-sheets/Pages/pharmacogenomics.aspx. Accessed February 24, 2021.
27. Dean L. Codeine therapy and CYP2D6 genotype. In: Pratt VM, Scott SA, Pirmohamed M, et al., eds. Medical genetics summaries. Bethesda, MD 2012. Available at: Available at: https://www.ncbi.nlm.nih.gov/books/NBK100662/.
28. Product information: codeine sulfate tablet. Eatontown, NJ: West-Ward Pharmaceutical Corp; 2019.
29. Ternant D, Bejan-Angoulvant T, Passot C, et al. Clinical pharmacokinetics and pharmacodynamics of monoclonal antibodies approved to treat rheumatoid arthritis. Clin Pharmacokinet 2015;54:1107–23.
30. Mould DR. The pharmacokinetics of biologics: a primer. Dig Dis 2015;33(Suppl 1):61–9.
31. Bartelds GM, Krieckaert CL, Nurmohamed MT, et al. Development of antidrug antibodies against adalimumab and association with disease activity and treatment failure during long-term follow-up. JAMA 2011;305:1460–8.
32. Bartelds GM, Wijbrandts CA, Nurmohamed MT, et al. Clinical response to adalimumab: relationship to anti-adalimumab antibodies and serum adalimumab concentrations in rheumatoid arthritis. Ann Rheum Dis 2007;66:921–6.
33. Chen DY, Chen YM, Tsai WC, et al. Significant associations of antidrug antibody levels with serum drug trough levels and therapeutic response of adalimumab and etanercept treatment in rheumatoid arthritis. Ann Rheum Dis 2015;74:e16.
34. Eng GP, Bouchelouche P, Bartels EM, et al. Anti-drug antibodies, drug levels, interleukin-6 and soluble TNF receptors in rheumatoid arthritis patients during the first 6 months of treatment with adalimumab or infliximab: a descriptive cohort study. PLoS One 2016;11:e0162316.
35. Wolbink GJ, Voskuyl AE, Lems WF, et al. Relationship between serum trough infliximab levels, pretreatment C reactive protein levels, and clinical response to infliximab treatment in patients with rheumatoid arthritis. Ann Rheum Dis 2005; 64:704–7.

36. Takeuchi T, Miyasaka N, Tatsuki Y, et al. Baseline tumour necrosis factor alpha levels predict the necessity for dose escalation of infliximab therapy in patients with rheumatoid arthritis. Ann Rheum Dis 2011;70:1208–15.
37. Maeda A, Iwayanagi Y, Haraya K, et al. Identification of human IgG1 variant with enhanced FcRn binding and without increased binding to rheumatoid factor autoantibody. MAbs 2017;9:844–53.
38. Product information: adalimumab injection, solution. North Chicago, IL: AbbVie Inc; 2018.
39. Product information: canakinumab injection, solution. Cambridge, MA: Novartis Pharmaceuticals Corporation; 2020.
40. Product information: etanercept solution. Thousand Oaks, CA: Immunex Corporation; 2018.
41. Ternant D, Ducourau E, Fuzibet P, et al. Pharmacokinetics and concentration-effect relationship of adalimumab in rheumatoid arthritis. Br J Clin Pharmacol 2015;79:286–97.
42. Yim DS, Zhou H, Buckwalter M, et al. Population pharmacokinetic analysis and simulation of the time-concentration profile of etanercept in pediatric patients with juvenile rheumatoid arthritis. J Clin Pharmacol 2005;45:246–56.
43. Nader A, Beck D, Noertersheuser P, et al. Population Pharmacokinetics and Immunogenicity of Adalimumab in Adult Patients with Moderate-to-Severe Hidradenitis Suppurativa. Clin Pharmacokinet 2017;56:1091–102.
44. Ternant D, Ducourau E, Perdriger A, et al. Relationship between inflammation and infliximab pharmacokinetics in rheumatoid arthritis. Br J Clin Pharmaco 2014;78:118–28.
45. Frey N, Grange S, Woodworth T. Population pharmacokinetic analysis of tocilizumab in patients with rheumatoid arthritis. J Clin Pharmacol 2010;50:754–66.
46. Sun H, Van LM, Floch D, et al. Pharmacokinetics and pharmacodynamics of canakinumab in patients with systemic juvenile idiopathic arthritis. J Clin Pharmacol 2016;56:1516–27.
47. Yang BB, Frazier J, McCabe D, et al. Population pharmacokinetics of recombinant interleukin-1 receptor antagonist (anakinra) in subjects with rheumatoid arthritis (RA). Arthritis Rheum 2000;43:S153–.
48. Li X, Roy A, Murthy B. Population pharmacokinetics and exposure-response relationship of intravenous and subcutaneous abatacept in patients with rheumatoid arthritis. J Clin Pharmacol 2019;59:245–57.
49. Sanmarti R, Inciarte-Mundo J, Estrada-Alarcon P, et al. Towards optimal cut-off trough levels of adalimumab and etanercept for a good therapeutic response in rheumatoid arthritis. Results of the INMUNOREMAR study. Ann Rheum Dis 2015;74:e42.
50. Benucci M, Meacci F, Grossi V, et al. Correlations between immunogenicity, drug levels, and disease activity in an Italian cohort of rheumatoid arthritis patients treated with tocilizumab. Biologics 2016;10:53–8.
51. Billiet T, Dreesen E, Cleynen I, et al. A genetic variation in the neonatal Fc-receptor affects anti-TNF drug concentrations in inflammatory bowel disease. Am J Gastroenterol 2016;111:1438–45.
52. Jancic I, Sefik-Bukilica M, Zivojinovic S, et al. Influence of Promoter Polymorphisms of the TNF-alpha (-308G/A) and IL-6 (-174G/C) genes on therapeutic response to etanercept in rheumatoid arthritis. J Med Biochem 2015;34:414–21.
53. Liu J, Dong Z, Zhu Q, et al. TNF-alpha promoter polymorphisms predict the response to etanercept more powerfully than that to infliximab/adalimumab in spondyloarthritis. Sci Rep 2016;6:32202.

54. Daien CI, Daien V, Parussini E, et al. Etanercept concentration in patients with rheumatoid arthritis and its potential influence on treatment decisions: a pilot study. J Rheumatol 2012;39:1533–8.
55. Jamnitski A, Krieckaert CL, Nurmohamed MT, et al. Patients non-responding to etanercept obtain lower etanercept concentrations compared with responding patients. Ann Rheum Dis 2012;71:88–91.
56. St Clair EW, Wagner CL, Fasanmade AA, et al. The relationship of serum infliximab concentrations to clinical improvement in rheumatoid arthritis: results from ATTRACT, a multicenter, randomized, double-blind, placebo-controlled trial. Arthritis Rheum 2002;46:1451–9.
57. Levi M, Grange S, Frey N. Exposure-response relationship of tocilizumab, an anti-IL-6 receptor monoclonal antibody, in a large population of patients with rheumatoid arthritis. J Clin Pharmacol 2013;53:151–9.
58. Ruiz-Esquide V, Zufferey P, Yague J, et al. Relationship between clinical remission and serum levels of tocilizumab in the treatment of rheumatoid arthritis. Ann Rheum Dis 2015;74:77.
59. Enevold C, Baslund B, Linde L, et al. Interleukin-6-receptor polymorphisms rs12083537, rs2228145, and rs4329505 as predictors of response to tocilizumab in rheumatoid arthritis. Pharmacogenet Genomics 2014;24:401–5.
60. Maldonado-Montoro M, Canadas-Garre M, Gonzalez-Utrilla A, et al. Influence of IL6R gene polymorphisms in the effectiveness to treatment with tocilizumab in rheumatoid arthritis. Pharmacogenomics J 2018;18:167–72.
61. Strik AS, Wang YC, Ruff LE, et al. Individualized dosing of therapeutic monoclonal antibodies-a changing treatment paradigm? AAPS J 2018;20:99.
62. Rahman MU, Strusberg I, Geusens P, et al. Double-blinded infliximab dose escalation in patients with rheumatoid arthritis. Ann Rheum Dis 2007;66:1233–8.
63. Dubinsky MC, Rosh J, Faubion WA Jr, et al. Efficacy and safety of escalation of adalimumab therapy to weekly dosing in pediatric patients with crohn's disease. Inflamm Bowel Dis 2016;22:886–93.
64. Mehta P, Cron RQ, Hartwell J, et al. Silencing the cytokine storm: the use of intravenous anakinra in haemophagocytic lymphohistiocytosis or macrophage activation syndrome. Lancet Rheumatol 2020;2:e358–67.
65. Singh R, Ivaturi VD, Penzenstadler J, et al. Response similarity assessment between polyarticular juvenile idiopathic arthritis and adult rheumatoid arthritis for biologics. Clin Pharmacol Ther 2021 Jul;110(1):98–107.
66. Vande Casteele N, Ferrante M, Van Assche G, et al. Trough concentrations of infliximab guide dosing for patients with inflammatory bowel disease. Gastroenterology 2015;148:1320–9.e3.
67. Syversen S, Goll G, Jørgensen K, et al. Therapeutic Drug Monitoring Compared to Standard Treatment of Patients Starting Infliximab: Results from a Multicenter Randomized Controlled Trial of 400 Patients [abstract]. Arthritis Rheumatol 2020; 72(suppl 10):13. Available at: https://acrabstracts.org/abstract/therapeutic-drug-monitoring-compared-to-standard-treatment-of-patients-starting-infliximab-results-from-a-multicenter-randomized-controlled-trial-of-400-patients/. Accessed October 19, 2021.
68. Neumann I, Fuhrmann H, Fang IF, et al. Association between mycophenolic acid 12-h trough levels and clinical endpoints in patients with autoimmune disease on mycophenolate mofetil. Nephrol Dial Transpl 2008;23:3514–20.
69. Croyle L, Morand EF. Optimizing the use of existing therapies in lupus. Int J Rheum Dis 2015;18:129–37.

70. Zahr N, Arnaud L, Marquet P, et al. Mycophenolic acid area under the curve correlates with disease activity in lupus patients treated with mycophenolate mofetil. Arthritis Rheum 2010;62:2047–54.
71. Lertdumrongluk P, Somparn P, Kittanamongkolchai W, et al. Pharmacokinetics of mycophenolic acid in severe lupus nephritis. Kidney Int 2010;78:389–95.
72. Sagcal-Gironella AC, Fukuda T, Wiers K, et al. Pharmacokinetics and pharmacodynamics of mycophenolic acid and their relation to response to therapy of childhood-onset systemic lupus erythematosus. Semin Arthritis Rheum 2011; 40:307–13.
73. Fukuda T, Goebel J, Cox S, et al. UGT1A9, UGT2B7, and MRP2 genotypes can predict mycophenolic acid pharmacokinetic variability in pediatric kidney transplant recipients. Ther Drug Monit 2012;34:671–9.
74. Kittanamongkolchai W, Rukrung C, Supasiri T, et al. Therapeutic drug monitoring of mycophenolate mofetil for the treatment of severely active lupus nephritis. Lupus 2013;22:727–32.
75. Woillard JB, Bader-Meunier B, Salomon R, et al. Pharmacokinetics of mycophenolate mofetil in children with lupus and clinical findings in favour of therapeutic drug monitoring. Br J Clin Pharmacol 2014;78:867–76.
76. Sagcal-Gironella AC, Fukuda T, Klein-Gitelman MS, et al. Pharmacokinetics and pharmacogenetics of mycophenolic acid and response to therapy in childhood-onset systemic lupus erythematosus. Arthritis Rheum 2014;66:S202.
77. Yap DYH, Tam CH, Yung S, et al. Pharmacokinetics and pharmacogenomics of mycophenolic acid and its clinical correlations in maintenance immunosuppression for lupus nephritis. Nephrol Dial Transpl 2020;35:810–8.
78. Chen Y, Sun L, Xu H, et al. PK/PD study of mycophenolate mofetil in children with systemic lupus erythematosus to inform model-based precision dosing. Front Pharmacol 2020;11:605060.
79. Godron-Dubrasquet A, Woillard JB, Decramer S, et al. Mycophenolic acid area under the concentration-time curve is associated with therapeutic response in childhood-onset lupus nephritis. Pediatr Nephrol 2021;36:341–7.
80. Zahr N, Urien S, Funck-Brentano C, et al. Evaluation of hydroxychloroquine blood concentrations and effects in childhood-onset systemic lupus erythematosus. Pharmaceuticals (Basel) 2021;14:273.
81. Munster T, Gibbs JP, Shen D, et al. Hydroxychloroquine concentration-response relationships in patients with rheumatoid arthritis. Arthritis Rheum 2002;46: 1460–9.
82. Costedoat-Chalumeau N, Amoura Z, Hulot JS, et al. Low blood concentration of hydroxychloroquine is a marker for and predictor of disease exacerbations in patients with systemic lupus erythematosus. Arthritis Rheum 2006;54:3284–90.
83. Costedoat-Chalumeau N, Amoura Z, Hulot JS, et al. Very low blood hydroxychloroquine concentration as an objective marker of poor adherence to treatment of systemic lupus erythematosus. Ann Rheum Dis 2007;66:821–4.
84. Ting TV, Kudalkar D, Nelson S, et al. Usefulness of cellular text messaging for improving adherence among adolescents and young adults with systemic lupus erythematosus. J Rheumatol 2012;39:174–9.
85. Jallouli M, Galicier L, Zahr N, et al. Determinants of hydroxychloroquine blood concentration variations in systemic lupus erythematosus. Arthritis Rheumatol 2015;67:2176–84.
86. Mok CC, Penn HJ, Chan KL, et al. Hydroxychloroquine serum concentrations and flares of systemic lupus erythematosus: a longitudinal cohort analysis. Arthritis Care Res (Hoboken) 2016;68:1295–302.

87. Balbi VSC, Pedrosa T, Pereira R, et al. Hydroxychloroquine Blood Levels Predicts 6-Months Disease Activity in Juvenile Lupus Nephritis [abstract]. Arthritis Rheumatol 2020;72(suppl 10). Available at: https://acrabstracts.org/abstract/hydroxychloroquine-blood-levels-predicts-6-months-disease-activity-in-juvenile-lupus-nephritis/. Accessed October 19, 2021.
88. Dervieux T, Furst D, Lein DO, et al. Polyglutamation of methotrexate with common polymorphisms in reduced folate carrier, aminoimidazole carboxamide ribonucleotide transformylase, and thymidylate synthase are associated with methotrexate effects in rheumatoid arthritis. Arthritis Rheum 2004;50:2766–74.
89. Dervieux T, Furst D, Lein DO, et al. Pharmacogenetic and metabolite measurements are associated with clinical status in patients with rheumatoid arthritis treated with methotrexate: results of a multicentred cross sectional observational study. Ann Rheum Dis 2005;64:1180–5.
90. Becker ML, van Haandel L, Gaedigk R, et al. Analysis of intracellular methotrexate polyglutamates in patients with juvenile idiopathic arthritis: effect of route of administration on variability in intracellular methotrexate polyglutamate concentrations. Arthritis Rheum 2010;62:1803–12.
91. Becker ML, Gaedigk R, van Haandel L, et al. The effect of genotype on methotrexate polyglutamate variability in juvenile idiopathic arthritis and association with drug response. Arthritis Rheum 2011;63:276–85.
92. Bulatovic M, Heijstek MW, Van Dijkhuizen EH, et al. Prediction of clinical nonresponse to methotrexate treatment in juvenile idiopathic arthritis. Ann Rheum Dis 2012;71:1484–9.
93. Pastore S, Stocco G, Moressa V, et al. 5-Aminoimidazole-4-carboxamide ribonucleotide-transformylase and inosine-triphosphate-pyrophosphatase genes variants predict remission rate during methotrexate therapy in patients with juvenile idiopathic arthritis. Rheumatol Int 2015;35:619–27.
94. Calasan MB, den Boer E, de Rotte MC, et al. Methotrexate polyglutamates in erythrocytes are associated with lower disease activity in juvenile idiopathic arthritis patients. Ann Rheum Dis 2015;74:402–7.
95. de Rotte MC, den Boer E, de Jong PH, et al. Methotrexate polyglutamates in erythrocytes are associated with lower disease activity in patients with rheumatoid arthritis. Ann Rheum Dis 2015;74:408–14.
96. Askanase AD, Wallace DJ, Weisman MH, et al. Use of pharmacognetics, enzymatic phenotyping, and metabolite monitoring to guide treatment with azathioprine in patients with systemic lupus erythematosus. J Rheumatol 2009;36(1):89–95. https://doi.org/10.3899/jrheum.070968.
97. Daniel LL, Dickson AL, Chung CP. Precision medicine for rheumatologists: lessons from the pharmacogenomics of azathioprine. Clin Rheumatol 2021;40:65–73.
98. Westervelt P, Cho K, Bright DR, et al. Drug-gene interactions: inherent variability in drug maintenance dose requirements. P T 2014;39:630–7.
99. Sherwin CM, Sagcal-Gironella AC, Fukuda T, et al. Development of population PK model with enterohepatic circulation for mycophenolic acid in patients with childhood-onset systemic lupus erythematosus. Br J Clin Pharmacol 2012;73:727–40.
100. Le Meur Y, Buchler M, Thierry A, et al. Individualized mycophenolate mofetil dosing based on drug exposure significantly improves patient outcomes after renal transplantation. Am J Transpl 2007;7:2496–503.

101. Djabarouti S, Duffau P, Lazaro E, et al. Therapeutic drug monitoring of mycophenolate mofetil and enteric-coated mycophenolate sodium in patients with systemic lupus erythematosus. Expert Opin Pharmacother 2010;11:689–99.
102. Jeong H, Kaplan B. Therapeutic monitoring of mycophenolate mofetil. Clin J Am Soc Nephrol 2007;2:184–91.
103. Lu YP, Zhu YC, Liang MZ, et al. Therapeutic drug monitoring of mycophenolic acid can be used as predictor of clinical events for kidney transplant recipients treated with mycophenolate mofetil. Transpl Proc 2006;38:2048–50.
104. Bergan S, Brunet M, Hesselink DA, et al. Personalized therapy for mycophenolate: consensus report by the international association of therapeutic drug monitoring and clinical toxicology. Ther Drug Monit 2021;43:150–200.
105. Polk BI, Becker ML. Pharmacogenomics in childhood rheumatic disorders: a foundation for future individualized therapy. Discov Med 2013;16:267–75.
106. Stamp LK, Barclay M. Therapeutic drug monitoring in rheumatic diseases: utile or futile? Rheumatology (Oxford) 2014;53:988–97.
107. Ravelli A, Di Fuccia G, Molinaro M, et al. Plasma levels after oral methotrexate in children with juvenile rheumatoid arthritis. J Rheumatol 1993;20:1573–7.
108. Albertioni F, Flato B, Seideman P, et al. Methotrexate in juvenile rheumatoid arthritis. Evidence of age dependent pharmacokinetics. Eur J Clin Pharmacol 1995;47:507–11.
109. Lafforgue P, Monjanel-Mouterde S, Durand A, et al. Lack of correlation between pharmacokinetics and efficacy of low dose methotrexate in patients with rheumatoid arthritis. J Rheumatol 1995;22:844–9.
110. Hinks A, Moncrieffe H, Martin P, et al. Association of the 5-aminoimidazole-4-carboxamide ribonucleotide transformylase gene with response to methotrexate in juvenile idiopathic arthritis. Ann Rheum Dis 2011;70:1395–400.
111. Moncrieffe H, Hinks A, Ursu S, et al. Generation of novel pharmacogenomic candidates in response to methotrexate in juvenile idiopathic arthritis: correlation between gene expression and genotype. Pharmacogenet Genomics 2010;20:665–76.
112. de Rotte MC, Bulatovic M, Heijstek MW, et al. ABCB1 and ABCC3 gene polymorphisms are associated with first-year response to methotrexate in juvenile idiopathic arthritis. J Rheumatol 2012;39:2032–40.
113. Pastore S, Stocco G, Favretto D, et al. Genetic determinants for methotrexate response in juvenile idiopathic arthritis. Front Pharmacol 2015;6:52.
114. de Rotte M, Pluijm SMF, de Jong PHP, et al. Development and validation of a prognostic multivariable model to predict insufficient clinical response to methotrexate in rheumatoid arthritis. PLoS One 2018;13:e0208534.
115. Ramsey LB, Moncrieffe H, Smith CN, et al. Association of SLCO1B1 *14 allele with poor response to methotrexate in juvenile idiopathic arthritis patients. ACR Open Rheumatol 2019;1:58–62.
116. Gearry RB, Barclay ML. Azathioprine and 6-mercaptopurine pharmacogenetics and metabolite monitoring in inflammatory bowel disease. J Gastroenterol Hepatol 2005;20:1149–57.
117. Evans WE, Horner M, Chu YQ, et al. Altered mercaptopurine metabolism, toxic effects, and dosage requirement in a thiopurine methyltransferase-deficient child with acute lymphocytic leukemia. J Pediatr 1991;119:985–9.
118. Relling MV, Hancock ML, Rivera GK, et al. Mercaptopurine therapy intolerance and heterozygosity at the thiopurine S-methyltransferase gene locus. J Natl Cancer Inst 1999;91:2001–8.

119. Chapdelaine A, Mansour AM, Troyanov Y, et al. Metabolite monitoring to guide thiopurine therapy in systemic autoimmune diseases. Clin Rheumatol 2017;36: 1341–8.
120. Bolia R, Rajanayagam J, Hardikar W. Lower 6-MMP/6-TG ratio may be a therapeutic target in pediatric autoimmune hepatitis. J Pediatr Gastroenterol Nutr 2018;67:695–700.
121. Frances C, Cosnes A, Duhaut P, et al. Low blood concentration of hydroxychloroquine in patients with refractory cutaneous lupus erythematosus: a French multicenter prospective study. Arch Dermatol 2012;148:479–84.
122. Costedoat-Chalumeau N, Houssiau F, Izmirly P, et al. A prospective international study on adherence to treatment in 305 patients with flaring SLE: assessment by drug levels and self-administered questionnaires. Clin Pharmacol Ther 2019 Aug;106(2):374–82.
123. Costedoat-Chalumeau N, Houssiau F, Izmirly P, et al. A prospective international study on adherence to treatment in 305 patients with flaring SLE: assessment by drug levels and self-administered questionnaires. Clin Pharmacol Ther 2018; 103:1074–82.
124. Balevic SJ, Becker ML, CohenWolkowiez M, et al, for the APPLE Investigators. Hydroxychloroquine levels and adherence in pediatric lupus. Poster at: Childhood Arthritis and Rheumatology Research Alliance Annual Meeting. April 2021.
125. Ter Haar NM, van Dijkhuizen EHP, Swart JF, et al. Treatment to target using recombinant interleukin-1 receptor antagonist as first-line monotherapy in new-onset systemic juvenile idiopathic arthritis: results from a five-year follow-up study. Arthritis Rheumatol 2019;71:1163–73.

Implementation Science in Pediatric Rheumatology: A Path to Health Equity

Emily A. Smitherman, MD, MSc[a,*], Ingrid Goh, PhD[b,c], Rajdeep Pooni, MD[d], Sheetal S. Vora, MD, MSc[e], Cagri Yildirim-Toruner, MD[f], Emily von Scheven, MD, MAS[g]

KEYWORDS

- Pediatric rheumatology • Implementation science • Health equity
- Evidence-based practice • Framework

KEY POINTS

- Although limited, initial studies demonstrate varied uptake of evidence-based clinical practices in pediatric rheumatology, which likely contributes to nonoptimal patient health outcomes including health disparities.
- Large-scale application of implementation science to promote uptake of evidence-based practice is needed in pediatric rheumatology to ensure consistent care delivery and reduce disparate health outcomes.
- The incorporation of health equity research principles into frameworks for implementation science and adaptation to the context of pediatric rheumatology practice holds promise both for improving evidence uptake and improving health equity for our patients.

INTRODUCTION

Despite advancements in the conduct and dissemination of scientific research, there remains a shocking 17-year lag in the time it takes to translate evidence into clinical practice, and only about half of evidence-based practices achieve widespread use.[1]

[a] Division of Pediatric Rheumatology, Department of Pediatrics, University of Alabama at Birmingham, 1601 4th Avenue South, Park Place North Suite G10, Birmingham, AL 35233, USA; [b] Division of Rheumatology, The Hospital for Sick Children, 686 Bay Street, Toronto, Ontario M5G 0A4, Canada; [c] Child Health Evaluative Sciences, SickKids Research Institute, Toronto, Ontario, Canada; [d] Division of Allergy, Immunology, and Rheumatology, Stanford University School of Medicine, Stanford Children's Health, 700 Welch Road, Suite 301, Palo Alto, CA 94304, USA; [e] Department of Pediatrics, Atrium Health Levine Children's Hospital, 1000 Blythe Boulevard, 4th Floor, Charlotte, NC 28203, USA; [f] Department of Pediatrics, Baylor College of Medicine, 6701 Fannin Street, 11th Floor, Houston, TX 77030, USA; [g] Division of Pediatric Rheumatology, University of California San Francisco, 550 16th Street, 5th Floor, #5453, San Francisco, CA, USA
* Corresponding author.
E-mail address: esmitherman@uabmc.edu

Rheum Dis Clin N Am 48 (2022) 331–342
https://doi.org/10.1016/j.rdc.2021.08.006
0889-857X/22/

For example, in pediatric practices across 12 cities, only 46.5% of care recommendations were delivered.[2] Thus, there is a critical need for development of implementation strategies to promote the timely and reliable delivery of evidence-based practices across our health care system, including in pediatric rheumatology clinical care.

Furthermore, disparities in health care access, delivery, and outcomes between groups of people based on characteristics such as race or ethnicity, sex, sexual identity, age, disability, socioeconomic status, and geographic location is a pervasive problem across our health system and society. Implementation science, integrated with a health disparities research approach, has been proposed as a strategy to address health disparities by studying determinants that impact care delivery at multiple levels.[3] Emerging conceptual frameworks are reframing the principles of implementation science by emphasizing the health equity lens and aiming to reduce or prevent increase in existing inequalities when implementing interventions.[4]

In this article, we will review the fundamental principles of implementation science, make a case for the need to conduct implementation studies in pediatric rheumatology, present a health equity-focused framework for implementation science in pediatric rheumatology, and propose next steps to take action.

IMPLEMENTATION SCIENCE: FUNDAMENTAL PRINCIPLES

Implementation science is a relatively new but rapidly progressing field, defined as "the scientific study of methods to promote the systematic uptake of research findings and other evidence-based practices into routine practice, and, hence, to improve the quality (effectiveness, reliability, safety, appropriateness, equity, efficiency) of health care."[5] Thus, implementation research is focused on evaluating the process of implementing clinical interventions with the goal of producing generalizable knowledge around implementation.[6] In addition, implementation research considers the contribution of multiple stakeholders and levels of health care, including providers, organizations, and policy, in contrast to the concentration on the patient-level in traditional clinical research.

Many theories, models, and frameworks around implementation have been described to guide the process of translating research into practice through process models; understand determinants of implementation outcomes through determinant frameworks, classic theories, and implementation theories; and evaluate implementation through evaluation frameworks.[7] There is also an increasing effort to clearly define the processes used to adopt evidence-based practices into clinical care, referred to as implementation strategies.[8] Key implementation outcomes include acceptability, adoption, appropriateness, feasibility, fidelity, implementation cost, penetration, and sustainability.[9] Hybrid effectiveness-implementation study designs have been proposed to further accelerate translation of research findings into practice while expanding knowledge of effective implementation strategies.[10]

CASE FOR IMPLEMENTATION SCIENCE WITHIN PEDIATRIC RHEUMATOLOGY

Pediatric rheumatology specializes in the care of chronic immune-mediated inflammatory conditions with onset during childhood. In recent decades, there has been a significant advancement in therapeutic options because of the rapid development and continued expansion of targeted biologic therapies[11]. However, available data for juvenile idiopathic arthritis (JIA) and childhood-onset systemic lupus erythematosus (cSLE) suggest there remain significant disparities in care delivery and patient outcomes. Implementation science studies aimed at evaluating strategies for improving use of practice guidelines may improve quality of care and health outcomes for children with rheumatic diseases.

Disparities in Care Delivery and Health Outcomes

Although long-term outcomes in JIA have improved in modern clinical practice, recent cohort studies have revealed that achieving and sustaining clinical remission remains a challenge for at least half of patients.[12–15] Moreover, racial and ethnic disparities exist in both severity of presentation and disease status, with African American and Southeast Asian children more likely to present with more severe subtypes of JIA[16–18] and Hispanic children more likely to have high disease activity, disability, and damage.[19] Higher use of systemic glucocorticoids was also observed in Hispanic compared to non-Hispanic children.[19] Globally, greater disease activity and damage have been observed in patients living in countries with lower GDP, and higher use of biologic agents was observed in North American and northern European countries.[18]

In cSLE, a disparity in disease status inherently exists compared to adult-onset SLE, including more active disease and irreversible organ damage,[20] higher prevalence of severe disease manifestations,[21–23] and increased use of glucocorticoids.[20,24,25] Survival has improved with the widespread use of glucocorticoids, but longitudinally, a substantial proportion of patients with cSLE have a relapsing disease activity course, associated with increased damage accrual.[26] Racial and ethnic disparities have been observed in acute care utilization including need for intensive care during hospitalization, morbidity from severe disease manifestations, and mortality especially of hospitalized patients.[27,28] In children with end-stage kidney disease due to cSLE nephritis, disparities in race and ethnicity, insurance status, and geographic location have been observed in placement on the kidney transplant wait-list, receipt of transplant, and overall mortality.[28,29]

Identifying Evidence-based Practices for Implementation

Similar to many pediatric chronic conditions, a barrier to the conduct of randomized controlled trials in pediatric rheumatology is low disease prevalence. Therefore, the field has largely relied on consensus methodology in combination with the best available evidence to develop treatment recommendations, consensus treatment plans (CTPs), and quality process measures that evaluate various aspects of care delivery.

Treatment Recommendations

The American College of Rheumatology (ACR) has sponsored the development of treatment recommendations for the management of JIA and associated conditions.[30–33] An initial benchmarking study revealed that while treatment escalation would have been recommended in 65% of treatment decisions according to the ACR guidelines, it was actually escalated in only 12%.[34] The "Single Hub and Access point for pediatric Rheumatology in Europe" consortium has published several recommendation statements across pediatric rheumatic diseases based on best-evidence and expert consensus,[35] though there is no published implementation to date.

Consensus Treatment Plans

The Childhood Arthritis and Rheumatology Research Alliance (CARRA) has established a program of CTP development to provide a limited set of standardized treatment pathways for clinical use and to support observational comparative effectiveness research by reducing treatment heterogeneity.[36] One pilot study of CTP use for proliferative lupus nephritis revealed poor adherence to treatment dosing recommendations.[37] Interestingly, most providers indicated that their treatment pathway decision was driven by alignment with typical practice, and there were observable patterns in treatment choice by pediatric rheumatology centers.

Quality Measures

The development of quality indicator measures that evaluate processes of care represent a method to define minimum standards of care[38] and have been proposed for both JIA and cSLE.[39–41] Initial benchmarking of the cSLE indicators in clinical practice at 7 international pediatric rheumatology centers revealed marked variation in uptake, including significant differences between large and small centers.[42–44] There is evidence of patient-level disparities in uptake from studies of adults with SLE, with lower uptake associated with younger age, minority race and ethnicity, poverty status, and lack of health insurance.[45]

In addition to evidence-based practices specifically for the management of pediatric rheumatic diseases, there are also evidence-based practices for the general management of pediatric chronic conditions that could benefit from an implementation science approach to enhance uptake. Examples include reliable transition of youth from pediatric to adult health care clinics[46] and optimizing mental health screenings and treatment.[47]

IMPLEMENTATION CHALLENGES IN PEDIATRIC RHEUMATOLOGY

Until now, a comprehensive research agenda for the study of implementation in pediatric rheumatology has not been established, evidenced by a lack of results within PubMed when searching "pediatric rheumatology" and "implementation science." However, increasing reports of quality improvement interventions in pediatric rheumatology point to the challenges of conducting studies using rigorous implementation science methodology.

Need for Multisite Studies

To date, there have been multiple efforts using quality improvement methodology to implement interventions in the pediatric rheumatology clinic, including cSLE quality measure screenings,[48,49] pneumococcal vaccinations,[50] medication toxicity counseling,[51] shared decision-making aids,[52] and clinical decision support.[53] Although these reports have shown improvement in intervention uptake with some improvement in patient outcomes, these studies have all been conducted using a single-center design and are limited in their ability to assess the contribution of context. Large-scale implementation studies with rigorous measurement of implementation outcomes at multiple system levels are needed to better understand how to scale-up and spread interventions across pediatric rheumatology centers.

The Pediatric Rheumatology Care and Outcomes Improvement Network (PR-COIN) provides an opportunity for this type of work as an established Learning Network comprised more than 20 pediatric centers in the United States and Canada.[54] The PR-COIN infrastructure includes longitudinal measurement of key variables in the care and outcomes of patients with JIA[55] and could be leveraged to evaluate both intervention effectiveness and implementation strategies and outcomes. Similarly, the CARRA Registry network, which includes more than 70 clinical sites and a patient registry for multiple rheumatic diseases,[56] could also be used as a platform to support implementation science studies.

Need for Health Equity–Focused Interventions

Another critical need to improve care delivery and outcomes in pediatric rheumatology is the design and implementation of health equity–focused interventions. In a post-hoc analysis of the implementation of a clinical decision support tool and disease activity target attestation in JIA, though rates of improvement in longitudinal disease activity did not differ by race, the average disease activity score remained higher for Black children.[57] This highlights the need to adapt existing interventions to address health equity when deployed in settings that serve vulnerable communities. For example, an intervention that improved time to access pediatric rheumatology care from an average of 65 to 23 business days via a referral triage tool is now being deployed at safety-net clinics within three of the lowest socioeconomic zip codes in that area.[58]

PROPOSED FRAMEWORK FOR HEALTH EQUITY–FOCUSED IMPLEMENTATION SCIENCE IN PEDIATRIC RHEUMATOLOGY

There is a rising call to action to not only focus on the identification of health care disparities but design interventions that implement evidence-based practices with a health equity focus and quickly adapt interventions to optimally address the needs of vulnerable populations.[59] New frameworks are emerging that integrate key elements of both health disparities research and implementation science.[4,60] The Health Equity Implementation Framework[61] is a determinant framework adapted from the Health Care Disparities Framework[62] and Integrated-Promoting Action on Research Implementation in Health Services (i-PARIHS).[63] Use of the framework to study hepatitis C treatment uptake among Black patients seeking care at the Veterans Administration was feasible and helped identify barriers and facilitators at multiple system levels and across elements of the framework.[61] To address the body of literature identifying disparities in care delivery and outcomes in our field, we have adapted the Health Equity Implementation Framework for use in pediatric rheumatology (**Fig. 1**).

Clinical Encounter is Key

The clinical encounter is the primary setting for most intervention implementation and largely determines whether the intervention will be delivered. In addition to patient-provider interaction and communication, the clinical encounter also involves the interaction of other key stakeholders who are affected by and influence the delivery of the intervention. The i-PARIHS framework refers to patients, providers, and other key stakeholders as "recipients" of the intervention, and considers the impact both individuals and teams can have in supporting or resisting an intervention. The i-PARIHS framework also highlights the importance of the characteristics of the intervention, such as strength of evidence, usability, support for the program, need, fit with initiatives, and capacity to implement.[64]

At the individual level, much of health services research has focused on individual race and ethnicity, socioeconomic status, and education level as potential determinants for disparities. However, there is increasing recognition for the importance of individual preferences as a determinant of care received and differentiating which preferences are grounded in an individual's culture. It is critical to acknowledge that the pediatric rheumatology clinical encounter involves a patient/caregiver dyad that is dynamic over time as children grow and mature. Once age appropriate, it is important to consider both perspectives as there is frequent discordance between patient and caregiver assessments of health.[65] Therefore, we emphasize the longitudinal nature of pediatric rheumatology care by highlighting the journey through time, including both the phase of the illness and the developmental stage of the pediatric patient.

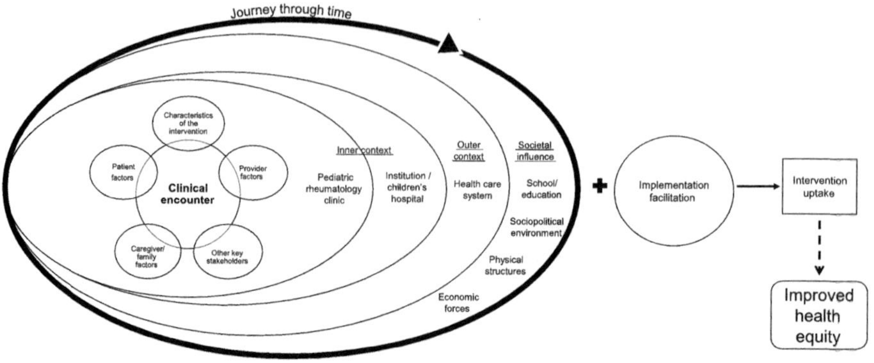

Fig. 1. Adaptation of the Health Equity Implementation Framework for Pediatric Rheumatology outlines possible determinants of implementation across multiple stakeholders and multiple system levels. The clinical encounter is the central setting of the intervention and consists of the interaction between pediatric patients, their caregivers and family, and providers, along with other key stakeholders. Multiple layers of context, including the pediatric rheumatology clinic, children's hospital or institution, and health care system, enveloped within societal influence, are also important to consider. We emphasize the effect of the longitudinal nature of pediatric rheumatology care on all other determinants, including the phase of the chronic condition (ie, recent diagnosis vs long-standing) and developmental stage of the pediatric patient. Implementation facilitation activates change through assessment of intervention characteristics and recipients within their contextual setting. Successful implementation facilitation through understanding determinants at each level leads to reliable intervention uptake and promotes improved health equity. (*Adapted from* Woodward EN, Matthieu MM, Uchendu US, Rogal S, Kirchner JE. The health equity implementation framework: proposal and preliminary study of hepatitis C virus treatment. *Implement Sci.* 2019;14(1):26. This article is distributed under the terms of the Creative Commons Attribution 4.0 International License (http://creativecommons.org/licenses/by/4.0/).)

Importance of Context and Societal Influence

Characteristics of the health care system, such as clinic structure, resources, and location, are important determinants of health disparities. Health care system factors are emphasized in the Health Care Disparities Framework, and the i-PARIHS framework further expands this construct by delineating the context of the inner system, referring to both the pediatric rheumatology clinic and the children's hospital or institution in our framework, and the outer health care system. Inclusion of these multiple levels of context allows distinction between disparities in access to care versus disparities in care processes.

The authors of the Health Equity Implementation Framework added a further outer level of societal influence which reflects social determinants of health[4] both at the community-level and broader society-level. All determinants within the framework are affected by societal influence. Key social determinants of health relevant to pediatric rheumatology include the influence of family, school, and the physical home environment. Although many of these constructs are not easily measurable, they should be kept in mind when studying health equity in the context of an implementation study.

Implementation Facilitation

Implementation facilitation is an evidence-based implementation strategy derived from the observation that change can be influenced by facilitators at each level.

Thus, implementation facilitation is positioned separately from the other framework constructs. Implementation facilitation consists of both a facilitator and a set of strategies and actions to activate implementation by assessing and responding to the intervention characteristics and recipients within the context. The process of implementation mapping can be used within implementation facilitation to improve adoption, implementation, and maintenance of the intervention.[66]

Study of Implementation

As mentioned earlier, there are key implementation outcomes that can be used to evaluate implementation strategies,[9] and hybrid effectiveness-implementation studies can be conducted to also measure impact on health outcomes.[10] With the availability of an integrated Health Equity and Implementation Science framework adapted for pediatric rheumatology, simultaneous study of implementation and health equity determinants can be achieved, eventually leading to acceleration of evidence-based practice dissemination to the most vulnerable populations. The potential for clinical impact through the integration of implementation science frameworks in pediatric rheumatology research cannot be underscored.

TAKING ACTION: LEVERAGING IMPLEMENTATION SCIENCE TO REDUCE DISPARITIES IN PEDIATRIC RHEUMATOLOGY

Achieving success in reducing observed disparities in care and outcomes in pediatric rheumatology through the use of implementation science methods will require a collaborative approach from researchers, clinicians, and patient/caregiver stakeholders. Our community is well-positioned to begin the tasks that we have outlined below.

Opportunities Through Collaborative Research

First, additional studies are needed to determine the best strategies for the implementation of evidence-based practices in pediatric rheumatology. Recognition of the need for infrastructure to facilitate the conduct of implementation science studies within pediatric rheumatology has driven members of the CARRA research organization to begin organizing an implementation science agenda. "Action" and "change-oriented"[67] implementation science terminology and taxonomies may be confusing to those without specific training,[68] and therefore difficult to apply without formal education. The CARRA Implementation Science workgroup was launched to promote implementation science education for pediatric rheumatologists, trainees, parent partners, and other members through organized lectures by experts and exposure through routine meetings. The Implementation Science workgroup will also work to identify disease-specific research appropriate for implementation science initiatives.

Quality Improvement in Clinical Practice

Application of quality improvement, especially around availability of data for population management, can help clinicians monitor for variation in care delivery and outcomes in their patients and uptake of evidence-based practices. Increased and earlier awareness could lead to accelerated improvement. Furthermore, incorporating key variables to identify disparities within local patient populations could drive significant impact.

Coproduction of Implementation Research with Patients and Caregivers

Of note, it is critical to identify representative patient and caregivers to participate with implementation efforts.[69,70] Implementation researchers need to engage a diverse group of patients and caregivers who represent the population who will receive the intervention.[71] The awareness of patients and caregivers of the social and cultural sensitivities and availability of resources in their communities can significantly impact implementation strategy selection for a study. Coproduced implementation efforts will likely result in faster uptake of evidence-based practices.

SUMMARY

Although implementation science is a nascent field with limited application in pediatric rheumatology to date, the community is actively organizing to support the study of context and dissemination within an implementation science structure. In this review, we propose a health equity–focused implementation science framework that can be applied to the design and analysis of implementation studies. The promotion of reliable evidence-based practice uptake is a critical step to work toward reducing known health disparities in care delivery and outcomes and achieving health equity in pediatric rheumatology.

DISCLOSURE

E.A. Smitherman is supported by grant funding from the Lupus Foundation of America and Childhood Arthritis and Rheumatology Research Alliance. E. von Scheven is supported by the Childhood Arthritis and Rheumatology Research Alliance and grant funding from the Patient-Centered Outcomes Research Institute. The authors have no commercial or financial conflicts to disclose.

REFERENCES

1. Balas EA, Boren SA. Managing clinical knowledge for health care improvement. Yearb Med Inform 2000;(1):65–70.
2. Mangione-Smith R, DeCristofaro AH, Setodji CM, et al. The quality of ambulatory care delivered to children in the United States. N Engl J Med 2007;357(15): 1515–23.
3. Baumann AA, Cabassa LJ. Reframing implementation science to address inequities in healthcare delivery. BMC Health Serv Res 2020;20(1):190.
4. Eslava-Schmalbach J, Garzon-Orjuela N, Elias V, et al. Conceptual framework of equity-focused implementation research for health programs (EquIR). Int J Equity Health 2019;18(1):80.
5. Eccles MP, Armstrong D, Baker R, et al. An implementation research agenda. Implement Sci 2009;4:18.
6. Bauer MS, Damschroder L, Hagedorn H, et al. An introduction to implementation science for the non-specialist. BMC Psychol 2015;3:32.
7. Nilsen P. Making sense of implementation theories, models and frameworks. Implement Sci 2015;10:53.
8. Powell BJ, Waltz TJ, Chinman MJ, et al. A refined compilation of implementation strategies: results from the Expert Recommendations for Implementing Change (ERIC) project. Implement Sci 2015;10:21.
9. Proctor E, Silmere H, Raghavan R, et al. Outcomes for implementation research: conceptual distinctions, measurement challenges, and research agenda. Adm Policy Ment Health 2011;38(2):65–76.
10. Curran GM, Bauer M, Mittman B, et al. Effectiveness-implementation hybrid designs: combining elements of clinical effectiveness and implementation research to enhance public health impact. Med Care 2012;50(3):217–26.

11. Stoll ML, Cron RQ. Treatment of juvenile idiopathic arthritis: a revolution in care. Pediatr Rheumatol Online J 2014;12:13.
12. Minden K. Adult outcomes of patients with juvenile idiopathic arthritis. Horm Res 2009;72(Suppl 1):20–5.
13. Guzman J, Oen K, Tucker LB, et al. The outcomes of juvenile idiopathic arthritis in children managed with contemporary treatments: results from the ReACCh-Out cohort. Ann Rheum Dis 2015;74(10):1854–60.
14. Guzman J, Oen K, Huber AM, et al. The risk and nature of flares in juvenile idiopathic arthritis: results from the ReACCh-Out cohort. Ann Rheum Dis 2016;75(6): 1092–8.
15. Shoop-Worrall SJW, Kearsley-Fleet L, Thomson W, et al. How common is remission in juvenile idiopathic arthritis: a systematic review. Semin Arthritis Rheum 2017;47(3):331–7.
16. Vilaiyuk S, Soponkanaporn S, Jaovisidha S, et al. A retrospective study on 158 Thai patients with juvenile idiopathic arthritis followed in a single center over a 15-year period. Int J Rheum Dis 2016;19(12):1342–50.
17. Fitzpatrick L, Broadaway KA, Ponder L, et al. Phenotypic characterization of juvenile idiopathic arthritis in African American children. J Rheumatol 2016;43(4): 799–803.
18. Consolaro A, Giancane G, Alongi A, et al. Phenotypic variability and disparities in treatment and outcomes of childhood arthritis throughout the world: an observational cohort study. Lancet Child Adolesc Health 2019;3(4):255–63.
19. Pelajo CF, Angeles-Han ST, Prahalad S, et al. Evaluation of the association between Hispanic ethnicity and disease activity and severity in a large cohort of patients with juvenile idiopathic arthritis. Rheumatol Int 2013;33(10):2549–54.
20. Brunner HI, Gladman DD, Ibanez D, et al. Difference in disease features between childhood-onset and adult-onset systemic lupus erythematosus. Arthritis Rheum 2008;58(2):556–62.
21. Bader-Meunier B, Armengaud JB, Haddad E, et al. Initial presentation of childhood-onset systemic lupus erythematosus: a French multicenter study. J Pediatr 2005;146(5):648–53.
22. Hiraki LT, Benseler SM, Tyrrell PN, et al. Clinical and laboratory characteristics and long-term outcome of pediatric systemic lupus erythematosus: a longitudinal study. J Pediatr 2008;152(4):550–6.
23. Groot N, Shaikhani D, Teng YKO, et al. Long-term clinical outcomes in a cohort of adults with childhood-onset systemic lupus erythematosus. Arthritis Rheumatol 2019;71(2):290–301.
24. Brunner HI, Silverman ED, To T, et al. Risk factors for damage in childhood-onset systemic lupus erythematosus: cumulative disease activity and medication use predict disease damage. Arthritis Rheum 2002;46(2):436–44.
25. Hersh AO, von Scheven E, Yazdany J, et al. Differences in long-term disease activity and treatment of adult patients with childhood- and adult-onset systemic lupus erythematosus. Arthritis Rheum 2009;61(1):13–20.
26. Lim LSH, Pullenayegum E, Feldman BM, et al. From childhood to adulthood: disease activity trajectories in childhood-onset systemic lupus erythematosus. Arthritis Care Res (Hoboken) 2018;70(5):750–7.
27. Son MB, Johnson VM, Hersh AO, et al. Outcomes in hospitalized pediatric patients with systemic lupus erythematosus. Pediatrics 2014;133(1):e106–13.
28. Hiraki LT, Lu B, Alexander SR, et al. End-stage renal disease due to lupus nephritis among children in the US, 1995-2006. Arthritis Rheum 2011;63(7): 1988–97.

29. Knight AM, Xie M, Mandell DS. Disparities in psychiatric diagnosis and treatment for youth with systemic lupus erythematosus: analysis of a National US Medicaid Sample. J Rheumatol 2016;43(7):1427–33.
30. Beukelman T, Patkar NM, Saag KG, et al. American College of Rheumatology recommendations for the treatment of juvenile idiopathic arthritis: initiation and safety monitoring of therapeutic agents for the treatment of arthritis and systemic features. Arthritis Care Res (Hoboken) 2011;63(4):465–82.
31. Ringold S, Weiss PF, Beukelman T, et al. update of the 2011 American College of Rheumatology recommendations for the treatment of juvenile idiopathic arthritis: recommendations for the medical therapy of children with systemic juvenile idiopathic arthritis and tuberculosis screening among children receiving biologic medications. Arthritis Care Res (Hoboken) 2013;65(10):1551–63.
32. Ringold S, Angeles-Han ST, Beukelman T, et al. American College of Rheumatology/arthritis foundation guideline for the treatment of juvenile idiopathic arthritis: therapeutic approaches for non-systemic polyarthritis, sacroiliitis, and enthesitis. Arthritis Care Res (Hoboken) 2019;71(6):717–34.
33. Angeles-Han ST, Ringold S, Beukelman T, et al. American College of rheumatology/arthritis foundation guideline for the screening, monitoring, and treatment of juvenile idiopathic arthritis-associated uveitis. Arthritis Care Res (Hoboken) 2019;71(6):703–16.
34. Swart JF, van Dijkhuizen EHP, Wulffraat NM, et al. Clinical juvenile arthritis disease activity score proves to be a useful tool in treat-to-target therapy in juvenile idiopathic arthritis. Ann Rheum Dis 2017;77(3):336–42.
35. Wulffraat NM, Vastert B, consortium S. Time to share. Pediatr Rheumatol Online J 2013;11(1):5.
36. Ringold S, Nigrovic PA, Feldman BM, et al. The childhood arthritis and rheumatology research alliance consensus treatment plans: toward comparative effectiveness in the pediatric rheumatic diseases. Arthritis Rheumatol 2018;70(5):669–78.
37. Cooper JC, Rouster-Stevens K, Wright TB, et al. Pilot study comparing the childhood arthritis and rheumatology research alliance consensus treatment plans for induction therapy of juvenile proliferative lupus nephritis. Pediatr Rheumatol Online J 2018;16(1):65.
38. Saag KG, Yazdany J, Alexander C, et al. Defining quality of care in rheumatology: the American College of Rheumatology white paper on quality measurement. Arthritis Care Res (Hoboken) 2011;63(1):2–9.
39. Lovell DJ, Passo MH, Beukelman T, et al. Measuring process of arthritis care: a proposed set of quality measures for the process of care in juvenile idiopathic arthritis. Arthritis Care Res (Hoboken) 2011;63(1):10–6.
40. Hollander MC, Sage JM, Greenler AJ, et al. International consensus for provisions of quality-driven care in childhood-onset systemic lupus erythematosus. Arthritis Care Res (Hoboken) 2013;65(9):1416–23.
41. Barber CEH, Twilt M, Pham T, et al. A Canadian evaluation framework for quality improvement in childhood arthritis: key performance indicators of the process of care. Arthritis Res Ther 2020;22(1):53.
42. Mina R, Harris JG, Klein-Gitelman MS, et al. Initial benchmarking of the quality of medical care in childhood-onset systemic lupus erythematosus. Arthritis Care Res (Hoboken) 2016;68(2):179–86.
43. Harris JG, Maletta KI, Kuhn EM, et al. Evaluation of quality indicators and disease damage in childhood-onset systemic lupus erythematosus patients. Clin Rheumatol 2017;36(2):351–9.

44. Basiaga ML, Burrows EK, Denburg MR, et al. Variation in preventive care in children receiving chronic glucocorticoid therapy. J Pediatr 2016;179:226–32.
45. Yazdany J, Trupin L, Tonner C, et al. Quality of care in systemic lupus erythematosus: application of quality measures to understand gaps in care. J Gen Intern Med 2012;27(10):1326–33.
46. White PH, Cooley WC. Transitions Clinical Report Authoring G, American Academy Of P, American Academy Of Family P, American College Of P. Supporting the Health Care Transition From Adolescence to Adulthood in the Medical Home. Pediatrics 2018;142(5).
47. Pickles DM, Lihn SL, Boat TF, et al. A roadmap to emotional health for children and families with chronic pediatric conditions. Pediatrics 2020;145(2):e20191324.
48. Smitherman EA, Huang B, Furnier A, et al. Quality of care in childhood-onset systemic lupus erythematosus: report of an intervention to improve cardiovascular and bone health screening. J Rheumatol 2019;47(10):1506–13.
49. AlAhmed O, Way A, Akoghlanian S, et al. Improving eye screening practice among pediatric rheumatology patients receiving hydroxychloroquine. Lupus 2021;30(2):269–79.
50. Harris JG, Maletta KI, Ren B, et al. Improving pneumococcal vaccination in pediatric rheumatology patients. Pediatrics 2015;136(3):e681–6.
51. Cooper AM, Horwitz M, Becker ML. Improving the safety of teratogen prescribing practices in a pediatric rheumatology clinic. Pediatrics 2019;143(4):e20180803.
52. Brinkman WB, Lipstein EA, Taylor J, et al. Design and implementation of a decision aid for juvenile idiopathic arthritis medication choices. Pediatr Rheumatol Online J 2017;15(1):48.
53. Buckley L, Ware E, Kreher G, et al. Outcome monitoring and clinical decision support in polyarticular juvenile idiopathic arthritis. J Rheumatol 2019;47(2):273–81.
54. Britto MT, Fuller SC, Kaplan HC, et al. Using a network organisational architecture to support the development of Learning Healthcare Systems. BMJ Qual Saf 2018; 27(11):937–46.
55. Harris JG, Bingham CA, Morgan EM. Improving care delivery and outcomes in pediatric rheumatic diseases. Curr Opin Rheumatol 2016;28(2):110–6.
56. Beukelman T, Kimura Y, Ilowite NT, et al. The new Childhood Arthritis and Rheumatology Research Alliance (CARRA) registry: design, rationale, and characteristics of patients enrolled in the first 12 months. Pediatr Rheumatol Online J 2017; 15(1):30.
57. Chang JC, Xiao R, Burnham JM, et al. Longitudinal assessment of racial disparities in juvenile idiopathic arthritis disease activity in a treat-to-target intervention. Pediatr Rheumatol Online J 2020;18(1):88.
58. Buitrago-Mogollon T, Vora SS. Creativity over capital: Using QI to ensure access. BMJ Open Qual 2019;8:A9.
59. Galaviz KI, Breland JY, Sanders M, et al. Implementation science to address health disparities during the coronavirus pandemic. Health Equity 2020;4(1): 463–7.
60. Napoles AM, Stewart AL. Transcreation: an implementation science framework for community-engaged behavioral interventions to reduce health disparities. BMC Health Serv Res 2018;18(1):710.
61. Woodward EN, Matthieu MM, Uchendu US, et al. The health equity implementation framework: proposal and preliminary study of hepatitis C virus treatment. Implement Sci 2019;14(1):26.

62. Kilbourne AM, Switzer G, Hyman K, et al. Advancing health disparities research within the health care system: a conceptual framework. Am J Public Health 2006; 96(12):2113–21.
63. Harvey G, Kitson A. PARIHS revisited: from heuristic to integrated framework for the successful implementation of knowledge into practice. Implement Sci 2016; 11:33.
64. Metz A, Louison L. The hexagon tool: exploring context. Chapel Hill, NC: National Implementation Research Network, Frank Porter Graham Child Development Institute, University of North Carolina; 2019. at Chapel Hill Based on Kiser, Zabel, Zachik, & Smith (2007) and Blase, Kiser, & Van Dyke (*2013*).
65. Brandon TG, Becker BD, Bevans KB, et al. Patient-reported outcomes measurement information system tools for collecting patient-reported outcomes in children with juvenile arthritis. Arthritis Care Res (Hoboken) 2017;69(3):393–402.
66. Fernandez ME, Ten Hoor GA, van Lieshout S, et al. Implementation mapping: using intervention mapping to develop implementation strategies. Front Public Health 2019;7:158.
67. Services UDoHaH. Qualitative methods in implementation science. National Institutes of Health Bethesda. National Cancer Institute; 2018. p. 1–20. Available at: https://cancercontrol.cancer.gov/sites/default/files/2020-09/nci-dccps-implementation science-whitepaper.pdf.
68. Mazza D, Bairstow P, Buchan H, et al. Refining a taxonomy for guideline implementation: results of an exercise in abstract classification. Implement Sci 2013; 8:32.
69. Domecq JP, Prutsky G, Elraiyah T, et al. Patient engagement in research: a systematic review. BMC Health Serv Res 2014;14:89.
70. Forsythe LP, Ellis LE, Edmundson L, et al. Patient and stakeholder engagement in the PCORI pilot projects: description and lessons learned. J Gen Intern Med 2016;31(1):13–21.
71. Lofters A, Virani T, Grewal G, et al. Using knowledge exchange to build and sustain community support to reduce cancer screening inequities. Prog Community Health Partnersh 2015;9(3):379–87.

The Role of Pediatric Rheumatologists in Autoimmune Brain Disease

Kathryn Taylor, DO[a,*], Eyal Muscal, MD, MS[b],
Heather Van Mater, MD, MSc[c]

KEYWORDS

• Autoimmune brain disease • Autoimmune encephalitis
• Central nervous system vasculitis • Encephalopathy • Vasculitis

KEY POINTS

- Autoimmune brain disease (ABD) encompasses a broad range of conditions, including central nervous system vasculitis, autoimmune encephalitis, and acquired demyelinating disease.
- Evaluation and optimal treatment of ABD require a thorough history, thoughtful testing, and consideration of potential alternative conditions to ensure accurate and timely diagnosis.
- Collaborative, multidisciplinary care is beneficial for children with ABD, given the breadth of the differential diagnosis, highly variable clinical presentations, and the opportunity for substantial improvement or reversibility of symptoms with timely diagnosis and treatment.

INTRODUCTION

Over the past decade, pediatric rheumatologists have become increasingly involved in the care of children with immune-mediated diseases of the central nervous system (CNS), reflecting the ongoing discovery of CNS involvement as a manifestation of classic rheumatic diseases and novel inflammatory CNS conditions.[1–5] Autoimmune brain disease (ABD) encompasses autoinflammatory, immune-mediated, and autoimmune etiologies of CNS pathologies, including CNS vasculitis, autoimmune encephalitis (AE), and acquired demyelinating syndromes. Patients with a primary rheumatic disease can have CNS involvement in any of these categories.[3,6–8]

The inherent complexity of ABD lends itself to collaboration among specialties to ensure accurate diagnosis and optimal treatment. As a result, there is an evolving

The authors have nothing to disclose.
[a] Pediatrics, Division of Neurology, Duke University, Durham, NC, USA; [b] Division of Rheumatology and Co-appointment in Neurology and Developmental Neuroscience, Baylor College of Medicine, Houston, TX, USA; [c] Pediatrics, Division of Rheumatology, Duke University, Durham, NC, USA
* Corresponding author.
E-mail address: kathryn.n.taylor@duke.edu

Rheum Dis Clin N Am 48 (2022) 343–369
https://doi.org/10.1016/j.rdc.2021.09.002 rheumatic.theclinics.com

role for pediatric rheumatologists in the evaluation and management of a broad spectrum of autoimmune and immune-mediated brain diseases. In some locations, pediatric rheumatologists are taking on a large role in the diagnosis, treatment, and long-term follow-up of these children. At other institutions, however, especially where additional neuroimmunology expertise is available, pediatric rheumatologists may serve in a primarily consultative role to exclude underlying rheumatic diseases and guide immunomodulatory therapy. In all cases, awareness of ABD and partnership with colleagues in neurology, psychiatry, and critical care are essential for accurate, timely diagnosis, and initiation of targeted therapies.

APPROACH

This review highlights the main clinical syndromes associated with ABD as well as common issues and important considerations that pediatric rheumatologists need to address. Because treatment recommendations vary based on the underlying diagnosis, the most critical step in the assessment and treatment of ABD is ensuring that complete evaluation and accurate diagnosis are made.

The goal of this article is to share a practical approach to the evaluation of both primary rheumatic conditions with CNS involvement and primary immune-mediated brain diseases, focusing on the most common clinical phenotypes and reflecting the experiences that pediatric rheumatologists encounter. The evaluation of ABD begins with a thorough history, including a complete rheumatologic review of systems, thoughtful discussion of any neuropsychiatric manifestations, and assessment for symptom evolution. Given the heterogeneity both within and across disease types, the authors recommend a standard baseline diagnostic work-up (**Table 1**) for all children with suspected ABD, which includes brain magnetic resonance imaging (MRI) with and without contrast, lumbar puncture, electroencephalogram (EEG), and serum antibody testing.[9] Additionally, vascular imaging, ophthalmologic evaluation, and formal neuropsychiatric testing often are part of the initial work-up based on the clinical presentation.

Currently, specific treatment choices, dosing, frequency, and duration of therapy vary by disease type, severity, and overall disease activity. There are limited evidence-based treatment recommendations at this time for most forms of ABD, and practices vary among providers and institutions. Therefore, this review focuses primarily on the clinical presentation and diagnosis of ABD with a brief overview of key treatment considerations (**Table 2**).

CLINICAL PHENOTYPES

Encephalopathic Presentations

Children with encephalopathy present with altered consciousness, confusion, and lethargy. They often have impaired ability to communicate; behavior changes, such as agitation or stupor; and seizures. Children with this presentation usually require hospitalization, often in a critical care unit. Pediatric neurologists should be consulted early in the evaluation because more common causes of encephalopathy, including infectious, metabolic, epileptic, and inherited conditions, are considered in addition to ABD. When pediatric rheumatology is involved, discussions with other pediatric subspecialists, including neurology and psychiatry, are crucial to ensure consideration of a robust differential, while utilizing specialized expertise to minimize unnecessary testing or treatment. The severity of illness, potential for further decompensation, and initial diagnostic uncertainty make the diagnosis challenging and the situation critical. Current recommendations highlight the importance of considering ABD early in

Table 1
Diagnostic work-up

Imaging	Cerebrospinal Fluid	Electroencephalogram	Serum[a]	Other
• MRI with/without gadolinium • Vascular imaging: MRA, CTA • Conventional angiogram, if high concern for CNS vasculitis	• Opening pressure • Cell counts • Protein • Oligoclonal bands • IgG index • Infectious testing per regional epidemiology • Antineuronal antibody testing	• Consider 24-h EEG to capture awake and asleep states • Assess for focal or generalized seizures, epileptiform discharges, changes in background activity	• Complete blood cell counts • Sedimentation rate • C-reactive protein • Ferritin • Metabolic testing per neurology/genetics; consider lactate • Thyroid function panel • Thyroid antibodies • Serum antineuronal antibodies (AE) • MOG/AQP4[a] demyelinating disease panel • Antinuclear antibodies, antiphospholipids, angiotensin-converting enzyme, complement, urinalysis • Infectious testing per regional epidemiology	• Urinalysis • Recreational substances • Neurocognitive testing • Obtain outside records for personal review

[a] Variable depending on presenting symptoms. AQP4, Aquaporin 4 antibody; MOG, Myelin oligodendrocyte glycoprotein.

Data from Hartman EAR, van Royen-Kerkhof A, Jacobs JWG, Welsing PMJ, Fritsch-Stork RDE. Performance of the 2012 Systemic Lupus International Collaborating Clinics classification criteria versus the 1997 American College of Rheumatology classification criteria in adult and juvenile systemic lupus erythematosus. A systematic review and meta-analysis. Autoimmun Rev. Mar 2018;17(3):316-322.

Table 2
Key clinical, diagnostic, and treatment considerations

Diagnosis	Key Clinical Features	Typical Laboratory Results/ Studies	Radiographic Findings	Important Notes	Treatment
Acute encephalopathy					
NMDAR AE	Psychosis Seizures Choreoathetoid movements Dyskinesia Autonomic instability	Abnormal EEG >70% Classic delta brush pattern rare LP can range from normal to leukocytosis, elevated protein, OCB, and/or elevated IgG index CSF NMDA antibody should be positive	Normal MRI in >50% Nonspecific MRI changes when MRI abnormal	Progression of symptoms to involve multiple domains over 4–8 wk	The following treatments are same for both NMDAR AE and GAD AE First line: IVIG, steroids, PLEX (no recommendations on timing, ideal combination; often all 3 used) Second line: rituximab, cyclophosphamide Other: MMF, azathioprine Refractory: additional treatment should be considered, but recommendations on specific treatment limited Tocilizumab Tofacitinib
GAD-associated syndromes	Stiff person syndrome	Electromyography with continuous motor unit activity even with attempted voluntary relaxation	MRI typically normal	Often treatment resistant Destructive inflammatory response; consider early escalation to second-line treatment.	
	Cerebellar ataxia	Requires CSF GAD antibody positivity	Cerebellar atrophy		
	Limbic encephalitis Seizures Severe memory Loss Psychiatric features	OCB present in 40%–70%	MRI changes variable		
HE	Seizures most common Strokelike episodes Cognitive impairment Psychosis	CSF with elevated protein (60%)	MRI normal	Need high titer–positive thyroid antibodies and clinical phenotype, given high healthy population prevalence of thyroid antibodies	Steroids are first line

NPSLE	Diffuse encephalopathy Confusion Seizures Cognitive decline Focal neurologic deficits	Usually with active SLE by disease activity measures Meet diagnostic criteria for SLE LP normal to leukocytosis, elevated protein, OCB and/or elevated IgG index	May be normal Parenchymal inflammation Ischemic lesions Abnormal vascular imaging (beading, narrowing)	Usually, evidence of systemic inflammation and organ dysfunction	IV steroids and cyclophosphamide Neurologic dysfunction in NPSLE may warrant rituximab (demyelination or thrombocytopenic purpura) or complement activation blockers (if thrombotic microangiopathies).
Angiography-negative primary CNS vasculitis	Focal deficits plus Diffuse deficits Cognitive decline Behavior changes Seizures (75%) Prominent headache	Elevated inflammatory markers (75%) and abnormal CSF studies (90%) Brain biopsy with lymphocytic infiltrate	Abnormal MRI (>90%) Leptomeningeal disease Ischemic lesions rare (8%) Normal angiography (100%)	By definition—negative angiography Brain biopsy required for definitive diagnosis Can have normal MRI (8%)	Induction: steroids and cyclophosphamide (monthly for 6 cycles) Maintenance: MMF (AZA may be less effective) Refractory disease: infliximab
Progressive angiography-positive primary CNS vasculitis	Focal deficits plus Diffuse deficits Cognitive decline Headache Seizure (30%)	May have elevated inflammatory markers CSF and serum	Abnormal MRI (>95%) Ischemic lesions common Angiography with multiple vascular beds, can be bilateral	Commonly bilateral disease, can be multifocal unilateral Progression of untreated disease by 3 mo	Anticoagulation Induction: steroids and cyclophosphamide Induction and/or maintenance: MMF

(*continued on next page*)

Table 2
(continued)

Diagnosis	Key Clinical Features	Typical Laboratory Results/ Studies	Radiographic Findings	Important Notes	Treatment
Granulomatosis with polyangiitis	Focal sensory or motor deficits Cranial neuropathy Delirium Severe headache Seizures	CSF elevated protein and/or WBC (60%) Typically, active systemic disease (elevated inflammatory parameters, nephritis, pulmonary infiltrate, sinus disease)	MRI usually abnormal (90%) Primary structures: pituitary, meninges, cerebral vasculature Normal angiography (small vessel disease)	Majority with systemic vasculitis CNS involvement can be extension of sinus disease	Steroids Rituximab Cyclophosphamide
Parenchymal neuro-Behçet disease	Ophthalmoparesis, cranial nerve deficits Dysarthria Sensory deficit/ hemiparesis Ataxia Headache Confusion/behavior changes Fever	Elevated CSF protein elevation and CSF WBC	Abnormal MRI (75%) Cerebellum lesions Brain stem atrophy White matter disease Basal ganglia Transverse myelitis (can be long segment) EEG normal	Definite diagnosis requires criteria for systemic Behçet disease Predilection for brainstem and hemispheres (less commonly periventricular and subcortical white matter) Mimics NMOSD when presenting with myelitis and optic neuritis	Steroids TNF inhibitor Cyclophosphamide Additional treatment recommendations limited (anakinra, tocilizumab, MMF, MTX)
Susac syndrome	Hearing loss Vision loss Encephalopathy Headache	BRAO CSF elevated protein (most), elevated WBC (45%) Brain biopsy: endothelial injury, microinfarcts, scant perivascular lymphocytic infiltration	Characteristic corpus callosum T2 or fluid-attenuated inversion recovery, hyperintense small round lesions (snowballs)	Classic triad of vision loss (BRAO), hearing loss, and encephalopathy may not be present at diagnosis.	Steroids IVIG Additional treatment recommendations limited (MMF, AZA, MTX, cyclophosphamide, rituximab)

Additional diagnosis for acute focal neurologic deficit without encephalopathy

Nonprogressive angiographic-positive primary CNS vasculitis	Focal neurologic deficit (motor or sensory)	Normal CSF Normal inflammatory markers	Abnormal MRI (100%) Ischemic lesions (89%) Unilateral disease	Consider varicella-zoster virus Requires no disease progression by 3 mo MRA misses 30% of cases detected on conventional angiogram.	Anticoagulation ± steroids
Anti-Phospholipid Syndrome	Thrombotic manifestations Thrombosis of cerebral vessels (stroke) Sinus venous thrombosis Nonthrombotic manifestations Movement disorders Seizures Cognitive deficits	Elevated anticardiolipin or b2-Gp1 antibodies Abnormal lupus anticoagulant	Often multifocal lesions that may be more prevalent in subcortical regions	Assess for concurrent SLE or if multiorgan dysfunction, catastrophic presentation.	Anticoagulation Steroids Rituximab (consider for initial presentation and for recurrent disease)
Nonparenchymal neuro-Behçet disease	Headache Vision changes Meningitis	Elevated opening pressure	Angiography: Venous thrombosis (most common) Arterial thrombosis		Steroids Anticoagulants Same as above for recurrent disease
Neurosarcoidosis	Rare (5% of patients with sarcoid) Optic neuritis Cranial nerve (hearing loss, facial palsy) Myelopathy Encephalopathy (uncommon)	Elevated ESR Biopsy with granulomatous inflammation CSF with elevated WBC, protein (60% each), oligoclonal bands (20%) Elevated serum ACE Elevated CSF ACE (elevation can be isolated CSF)	MRI abnormalities common: Parenchymal (most common) Pituitary Hypothalamus Cranial nerves Meningeal	Neurosarcoidosis may be the presenting symptom of systemic disease Can have isolated neurosarcoidosis Diagnostic criteria by Neurosarcoidosis Consortium Consensus Group[4] Mimics NMOSD with optic neuritis and myelitis	Steroids TNF inhibitors (may require higher dose for CNS disease) MMF, AZA, MTX also reported

(*continued on next page*)

Table 2
(continued)

Diagnosis	Key Clinical Features	Typical Laboratory Results/ Studies	Radiographic Findings	Important Notes	Treatment
DADA2	Fever Focal deficits Livedo reticularis rash	Variable Elevated ESR Cytopenia	Acute and chronic lacunar strokes (brainstem and deep gray matter) Diffuse cerebral volume loss	May mimic PAN Strokes most common before 5 y Dramatic variability in phenotypes	Consider TNF inhibitors
RCVS	Thunderclap headache, with or without focal neurologic deficits	Normal serum and CSF studies	Abnormal (80%) with subarachnoid hemorrhage, ischemia, edema Angiography with reversible multifocal narrowing	Important mimic of primary angiitis of the CNS Monophasic with vasoactive trigger Resolves in 1–3 mo SLE patients at higher risk	No treatment recommendations
Demyelinating disease					
NMOSD	Optic neuritis Myelitis Brainstem syndromes (ie, area postrema syndrome)	AQP4 IgG antibody positive (serum cell-based assay) CSF may have oligoclonal bands, pleocytosis with >50 WBC/mm and lymphocytic predominance common	Large confluent T2-hyperintense, T1 hypointense and cloudlike contrast-enhancing lesions involving periaqueductal gray matter, thalamus or hypothalamus Lesions of optic nerve often involving optic chiasm	Established diagnostic criteria by the International Panel for NMO Diagnosis[23]	Induction: PLEX, high-dose steroids, and rituximab Maintenance: rituximab, azathioprine, or MMF Several monoclonal antibodies now approved in adults

			Transverse myelitis (>3 contiguous spinal segments) often with cervicothoracic predominance		
MOGAD	Optic neuritis (often bilateral) Myelitis Younger children (<8 y) have ADEM-like presentation with associated encephalopathy	MOG IgG antibody positive (serum cell-based assay) May have oligo clonal bands in CSF	Supratentorial T2 hyperintense lesions, often bilateral with poorly demarcated fluffy appearance Lesions involving deep gray matter or cerebellar peduncles common Leukodystrophy-like pattern with extensive periventricular white matter lesions Optic nerve lesions with anterior optic nerve involvement transverse myelitis (>3 contiguous spinal segments) with thoracolumbar and conus predominance	Children > adults, represents approximately one-third of pediatric acquired demyelinating syndromes	Induction: IV steroids followed by prolonged taper, IVIG. Consider PLEX. Relapsing: rituximab, azathioprine, MMF, monthly IVIG

(*continued on next page*)

Table 2
(*continued*)

Diagnosis	Key Clinical Features	Typical Laboratory Results/ Studies	Radiographic Findings	Important Notes	Treatment
POMS	Monofocal or polyfocal neurologic deficits Relapsing remitting course	Typically, oligoclonal bands in CSF	T2 hyperintense lesions that contrast enhance, involving periventricular white matter ± T1 hypointense lesions Spinal cord lesions involve dorsolateral tracts and short segments	2017 McDonald diagnostic criteria[65] Requires evidence of dissemination in time and dissemination of space of neurologic symptoms	Typically managed by neurologists Maintenance: rituximab, natalizumab, ocrelizumab, interferon-β, fingolimod
Additional diagnoses to consider					
PANS/PANDAS	Acute onset of neuropsychiatric dysfunction	Normal serum and CSF studies	Normal brain MRI	Diagnosis of exclusion after ruling out primary psychiatric and inflammatory disorders	Treatment not standardized: cognitive-behavior therapy, psychotropics, antibiotics (acute or chronic) under special consideration AE treatment approaches controversial; consider in life-threatening disease, presence of AE features, or initial response to corticosteroids/IVIG.

FIRES/NORSE	Acute onset of cognitive changes, explosive and difficult to control seizures after febrile illness	Standard work-up for systemic or CNS inflammation is unrevealing. Unclear role of CSF cytokine panels	Initial normal MRI. Atrophy and signs of damage in longitudinal studies	Mimics CNS infections and metabolic conditions	Consider ketogenic diet in addition to multimodal antiseizure medications. Role of innate immunomodulation with targeted agents unclear (anakinra and tocilizumab)

Abbreviations: AZA, azathioprine, BRAO, branch retinal artery occlusion; ESR, erythrocyte sedimentation rate; LP, lumbar puncture; MMF, mycophenolate mofetil; MOG, myelin-oligodendrocyte; MTX, methotrexate; OCB, oligoclonal band; WBC, white blood cells.

Table 3
Pediatric autoimmune encephalitis classification criteria

Diagnosis of all classifications require:
- Acute to subacute onset (<3 mo) of neurologic and/or psychiatric symptoms in otherwise healthy child
- Two or more clinical features of neurologic dysfunction:
  - Altered mental status/level of consciousness or slowing or epileptiform activity
  - Focal neurologic deficits
  - Cognitive difficulties (severe cognitive dysfunction that is not attributable to a psychiatric syndrome as documented by a qualified clinical), or significant drop in IQ >20 points.
  - Acute developmental regression
  - Movement disorder (except tics)
  - Psychiatric symptoms
  - Seizures not explained by previously known seizure disorder/other condition
- Exclusion of other etiologies

Diagnostic Category	Paraclinical Evidence of Neuroinflammation[a]	Antineuronal Antibodies
Possible AE	Not available (perform AE testing if meets above criteria)	Unknown
Probable antibody-negative AE	≥1 paraclinical feature	Negative
Definite antibody-positive AE	≥1 paraclinical feature	Positive (NMDA and GAD AE require CSF to be positive)

[a] CSF greater than 5 white blood cells and/or oligoclonal bands; MRI features of encephalitis; brain biopsy with inflammatory infiltrates.

the evaluation of children with progressive encephalopathy and consideration of empiric treatment while awaiting results of diagnostic testing.

Neuropsychiatric systemic lupus erythematosus

Neuropsychiatric systemic lupus erythematosus (NPSLE) syndromes are reported in 20% to 95% of pediatric systemic lupus erythematosus (SLE) patients, with 15% to 81% of cases present at initial SLE diagnosis.[6,7,10] The apparent epidemiologic variability is related to differing definitions, with higher incidence reported when headache or depression are included in the criteria. Although a diagnosis of NPSLE is associated with higher morbidity and mortality, it is more common in children than in adults.[6,7,10] Neurologic complications include seizures, stroke, psychosis, headaches, changes in mood, and cognitive issues. The pathophysiology of NPSLE involves small vessel vasculopathy, thrombosis, and parenchymal damage related to antineuronal antibodies and complement/cytokine-mediated inflammation.[11,12] NPSLE rarely is an isolated feature. Most children with significant lupus neurologic involvement also have other organ system involvement and meet American College of Rheumatology and/or Systemic Lupus International Collaborating Clinics criteria, which differentiate NPSLE from other conditions that cause encephalopathy, such as AE or primary CNS vasculitides.[13,14] For many pediatric rheumatologists, NPSLE serves as a way to conceptualize ABD, because NPSLE also presents as a vasculitis, encephalitis, or demyelinating disease. NPLSE is an example of an autoimmune CNS process that can have widely variable clinical presentations, with symptoms ranging from a focal neurologic deficit or encephalopathy to psychiatric manifestations, such as psychosis or catatonia (psychomotor retardation, paucity of speech, and rigidity).[15] Although typically an acute to subacute process, NPSLE also can present with insidious symptoms, exemplifying the range of onset and progression that are possible with ABD.

Autoimmune encephalitis

AE classically presents as acute to subacute encephalopathy, with rapid progression over days to weeks of memory impairment (in particular, short-term memory), seizures, movement disorders, and behavioral changes[9,16–19] Pediatric specific classification criteria have been proposed, covering the spectrum of potential diagnosis from possible AE (where the diagnosis is considered) to definite antibody-positive disease (**Table 3**). Depending on the institution, rheumatologists may be consulted only for atypical presentations of AE, to rule out other conditions, or to assist with immunotherapy. A key feature to differentiate AE from other conditions is the presence of symptoms across multiple domains (seizures, psychiatric, movement disorders, memory loss, changes in speech, and decreased level of consciousness or autonomic instability). Although patients may present with 1 primary manifestation initially, the hallmark of AE is diffuse inflammation affecting multiple locations in the brain. This results in a range of symptoms dependent on the breadth and heterogeneity of CNS involvement. Patients with AE classically display abnormalities in several domains within 1 month to 2 months of onset.[9,16–19] A lack of symptom progression should raise speculation for an alternate diagnosis.

At times, pediatric rheumatologists may direct antibody testing and determine diagnostic testing to differentiate between AE and other conditions. Given the potential for both false-positive and false-negative antibody testing, careful clinical history and examination are vital to estimate the probability of AE and guide testing. It also is important to recognize the relative prevalence of specific antibodies in the normal population (glutamic acid decarboxylase [GAD65], 8%; thyroid, 2%–20%) when interpreting antibody testing results. Overemphasis on antibody results can lead to unnecessary treatments and delay accurate diagnosis, especially in patients with isolated neuropsychiatric symptoms or if there is low suspicion for AE.[17,20,21] It is important to confirm that a patient meets the criteria for the syndrome associated with that antibody before attributing the patient's symptoms to an autoimmune encephalopathy.[17,20,21] It is in part because of the lack of specificity of many antibodies that the diagnostic criteria for AE depend on both the typical clinical presentation and greater than or equal to 2 specific abnormalities on work-up (MRI changes consistent with AE [per neuroradiology assessment], new-onset seizures/EEG abnormalities, inflammatory changes in cerebrospinal fluid [CSF], or a positive antineuronal antibody; see **Table 3**).[9,18] An important additional caveat to antibody testing is the need for CSF antibody positivity in several of the more common pediatric AE syndromes. To make a diagnosis of *N*-methyl-D-aspartate (NMDA) and GAD AE, patients require CSF antibody positivity because both NMDA and GAD65 antibodies can be seen in the serum of healthy individuals.[17] The proposed pediatric classification criteria for AE guide providers through the work-up and diagnosis. Once the work-up is complete, the current recommendations are to initiate treatment with first-line therapy for those meeting "possible AE" criteria, similar to adult criteria[9,18] (see **Table 3**).

Although it is outside the scope of this article to discuss each AE subtype, seronegative AE deserves special attention. Pediatric rheumatologists may be consulted when seronegative AE is considered. Seronegative AE is diagnosed when a child has a clinical history consistent with AE and signs of CNS inflammation, with greater than or equal to 2 of the following: MRI changes consistent with AE, new-onset seizures/EEG abnormalities, or inflammatory changes in CSF.[9] The 1 and only defining difference from seropositive disease is the lack of an identified antineuronal antibody. For children with symptoms concerning for AE who do not meet the established classification criteria (**Table 3**) and do not have findings consistent with other autoimmune or rheumatic disease, alternate diagnoses should be evaluated thoroughly before making a presumed diagnosis of seronegative AE and initiating treatment. In these situations, having the patient seen by a neuroimmunology team with expertise in AE may be helpful, even if this requires referral to another medical center. This is true especially in younger patients, in those with baseline neurodevelopmental differences, with imaging changes that could suggest metabolic disorders, or with chronic disease states.

Central nervous system vasculitis

CNS vasculitis can be either a primary process, isolated to the CNS vasculature, or secondary to another inflammatory or autoimmune condition with systemic involvement, as in NPSLE or neuro-Behçet disease.[27–30] CNS vasculitis can present with a wide variety of symptoms from an isolated focal neurologic deficit to a diffuse encephalopathy.[2,31–35] Both angiographic-negative and diffuse progressive angiographic-positive primary CNS vasculitis can present as acute encephalopathy, typically with a prodromal illness concurrent with other signs of systemic inflammation, including malaise and fever. Neurologic deficits may be mild or intermittent early in the course of disease but progress to more severe and sustained symptoms over weeks to months. Both angiographic-negative and progressive primary CNS vasculitis result in diffuse brain inflammation and a broad range of CNS symptoms, often overlapping those seen in AE. The most common presenting symptom is headache, which can become severe and disabling. Cognitive deficits, seizures, altered level of consciousness, and focal neurologic deficits are common.

Encephalopathy with focal strokelike features should alert providers to consider CNS vasculitis. MRI changes are present in more than 95% of primary CNS vasculitis patients, including multifocal, leptomeningeal, and parenchymal enhancing lesions.[36] Magnetic resonance angiogram (MRA) may be the initial imaging modality, often acquired at the time of the brain MRI. Given the variable sensitivity of MRA, however, computed topography angiogram (CTA) or conventional angiogram may be necessary to identify vasculitic changes. In cases of possible CNS vasculitis, pediatric rheumatologists may recommend more invasive studies, including conventional angiograms or brain biopsies. Conventional angiogram is the most sensitive study and still considered the gold standard for diagnosing angiographic-positive CNS vasculitis. Conventional angiogram may be especially useful for evaluation of the posterior cerebral circulation and more distal, and therefore smaller, intracranial vessels.[37–39] When there is a high suspicion for CNS vasculitis, it is reasonable to proceed to conventional angiogram if other imaging is nondiagnostic to fully exclude an angiographic-positive vasculitis, before proceeding to a brain biopsy to evaluate for angiographic-negative disease.

Systemic rheumatic diseases also can involve the CNS vasculature. Antineutrophil cytoplasmic antibody–associated CNS vasculitis, a small vessel vasculitis with normal vascular imaging, may show ischemic lesions on MRI and a predilection for the pituitary gland, pachymeninges (rather than leptomeninges), and intracranial dura.[40] Intracranial dura involvement can result in cranial neuropathies.[3] Neuro-Behçet disease classically involves the brainstem, especially around the cerebral peduncles and pons, with brainstem atrophy. Prompt consultation with pediatric rheumatology and consideration of neuro-Behçet disease are recommended strongly for patients with neuroimaging that demonstrates unexplained abnormalities in the brainstem[41,42]

Table 4
Acquired demyelinating syndromes classification criteria[22–26]

Acute Disseminated Encephalomyelitis	Neuromyelitis Optica Spectrum Disorders with Aquaporin-4	Neuromyelitis Optica Spectrum Disorder without Aquaporin-4/or Unknown Aquaporin-4
Must meet all 4: 1. Presence of encephalopathy that cannot be explained by fever 2. First multifocal clinical CNS event with presumed inflammatory cause 3. MRI shows diffuse, poorly demarcated, large >1–2 cm lesions involving predominantly cerebral white matter. T1 hypointense white matter lesions are rare; deep gray matter lesions (thalamus and basal ganglia) can be present 4. No new symptoms, signs, or MRI findings after 3 mo of initial presentation Multiphasic AEM New ADEM event 3 mo or more after initial event associated with new or re-emergence of prior clinical and MRI findings. Timing in relation to steroids no longer is pertinent.	1. At least 1 core clinical characteristic: a. Optic neuritis b. Acute myelitis c. Area postrema syndrome: episode of otherwise unexplained hiccups or nausea and vomiting d. Acute brainstem syndrome e. Symptomatic narcolepsy or acute diencephalic clinical syndrome with NMOSD-typical diencephalic MRI lesions f. Symptomatic cerebral syndrome with NMOSD-typical brain lesions 2. Positive AQP4-IgG antibody using best available detection method (cell-based assay strongly recommended) 3. Exclusion of alternative diagnoses	1. At least 2 core NMOSDs with AQP4 clinical characteristics with ≥1 clinical attacks and meeting all of the following: a. 1 core clinical characteristic must be optic neuritis, acute myelitis with >3 contiguous segments, or area postrema syndrome b. Dissemination in space (≥2 different core clinical characteristics) c. MRI findings for the core clinical characteristic: i. Acute optic neuritis: (a) brain MRI with normal findings or only nonspecific white matter lesions, OR (b) optic nerve MRI with T2-hyperintense lesion or T1-weighted gadolinium-enhancing lesion extending over 1/2 optic nerve length or involving optic chiasm ii. Acute myelitis: requires associated intramedullary MRI lesion extending over 3 contiguous segments iii. Area postrema syndrome with dorsal medulla/area postrema lesions iv. Acute brainstem syndrome with periependymal brainstem lesions 2. Negative tests for AQP4-IgG antibody using best available detection method (cell-based assay strongly recommended), or testing unavailable 3. Exclusion of alternative diagnoses

Neurosarcoidosis can present with encephalopathy and seizures, especially in younger children. Classic areas of involvement include the pituitary, hypothalamus, cranial nerves, and meninges.[4,43] When classic abnormalities are seen with neuroimaging or when a diagnosis of neuro-Behçet disease or neurosarcoidosis is suspected, a thorough evaluation for systemic rheumatic disease is warranted. Although neurologic symptoms may be the presenting feature of neuro-Behçet disease or neurosarcoidosis, few have isolated CNS involvement.

Acute disseminated encephalomyelitis

Acute disseminated encephalomyelitis (ADEM) is defined by the presence of encephalopathy as evidenced by alteration in consciousness or behavioral abnormality not explained by fever.[44] ADEM is more common in children than in adults, often presenting between ages 5 years to 8 years of age.[45] In ADEM, encephalopathy coexists with polyfocal neurologic symptoms, such as motor or sensory deficits, ataxia, cranial neuropathies, urinary retention, seizures, and myelitis. Evaluation for children presenting with ADEM includes neurologic assessment, MRI with and without contrast of the brain, orbits and spinal cord, lumbar puncture, and serum testing for both aquaporin-4 (AQP4) antibodies and myelin oligodendrocyte glycoprotein antibodies.[46] Brain MRI often demonstrates large, poorly demarcated white matter lesions but also can show involvement of the basal ganglia or thalamus.[44] Clinical symptoms and neuroimaging findings may wax and wane over the initial 3 months after disease onset.[22,44,45] ADEM also may be the first clinically recognized event of a distinct multiphasic demyelinating illness. With the exception of myelin-oligodendrocyte GAD (MOGAD), encephalopathy is an uncommon presentation for acquired demyelinating syndromes, such as multiple sclerosis or neuromyelitis optica.

Hashimoto encephalopathy

Children with Hashimoto encephalopathy (HE) classically present with seizures, myoclonus, hallucinations, or strokelike episodes.[9,18,47,48] There are 2 described patterns of HE, 1 with focal neurologic deficits from strokelike events with cognitive decline and the other a more progressive encephalopathy presenting with insidious progression of altered mental status, psychosis, and confusion. The most common symptom in children is seizure. Thyroid antibodies to either antithyroglobulin or antiperoxidase antibodies must be present to make a diagnosis. Thyroid antibodies are present in 2% to 20% of the general population so are not sufficient to make a diagnosis of HE.[17,20,21,49,50] Therefore, caution is recommended before making a diagnosis of HE in children with nonspecific neuropsychiatric symptoms based on antibody positivity alone. Evidence of CNS inflammation is needed to support the diagnosis of HE and may be found via lumbar puncture and EEG. Electrographic abnormalities, such as generalized slowing and electrographic seizures, are common. An elevated CSF protein is present in 60% of pediatric cases.[18,47,49,50] HE also is called steroid-responsive encephalopathy associated with autoimmune thyroiditis, given the strong response to treatment with steroids. Approximately 80% of children with HE respond to steroids; however, half of these patients require additional agents for more robust recovery.[51,52]

Acute Focal Neurologic Deficit Presentations

ABD also can present with acute focal neurologic deficits without an associated encephalopathy. This presentation may include clinical symptoms, such as acute vision loss, weakness or sensory changes, changes in speech, and abnormal movements.

Autoimmune encephalitis

AE typically presents with diffuse symptoms, as discussed previously. AE also must be included, however, on the differential diagnosis for ABD presenting with acute focal neurologic deficits, especially early in the disease course. Children may present with 1 prominent symptom, such as dyskinesias or choreoathetoid movements, focal loss of language, or psychosis.[9,16,18,19] Although typically AE progresses to additional symptoms spanning multiple domains over the first few weeks to months, if there is prompt diagnosis and early effective treatment, it is possible for the disease to remain isolated to 1 domain. It is unusual for AE to remain limited to 1 domain for more than a month after symptom onset without treatment. Therefore, a prolonged course with symptoms in only 1 of the domains makes AE less likely.

Angiographic-positive central nervous system vasculitis

Children with angiographic-positive or large vessel CNS vasculitis may have disease limited to 1 vascular bed, resulting in more focal deficits compared with the encephalopathy seen with more diffuse vessel involvement.[2,27,53–55] Headache is a prominent symptom, which may start as mild and intermittent, with severity and persistence worsening over time. Both the anterior and posterior circulation can be affected, although classically the anterior circulation (anterior and middle cerebral arteries) is more likely to be involved with primary angiographic-positive disease. Evaluation for underlying etiology should include testing for parainfectious processes, such as varicella-zoster virus; classic systemic vasculitides, such as polyarteritis nodosa (PAN); and deficiency of adenosine deaminase 2 (DADA2) in children presenting with a PAN-like phenotype.[56–59] Children with DADA2 can present with strokes, classically recurrent lacunar strokes, or other findings of a systemic vasculopathy, such as recurrent fever or livedo rash.

Classic rheumatic diseases

Systemic vasculitides can present with acute focal neurologic deficits in addition to more diffuse manifestations (see **Table 2**). When patients with SLE present with sudden onset of a severe headache (thunderclap headache) and imaging changes consistent with vasculitis, it also is important to consider a diagnosis of reversible cerebral vasoconstriction syndrome (RCVS), because this can mimic vasculitis. RCVS is more common in SLE patients on high-dose steroids or with hypertension.[60–62] Similarly, patients with SLE are at increased risk for acquired endothelial damage, as seen in posterior reversible encephalopathy syndrome, with added risk from concurrent hypertension. Antiphospholipid syndrome (APS) is on differential diagnosis in a child presenting with strokelike features or chorea. Primary APS as well as APS-associated with SLE can cause CNS injury either through the associated coagulopathy and stroke or through direct antibody-mediated neuronal injury.[8]

Acquired demyelinating syndromes

Acquired demyelinating syndromes encompass several diseases with immune-mediated destruction of CNS targets, including myelin, oligodendrocyte, and astrocytes. These conditions include pediatric-onset multiple sclerosis (POMS), neuromyelitis optica spectrum disorder (NMOSD), and MOGAD (**Table 4**).[23,63–65]

NMOSD is a multiphasic immune-mediated demyelinating disorder classically involving the optic nerves and spinal cord.[66,67] NMOSD is associated with antibodies to astrocytic AQP4 channels, although antibody detection is not required for diagnosis.[23] AQP4 channels are expressed in higher concentrations in the optic nerves, hypothalamus, periaqueductal gray matter, area postrema, and spinal cord, correlating with the characteristic symptoms and imaging findings of NMOSD.[64,68,69] AQP4-positive NMOSD presents most commonly with optic neuritis, often bilateral in the pediatric population, myelitis, or both.[66,70] Many cases previously classified as seronegative NMOSD now are recognized as secondary to MOG antibodies, particularly in children.[24] There is a broad range of symptoms reflecting the extensive areas of involvement, including the area of postrema, brainstem, and hypothalamus.

In AQP4 antibody–positive disease, plasma exchange (PLEX) within 5 days of presentation can improve outcomes. High relapse risk and resulting disability accrual in pediatric patients prompt early and often prolonged treatment courses.[71] AQP4 IgG-seropositive NMOSD may coexist with other autoimmune disorders, in particular SLE and Sjögren syndrome. Serum testing for both AQP4 antibodies and MOG antibodies should be considered when these patients present with new-onset neurologic deficits.[23,25,66,72,73]

MOGAD accounts for approximately one-third of pediatric acute demyelinating syndromes[26,74] Although younger children tend to present with ADEM, children over 9 years of age are more likely to present with focal symptoms, such as optic neuritis or myelitis.[26] It is important for pediatric rheumatologists to be aware of MOGAD because it mimics CNS vasculitis.[75] It now is recognized that children previously diagnosed with angiographic-negative CNS vasculitis likely had MOG encephalitis, because the inflammatory response to MOG antibodies induces a vasculopathy with perivascular and parenchymal infiltrate and necrosis similar to those reported in angiographic-negative vasculitis.[76–78] The reported frequency of relapsing MOGAD in pediatrics is variable, with both monophasic and multiphasic courses described. Both older patients and those who remain MOG antibody seropositive at follow-up have an increased risk of relapse, prompting treatment with similar medication regimens to NMOSD.[26,79]

Pediatric-onset multiple sclerosis

POMS is a multiphasic disease characterized by inflammatory demyelination and neuronal injury.[80–82] Almost all cases of POMS present with a relapsing and remitting form of disease.[67,83–85] Common presenting symptoms include optic neuritis, weakness, sensory deficit, discoordination, bowel or bladder dysfunction, and hearing impairment. Fatigue, depression, and cognitive impairment also are prominent features.[84,85] Diagnosis, based on the 2017 McDonald criteria, largely is dependent on clinical features supported by MRI and CSF findings.[65,86] Brain MRI typically reveals T2-bright lesions involving the periventricular white matter and potentially evidence of dissemination over time with hypointense lesions on T1 imaging.[87] CSF may reveal mild pleocytosis, elevated protein, elevated IgG index, and oligoclonal bands. Although the presence of oligoclonal bands supports the diagnosis of POMS, this is a nonspecific finding present in many inflammatory CNS conditions.[70,84–88]

Central demyelinating syndromes associated with tumor necrosis factor α inhibitors

A demyelinating syndrome is recognized as a rare but serious complication of tumor necrosis factor (TNF)-α inhibitors[89,90] Demyelinating neuropathies and central demyelinating syndromes following treatment with etanercept and infliximab represent the vast majority of reported cases.[45,89,90] The use of infliximab or etanercept for patients with multiple sclerosis was associated with significant worsening of patient symptoms.[91,92] Given the correlation between TNF-α inhibitors and demyelinating events, these medications should be avoided in patients with multiple sclerosis or a history of prior demyelinating event. Providers should monitor for the development of neurologic deficits in patients treated with TNF inhibition.[45]

Acute-onset Neuropsychiatric Symptoms

Some of the most challenging ABD cases involve the acute onset of neuropsychiatric symptoms with tics or psychiatric symptoms as prominent manifestations. Assessment of cognitive and behavioral symptoms is a challenging aspect of the history collection. Evaluating cognitive function in children may be difficult, depending on age at presentation, severity of impairment, and presence of comorbid psychiatric symptoms. Formal neurocognitive assessments are instrumental in differentiating cognitive decline related to encephalopathy from other neuropsychiatric conditions.[93–95] Comprehensive testing can help distinguish between primary psychiatric disease, often associated with an IQ decline of 10 points to 20 points, and encephalopathy, which tends to cause more profound changes in cognitive performance. Obtaining records from previous primary care evaluations, academic testing, and especially previous cognitive evaluations is particularly helpful to establishing prior performance, given the potential for recall limitations of providers, patients, and families. Similarly, videos and behavior logs documenting the frequency, environment, and triggers for behavior changes or movement disorders also provide valuable information in the assessment of ABD.

Pediatric acute-onset neuropsychiatric syndrome (PANS)/pediatric autoimmune neuropsychiatric disorder associated with streptococcal infection (PANDAS) (hereafter referred to as PANS) is a controversial syndrome characterized by abrupt onset of obsessive-compulsive disorder (OCD) or restrictive eating and 2 additional psychiatric or cognitive symptoms.[96] Streptococcal infection precedes PANS, which is characterized by explosive onset of motor and vocal tics, change in behavior, and occasionally abnormal nontic movements.[97] Classically, imaging and systemic inflammatory testing are normal in PANS. There are no reliable specific biomarkers for PANS.[98] The primary treatment recommendations are for symptomatic management of the psychiatric symptoms with cognitive-behavior therapy or psychotropics. Immunomodulatory regimens have been described in consensus opinions; however, the role of agents, such as intravenous immunoglobulin (IVIG), is less clear because randomized trials of IVIG have not shown improvement over placebo.[99,100] When considering PANS, it is important to remember that anxiety is the most common childhood mental health disorder, with generalized anxiety disorder occurring in approximately 10% of all children. Although severe anxiety and OCD can be part of the symptom complex of children with ABD, based on prevalence alone, these symptoms are significantly more likely to result from a primary psychiatric disorder, even when severe, rather than ABD. Severe and/or refractory anxiety and/or OCD is not sufficient to make a diagnosis of ABD.[101]

New-onset Refractory Seizures

Sudden-onset refractory seizures are present in many forms of ABD, including AE and CNS vasculitis. There also are other acute-onset epileptic syndromes where primary immune dysregulation is the suspected underlying etiology.

Febrile infection–related epilepsy syndrome (FIRES) or other new-onset refractory status epilepticus (NORSE) syndromes are conditions described in children with refractory and super-refractory status epilepticus.[102] These conditions may present with acute cognitive changes due to the increase in clinical seizures. Research regarding the utility of immunomodulation in NORSE is ongoing. Experts in the field advocate for early diagnosis and modulation of immune activation in both adults and children with NORSE. Unlike traditional rheumatic disorders and AE, there are no overt signs of systemic inflammation and a less pronounced neurologic or neuropsychiatric prodrome. Initial neuroimaging may be normal and worsen over time, with evidence of atrophy and cytotoxicity, as can be seen in persistent status epilepticus.

TREATMENT

The treatment of ABD varies by disease type, severity, and comorbidities. Therefore, a thorough diagnostic evaluation to ensure an accurate diagnosis is of paramount importance and is the primary determinant of treatment approach. There are few clinical trials to inform medication initiation, treatment escalation, or optimal dosing, timing, or duration of treatment of most ABDs. Given the lack of evidence-based treatment guidelines, this section focuses on the treatment by broad disease categories (see **Table 2**).

Recently proposed best practices for AE defined severity of disease as the first consideration when choosing treatment.[103,104] Steroids, both oral and intravenous (IV), IVIG, and PLEX/plasmapheresis all are considered first-line therapies, with PLEX/plasmapheresis reserved for more severe disease or the presence of contraindications to steroids or IVIG. For patients who fail to respond fully to first-line treatments, rituximab is the most common second-line agent, although cyclophosphamide also is a consideration. Rituximab is dosed at either 750 mg/m^2 (maximum dose, 1000 mg), every 2 weeks for 2 doses, or 375 mg/m^2, weekly for 4 doses. Cyclophosphamide may be given concurrently or in series if rituximab does not result in improvement. How long to wait for response to first-line or second-line treatments before therapy escalation is not defined clearly, but surveys of clinicians suggest 7 days to 10 days for first-line treatments and 1 month to 2 months for second-line agents, with neurologists expecting response within 1 month and rheumatologists after 2 months to 3 months. Continuing IVIG and steroids for the first few months after beginning rituximab or cyclophosphamide is important, given their delayed onset of action in many patients and the potential additive benefits of first-line and second-line treatments to reduce disease progression, even in patients without a clear response to the first-line agents alone. There has been a recent shift by providers to prescribe tocilizumab prior to cyclophosphamide, given the reduced potential toxicity, especially in pediatric populations.[105] There are no studies, however, directly comparing tocilizumab and cyclophosphamide efficacy or safety.

Similar to AE, the treatment of acquired demyelinating syndromes varies based on underlying etiology and severity.[106,107] Many children with ADEM require only a brief course of steroids, including those with positive MOG antibodies, whereas others require longer courses of steroids and IVIG or escalation to second-line agents, including rituximab, mycophenolic acid, and azathioprine. In contrast, AQP4-mediated NMOSD requires more aggressive initial therapy with PLEX, steroids, and rituximab along with long-term maintenance therapy due to the destructive nature of the antibody and high rates of relapse.

CNS disease secondary to primary rheumatic disease, such as SLE, sarcoidosis, or Behçet disease, often requires escalation to potent immunosuppressant treatments options employed to treat the systemic diseases. Cyclophosphamide still is the recommended treatment of CNS vasculitis, both for primary progressive and angiographic-negative disease as well as vasculitis related to SLE, with mycophenolic acid preferred for maintenance therapy over azathrioprine.[108–110] TNF inhibitors may be more efficacious in sarcoidosis and neuro-Behçet disease but may require higher doses than routinely used for general systemic disease.[110]

SUMMARY

The spectrum of ABD continues to evolve, with medical advancements that facilitate both detection of CNS inflammation and the discovery of novel mechanisms of disease. Given the clinical overlap with many primary rheumatic diseases and the efficacy of immunotherapy, multidisciplinary partnerships among subspecialty providers, including pediatric rheumatologists, neurologists, and psychiatrists, optimize care and improve outcomes for children with these disorders.

CLINICS CARE POINTS

- A thorough evaluation is required to accurately diagnose autoimmune brain diseases given the overlap in clinical features and diagnostic testing.
- Given medications treatments and duration of therapy vary based on underlying disease, assuring an accurate diagnosis is essential.
- There are few clinical trials in pediatric autoimmune brain diseases to guide treatment recommendations. Current treatment recommendations include therapies to both decrease the autoimmune/inflammatory process and provide symptomatic management.

REFERENCES

1. Lim M, Hacohen Y, Vincent A. Autoimmune encephalopathies. Pediatr Clin North Am 2015;62(3):667–85.
2. Twilt M, Benseler SM. The spectrum of CNS vasculitis in children and adults. Nat Rev Rheumatol 2012;8(2):97–107.
3. Graf J. Central nervous system disease in antineutrophil cytoplasmic antibodies-associated vasculitis. Rheum Dis Clin North Am 2017;43(4):573–8.
4. Stern BJ, Royal W 3rd, Gelfand JM, et al. Definition and consensus diagnostic criteria for neurosarcoidosis: from the neurosarcoidosis consortium consensus group. JAMA Neurol 2018. https://doi.org/10.1001/jamaneurol.2018.2295.
5. Meyts I, Aksentijevich I. Deficiency of adenosine deaminase 2 (DADA2): updates on the phenotype, genetics, pathogenesis, and treatment. J Clin Immunol 2018;38(5):569–78.
6. Shaban A, Leira EC. Neurological complications in patients with systemic lupus erythematosus. Curr Neurol Neurosci Rep 2019;19(12):97.
7. Yu HH, Lee JH, Wang LC, et al. Neuropsychiatric manifestations in pediatric systemic lupus erythematosus: a 20-year study. Lupus 2006;15(10):651–7.
8. Garcia D, Erkan D. Diagnosis and management of the antiphospholipid syndrome. N Engl J Med 2018;379(13):1290.
9. Cellucci T, Van Mater H, Graus F, et al. Clinical approach to the diagnosis of autoimmune encephalitis in the pediatric patient. Neurol Neuroimmunol Neuroinflamm 2020;7(2):e730.
10. Hanly JG, Li Q, Su L, et al. Cerebrovascular events in systemic lupus erythematosus: results from an international inception cohort study. Arthritis Care Res (Hoboken) 2018;70(10):1478–87.
11. Schwartz N, Stock AD, Putterman C. Neuropsychiatric lupus: new mechanistic insights and future treatment directions. Nat Rev Rheumatol 2019;15(3):137–52.
12. Govoni M, Hanly JG. The management of neuropsychiatric lupus in the 21st century: still so many unmet needs? Rheumatology (Oxford) 2020;59(Suppl5):v52–62.
13. Hartman EAR, van Royen-Kerkhof A, Jacobs JWG, et al. Performance of the 2012 Systemic Lupus International Collaborating Clinics classification criteria versus the 1997 American College of Rheumatology classification criteria in

adult and juvenile systemic lupus erythematosus. A systematic review and meta-analysis. Autoimmun Rev 2018;17(3):316–22.
14. Ahn GY, Kim D, Won S, et al. Prevalence, risk factors, and impact on mortality of neuropsychiatric lupus: a prospective, single-center study. Lupus 2018;27(8): 1338–47.
15. Rasmussen SA, Mazurek MF, Rosebush PI. Catatonia: our current understanding of its diagnosis, treatment and pathophysiology. World J Psychiatry 2016; 6(4):391–8.
16. Armangue T, Titulaer MJ, Malaga I, et al. Pediatric anti-N-methyl-D-aspartate receptor encephalitis-clinical analysis and novel findings in a series of 20 patients. J Pediatr 2013;162(4):850–6.e2.
17. Graus F, Saiz A, Dalmau J. GAD antibodies in neurological disorders - insights and challenges. Nat Rev Neurol 2020;16(7):353–65.
18. Graus F, Titulaer MJ, Balu R, et al. A clinical approach to diagnosis of autoimmune encephalitis. Lancet Neurol 2016;15(4):391–404.
19. Titulaer MJ, McCracken L, Gabilondo I, et al. Treatment and prognostic factors for long-term outcome in patients with anti-NMDA receptor encephalitis: an observational cohort study. Lancet Neurol 2013;12(2):157–65.
20. Bjoro T, Holmen J, Kruger O, et al. Prevalence of thyroid disease, thyroid dysfunction and thyroid peroxidase antibodies in a large, unselected population. The Health Study of Nord-Trondelag (HUNT). Eur J Endocrinol 2000; 143(5):639–47.
21. Hollowell JG, Staehling NW, Flanders WD, et al. Serum TSH, T(4), and thyroid antibodies in the United States population (1988 to 1994): National Health and Nutrition Examination Survey (NHANES III). J Clin Endocrinol Metab 2002; 87(2):489–99.
22. Cole J, Evans E, Mwangi M, et al. Acute disseminated encephalomyelitis in children: an updated review based on current diagnostic criteria. Pediatr Neurol 2019;100:26–34.
23. Wingerchuk DM, Banwell B, Bennett JL, et al. International consensus diagnostic criteria for neuromyelitis optica spectrum disorders. Neurology 2015; 85(2):177–89.
24. Jarius S, Paul F, Aktas O, et al. MOG encephalomyelitis: international recommendations on diagnosis and antibody testing. J Neuroinflammation 2018; 15(1):134.
25. Borisow N, Mori M, Kuwabara S, et al. Diagnosis and treatment of NMO spectrum disorder and MOG-encephalomyelitis. Front Neurol 2018;9:888.
26. Bruijstens AL, Lechner C, Flet-Berliac L, et al. E.U. paediatric MOG consortium consensus: Part 1 - Classification of clinical phenotypes of paediatric myelin oligodendrocyte glycoprotein antibody-associated disorders. Eur J Paediatr Neurol 2020;29:2–13.
27. Benseler S, Pohl D. Childhood central nervous system vasculitis. Handb Clin Neurol 2013;112:1065–78.
28. Kleffner I, Dorr J, Ringelstein M, et al. Diagnostic criteria for Susac syndrome. J Neurol Neurosurg Psychiatry 2016;87(12):1287–95.
29. Vodopivec I, Venna N, Rizzo JF 3rd, et al. Clinical features, diagnostic findings, and treatment of Susac syndrome: a case series. J Neurol Sci 2015; 357(1–2):50–7.
30. Van Mater H. Pediatric inflammatory brain diseases: a diagnostic approach. Curr Opin Rheumatol 2014;26(5):553–61.

31. Calabrese LH, Furlan AJ, Gragg LA, et al. Primary angiitis of the central nervous system: diagnostic criteria and clinical approach. Cleve Clin J Med 1992;59(3): 293–306.
32. Hajj-Ali RA, Calabrese LH. Diagnosis and classification of central nervous system vasculitis. J Autoimmun 2014;48-49:149–52.
33. Benseler SM. Central nervous system vasculitis in children. Curr Rheumatol Rep 2006;8(6):442–9.
34. Benseler SM, deVeber G, Hawkins C, et al. Angiography-negative primary central nervous system vasculitis in children: a newly recognized inflammatory central nervous system disease. Arthritis Rheum 2005;52(7):2159–67.
35. Cellucci T, Benseler SM. Central nervous system vasculitis in children. Curr Opin Rheumatol 2010;22(5):590–7.
36. Beuker C, Schmidt A, Strunk D, et al. Primary angiitis of the central nervous system: diagnosis and treatment. Ther Adv Neurol Disord 2018;11. 1756286418785071.
37. Edgell RC, Sarhan AE, Soomro J, et al. The role of catheter angiography in the diagnosis of central nervous system vasculitis. Interv Neurol 2016;5(3–4): 194–208.
38. Eleftheriou D, Cox T, Saunders D, et al. Investigation of childhood central nervous system vasculitis: magnetic resonance angiography versus catheter cerebral angiography. Dev Med Child Neurol 2010;52(9):863–7.
39. Smitka M, Bruck N, Engellandt K, et al. Clinical perspective on primary angiitis of the central nervous system in childhood (cPACNS). Front Pediatr 2020;8:281.
40. Fragoulis GE, Lionaki S, Venetsanopoulou A, et al. Central nervous system involvement in patients with granulomatosis with polyangiitis: a single-center retrospective study. Clin Rheumatol 2018;37(3):737–47.
41. Peno IC, De las Heras Revilla V, Carbonell BP, et al. Neurobehcet disease: clinical and demographic characteristics. Eur J Neurol 2012;19(9):1224–7.
42. Houman MH, Bellakhal S, Ben Salem T, et al. Characteristics of neurological manifestations of Behcet's disease: a retrospective monocentric study in Tunisia. Clin Neurol Neurosurg 2013;115(10):2015–8.
43. Pawate S, Moses H, Sriram S. Presentations and outcomes of neurosarcoidosis: a study of 54 cases. QJM 2009;102(7):449–60.
44. Krupp LB, Tardieu M, Amato MP, et al. International Pediatric Multiple Sclerosis Study Group criteria for pediatric multiple sclerosis and immune-mediated central nervous system demyelinating disorders: revisions to the 2007 definitions. Mult Scler 2013;19(10):1261–7.
45. Kristensen LB, Lambertsen KL, Nguyen N, et al. The role of non-selective TNF inhibitors in demyelinating events. Brain Sci 2021;11(1):38.
46. Chitnis T. Pediatric central nervous system demyelinating diseases. Continuum (Minneap Minn) 2019;25(3):793–814.
47. Laurent C, Capron J, Quillerou B, et al. Steroid-responsive encephalopathy associated with autoimmune thyroiditis (SREAT): Characteristics, treatment and outcome in 251 cases from the literature. Autoimmun Rev 2016;15(12): 1129–33.
48. Zhou JY, Xu B, Lopes J, et al. Hashimoto encephalopathy: literature review. Acta Neurol Scand 2017;135(3):285–90.
49. Ferracci F, Bertiato G, Moretto G. Hashimoto's encephalopathy: epidemiologic data and pathogenetic considerations. J Neurol Sci 2004;217(2):165–8.

50. Ferracci F, Moretto G, Candeago RM, et al. Antithyroid antibodies in the CSF: their role in the pathogenesis of Hashimoto's encephalopathy. Neurology 2003;60(4):712–4.
51. Kirshner HS. Hashimoto's encephalopathy: a brief review. Curr Neurol Neurosci Rep 2014;14(9):476.
52. Mamoudjy N, Korff C, Maurey H, et al. Hashimoto's encephalopathy: identification and long-term outcome in children. Eur J Paediatr Neurol 2013;17(3):280–7.
53. Cellucci T, Tyrrell PN, Twilt M, et al. Distinct phenotype clusters in childhood inflammatory brain diseases: implications for diagnostic evaluation. Arthritis Rheumatol 2014;66(3):750–6.
54. Benseler SM, Silverman E, Aviv RI, et al. Primary central nervous system vasculitis in children. Arthritis Rheum 2006;54(4):1291–7.
55. Cellucci T, Benseler SM. Diagnosing central nervous system vasculitis in children. Curr Opin Pediatr 2010;22(6):731–8.
56. Amlie-Lefond C, Gilden D. Varicella zoster virus: a common cause of stroke in children and adults. J Stroke Cerebrovasc Dis 2016;25(7):1561–9.
57. Zhou Q, Yang D, Ombrello AK, et al. Early-onset stroke and vasculopathy associated with mutations in ADA2. N Engl J Med 2014;370(10):911–20.
58. Navon Elkan P, Pierce SB, Segel R, et al. Mutant adenosine deaminase 2 in a polyarteritis nodosa vasculopathy. N Engl J Med 2014;370(10):921–31.
59. Caorsi R, Penco F, Grossi A, et al. ADA2 deficiency (DADA2) as an unrecognised cause of early onset polyarteritis nodosa and stroke: a multicentre national study. Ann Rheum Dis 2017;76(10):1648–56.
60. Cui HW, Lei RY, Zhang SG, et al. Clinical features, outcomes and risk factors for posterior reversible encephalopathy syndrome in systemic lupus erythematosus: a case-control study. Lupus 2019;28(8):961–9.
61. Durrleman C, Naggara O, Grevent D, et al. Reversible cerebral vasoconstriction syndrome in paediatric patients with systemic lupus erythematosus: implications for management. Dev Med Child Neurol 2018. https://doi.org/10.1111/dmcn.14031.
62. Vieira RM, do Nascimento FBP, Barbosa Junior AA, et al. Spectrum of central nervous system involvement in rheumatic diseases: pictorial essay. Radiol Bras 2018;51(4):262–7.
63. Bar-Or A, Hintzen RQ, Dale RC, et al. Immunopathophysiology of pediatric CNS inflammatory demyelinating diseases. Neurology 2016;87(9 Suppl 2):S12–9.
64. Tenembaum S, Chitnis T, Nakashima I, et al. Neuromyelitis optica spectrum disorders in children and adolescents. Neurology 2016;87(9 Suppl 2):S59–66.
65. Thompson AJ, Banwell BL, Barkhof F, et al. Diagnosis of multiple sclerosis: 2017 revisions of the McDonald criteria. Lancet Neurol 2018;17(2):162–73.
66. McKeon A, Lennon VA, Lotze T, et al. CNS aquaporin-4 autoimmunity in children. Neurology 2008;71(2):93–100.
67. Chitnis T, Krupp L, Yeh A, et al. Pediatric multiple sclerosis. Neurol Clin 2011; 29(2):481–505.
68. Tenembaum S, Yeh EA, Guthy-Jackson Foundation International Clinical C. Pediatric NMOSD: a review and position statement on approach to work-up and diagnosis. Front Pediatr 2020;8:339.
69. Verkman AS, Phuan PW, Asavapanumas N, et al. Biology of AQP4 and anti-AQP4 antibody: therapeutic implications for NMO. Brain Pathol 2013;23(6): 684–95.
70. Matricardi S, Farello G, Savasta S, et al. Understanding childhood neuroimmune diseases of the central nervous system. Front Pediatr 2019;7:511.

71. Paolilo RB, Hacohen Y, Yazbeck E, et al. Treatment and outcome of aquaporin-4 antibody-positive NMOSD: a multinational pediatric study. Neurol Neuroimmunol Neuroinflamm 2020;7(5):e837.
72. Moraitis E, Stathopoulos Y, Hong Y, et al. Aquaporin-4 IgG antibody-related disorders in patients with juvenile systemic lupus erythematosus. Lupus 2019;28(10):1243–9.
73. Martin-Nares E, Hernandez-Molina G, Fragoso-Loyo H. Aquaporin-4-IgG positive neuromyelitis optica spectrum disorder and systemic autoimmune diseases overlap syndrome: a single-center experience. Lupus 2019;28(11):1302–11.
74. Reindl M, Waters P. Myelin oligodendrocyte glycoprotein antibodies in neurological disease. Nat Rev Neurol 2019;15(2):89–102.
75. Patterson K, Iglesias E, Nasrallah M, et al. Anti-MOG encephalitis mimicking small vessel CNS vasculitis. Neurol Neuroimmunol Neuroinflamm 2019;6(2):e538.
76. Chitnis T, Ness J, Krupp L, et al. Clinical features of neuromyelitis optica in children: US Network of Pediatric MS Centers report. Neurology 2016;86(3):245–52.
77. Hoftberger R, Guo Y, Flanagan EP, et al. The pathology of central nervous system inflammatory demyelinating disease accompanying myelin oligodendrocyte glycoprotein autoantibody. Acta Neuropathol 2020;139(5):875–92.
78. Elbers J, Halliday W, Hawkins C, et al. Brain biopsy in children with primary small-vessel central nervous system vasculitis. Ann Neurol 2010;68(5):602–10.
79. Waters P, Fadda G, Woodhall M, et al. Serial anti-myelin oligodendrocyte glycoprotein antibody analyses and outcomes in children with demyelinating syndromes. JAMA Neurol 2020;77(1):82–93.
80. Alroughani R, Boyko A. Pediatric multiple sclerosis: a review. BMC Neurol 2018;18(1):27.
81. Nourbakhsh B, Mowry EM. Multiple sclerosis risk factors and pathogenesis. Continuum (Minneap Minn) 2019;25(3):596–610.
82. Thompson AJ, Baranzini SE, Geurts J, et al. Multiple sclerosis. Lancet 2018;391(10130):1622–36.
83. Waldman AT, Gorman MP, Rensel MR, et al. Management of pediatric central nervous system demyelinating disorders: consensus of United States neurologists. J Child Neurol 2011;26(6):675–82.
84. Banwell B, Krupp L, Kennedy J, et al. Clinical features and viral serologies in children with multiple sclerosis: a multinational observational study. Lancet Neurol 2007;6(9):773–81.
85. Nikolic B, Ivancevic N, Zaletel I, et al. Characteristics of pediatric multiple sclerosis: a tertiary referral center study. PLoS One 2020;15(12):e0243031.
86. Hacohen Y, Brownlee W, Mankad K, et al. Improved performance of the 2017 McDonald criteria for diagnosis of multiple sclerosis in children in a real-life cohort. Mult Scler 2020;26(11):1372–80.
87. Banwell B, Arnold DL, Tillema JM, et al. MRI in the evaluation of pediatric multiple sclerosis. Neurology 2016;87(9 Suppl 2):S88–96.
88. Tardieu M, Banwell B, Wolinsky JS, et al. Consensus definitions for pediatric MS and other demyelinating disorders in childhood. Neurology 2016;87(9 Suppl 2):S8–11.
89. Pavlakis PP. Rheumatologic Disorders and the Nervous System. Continuum (Minneap Minn) 2020;26(3):591–610.
90. Kemanetzoglou E, Andreadou E. CNS demyelination with TNF-alpha blockers. Curr Neurol Neurosci Rep 2017;17(4):36.

91. van Oosten BW, Barkhof F, Truyen L, et al. Increased MRI activity and immune activation in two multiple sclerosis patients treated with the monoclonal anti-tumor necrosis factor antibody cA2. Neurology 1996;47(6):1531–4.
92. TNF neutralization in MS: results of a randomized, placebo-controlled multicenter study. The Lenercept Multiple Sclerosis Study Group and The University of British Columbia MS/MRI Analysis Group. Neurology 1999;53(3):457–65.
93. Castaneda AE, Tuulio-Henriksson A, Marttunen M, et al. A review on cognitive impairments in depressive and anxiety disorders with a focus on young adults. J Affect Disord 2008;106(1–2):1–27.
94. Cohen LJ, Hollander E, DeCaria CM, et al. Specificity of neuropsychological impairment in obsessive-compulsive disorder: a comparison with social phobic and normal control subjects. J Neuropsychiatry Clin Neurosci 1996;8(1):82–5.
95. Ferreri F, Lapp LK, Peretti CS. Current research on cognitive aspects of anxiety disorders. Curr Opin Psychiatry 2011;24(1):49–54.
96. Wilbur C, Bitnun A, Kronenberg S, et al. PANDAS/PANS in childhood: controversies and evidence. Paediatr Child Health 2019;24(2):85–91.
97. Swedo SE, Seidlitz J, Kovacevic M, et al. Clinical presentation of pediatric autoimmune neuropsychiatric disorders associated with streptococcal infections in research and community settings. J Child Adolesc Psychopharmacol 2015;25(1):26–30.
98. Hesselmark E, Bejerot S. Biomarkers for diagnosis of Pediatric Acute Neuropsychiatric Syndrome (PANS) - Sensitivity and specificity of the Cunningham Panel. J Neuroimmunol 2017;312:31–7.
99. Sigra S, Hesselmark E, Bejerot S. Treatment of PANDAS and PANS: a systematic review. Neurosci Biobehav Rev 2018;86:51–65.
100. Swedo SE, Frankovich J, Murphy TK. Overview of treatment of pediatric acute-onset neuropsychiatric syndrome. J Child Adolesc Psychopharmacol 2017;27(7):562–5.
101. Walkup JT, Friedland SJ, Peris TS, et al. Dysregulation, catastrophic reactions, and the anxiety disorders. Child Adolesc Psychiatr Clin N Am 2021;30(2):431–44.
102. Hirsch LJ, Gaspard N, van Baalen A, et al. Proposed consensus definitions for new-onset refractory status epilepticus (NORSE), febrile infection-related epilepsy syndrome (FIRES), and related conditions. *Epilepsia* Apr 2018;59(4):739–44.
103. Abboud H, Probasco JC, Irani S, et al. Autoimmune encephalitis: proposed best practice recommendations for diagnosis and acute management. J Neurol Neurosurg Psychiatry 2021. https://doi.org/10.1136/jnnp-2020-325300.
104. Abboud H, Probasco J, Irani SR, et al. Autoimmune encephalitis: proposed recommendations for symptomatic and long-term management. J Neurol Neurosurg Psychiatry 2021. https://doi.org/10.1136/jnnp-2020-325302.
105. Thong KM, Chan TM. Infectious complications in lupus nephritis treatment: a systematic review and meta-analysis. Lupus 2019;28(3):334–46.
106. Whittam DH, Karthikeayan V, Gibbons E, et al. Treatment of MOG antibody associated disorders: results of an international survey. J Neurol 2020;267(12):3565–77.
107. Velasco M, Zarco LA, Agudelo-Arrieta M, et al. Effectiveness of treatments in Neuromyelitis optica to modify the course of disease in adult patients. Systematic review of literature. Mult Scler Relat Disord 2021;50:102869.

108. Quan AS, Brunner J, Rose B, et al. Diagnosis and treatment of angiography positive medium to large vessel childhood primary angiitis of central nervous system (p-cPACNS): an international survey. Front Pediatr 2021;9:654537.
109. Nikolopoulos D, Fanouriakis A, Bertsias G. Treatment of neuropsychiatric systemic lupus erythematosus: clinical challenges and future perspectives. Expert Rev Clin Immunol 2021;17(4):317–30.
110. Lapides DA, McDonald MM. Inflammatory manifestations of systemic diseases in the central nervous system. Curr Treat Options Neurol 2020;22(9):26.

Systemic Autoinflammatory Diseases

A Growing Family of Disorders of Overlapping Immune Dysfunction

Maria J. Gutierrez, MD, MHS[a], Sivia K. Lapidus, MD[b,*]

KEYWORDS

- Autoinflammatory disease • Systemic autoinflammatory disease
- Immune dysfunction • Periodic fevers • Immune dysregulation
- Inborn errors of immunity

KEY POINTS

- Systemic autoinflammatory diseases (SAIDs) are conditions that, with autoinflammation as their mainstay, overlap with other types of immune dysfunction.
- A thorough clinical evaluation remains the cornerstone in the initial assessment of a patient with suspected immune dysfunction and provides the framework for subsequent studies and management.
- Genetically defined SAIDs are the minority of SAIDs, but genetic testing increasingly is used in diagnosis.
- Phenotypic-molecular characterization of SAIDs guides targeted therapeutics.
- Emerging targeted treatments can be curative, control flares, and minimize sequelae.

INTRODUCTION

The first known systemic autoinflammatory disease (SAID), familial Mediterranean fever (FMF), was described in 1945,[1] and the term, *autoinflammatory*, was coined in 1999 to distinguish a family of inflammatory disorders characterized by dysregulation of the innate immune response independent from the adaptive immune system.[2] Since

Funding: M.J. Gutierrez receives support from the American Academy of Allergy, Asthma, and Immunology (AAAAI) Foundation Faculty Development Award and the National Institutes of Health (NIH) (grant 1K23HD104933). The funding agencies had no involvement in the writing of this review or in the decision to submit the article for publication.
[a] Division of Pediatric Allergy, Immunology and Rheumatology, Johns Hopkins University School of Medicine, 600 North Wolfe Street CMSC 1102, Baltimore, MD 21287, USA; [b] Division of Pediatric Rheumatology, Joseph M. Sanzari Children's Hospital, Hackensack University Medical Center and Hackensack Meridian School of Medicine, 3WFAN 30 Prospect Avenue, Hackensack, NJ 07601, USA
* Corresponding author.
E-mail address: sivia.lapidus@hmhn.org

Rheum Dis Clin N Am 48 (2021) 371–395
https://doi.org/10.1016/j.rdc.2021.07.011
rheumatic.theclinics.com

then, more than 40 disorders have been discovered,[2,3] unraveling essential mechanisms in human immunity. Nowadays, SAIDs are a group of conditions that, with autoinflammation as their central mechanism, also may overlap with autoimmunity, immunodeficiency, and allergy.[4] Accordingly, in light of the SAID family's complexity, this article aims to provide a framework for the clinical approach to patients with these disorders. Major categories and clinical features of SAIDs are summarized, practical molecular-clinical-therapeutic correlations reviewed, and an overview of overlapping features of immune dysfunction and key aspects of SAID's diagnosis and treatment presented.

AGE AND INHERITANCE OF SYSTEMIC AUTOINFLAMMATORY DISEASES

A large number of SAIDs are inborn errors of immunity (IEIs),[3] with varying prevalence by disease.[5] The SAID family also includes polygenic disorders, such as periodic fever, aphthous stomatitis, pharyngitis, and adenitis (PFAPA) syndrome; systemic juvenile idiopathic arthritis (sJIA); adult-onset Still disease (AOSD), ; and Behçet disease. Remarkably, some adult-onset SAIDs, such as Schnitzler syndrome[6] and the recently described vacuoles, E1 enzyme, X-linked, autoinflammatory, and somatic (VEXAS) syndrome,[7] may arise from somatic mutations, underscoring that age-related genetic abnormalities may underlie nonmalignant adult-onset autoinflammatory disorders.

An intriguing diagnostic feature of SAIDs is the presence of age-associated patterns of disease (**Fig. 1**). For instance, PFAPA, the most common SAID in North America, is a predominantly pediatric disease that ultimately is outgrown, with rare reports in adults.[8] Age-related improvement also is seen in monogenic SAIDs, such as mevalonate kinase deficiency (MKD) and sideroblastic anemia, B-cell deficiency, and developmental delay (SIFD).[9,10] Furthermore, the age of onset is characteristic in several SAIDs. For instance, severe inflammasomopathies and disorders of interleukin (IL)-1 overactivation, type I interferon (IFN), and nuclear factor (NF)-κB signaling defects present in early infancy or even in utero,[9–12] whereas others (e.g., milder inflammasomopathies or polygenic disorders, such as sJIA and PFAPA) present later in childhood.[8,13,14] A spectrum of age of onset is reported in TNF receptor–associated periodic syndrome (TRAPS)[15] and some diseases (e.g., VEXAS syndrome and Schnitzler syndrome) occur only in adulthood. Whether genetic modifiers, environment-gene interactions, and aging of the immune system drive age-related differences in SAIDs remains poorly understood.[16]

MECHANISMS OF DISEASE AND MOLECULAR CLINICAL CORRELATIONS IN SYSTEMIC AUTOINFLAMMATORY DISEASES

The description of periodic fever syndromes stemming from overactivation of the NLRP3 inflammasome and IL-1 activity prompted treatment with IL-1 blockade. Subsequently, IL1 inhibition expanded to treat additional inflammasomopathies (NLRC4, NLRP1, and NLRP12 defects) and dysregulation of IL-1 family cytokines (IL-18 and IL-36).[17–19] More recently, mutations in transcription factors (e.g., *CEBPE*) have been shown to cause autoinflammation with immunodeficiency from overactivation of the noncanonical caspase 4/5 inflammasome and IFN pathways.

Abnormalities in tumor necrosis factor (TNF) signaling represent a distinct category of SAIDs characterized by defects in the TNF receptor 1 (TNFR1),[15] its associated cleaving enzyme (ADAM17),[20] the receptor-interacting serine/threonine protein kinase 1 (RIPK1),[21] and downstream mediators and regulatory proteins in NF-κB pathways.[12,17,22,23] Together, this SAID group presents with fever, systemic inflammation, and frequent mucosal, gastrointestinal, and articular involvement. In this group, TRAPS,

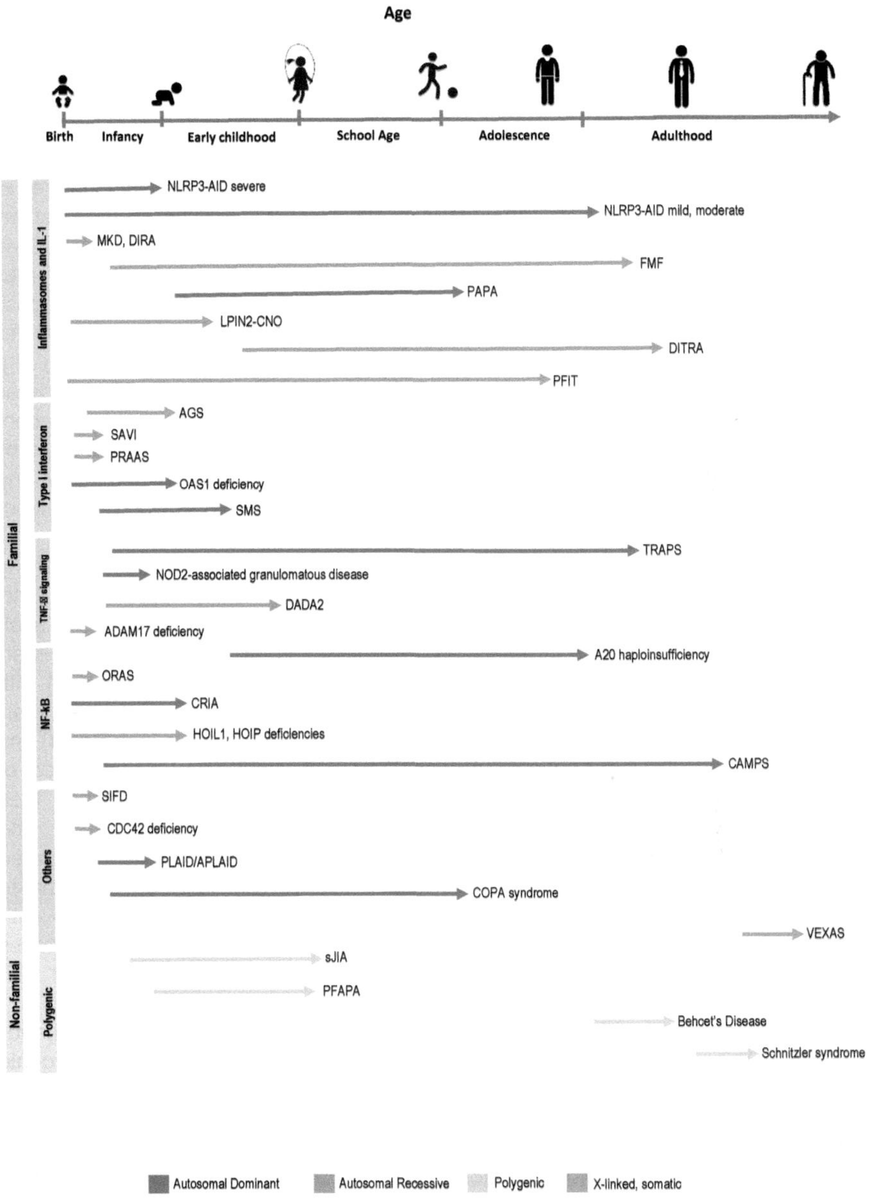

Fig. 1. Age of onset and inheritance of SAIDs. The age of disease onset is characteristic of several SAIDs. *Abbreviations:* NLRP3-AID, NLRP3-associated autoinflammatory disease; MKD, Mevalonate Kinase Deficiency; FMF, Familial Mediterranean Fever; PAPA, Pyogenic arthritis, pyoderma gangrenosum and acne; LPIN2-CNO, LPIN2-chronic non-bacterial osteomyelitis; DITRA, Deficiency of the IL36 receptor antagonist; PFIT, Periodic fever, immunodeficiency and thrombocytopenia; AGS, Aicardi-Goutieres syndrome; SAVI, STING-associated vasculopathy with onset in infancy; PRAAS; Proteosome-associated autoinflammatory syndromes; OAS1 Oligoadenylate Synthetase 1; SMS Singleton-Merten syndrome; TRAPS, Tumor Necrosis Factor Receptor-associated periodic syndrome; DADA2, Deficiency of Adenosine Deaminase 2; HA20, A20 haploinsufficiency; ORAS, OTULIN-related

caused by mutations in the TNFR1 gene (*TNFRSF1A*), is characterized by sustained NF-κB and mitogen-activated protein kinase activation.[15] A related disorder, ADAM17 deficiency, impairs TNF cleavage from cells[20] and RIPK1 deficiency features increased cell death.[21] Downstream, A20 haploinsufficiency (HA20) and OTULIN-related autoinflammatory syndrome (ORAS) cause increased activation of NF-κB and activator protein 1 (AP-1) via defective cleavage of ubiquitination proteins from RIPK1, an NF-κB negative regulatory mechanism.[12,17] Clinically, HA20 resembles Behçet disease, featuring recurrent fever, arthritis, oral, genital, and gastrointestinal ulcers,[17] and ORAS is characterized by neonatal onset systemic inflammation, arthritis, diarrhea, neutrophilia, and lipodystrophy.[12] Conversely, defects in linear ubiquitin chain assembly complex (LUBAC) proteins (HOIL1 and HOIP) result in decreased NF-κB activation in response to IL-1β and cytokines of the TNF superfamily (e.g., TNF-α and CD40), with critical roles in immune cell development and function.[22,23] Mutations in the nucleotide-binding oligomerization domain-containing protein 2 (NOD2), a LUBAC target, underlie a disease characterized by arthritis, uveitis, and skin granulomas,[18] and biallelic defects of adenosine deaminase 2 *(ADA2)* (**Box 1**) causes a heterogeneous syndrome characterized by autoinflammation, cytopenias, PAN-like vasculitis, strokes with partial deficiency, and severe immunodeficiency with a profound hematologic compromise when ADA2 function is abrogated.[19,46]

Additional autoinflammatory mechanisms were discovered through identifying SAIDs refractory to IL-1 inhibition. For example, the dysregulation of type I IFN activity from defects in nucleic acid RNA sensing and processing, IFN signaling, or intracellular protein accumulation (disorders of proteasome function) characterize type I interferonopathies.[34,35,57] Type I interferonopathies present early in life (see **Fig. 1**) with clinical heterogeneity, including cerebral calcifications, myositis, lipodystrophy, interstitial lung disease, skin vasculitis, and production of autoantibodies (see **Box 1**) and may be treated with Janus kinase (JAK) inhibitors that block type I IFN signaling, or agents that limit the production of endogenous nucleic acids or enhance their removal.[35] Defects in actin assembly and polymerization (ARPC1B, CDC42, and NCKAP1L deficiencies),[48–50] endoplasmic reticulum (ER) stress (cotamer associated protein-alpha (COPA) syndrome),[53] intracellular calcium signaling (*PLCγ2*-associated antibody deficiency and immune dysregulation [PLAID] and autoinflammation antibody deficiency and immune dysregulation syndrome [APLAID])[51,52] are diseases resulting in autoinflammation frequently overlapping with immunodeficiency with poor responses to IL-1 blockade (see **Box 1**).

Importantly, the elucidation of innate immune pathways associated with monogenic SAIDs has informed the classification, diagnosis, and treatment of polygenic disorders involving similar immunologic mechanisms. IL-1 inhibition in more complex disorders exemplifies this concept with the recognition of the central role of inflammasomes and the IL-1 family of cytokines in disorders, such as sJIA, gout, Behçet disease, macrophage activation syndrome, and cytokine storm

autoinflammatory syndrome; CRIA Cleavage-resistant RIPK1-induced autoinflammatory syndrome; CAMPS CARD14-mediated psoriasis; SFID, Sideroblastic anemia with B-cell immunodeficiency; PLAID, PLCG2-associated antibody deficiency and immune dysregulation; APLAID, Autoinflammation and PLCG2-associated antibody deficiency and immune dysregulation; VEXAS Vacuoles, E1 enzyme, X-linked, autoinflammatory, somatic syndrome; sJIA, Systemic Juvenile Idiopathic Arthritis; PFAPA, Periodic Fever, Aphthous Stomatitis, Pharyngitis, Adenitis.

Box 1
Disease mechanism, causative genes, heritability, and main clinical characteristics of systemic autoinflammatory diseases

IL-1 and inflammasome disorders
- Pyrin activation
  - Familial Mediterranean Fever (FMF). AR with one-third AD (*MEFV*)
    - Short (<72 h), irregular fevers, polyserositis, abdominal pain, arthritis, erysipelas-like rash, amyloidosis. More prevalent among individuals from Middle Eastern or Mediterranean ancestry[13]
  - Pyrin-associated autoinflammation with neutrophilic dermatosis. AD (*MEFV*)
    - Recurrent long-lasting fevers, sterile skin abscesses, maculopapular rashes, abdominal pain, myalgia, myositis, anemia, failure to thrive[13]
  - Mevalonate Kinase Deficiency (MKD). AR (*MVK*)
    - MKD mild: regularly recurrent fevers, cervical adenopathy, oral ulcers, diarrhea, rash, arthralgias/arthritis, triggered by immunizations or stress[26]
    - MKD severe: neonatal fevers, hypertelorism, frontal bossing, triangularly shaped face, developmental delay, seizures. Also known as mevalonate aciduria[2]
  - PSTPIP1-associated arthritis, pyoderma gangrenosum, acne (PAPA) syndrome. AD (*PSTPIP1*)
    - Early-onset, painful, deforming arthritis, severe cystic acne, pyoderma gangrenosum[27]
  - Hyperzincemia and hypercalprotectinemia. AD (*PSTPIP1*)
    - Early-onset cutaneous inflammation, arthritis, hepatosplenomegaly, lymphadenopathies, cytopenia (anemia, neutropenia, and thrombocytopenia), failure to thrive[2]
  - Periodic fevers with immunodeficiency and thrombocytopenia (PFIT). AR (*WDR1*)
    - Oral and perianal ulcerations, frequent infections, moderate thrombocytopenia, IL-18–driven inflammation, independent of IL-1[28]
- Cryopyrin activation
  - NLRP3-associated autoinflammatory disease. AD (*NLRP3*)[2,4,24]
    - Encompasses 3 clinical entities:
      - NLRP3 mild/familial cold autoinflammatory syndrome (FCAS): infantile-onset cold urticaria (ice cube test negative), chills, fever (may be low grade or absent), arthritis, conjunctivitis
      - NLRP3 moderate/Muckle-Wells syndrome: infantile-onset low-grade fevers, urticaria, conjunctivitis, oral ulcers, abdominal pain with deafness in adolescence, and potential amyloidosis
      - Neonatal Onset Multisystem Inflammatory Disease/chronic infantile neurologic cutaneous and articular syndrome (NOMID/CINCA): neonatal-onset urticaria, continuous fever, seizures, spasticity, developmental delay. Frontal bossing, saddle nose, shortened digits, optic nerve atrophy/uveitis, deforming arthropathy, anemia, neutrophilia, leukocytosis, thrombocytosis, eosinophilia
  - LPIN2-chronic nonbacterial osteomyelitis (LPIN2-CNO)/Majeed syndrome. AR (*LPIN2*)[2]
    - Congenital dyserythropoietic anemia with neonatal or early childhood onset of chronic multifocal osteomyelitis, soft tissue swelling, anemia, neutrophilic dermatosis in flares occurring every 2 weeks to 4 weeks.
- Receptor antagonist deficiency
  - Deficiency of the interleukin 1 receptor antagonist (DIRA). AR (*IL1RN*)
    - Neonatal-onset pustular dermatitis, multifocal osteomyelitis, CNS vasculitis, severe systemic inflammation[11]
  - Deficiency of the interleukin-36 receptor antagonist (DITRA). AR (*IL36RN*)
    - Episodes of childhood-onset, life-threatening, multisystem inflammatory disease with pustular psoriasis. Infections may trigger symptoms.[25]
- Other inflammasomes activation
  - NLRC4-associated autoinflammatory disease. AD (*NLRC4*)
    - Heterogeneous clinical spectrum, including cold urticaria (mild disease), very-early-onset inflammatory bowel disease (IBD), NOMID-like (CNS inflammation), severe HLH/MAS. Severe disease may start in utero (systemic inflammation and coagulopathy)[30]
  - NLRP1-associated autoinflammatory disease. AD (*NLRP1*)

Dyskeratosis, fever, arthritis, urticaria[31]
NLRP12-associated autoinflammatory disease/FCAS2. AD (*NLRP12*)
Episodic urticaria (may be cold-induced), arthralgia, myalgia, fever, elevated markers of inflammation[4]
Polygenic disorders
Periodic fever, aphthous stomatitis, pharyngitis and adenitis (PFAPA)
Regular, periodic fevers lasting 3 days to 5 days and at least 1 of the following: aphthous stomatitis, cervical lymphadenitis, and pharyngitis.[8]
Systemic juvenile idiopathic arthritis (sJIA)
Fevers, salmon-colored rash, serositis, lymphadenopathy, arthritis, anemia[14]
Behçet disease
Oral and genital ulcers, uveitis, skin lesions, pathergy, arthritis[29]
Schnitzler syndrome
Adult-onset, chronic, recurrent irregular urticarial rash with fevers, joint and bone pain, hepatosplenomegaly, adenopathy, leukocytosis, elevated inflammatory markers, monoclonal gammopathy. It may progress to Waldenström macroglobulinemia.[6]

Type I interferonopathies
Nucleic acid processing
Aicardi-Goutieres syndromes (AGS). AR (*TREX1*, *ADAR1*, *RNASEH2A/B/C*, *SAMHD1*) or AD (*IFIH1*)
Leukoencephalopathy with basal ganglia calcifications, cerebral atrophy, leukocytosis, and elevated IFN-α in CSF. Hepatitis, arthritis, chilblains, cytopenia, autoantibodies[32,33]
Monogenic SLE. AR (*DNASE2, DNA1L3, C1Q, C1S*) or AD (*DNASE1*)
Very-early-onset SLE, hypocomplementemia[32,34]
Nucleic acid sensing
STING-associated vasculopathy, infantile-onset. AD (*TMEM173*)
Systemic autoinflammation, skin vasculitis, chilblains, hepatosplenomegaly, cytopenia, inflammatory lung disease, autoantibodies[35]
Singleton-Merten syndrome. AD (*IFIH1*, *DDX58C*)
Calcification of the aorta, muscle weakness/atrophy, glaucoma, osteoporosis, skeletal changes, dental abnormalities[33]
Type I IFN signaling
Aicardi-Goutières syndrome–like AD (*USP18, STAT2, ISG15*)
TORCH-like (CNS calcifications and microcephaly), respiratory insufficiency in infancy. Mycobacterial disease (*ISG15*)[36–38]
X-linked reticulate pigmentary disorder (XLPDR). XL (*POLA1*)
Skin hyperpigmentation with amyloid-like material, characteristic facies, recurrent infections, severe colitis, corneal inflammation/scarring, hypohidrosis[39]
SOCS1 haploinsufficiency. AD (*SOCS1*)
Recurrent bacterial infections and severe, early-onset multisystem autoimmunity (hepatosplenomegaly, cytopenia, glomerulonephritis, arthritis, thyroiditis, hepatitis), autoantibody production[40]
Proteosome disorders
Proteosome-associated autoinflammatory syndromes (PRAAS). AR (*PSMB8*), digenic (*PSMA4/PSMB9, PSMB4/PSMB9, PSMA3/PSMG8*), AD (*POMP*)[2,41,42]
Recurrent fevers, arthritis, lipodystrophy,[41] hepatosplenomegaly, lymphadenopathy, annular plaques, eyelid swelling, anemia. Also known as chronic atypical neutrophilic dermatosis with lipodystrophy and elevated temperature (CANDLE); Nakajo-Nishimura syndrome; and joint contractures, muscle atrophy, microcytic anemia, and panniculitis-induced lipodystrophy.
Other
Oligoadenylate Synthetase 1 (OAS1) deficiency. AD (*OAS1*)
Pulmonary alveolar proteinosis, hypogammaglobulinemia[43]
Spondyloenchondrodysplasia with immune dysregulation (SPENCDI). AR (*ACP5*)
Short stature, skeletal dysplasia, cerebral calcifications, cytopenia, autoimmunity (Sjögren syndrome, hypothyroidism, myositis, vitiligo), recurrent viral and bacterial infections[44]
C/EBPε-associated autoinflammation and immune impairment of neutrophils. AR (*CEBPE*)

Periodic fevers, abdominal pain, ileitis, oral ulcers, lymphangitis, myalgia, granulomas, bleeding diathesis, immunodeficiency[45]

Dysregulation of TNF and NF-κB signaling

TNF signaling

Tumor Necrosis Factor Receptor-associated Periodic Syndrome (TRAPS). AD (*TNFRSF1A*)

Irregular, prolonged fevers (>7 days), serositis (abdominal pain, pleuritic chest pain), periorbital edema, conjunctivitis, migratory myalgias with overlying painful erythematous rash, arthritis. Amyloidosis[15]

ADAM17 deficiency. AR (*ADAM17*)

Neonatal-onset inflammatory and bowel disease, bacteremia, defective TNF-α production[20]

NOD2-associated granulomatous disease

Minimal fever, uveitis, granulomatous inflammation of the skin, joints, and internal organs (noncaseating), arthritis, cranial neuropathies, ichthyosis-like rash, Crohn's Disease. Also known as Blau syndrome or early-onset sarcoidosis.[18]

Deficiency of Adenosine Deaminase 2 (DADA2). AR (*ADA2*)

Recurrent fevers, hepatosplenomegaly, vasculitis (PAN-like), early-onset strokes, cytopenia, and hypogammaglobulinemia[46]

NF-κB signaling

RelA haploinsufficiency. AD (*RELA)*

Chronic mucocutaneous ulcerations, cytopenia, colitis, lymphoproliferation[47]

Cleavage-resistant *RIPK1*-induced autoinflammatory syndrome (CRIA). AD (*RIPK1*)

Fever, early-onset IBD, lymphoproliferation, progressive polyarthritis, and severe immunodeficiency[21]

CARD14-associated disease. AD *(PSORS2)*

Includes 2 syndromes: CARD14-mediated psoriasis (CAMPS), characterized by childhood-onset fevers with generalized pustular psoriasis, palmoplantar pustulosis, or hyperkeratosis[3]; and familial pityriasis rubra pilaris, characterized by reddish, scaly patches of the skin and palmoplantar keratoderma[2]

NF-κB ubiquitination/deubiquitination system

A20 haploinsufficiency (HA20). AD(*TNFAIP3*)

Autoinflammatory, Behçet-like disease with recurrent oral/genital ulcers, polyarthritis, cutaneous lesions, ocular inflammation, autoantibodies, combined immunodeficiency[17]

LUBAC deficiency. AR (*HOIL1* and *HOIP*)

Fever, recurrent infections, combined immunodeficiency, amylopectinosis, lymphangiectasia[22,23]

OTULIN-related autoinflammatory syndrome (ORAS). AR (*OTULIN*)

Neonatal-onset fever, diarrhea, elevated inflammatory markers, panniculitis, neutrophilic dermatitis, vasculitis, gastrointestinal inflammation, and arthritis[12]

Other mechanisms

Actin polymerization/assembly

CDC42 deficiency. AR (*CDC42*)

Macrothrombocytopenia, facial dysmorphism, developmental delay, lymphedema, and camptodactyly (Takenouchi-Kosaki syndrome). Also, neonatal-onset recurrent fevers, transaminitis, lymphoproliferation, cytopenias, urticaria-like rashes, increased inflammatory markers, immunodeficiency. May develop HLH and malignancy (non-Hodgkin lymphoma)[48]

ARPC1B deficiency. AR (*ARPC1B*)

Platelet abnormalities, small vessel vasculitis, arthritis, recurrent infections, moderate to severe eczema, allergy (food allergy and asthma)[49]

Nck-associated protein 1-like (NCKAP1L) deficiency. AR (*NCKAP1L*)

Immunodeficiency, lymphoproliferation, and hyperinflammation with features of hemophagocytic lymphohistiocytosis[50]

Intracellular calcium signaling

PLCg2-associated antibody deficiency and immune dysregulation (PLAID). AD (*PLCG2*)

Neonatal or infantile-onset cold urticaria (ice cube test negative), atopy, skin granulomas, immunodeficiency (infections, hypogammaglobulinemia), autoimmunity (thyroiditis and vitiligo), autoantibodies[51]

Autoinflammation and PLCg2-associated antibody deficiency and immune dysregulation (APLAID). AD (*PLCG2*)
Recurrent skin blisters, interstitial lung disease, bronchiolitis, eye inflammation, colitis, humoral immunodeficiency[52]
ER stress
Cotamer associated protein-alpha (COPA) syndrome. AD (*COPA*)
Arthritis, interstitial lung disease, and lung hemorrhage in early childhood, renal disease, autoantibody production[53]
Other
Vacuoles, E1 enzyme, X-linked, autoinflammatory, somatic (VEXAS) syndrome. X-linked (*UBA1*) somatic mutations.
Fever, skin rash, pulmonary infiltrates, ear and nose chondritis, venous thromboembolism, macrocytic anemia, and bone marrow vacuoles[7]
SH3BP2 deficiency with multilocular cystic disease of the mandibles (SDCM). AD (*SH3BP2*)
Bone degeneration of the jaw. It begins to regress in puberty. Also known as cherubism[54]
Adaptor Related Protein Complex 1 Subunit Sigma 3 (APS1S3) deficiency. AR (*AP1S3*)
Recurrent pustular psoriasis (painful, skin pustules), sometimes with arthritis[55]
Laccase Domain Containing 1 (LACC) deficiency. AR (*LACC/FAMIN*)
Fever and features of systemic, oligoarticular, or polyarticular juvenile idiopathic arthritis[56]
Sideroblastic anemia with B-cell immunodeficiency, periodic fevers and developmental delay (SIFD). AR (*TRNT1*)
Congenital sideroblastic anemia, and the early-life onset of antibody immunodeficiency, periodic fevers, seizures, sensorineural deafness, and developmental delay.[10]

Abbreviations: AD, autosomal dominant; AR, autosomal recessive; CNS, central nervous system; CSF, cerebral spinal fluid; ER, endoplasmic reticulum; HLH, hemophagocytic lymphohistiocytosis; MAS, macrophage activation syndrome; NOMID, NLRP3 severe/neonatal-onset multisystem inflammatory disease.

syndromes.[4,58] The discovery that polygenic autoimmune disorders (e.g., systemic lupus erythematosus [SLE]) feature type I IFN overactivation has triggered the investigation of IFN inhibition in their treatment.[59] In addition, the localized manifestations of SAIDs involving dysregulation of the IL-1 family in diseases, such as deficiency of IL-1 receptor antagonist (DIRA), deficiency of IL-36 receptor antagonist (DITRA), Majeed syndrome, and CARD 14–mediated pustular psoriasis (CAMPS), also have provided important insights into the role of those mediators in the homeostasis of local tissues (e.g., keratinocytes and epithelia),[25] and, remarkably, the discovery of IL-1 dysregulation in atherosclerosis has triggered investigations of the role of IL-1 in cardiovascular diseases.[42]

AUTOINFLAMMATORY DISEASES IN THE LARGER SPECTRUM OF HUMAN IMMUNOLOGIC DISORDERS

The first SAIDs initially were termed, *periodic fever syndromes*.[4] With emerging phenotypes and molecular defects, however, the clinical spectrum of SAIDs has evolved to encompass a diverse group of disorders with overlapping types of immune dysfunction (**Fig. 2**).

Interferonopathies and disorders, such as COPA syndrome, DADA2 (see **Fig 2**), and other SAIDs, feature autoantibodies as well as clinical manifestations of autoimmune diseases (cytopenia, myositis, nephritis, arthritis, vasculitis, and interstitial lung disease)[4,60,61] and variable degrees of immunodeficiency present in several SAIDs (see **Fig. 2**; **Table 1**).

Conversely, autoinflammatory symptoms may mimic those of autoimmune, immunodeficiency, and allergic diseases. For example, recurrent oral ulcers and

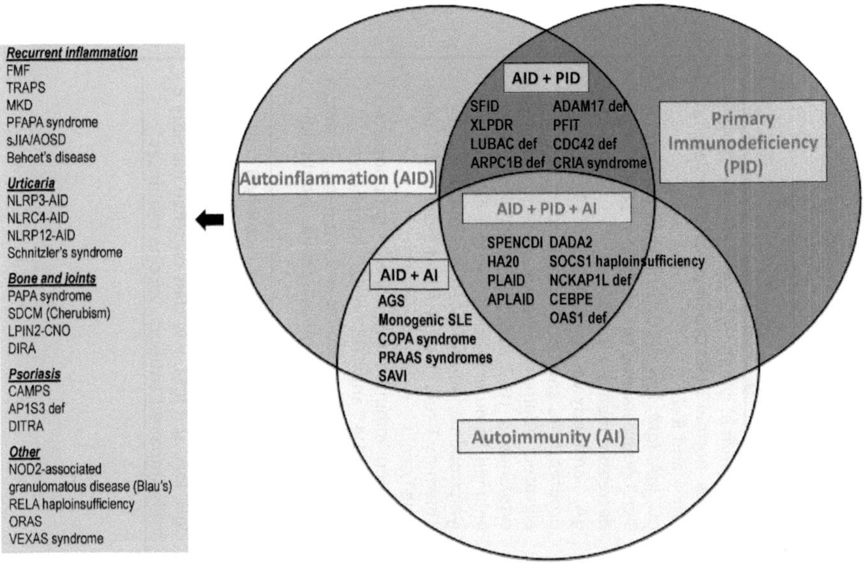

Fig. 2. Autoinflammation in the spectrum of immunologic diseases. A growing number of autoinflammatory disorders present with overlapping types of immune dysfunction. *Abbreviations*: FMF, Familial Mediterranean Fever; TRAPS, Tumor Necrosis Factor Receptor-associated periodic syndrome; PFAPA, Periodic Fever, Aphthous Stomatitis, Pharyngitis, Adenitis; sJIA, Systemic Juvenile Idiopathic Arthritis; AOSD, Adult-onset Still's Disease; NLRP3-AID, NLRP3-associated autoinflammatory disease; NLRC4-AID, NLRC4-associated autoinflammatory disease; NLRP12-AID, NLRP12-associated autoinflammatory disease, PAPA, Pyogenic arthritis, pyoderma gangrenosum and acne; SDCM, SH3BP2 deficiency with multilocular cystic disease of the mandibles; LPIN2-CNO, LPIN2-chronic non-bacterial osteomyelitis; DIRA, Deficiency of the Interleukin-1 receptor antagonist; CAMPS, CARD14-mediated psoriasis syndrome; DITRA, Deficiency of the IL36 receptor antagonist; ORAS, OTULIN-related autoinflammatory syndrome; SIFD, Sideroblastic anemia with B-cell immunodeficiency, periodic fevers, and developmental delay; XLPDR, X-linked reticulate pigmentary disorder; PFIT, Periodic fever, immunodeficiency and thrombocytopenia; SPENCDI, Spondyloenchondroplasia with immune dysregulation syndrome; HA20, A20 haploinsufficiency; PLAID, PLCG2-associated antibody deficiency and immune dysregulation; APLAID, Autoinflammation and PLCG2-associated antibody deficiency and immune dysregulation; DADA2, Deficiency of Adenosine Deaminase 2; CEBPE, C/EBPε-associated autoinflammation and immune impairment of neutrophils; AGS, Aicardi-Goutieres syndrome; SLE, Systemic Lupus Erythematosus; SAVI, STING-associated vasculopathy with onset in infancy; def, deficiency.

adenopathy, typical in many SAIDs, may accompany disorders as diverse as SLE (autoimmune disorder) or chronic granulomatous disease (primary immunodeficiency disorder).[60] Urticaria in SAIDs resembles allergic (e.g., cold urticaria and mast cell disorders) or autoimmune diseases (e.g., urticarial vasculitis).[61] Inflammasomopathies, immunodeficiencies (Omenn syndrome), and immune dysregulation (immune dysregulation, polyendocrinopathy, enteropathy, X-linked, or familial hemophagocytic lymphohistiocytosis) may present in infancy with systemic inflammation and severe skin rashes. Likewise, SAIDs presenting with hypogammaglobulinemia or combined immunodeficiency (see **Table 1**) are distinct from other IEIs.[3]

DIAGNOSTIC APPROACH TO SYSTEMIC AUTOINFLAMMATORY DISORDERS

In the evaluation of patients with suspected SAIDs, initially excluding malignancies, infections, autoimmunity, immunodeficiency and immune dysregulation,

Table 1
Summary of immunodeficiency manifestations in systemic autoinflammatory diseases

Pathway affected	Autoinflammatory Disorder	Infectious Manifestations	Immunodeficiency Features
TNF and NF-κB	ADAM17 deficiency[20]	Neonatal or early infancy onset, sepsis, severe RSV, skin rash, diarrhea, weight loss	↑ WBC, normal lymphocyte phenotype including Tregs, normal T-cell proliferation, ↓ intracellular TNF-α and IL-2
	DADA2[19,46]	Upper and lower respiratory infections, herpes, intestinal, urinary, and CNS infections	↓IgG, IgA, IgM, low WBC, lymphopenia, normal T-cell numbers, and proliferation, ↓B cells with decreased memory B cells
	HA20[17]	Sinopulmonary and skin infections, oral thrush, chronic EBV	↓IgA, ↓antibody vaccine responses, ↓T-cell proliferation, and NK function, minimally elevated inflammatory markers, ↑ inflammatory cytokines (IL-1β, 2, 4, 6,12,13,17, TNF-α, IFN-γ)
	CRIA[62]	Diarrhea, perianal disease, and VEO-IBD may present before infections (neonatal or early infancy). Recurrent bacterial and/or viral infections	Combined immunodeficiency with T-cell and B-cell lymphopenia, normal T-cell proliferation, ↓memory T-cell, class-switched B-cell and T-helper type17 cells
	LUBAC deficiency (HOIL1 and HOIP deficiencies)[63]	Recurrent viral and bacterial infections	Combined immunodeficiency with lymphopenia, ↓naïve $CD4^+$ and $CD8^+$ cells, ↓lymphocyte proliferation to mitogens and antigens, ↓memory B cells, hypogammaglobulinemia, ↓ antibody vaccine responses
IC calcium	PLAID[51]	Recurrent sinopulmonary infections, early-onset shingles, onychomycosis	↓IgG, IgA, and IgM, ↓switched memory B cells (IgM^-, IgD^-, $CD27^+$) and NK cells, ↓antibody responses to pneumococcal vaccines, ↑ ESR and CRP, ANA^+
	APLAID[52]	Recurrent sinopulmonary infections	↓ IgG, IgA, and IgM, low class-switched memory B cells, impaired antibody vaccine responses

Type I IFN	SPENCDI[44]	Recurrent respiratory tract infections, severe varicella infections,	↓ $CD4^+$ and $CD8^+$ T cells, ↓ T-cell proliferation to mitogens, normal or ↓ immunoglobulins, ↓ antibody vaccine responses, ANA + frequent
	XLPDR[39]	Recurrent upper and lower respiratory tract infections, some have mycobacterial and staphylococcal infections	Variable lymphopenia and neutrophilia, IgE elevation, defective NK function
	OAS1 deficiency[43]	Early-life viral lower respiratory tract infections, lung CMV	↓ IgG, IgA, IgM
	SOCS1 haploinsufficiency[40]	Recurrent bacterial infections	↓ IgG, IgM, and IgA with normal specific antibody responses, ↓ CD4, CD8, and switched memory B cells, ↑ serum BAFF, autoantibody production
	C/EBPε-associated autoinflammation and immune impairment of neutrophils[45]	Paronychia, skin and mucosal abscesses, respiratory tract infections	Mild lymphopenia, ↓ naïve T cells and increased T_{EMRA} cells, neutrophil dysfunction
Others	SIFD[10]	Anemia may be present before infections (neonatal or early infancy), respiratory tract infections	B-cell lymphopenia, panhypogammaglobulinemia (may not be detected in young infants due to maternally transferred IgG and age-related IgA decreases), ↓ antibody vaccine responses. T-cell and NK-cell numbers may be normal at onset and decline later in the disease course.
	PFIT[28]	Recurrent fevers, recurrent respiratory infections, skin and other bacterial infections, PJP pneumonia	Thrombocytopenia, B-cell lymphopenia with low memory B cells (switched and nonswitched), hypogammaglobulinemia, ↓ antibody vaccine responses, ↓ neutrophil migration
	CDC42 deficiency[48]	Early-onset recurrent sinopulmonary infections, skin infections, severe varicella, chronic EBV	↓ IgG and IgM, decreased memory B cells, ↓ NK function, elevated soluble CD25 levels

(continued on next page)

Table 1
(*continued*)

Pathway affected	Autoinflammatory Disorder	Infectious Manifestations	Immunodeficiency Features
	ARPC1B deficiency[49]	Very-early-onset gastrointestinal bleeding, severe eczema, viral and bacterial infections, allergies (food allergy and asthma), thrombocytopenia, skin vasculitis, arthritis	↓ $CD19^+$ B cells, ↓ $CD4^+$ and $CD8^+$ T cells, ↑ IgA and IgE levels. Normal T-cell proliferation to mitogens but defective Treg function. Normal humoral response to polysaccharide vaccines, NK-cell degranulation, and migration impaired
	NCKAP1L deficiency[50]	Recurrent respiratory infections, skin rashes/ abscesses, BCG lymphadenitis, HLH	Normal $CD4^+$ T-cell and B-cell numbers, ↑ $CD8^+$, central and effector memory T cells, ↑ expression of T-cell senescence markers, ↑ NK cells. ↑ Ig levels and autoantibody production (high-titer ANA)

Abbreviations: DADA2, Deficiency of Adenosine Deaminase 2; HA20, A20 haploinsufficiency; CRIA, Cleavage-resistant RIPK1-induced autoinflammatory syndrome; PLAID, PLCG2-associated antibody deficiency and immune dysregulation; APLAID, Autoinflammation and PLCG2-associated antibody deficiency and immune dysregulation; SPENCDI, Spondyloenchondroplasia with immune disregulation; XLPDR, X-linked reticulate pigmentary disorder; SIFD, Sideroblastic anemia with B-cell immunodeficiency, periodic fevers and developmental delay; PFIT, Periodic fever immunodeficiency and thrombocytopenia; ANA, Antinuclear antibodies; BAFF, B-cell activating factor; BCG, Bacillus Calmette-Guerin,;NK, Natural Killer; C/EBPe, CCAAT/enhancer binding protein epsilon; CNS, Central Nervous System; EBV, Epstein-Barr virus; ESR, Erythrocyte Sedimentation Rate; HLH, Hemophagocytic Lymphohistiocytosis IBD, Inflammatory Bowel Disease; PJP, Pneumocystis jirovecii; RSV, Respiratory Sincitial Virus; TEMRA cells, T effector memory re-expressing CD45RA cells; Treg, Regulatory T-cells; VEO-IBD, Very early onset inflammatory Bowel Disease; WBC, White blood cells.

and drug hypersensitivity as etiologies for fever is key (**Fig. 3**). Pertinent family history includes information about ancestry, consanguinity, family deaths, immunologic diseases (other IEIs, malignancy, and autoimmunity), and specific stigmata of SAIDs (arthritis, urticaria, hearing loss, renal disease, and recurrent tonsillitis). Important fever details involve onset, frequency, regularity, triggers (vaccines, stress, and cold), duration, and severity.[63,64] Accompanying symptoms' characteristics and timing (intermittent vs persistent, regular vs irregular, and frequency) offer critical clues to the differential diagnosis. Pediatric growth and development impairment is an indicator of disease severity. Characterization of mouth lesions, rashes, lymphadenopathy, organomegaly, joint abnormalities, and other organ involvement facilitates diagnosis. Medication response to corticosteroids, cimetidine, colchicine, IL-1, or TNF inhibitors also may be informative regarding the underlying disorder.

Laboratory investigations for inflammation (blood cell counts and acute-phase reactants) should be clinically correlated closely with flares and nonflares. Alternative causes of prolonged and recurrent fever (infections and malignancy) should be evaluated (cultures, serologies, and imaging studies) as necessary, especially if inflammatory markers do not correlate with flares. Evaluation of autoantibodies if autoimmunity is suspected, narrows the differential. An ice cube challenge differentiates SAIDs with urticaria (NLRP3-associated autoinflammatory disease NLRP3-AID]) from cold urticaria.[61] An initial immunologic evaluation comprising blood cell counts, quantitative immunoglobulins, antibody levels to prior vaccines, and lymphocyte phenotyping/function is indicated if other types of IEI (e.g., predominantly antibody immunodeficiencies, combined immunodeficiency or immunedysregulation disorders) are suspected. Importantly, in newborns and young children with primary immunodeficiency and immune dysregulation disorders, unusual patterns of infections may not be evident until later in life. Hence, in this population, inflammatory manifestations, such as erythroderma, severe eczema, lymphoproliferation, granulomatous disorders, chronic diarrhea and colitis, cytopenias, TORCH-like symptoms, early-onset autoimmunity, failure to thrive, and systemic inflammation, may be the initial sign of these disorders,[65] underscoring the need to characterize the type and extent of immune dysfunction comprehensively in infants with these clinical manifestations.

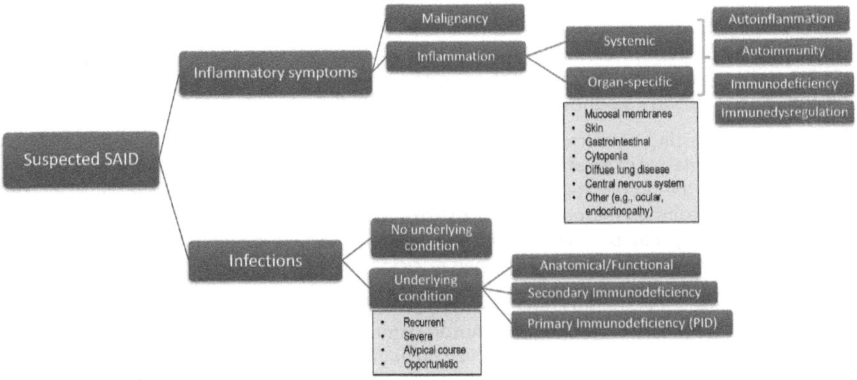

Fig. 3. Approach to the patient with suspected SAID.

THE ROLE OF GENETIC TESTING

The availability of next-generation sequencing (NGS) has revolutionized the diagnosis of human immunologic diseases.[66] In evaluating individuals afflicted with autoinflammatory diseases, the objectives of genetic testing are to determine whether a molecular defect underlies a clinical phenotype, because early molecular diagnosis may alter treatment, help prevent sequelae of severe inflammation, and have future implications for patients and their families. To guide the selection and interpretation of genetic studies in SAIDs, the International Society of Systemic Auto-Inflammatory Diseases (ISSAID) and European Molecular Genetics Quality Network have developed "Best Practice Guidelines for the Genetic Diagnosis of Monogenic Autoinflammatory Diseases"[67] providing general principles and indications for genetic testing (**Box 2**).

Selection of Genetic Studies in Systemic Autoinflammatory Disease Diagnosis

The characteristics of available testing modalities are important for the selection and proper interpretation of genetic studies in immunologic disorders. Single or targeted gene sequencing may be used if clinical characteristics of a specific SAID are suspected. If one specific SAID is not suggested clinically or if individuals remain undiagnosed after targeted testing, a wider net of genes may be interrogated using whole-exome sequencing (WES) or whole-genome sequencing (WGS). Currently, WES is widely available in clinical settings. Considering the limitations of WES to detect variants in intronic regions of the genome, well-documented in other IEIs,[66] WGS should be used when defects not covered by WES platforms are suspected or in undiagnosed patients after other methods have been used.[66] In general, NGS methods should be paired with the assessment of copy number variants (CNVs) when evaluating SAIDs and other IEIs. This is important particularly if the clinical phenotype appears syndromic or is nonspecific. In SAIDs, evaluation of CNVs should

Box 2
Indications for genetic studies in systemic autoinflammatory diseases

Indications for individual genetic testing

1. Case fulfilling clinical criteria for a known monogenic autoinflammatory disease
2. Patients with partial presentations who present with a family history of monogenic autoinflammatory disease
3. Suspicion for SAIDs that cause irreversible damage (severe NLRP3-associated autoinflammatory disease and DADA2)
4. If clinical criteria for specific disorders are not fulfilled, but a SAID is suspected, an expanded panel may be performed, followed WES or WGS if the initial test is nonconfirmatory.
5. Prenatal or newborn testing is not indicated unless there is a striking family history or suspicion, and early diagnosis may change the infant's outcome.

Indications for testing of asymptomatic relatives

1. First-degree relative of an affected person with a known hereditary periodic fever syndrome to determine the predictability of high-risk diseases, such as CNS involvement in NLRP3-associated autoinflammatory disease or stroke in DADA2
2. Parental testing may be used to confirm whether a variant is familial or de novo and to evaluate if inherited in *cis* or *trans* when relevant.

Data from Shinar Y, Ceccherini I, Rowczenio D, et al. ISSAID/EMQN Best Practice Guidelines for the Genetic Diagnosis of Monogenic Autoinflammatory Diseases in the Next-Generation Sequencing Era. Clinical Chemistry. 2020;66(4):525-536. https://doi.org/10.1093/clinchem/hvaa024.

be pursued if initial testing is negative and HA20, MKD, or DADA2 are suspected. Additionally, in classical presentations of NOD2-associated granulomatous disease, cryopyrin-associated periodic fever syndrome (CAPS), and TRAPS with negative exon sequencing, mosaicism should be evaluated.[67]

Diagnostic Interpretation of Genetic Studies in Systemic Autoinflammatory Diseases

Guidelines from the American College of Medical Genetics and Genomics and the Association for Molecular Pathology, based on computational predictions, population data, functional studies, and roles of inheritance and segregation, help to determine the pathogenicity of a variant. In SAIDs, ISSAID classified genetic variants associated with FMF, TRAPS, MKD, and CAPS. The list of available classified variants is in the database (https://infevers.umai-montpellier.fr/).[68] A tool to determine the significance of genetic findings in hereditary periodic fevers through the development of a genotype-phenotype association in the Eurofever Registry also was proposed.[69] The methodology included stratifying Eurofever patients based on disease patterns, including recurrent attacks, chronic inflammation, or chronic inflammatory states with flares. There was a group of expert clinicians selected by the Eurofever Steering Committee, who reviewed the clinical and genetic information from the enrolling physician to determine if modification of the diagnosis is needed. These data parallel findings in the Infevers database.[69]

Limitations of Genetic Studies in Systemic Autoinflammatory Diseases

One of the main limitations of most genetic studies used in the diagnosis of SAIDs is their limited yield. When targeted gene testing is employed, 20% of samples from SAID patients yield an explanatory result, and WES or WGS may increase this number by 5% to 10%.[67] All exon sequencing methods (single gene, targeted panels, and WES) fail to detect defects located in noncoding regions of the genome and feature poor detection of sequences shared with pseudogenes and CNVs. In addition, coverage of certain exons or regions may be limited (e.g., guanosine-cytosine–rich regions with WES).[66] Most of these limitations are overcome by WGS, which features better CNV coverage and may detect variants in intronic regions. Nonetheless, cost, accessibility, requirements for large storage capacity, and long process times remain an obstacle for more widespread WGS use. In addition, a greater frequency of sequencing errors, secondary findings, and variants of unknown significance should be considered in the interpretation of WGS results[66] (**Fig. 4**).

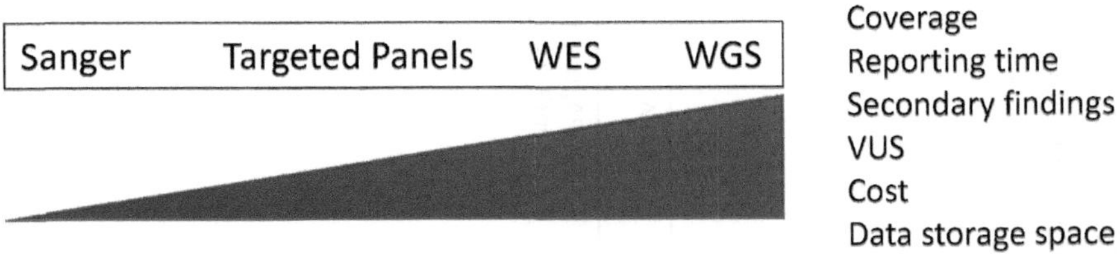

Fig. 4. Comparison of sequencing methods employed in the diagnosis of SAIDs. Nontargeted approaches, such as WES and WGS, provide increased coverage of genomic regions and may identify pathogenic variants in known or novel-disease associated genes. Nonetheless, cost, reporting time, need for storage space, frequency of secondary findings, and detection of variables of unknown significance (VUS) parallels the number of genomic regions examined.

Table 2
Medications and therapeutic considerations in the treatment of systemic autoinflammatory diseases

Therapy	Common Clinical Use	Special Considerations	Monitoring
Colchicine	FMF[a], gout[a], Behçet Disease, PFAPA, low penetrance variants of the *TNFRSF1A* gene, undifferentiated recurrent fever syndromes[72]	Pediatric dosing from EULAR recommendations 1. ≤0.5 or ≤0.6 mg/d for <5 y, 0.5–1.0 or 1.2 mg/d for 5–10 y, 1.0–1.5 or 1.8 mg/d in >10 y 2. Can be titrated up to maximum dosing if needed to 2 mg (children) and 3 mg (adults)[73] 3. Colchicine has been found to be safe in children with FMF.[74]	Complete blood cell count, renal function, liver function every 6 mo; CK if toxicity is suspected[73]
Cimetidine	PFAPA	Effective in less than one-third of PFAPA patients 20–40 mg/kg/d[75]	N/A
Tonsillectomy	PFAPA, undifferentiated recurrent fever syndrome[72]	Effective in a majority of PFAPA patients with complete tonsillectomy and adenoidectomy with regrowth associated with palatine tonsillar regrowth[76] The American Academy of Otolaryngology-Head and Neck Surgery Foundation guidelines: PFAPA is a modifying factor to consider for tonsillectomy.[77] Undifferentiated recurrent fever syndromes with more gastrointestinal symptoms had resolution to tonsillectomy with an IL-1 signature on extracted tonsils (n = 15 patients)[72]	N/A

IL-1 inhibition a. Rilonacept b. Anakinra c. Canakinumab	a. Rilonacept: Recurrent pericarditis[a], CAPS (including MWS and FCAS)[a], and DIRA[a] b. Anakinra: NOMID[a], (continuously or intermittent) refractory Behçet disease and refractory PFAPA[78] c. Canakinumab Colchicine-resistant FMF[a], CAPS[a], MKD/HIDS[a], TRAPS[a], HA 20, Behçet disease.	Anakinra is Food and Drug Administration approved For NOMID, 1–2 mg/kg with escalation to > 8 mg/kg[79] Dose intensification variable depending on condition (FMF/TRAPS relatively less and HIDS/CAPS relatively more) in JIR cohort[80] IL-1 inhibition (canakinumab and anakinra) in longstanding Behçet disease and uveitis[81] TRAPS patients receiving IL-1 inhibition vs TNF inhibition as initial biologic with a statistically significant increase in clinical and biochemical response[82]	Monthly for 3 mo and then every 3 mo: CBC (mostly) and renal function, liver function[79]
TNF inhibition	TNF and NF-κB dysregulation disorders: Pediatric granulomatous arthritis, TRAPS, DADA2, HA 20/Behçet disease, NLRP12-associated AID	Avoidance of monoclonal antibody TNF inhibition in TRAPS (etanercept can be used)[83] Some response in Blau arthritis but suboptimal for ocular inflammation[84] Inconsistent response in MKD,[85] response in FMF patients with chronic arthritis or sacroiliitis[86] DADA2 responsive to TNF inhibition[87]	Tuberculosis testing prior to treatment and annually Blood counts and comprehensive metabolic panel every 3–6 mo[88]

(*continued on next page*)

Table 2
(*continued*)

Therapy	Common Clinical Use	Special Considerations	Monitoring
JAK inhibition	Interferonopathies	Baricitinib reduced signs and symptoms of CANDLE, SAVI, and other interferonopathies (panniculitis and lipoatrophy).[89] CANDLE with remission on baricitinib with reduction in biomarkers of IFN signaling, IP-10 and IFN response gene score with residual increased inflammatory markers in SAVI[89] Constitutional growth with steroid taper to <0.16 mg/kg/d on baricitinib Careful monitoring of infections (especially BK virus and herpes)[89]	Monitor liver enzyme, renal parameters, and blood counts. Lipid panel prior to inception and 12 wk after initiation. BK virus titers and BK virus measurement in urine were done in clinical trial.[89]
Vitamin D	PFAPA, FMF, and NLRP3-associated AID	Vitamin D levels >30 are associated with fewer PFAPA flares[90] Vitamin D levels are lower in FMF and can interfere with sleep[91] Vitamin D inhibits *NLRP3* activation via the vitamin D receptor[92]	Every 6 months monitoring showed hypovitaminosis D as a risk factor for PFAPA febrile attacks[90]

[a] Food and Drug Administration–approved indications; all other indications are off label. CANDLE, chronic atypical neutrophilic dermatosis with lipodystrophy and elevated temperature; CK, creatinine Kinase; FCAS, familial cold autoinflammatory syndrome; MWS, muckle-wells syndrome; NOMID, neonatal-onset multisystem inflammatory disease; SAVI, STING-associated vasculopathy with onset in infancy.

The Role of Genetic Studies in Polygenic Systemic Autoinflammatory Diseases

Deepening the molecular understanding of polygenic SAIDs may advance the understanding of these disorders and ultimately inform treatment. For instance, PFAPA is a complex genetic disease often cited as a paradigm illustrating how genetic discovery directs the characterization of polygenic immunologic disorders. Specifically, European-American and Turkish populations with PFAPA had a strong association with a variant upstream of *IL12 A* as well as variants near *STAT4*, *IL10*, and *CCR1-CCR3,* similarly to susceptibility variants of Behçet and recurrent aphthous stomatitis. Similar genetic underpinnings for Behçet, PFAPA, and recurrent aphthous stomatitis now are recognized as part of a continuum that can be termed, *Behçet spectrum disorders*.[70] Furthering understanding of molecular mechanisms underlying polygenic autoinflammatory diseases as well as disease-modifying factors (epigenetic and environment-gene interactions) may point to more precise clinical definitions of disease and targeted therapies.

APPROACH TO THERAPY

Therapeutic advances have significantly improved the outcome and prognosis for SAIDs. Implementing robust, evidence-based targeted therapies personalized to individual conditions based on their known specific mechanisms, although ideal, has been limited by the rarity of these disorders and limitation with confirming genetic diagnoses in the majority of SAIDs. The explosion of knowledge on therapeutics largely stems from targeted therapy guided by molecular defects discovered that might be a potential target of currently available medications. Additionally, systematic literature reviews with evidence grading followed by expert-driven guidelines have occurred for the most common monogenic SAIDs/hereditary periodic fever syndromes (FMF, TRAPS, CAPS, and MKD) in addition to the development of a consensus treatment plan for complex polygenic disorders, such as PFAPA.[71] A brief overview of the management of these disorders is the focus of this section (**Table 2**).

The PROKIND CAPS/TRAPS/MKD/hyper-IgD syndrome (HIDS) treatment plans adopted a treat-to-target approach with stratified treatment founded on the severity of disease accounting for patient/parental input, physician evaluation, and laboratory parameters. An example is for younger children with CAPS, recognizing that IL-1 inhibition likely will be needed at relatively higher doses.[93] The 2016 European Alliance of Associations for Rheumatology (EULAR) recommendations for treatment of FMF proposes indications for treatment, details of management with colchicine, approach to colchicine-refractory FMF, and other essential components of disease management.[73] Additionally, EULAR created recommendations for the management of Behçet disease based on a systematic literature review and Delphi procedure among Behçet experts.[81] One therapeutic strategy recently described in PFAPA illustrates the use of comparative effectiveness research through the development of consensus treatment plans reflective of current common practices in PFAPA management to elucidate optimum future therapies.[94]

SUMMARY

Nearly one-quarter of a century after molecularly characterizing FMF, the ever-expanding lattice of genetic discovery in autoinflammatory disorders has unraveled essential mechanisms of innate immunity. Elucidating novel networks of immune dysfunction in SAIDs has exposed that intertwined innate and adaptive elements of the immune response result in overlapping immune dysregulation between autoinflammation, autoimmunity, allergy, and/or immune deficiency. Despite the discovery that many autoinflammatory disorders are IEIs, facilitated by burgeoning genetic technology, a majority of autoinflammatory disorders remain genetically undefined, emphasizing the need for continued development of innovative diagnostic strategies to establish earlier diagnoses, thereby advancing personalized therapeutics. Elucidating predisposing factors for exaggerated inflammatory responses has the potential to unveil critical clues into the origin of hyperinflammation.

CLINICS CARE POINTS

- A growing number of autoinflammatory disorders present with multiple signs of immune dysfunction, including allergic, autoimmune and immunodeficiency features. Monogenic causes of autoinflammation as well as other IEIs (e.g., primary immunodeficiency and immune dysregulation disorders) need to be considered in patients presenting with these overlapping manifestations.
- Molecular diagnosis should be considered early in the evaluation of patients with suspected monogenic causes of autoinflammation, and expert advice is required for appropriate test selection and interpretation.
- Personalized therapeutics in SAID patients can be achieved through molecular diagnostics, optimization of medication dosing, and guidance provided based on evidence grading of available literature in addition to expert opinion.

DISCLOSURE

The authors have nothing to disclose.

REFERENCES

1. Siegal S. Benign paroxysmal peritonitis. Ann Intern Med 1945;23:1–21.
2. Ben-Chetrit E, Gattorno M, Gul A, et al. Consensus proposal for taxonomy and definition of the autoinflammatory diseases (AIDs): a Delphi study. Ann Rheum Dis 2018;77(11):1558–65.
3. Bousfiha A, Jeddane L, Picard C, et al. Human inborn errors of immunity: 2019 update of the IUIS phenotypical classification. J Clin Immunol 2020;40(1): 66–81.
4. Manthiram K, Zhou Q, Aksentijevich I, et al. The monogenic autoinflammatory diseases define new pathways in human innate immunity and inflammation. Nat Immunol 2017;18(8):832–42.
5. Jamilloux Y, Belot A, Magnotti F, et al. Geoepidemiology and immunologic features of autoinflammatory diseases: a comprehensive review. Clin Rev Allergy Immunol 2018;54(3):454–79.
6. de Koning HD, van Gijn ME, Stoffels M, et al. Myeloid lineage–restricted somatic mosaicism of NLRP3 mutations in patients with variant Schnitzler syndrome. J Allergy Clin Immunol 2015;135(2):561–4.e4.
7. Beck DB, Ferrada MA, Sikora KA, et al. Somatic mutations in *UBA1* and severe adult-onset autoinflammatory disease. N Engl J Med 2020;383(27):2628–38.
8. Feder HM, Salazar JC. A clinical review of 105 patients with PFAPA (a periodic fever syndrome). Acta Paediatr 2010;99(2):178–84.
9. van der Hilst JCH, Bodar EJ, Barron KS, et al. Long-term follow-up, clinical features, and quality of life in a series of 103 patients with hyperimmunoglobulinemia D syndrome. Medicine (Baltimore) 2008;87(6):301–10.

10. Barton C, Kausar S, Kerr D, et al. SIFD as a novel cause of severe fetal hydrops and neonatal anaemia with iron loading and marked extramedullary haemopoiesis. J Clin Pathol 2018;71(3):275–8.
11. Altiok E, Aksoy F, Perk Y, et al. A novel mutation in the interleukin-1 receptor antagonist associated with intrauterine disease onset. Clin Immunol 2012; 145(1):77–81.
12. Damgaard RB, Elliott PR, Swatek KN, et al. OTULIN deficiency in ORAS causes cell type-specific LUBAC degradation, dysregulated TNF signalling and cell death. EMBO Mol Med 2019;11(3).
13. Touitou I. The spectrum of Familial Mediterranean Fever (FMF) mutations. Eur J Hum Genet 2001;9(7):473–83.
14. Lee JJY, Schneider R. Systemic juvenile idiopathic arthritis. Pediatr Clin North Am 2018;65(4):691–709.
15. Gaggiano C, Vitale A, Obici L, et al. Clinical features at onset and genetic characterization of pediatric and adult patients with TNF- α Receptor—Associated Periodic Syndrome (TRAPS): A series of 80 cases from the AIDA Network. Mediators Inflamm 2020;2020:1–12.
16. Álvarez-Errico D, Vento-Tormo R, Ballestar E. Genetic and epigenetic determinants in autoinflammatory diseases. Front Immunol 2017;8. https://doi.org/10.3389/fimmu.2017.00318.
17. Zhou Q, Wang H, Schwartz DM, et al. Loss-of-function mutations in TNFAIP3 leading to A20 haploinsufficiency cause an early-onset autoinflammatory disease. Nat Genet 2016;48(1):67–73.
18. Rosé CD, Pans S, Casteels I, et al. Blau syndrome: cross-sectional data from a multicentre study of clinical, radiological and functional outcomes. Rheumatology 2015;54(6):1008–16.
19. Schepp J, Proietti M, Frede N, et al. Screening of 181 patients with antibody deficiency for deficiency of adenosine deaminase 2 sheds new light on the disease in adulthood: DADA2 in patients with antibody deficiency. Arthritis Rheumatol 2017; 69(8):1689–700.
20. Bandsma RHJ, van Goor H, Yourshaw M, et al. Loss of ADAM17 is associated with severe multiorgan dysfunction. Hum Pathol 2015;46(6):923–8.
21. Lalaoui N, Boyden SE, Oda H, et al. Mutations that prevent caspase cleavage of RIPK1 cause autoinflammatory disease. Nature 2020;577(7788):103–8.
22. Boisson B, Laplantine E, Prando C, et al. Immunodeficiency, autoinflammation and amylopectinosis in humans with inherited HOIL-1 and LUBAC deficiency. Nat Immunol 2012;13(12):1178–86.
23. Boisson B, Laplantine E, Dobbs K, et al. Human HOIP and LUBAC deficiency underlies autoinflammation, immunodeficiency, amylopectinosis, and lymphangiectasia. J Exp Med 2015;212(6):939–51.
24. Goldbach-Mansky R, Gelabert A, Kim HJ, et al. Neonatal-onset multisystem inflammatory disease responsive to interleukin-1beta inhibition. N Engl J Med 2006;355(6):581–92.
25. Cowen EW. DIRA, DITRA, and new insights into pathways of skin inflammation: what's in a name? Arch Dermatol 2012;148(3):381.
26. Lainka E, Neudorf U, Lohse P, et al. Incidence and clinical features of hyperimmunoglobulinemia D and periodic fever syndrome (HIDS) and spectrum of mevalonate kinase (MVK) mutations in German children. Rheumatol Int 2012;32(10): 3253–60.

27. Lindor NM, Arsenault TM, Solomon H, et al. A new autosomal dominant disorder of pyogenic sterile arthritis, pyoderma gangrenosum, and acne: PAPA syndrome. Mayo Clin Proc 1997;72(7):611–5.
28. Standing ASI, Malinova D, Hong Y, et al. Autoinflammatory periodic fever, immunodeficiency, and thrombocytopenia (PFIT) caused by mutation in actin-regulatory gene WDR1. J Exp Med 2017;214(1):59–71.
29. Bettiol A, Silvestri E, Di Scala G, et al. The right place of interleukin-1 inhibitors in the treatment of Behçet's syndrome: a systematic review. Rheumatol Int 2019; 39(6):971–90.
30. Canna SW, de Jesus AA, Gouni S, et al. An activating NLRC4 inflammasome mutation causes autoinflammation with recurrent macrophage activation syndrome. Nat Genet 2014;46(10):1140–6.
31. Fenini G, Karakaya T, Hennig P, et al. The NLRP1 inflammasome in human skin and beyond. Int J Mol Sci 2020;21(13). https://doi.org/10.3390/ijms21134788.
32. Kim H, Sanchez GAM, Goldbach-Mansky R. Insights from mendelian interferonopathies: comparison of CANDLE, SAVI with AGS, monogenic lupus. J Mol Med 2016;94(10):1111–27.
33. Rice GI, del Toro Duany Y, Jenkinson EM, et al. Gain-of-function mutations in IFIH1 cause a spectrum of human disease phenotypes associated with upregulated type I interferon signaling. Nat Genet 2014;46(5):503–9.
34. de Jesus AA, Hou Y, Brooks S, et al. Distinct interferon signatures and cytokine patterns define additional systemic autoinflammatory diseases. J Clin Invest 2020;130(4):1669–82.
35. Liu Y, Jesus AA, Marrero B, et al. Activated STING in a vascular and pulmonary syndrome. N Engl J Med 2014;371(6):507–18.
36. Gruber C, Martin-Fernandez M, Ailal F, et al. Homozygous STAT2 gain-of-function mutation by loss of USP18 activity in a patient with type I interferonopathy. J Exp Med 2020;217(5):e20192319.
37. Duncan CJA, Thompson BJ, Chen R, et al. Severe type I interferonopathy and unrestrained interferon signaling due to a homozygous germline mutation in *STAT2*. Sci Immunol 2019;4(42):eaav7501.
38. Meyts I, Casanova J-L. A human inborn error connects the α's. Nat Immunol 2016; 17(5):472–4.
39. Starokadomskyy P, Gemelli T, Rios JJ, et al. DNA polymerase-α regulates the activation of type I interferons through cytosolic RNA:DNA synthesis. Nat Immunol 2016;17(5):495–504.
40. Hadjadj J, Castro CN, Tusseau M, et al. Early-onset autoimmunity associated with SOCS1 haploinsufficiency. Nat Commun 2020;11(1):5341.
41. Torrelo A. CANDLE syndrome as a paradigm of proteasome-related autoinflammation. Front Immunol 2017;8:927.
42. Brehm A, Liu Y, Sheikh A, et al. Additive loss-of-function proteasome subunit mutations in CANDLE/PRAAS patients promote type 1 IFN production. J Clin Invest 2016;126(2):795.
43. Cho K, Yamada M, Agematsu K, et al. Heterozygous mutations in OAS1 cause infantile-onset pulmonary alveolar proteinosis with hypogammaglobulinemia. Am J Hum Genet 2018;102(3):480–6.
44. Roifman C, Melamed I. A novel syndrome of combined immunodeficiency, autoimmunity and spondylometaphyseal dysplasia: a novel syndrome of combined immunodeficiency, autoimmunity and spondylometaphyseal dysplasia. Clin Genet 2003;63(6):522–9.

45. Göös H, Fogarty CL, Sahu B, et al. Gain-of-function CEBPE mutation causes non-canonical autoinflammatory inflammasomopathy. J Allergy Clin Immunol 2019; 144(5):1364–76.
46. Zhou Q, Yang D, Ombrello AK, et al. Early-onset stroke and vasculopathy associated with mutations in ADA2. N Engl J Med 2014;370(10):911–20.
47. Badran YR, Dedeoglu F, Leyva Castillo JM, et al. Human RELA haploinsufficiency results in autosomal-dominant chronic mucocutaneous ulceration. J Exp Med 2017;214(7):1937–47.
48. Gernez Y, de Jesus AA, Alsaleem H, et al. Severe autoinflammation in 4 patients with C-terminal variants in cell division control protein 42 homolog (CDC42) successfully treated with IL-1β inhibition. J Allergy Clin Immunol 2019;144(4): 1122–5.e6.
49. Volpi S, Cicalese MP, Tuijnenburg P, et al. A combined immunodeficiency with severe infections, inflammation, and allergy caused by ARPC1B deficiency. J Allergy Clin Immunol 2019;143(6):2296–9.
50. Castro CN, Rosenzwajg M, Carapito R, et al. NCKAP1L defects lead to a novel syndrome combining immunodeficiency, lymphoproliferation, and hyperinflammation. J Exp Med 2020;217(12):e20192275.
51. Ombrello MJ, Remmers EF, Sun G, et al. Cold urticaria, immunodeficiency, and autoimmunity related to PLCG2 deletions. N Engl J Med 2012;366(4):330–8.
52. Zhou Q, Lee G-S, Brady J, et al. A hypermorphic missense mutation in PLCG2, encoding phospholipase Cγ2, causes a dominantly inherited autoinflammatory disease with immunodeficiency. Am J Hum Genet 2012;91(4):713–20.
53. Watkin LB, Jessen B, Wiszniewski W, et al. COPA mutations impair ER-Golgi transport and cause hereditary autoimmune-mediated lung disease and arthritis. Nat Genet 2015;47(6):654–60.
54. Mehrotra D, Kesarwani A, Nandlal. Cherubism: case report with review of literature. J Maxillofac Oral Surg 2011;10(1):64–70.
55. Satveer M, Twelves S, Farkas K, et al. AP1S3 Mutations Cause Skin Autoinflammation by Disrupting Keratinocyte Autophagy and Up-Regulating IL-36 Production. J Invest Dermatology 2016; 136(11) 2251-2259.
56. Rabionet R, Remesal A, Mensa-Vilaró A, et al. Biallelic loss-of-function LACC1/FAMIN Mutations Presenting as Rheumatoid Factor-Negative Polyarticular Juvenile Idiopathic Arthritis. Sci Rep 2019;9(1):4579.
57. Sanchez GAM, Reinhardt A, Ramsey S, et al. JAK1/2 inhibition with baricitinib in the treatment of autoinflammatory interferonopathies. J Clin Invest 2018;128(7): 3041–52.
58. Canna SW, Cron RQ. Highways to hell: mechanism-based management of cytokine storm syndromes. J Allergy Clin Immunol 2020;146(5):949–59.
59. Yuan K, Huang G, Sang X, et al. Baricitinib for systemic lupus erythematosus. Lancet 2019;393(10170):402.
60. Siu A, Landon K, Ramos D. Differential diagnosis and management of oral ulcers. Semin Cutan Med Surg 2015;34(4):171–7.
61. Davis MDP, van der Hilst JCH. Mimickers of urticaria: urticarial vasculitis and autoinflammatory diseases. J Allergy Clin Immunol Pract 2018;6(4):1162–70.
62. Cuchet-Lourenço D, Eletto D, Wu C, et al. Biallelic *RIPK1* mutations in humans cause severe immunodeficiency, arthritis, and intestinal inflammation. Science 2018;361(6404):810–3.
63. Long SS. Distinguishing among prolonged, recurrent, and periodic fever syndromes: approach of a pediatric infectious diseases subspecialist. Pediatr Clin North Am 2005;52(3):811–35.

64. Hashkes PJ, Barron KS, Laxer RM. Clinical approach to the diagnosis of autoinflammatory diseases. In: Hashkes PJ, Laxer RM, Simon A, editors. Textbook of autoinflammation. Cham, Switzerland: Springer International Publishing; 2019. p. 203–23.
65. O'Connell AE. Primary immunodeficiency in the NICU. Neoreviews 2019;20(2): e67–78.
66. Chinn IK, Chan AY, Chen K, et al. Diagnostic interpretation of genetic studies in patients with primary immunodeficiency diseases: a working group report of the Primary Immunodeficiency Diseases Committee of the American Academy of Allergy, Asthma & Immunology. J Allergy Clin Immunol 2020;145(1):46–69.
67. Shinar Y, Ceccherini I, Rowczenio D, et al. ISSAID/EMQN best practice guidelines for the genetic diagnosis of monogenic autoinflammatory diseases in the next-generation sequencing era. Clin Chem 2020;66(4):525–36.
68. Gijn MEV, Ceccherini I, Shinar Y, et al. New workflow for classification of genetic variants' pathogenicity applied to hereditary recurrent fevers by the International Study Group for Systemic Autoinflammatory Diseases (INSAID). J Med Genet 2018;55(8):530–7.
69. Papa R, Doglio M, et al, Paediatric Rheumatology International Trials Organisation (PRINTO) and the Eurofever Project. A web-based collection of genotype-phenotype associations in hereditary recurrent fevers from the Eurofever registry. Orphanet J Rare Dis 2017;12(1):167.
70. Manthiram K, Preite S, Dedeoglu F, et al. Common genetic susceptibility loci link PFAPA syndrome, Behçet's disease, and recurrent aphthous stomatitis. Proc Natl Acad Sci U S A 2020;117(25):14405–11.
71. Soriano A, Soriano M, Espinosa G, et al. Current Therapeutic Options for the Main Monogenic Autoinflammatory Diseases and PFAPA Syndrome: Evidence-Based Approach and Proposal of a Practical Guide. Front Immunol 2020;11:865.
72. Luu I, Nation J, Page N, et al. Undifferentiated recurrent fevers in pediatrics are clinically distinct from PFAPA syndrome but retain an IL-1 signature. Clin Immunol 2021;226:108697.
73. Ozen S, Demirkaya E, Erer B, et al. EULAR recommendations for the management of familial Mediterranean fever. Ann Rheum Dis 2016;75(4):644–51.
74. Padeh S, Gerstein M, Berkun Y. Colchicine is a safe drug in children with familial Mediterranean fever. J Pediatr 2012;161(6):1142–6.
75. Feder HM, Salazar JC. A clinical review of 105 patients with PFAPA (a periodic fever syndrome). Acta Pædiatrica 2010;99(2):178–84.
76. Lantto U, Koivunen P, Tapiainen T, et al. Periodic Fever, Aphthous Stomatitis, Pharyngitis, and Cervical Adenitis Syndrome: Relapse and Tonsillar Regrowth After Childhood Tonsillectomy. Laryngoscope 2021;00:1–4.
77. Mitchell R, Archer S, Ishman S, et al. Clinical Practice Guideline: Tonsillectomy in Children (Update)—Executive Summary. Otolaryngol Head Neck Surg 2019; 160(2):187–205.
78. Stojnaov S, Lapidus S, Chitkara P, et al. Periodic fever, aphthous stomatitis, pharyngitis, and adenitis (PFAPA) is a disorder of innate immunity and Th1 activation responsive to IL-1 blockade. *Proc Natl Acad Sci* U S A 2011;108(17):7148–53.
79. Available at: https://www.fda.gov/media/124784/download.
80. Hentgen V, Koné-Paut I, Belot A, et al. Long-term follow-up and optimization of interleukin-1 inhibitors in the management of monogenic autoinflammatory diseases: real-life data from the jir cohort. Front Pharmacol 2021;11:568865.

81. Hatemi G, Christensen R, Bang D, et al. 2018 update of the EULAR recommendations for the management of Behçet's syndrome. Ann Rheum Dis 2018;77(6): 808–18.
82. Ozen S, Kuemmerle-Deschner JB, Cimaz R, et al. International Retrospective Chart Review of Treatment Patterns in Severe Familial Mediterranean Fever, Tumor Necrosis Factor Receptor-Associated Periodic Syndrome, and Mevalonate Kinase Deficiency/Hyperimmunoglobulinemia D Syndrome. Arthritis Care Res 2017;69(4):578–86.
83. Nedjai B, Hitman G, Quillinan N, et al. Proinflammatory action of the anti-inflammatory drug infliximab in tumor necrosis factor receptor-associated periodic syndrome. Arthritis Rheum 2009;60(2):619–25.
84. Rosé CD, Pans S, Casteels I, et al. Blau syndrome: cross-sectional data from a multicentre study of clinical, radiological and functional outcomes. Rheumatology 2015;54(6):1008–16.
85. Ter Haar NM, Jeyaratnam J, Lachmann HJ, et al. The Phenotype and Genotype of Mevalonate Kinase Deficiency: A Series of 114 Cases From the Eurofever Registry. Arthritis Rheumatol 2016;68(11):2795–805.
86. Bilgen SA, Kilic L, Akdogan A, et al. Effects of anti-tumor necrosis factor agents for familial mediterranean fever patients with chronic arthritis and/or sacroiliitis who were resistant to colchicine treatment. J Clin Rheumato 2011;17(7):358–62.
87. Nanthapisal S, Murphy C, Omoyinmi E, et al. Deficiency of Adenosine Deaminase Type 2: A Description of Phenotype and Genotype in Fifteen Cases. Arthritis Rheumatol 2016;68(9):2314–22.
88. Emer JJ, Frankel A, Zeichner JA. A practical approach to monitoring patients on biological agents for the treatment of psoriasis. J Clin Aesthet Dermatol 2010; 3(8):20–6.
89. Montealegre Sanchez G, Reinhardt A, Ramsey S, et al. JAK1/2 inhibition with baricitinib in the treatment of autoinflammatory interferonopathies. J Clin Invest 2018; 128(7):3041–52.
90. Nalbantoğlu A, Nalbantoğlu B. Vitamin D deficiency as a risk factor for PFAPA syndrome. Int J Pediatr Otorhinolaryngol 2019;121:55–7.
91. Onur H, Kasapcopur. Vitamin D levels in children with familial Mediterranean fever. Clin Exp Rheumatol 2017;35:8. Suppl 104(2).
92. Zebing R, Chen X, Wu J, et al. Vitamin D Receptor Inhibits NLRP3 Activation by Impeding Its BRCC3-Mediated Deubiquitination. Front Immunol 2019;10:2783.
93. Hansmann S, Lainka E, Horneff G, et al. Consensus protocols for the diagnosis and management of the hereditary autoinflammatory syndromes CAPS, TRAPS and MKD/HIDS: a German PRO-KIND initiative. Pediatr Rheumatol Online J 2020;18:17.
94. Amarilyo G, Rothman D, Manthiram K, et al. Consensus treatment plans for periodic fever, aphthous stomatitis, pharyngitis and adenitis syndrome (PFAPA): a framework to evaluate treatment responses from the childhood arthritis and rheumatology research alliance (CARRA) PFAPA work group. Pediatr Rheumatol 2020;18(1):31.

9780323848800